Mesothelioma

Giovanni Luca Ceresoli
Emilio Bombardieri • Maurizio D'Incalci
Editors

Mesothelioma

From Research to Clinical Practice

Springer

Editors
Giovanni Luca Ceresoli
Department of Medical Oncology
Humanitas Gavazzeni Hospital
Bergamo
Italy

Emilio Bombardieri
Scientific Direction
Humanitas Gavazzeni Hospital
Bergamo
Italy

Maurizio D'Incalci
Department of Oncology
Istituto di Ricerche Farmacologiche
Mario Negri IRCCS
Milano
Italy

ISBN 978-3-030-16886-5 ISBN 978-3-030-16884-1 (eBook)
https://doi.org/10.1007/978-3-030-16884-1

This Springer imprint is published by the registered company Springer Nature Switzerland AG.
The registered company address is: Gewerbestrasse 11, 6330 Cham, Switzerland

Foreword

This book is a comprehensive—and therefore welcome—text dealing with one of the most malignant tumors, mesothelioma, fortunately relatively rare. The cause of this tumor, as stated by the International Agency for Research on Cancer (IARC), is asbestos, a generic name for a family of magnesium or other minerals and fibrous silicate minerals. In fact asbestos, which is made up of fibers, can be divided into serpentine and amphibole structures. Chrysotile is a serpentine type of asbestos with magnesium as the main element, while the group of amphiboles includes crocidolite, amosite, anthophyllite, tremolite, and actinolite. In addition to magnesium, the components may also include calcium, iron, and/or sodium.

There are other fibers besides asbestos that can induce mesotheliomas, such as erionite belonging to the zeolite family, found in three villages in southeast Turkey. Some studies suggest that predisposition to the development of erionite mesothelioma is genetically transmitted as an autosomal dominant characteristic. The possible relation between cosmetic talc and mesothelioma is still debated. However, in several cases the products utilized are made up of a mixture of components.

In nature, asbestos is present in various areas of the world. For instance, chrysotile is predominant in Quebec (Canada) and in the Ural Mountains (Russia), and much less in Italy. In South Africa, crocidolite and amosite are predominant while in Finland there are deposits of anthophyllite.

The production of the various forms of asbestos increased 80,000 times over the course of a century (1880–1980), reaching the figure of four million tons per year. Given its resistance to heat and its insulation properties, asbestos has been employed for a wide variety of industrial products: from textile manufacturing to cement products, construction, and insulation for steam engines.

The widespread use of asbestos products results in the presence of mineral fibers in the lungs of the general population to a greater extent than in the rural population but with broad variability among subjects. Scanning electron microscopy shows a range of fibers that varies from fewer than 100–2500 fibers per gram of wet tissue. Within the asbestos bodies, fiber aggregates may be observed. The Helsinki Report indicates that attention should be paid to individuals with more than 100,000 amphibole fibers longer than 5 μm/gram of dry lung or more than one asbestos body per milliliter of bronchial alveolar lavage.

Epidemiology distinguishes occupational and nonoccupational exposure, and for nonoccupational exposure a distinction is made between household and neighborhood exposure. The percentages are higher for occupational than nonoccupational exposure but vary widely depending on the type of observational study considered. Eighty to ninety percent of mesotheliomas are found in the pleura, 10–15% are peritoneal and less than 5% are located in the pericardium. The median age of onset is 74 years.

Chrysotile seems to be less carcinogenic than amphibole fibers, but not all types have been studied in detail, partly because of the mixtures of various fibers. The carcinogenic properties of these materials need to be further investigated to better define the genomic heterogeneity, the localization, and the morphological characteristics of the derived mesotheliomas.

The book describes the process of asbestos-dependent carcinogenesis in detail, considering not only the cancer cell but also the tumor microenvironment, with particular reference to the immunological aspects. Early diagnosis is important. In this field, the recent identification of miRNAs, designated as "mesomiRNAs," as potential biomarkers of the disease is of particular interest although confirmatory data based on large trials are necessary. In this context, the development of liquid biomarkers will be of particular value.

The prognosis of mesothelioma is particularly negative because of the lack of specific treatments. Hence, the development of efficacious and innovative treatment strategies is a priority. This process requires the conduction of preclinical studies, which are likely to benefit from the variety of preclinical tests available. A chapter of this book contains a comprehensive description of the preclinical tests in use along with a detailed discussion of their advantages and limitations. The current panel of in vitro tests available is based on the use of primary cell cultures, immortalized cell lines, and derived spheroid cultures. Several in vivo models have also been developed and they consist of mouse xenografts of human cell lines and patient-derived tissues or primary tumor cells. There is a need for the development of asbestos-induced mouse models of mesothelioma that may be transplanted subcutaneously or orthotopically in the pleura.

Due to the long latency of this tumor—estimated at 30 years or more—there is ample time for intervention to block its progression and dissemination in man. This long latency means that asbestos-related cancers are likely to peak in the next decade. The therapy of mesothelioma is still in its infancy. Classical chemotherapy, with cisplatin and pemetrexed, is not very effective, so ongoing trials include combinations of drugs targeting angiogenesis such as bevacizumab or antibodies acting as checkpoint inhibitors. Clearly, prevention is another major issue and a straightforward measure to be implemented is banning the production and all sorts of products containing asbestos.

To conclude, I believe this very easy readable book is a careful update of the current literature on asbestos. The chapters are presented in a clear form with appropriate tables and figures. The book will serve as a reference for all physicians and researchers dealing with the research and care of patients with mesothelioma.

Silvio Garattini,
Istituto di Ricerche Farmacologiche
Mario Negri IRCCS
Milan, Italy

Preface

Why a Book on Mesothelioma?

Recent advances in the diagnosis, characterization, and therapy of many hematological and solid malignancies are certainly extraordinary and have significantly improved the survival of patients with cancer. However, for some human malignancies like mesothelioma, although there have been remarkable increases in our knowledge of the main cause(s), and improvements in clinical management, the overall survival is still short. This book provides an authoritative overview of the latest validated clinical results on the diagnosis and therapy of mesothelioma, with special emphasis on open questions and preclinical and clinical research.

Much interesting research on mesothelioma is going on in different parts of the world so we have selected the authors of the various chapters not only on the basis of their internationally recognized outstanding expertise in mesothelioma but also considering their experience and involvement in research. Therefore, the chapters present not only the "state of the art" but also report novel ideas and hypotheses currently under investigation. An important part of the book is devoted to preclinical and translational research that—everybody hopes—will have an impact on clinical research and practice in the near future.

Growing evidence that the tumor microenvironment and immune response are key factors in the onset and progression of human malignancies is of particular importance for mesothelioma because chronic inflammation caused by exposure to asbestos is a hallmark of the disease. Several chapters therefore highlight the influence of the host mechanisms, as important for novel therapeutic approaches.

Mesothelioma is a complex and heterogeneous disease and clinicians need to keep up to date on new, rapidly expanding findings from biological, pharmacological, and immunological research. Obviously, though, information from pathological, surgical, and clinical experience is equally important to direct preclinical research towards clinically relevant objectives.

We sincerely hope this book will contribute to enhancing communication and boosting the integration of knowledge among scientists and clinicians with different expertise.

Bergamo, Italy — Giovanni Luca Ceresoli
Bergamo, Italy — Emilio Bombardieri
Milano, Italy — Maurizio D'Incalci

Acknowledgments

The editors are grateful to Ms. Anna Luisa De Simone Sorrentino (Milano) for her valid collaboration in connecting authors and for her secretarial help.

Contents

Epidemiology of Mesothelioma

1

Dario Mirabelli, Alessandro Marinaccio,
Pietro Comba, and Corrado Magnani

1.1 Introduction

In 1960, Richard Wagner and colleagues first presented a large case series of malignant mesothelioma (MM), with clear description of the clinical and diagnostic aspects and of the association with asbestos exposure, both occupational and nonoccupational [1]. Until then the existence of a primary malignancy from the mesothelium was debated and even denied by some authors. In the following years, the evidence on the association of MM and asbestos exposure was confirmed by several cohort studies on occupational exposure in different industrial sectors [2–6]. In the early studies, a special attention was given, as expected, to the asbestos mining [7], to the transformation of raw asbestos in industrial products and to the main industrial uses, such as lagging and insulation [6], asbestos textile [5] or asbestos cement [8]. Most of the studies regarded cohorts exposed either to the amphibole asbestos (in particular crocidolite and amosite), the type of fibres that present the greater carcinogenic potency for the mesothelium, or to mixed (chrysotile and amphiboles) asbestos types. The epidemiological cohort studies on the effects of chrysotile asbestos followed in the 1970s, with the cohorts of Canadian [7] and Italian chrysotile miners [9]. The first studies on chrysotile and MM did not show a strong association, but were accompanied by a strong evidence of association from animal studies [10], showing similar results for amphiboles and chrysotile asbestos. A long-lasting debate followed on carcinogenic potency of the different asbestos fibres [11] and on the effect of the different durability in biological tissues of chrysotile (short duration) compared to amphiboles (long). The accumulating scientific evidence led to the formal assessment of carcinogenic risk of asbestos and of other mineral fibres with similar mineralogic properties, with evidence of association for the MM as well as for the cancer of the lung and of other organs [2, 3, 12].

In the 1980s and 1990s, epidemiological research started investigating more systematically the occurrence of MM in relation to asbestos-

D. Mirabelli
Cancer Epidemiology, CPO Piemonte,
University of Turin, Turin, Italy

A. Marinaccio
Department of Occupational and Environmental Medicine, Epidemiology and Hygiene, Unit of Occupational and Environmental Epidemiology, INAIL, Italian National Institute for Insurance Against Accidents at Work, Rome, Italy
e-mail: a.marinaccio@inail.it

P. Comba
Unit of Environmental and Social Epidemiology, Department of Environment and Health, Istituto Superiore di Sanità, Rome, Italy
e-mail: pietro.comba@iss.it

C. Magnani (✉)
Department of Translational Medicine, University of Eastern Piedmont, and Cancer Epidemiology Unit, Maggiore Hospital and CPO Piedmont, Novara, Italy
e-mail: corrado.magnani@med.uniupo.it

G. L. Ceresoli et al. (eds.), *Mesothelioma*, https://doi.org/10.1007/978-3-030-16884-1_1

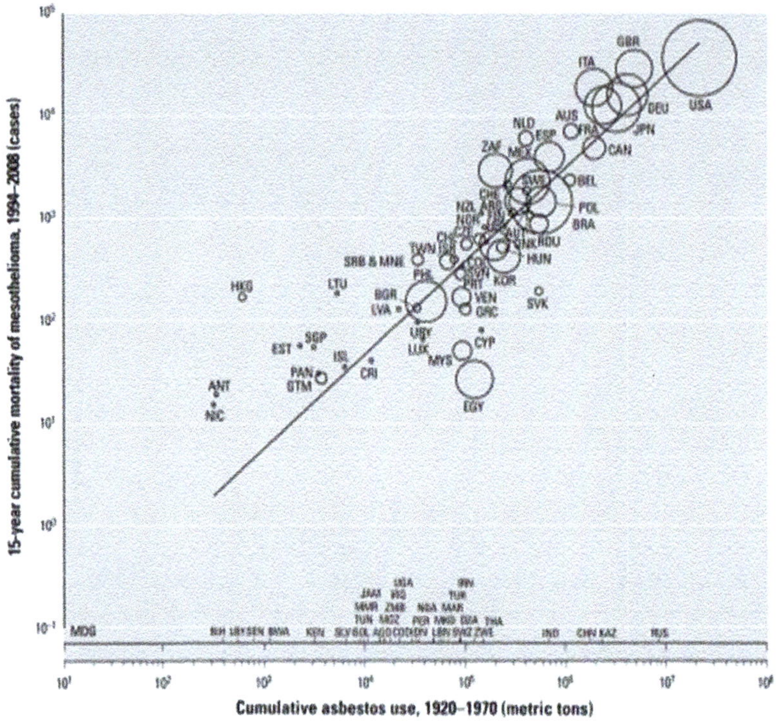

Fig. 1.1 From Park et al. [28]. Reproduced with permission from Environ Health Perspect. 2011;119:514–518. doi: https://doi.org/10.1289/ehp.1002845

containing products in place, the so-called 'third wave of asbestos diseases' [13], and also the first studies on MM in subjects with domestic exposure to asbestos were presented [14, 15]. The evidence on nonoccupational asbestos exposure and mesothelioma was completed by the studies regarding the environmental exposure to asbestos [16–20].

The issues regarding epidemiology and public health aspects of asbestos exposure and mesothelioma have been considered in several reviews [12, 21–25].

1.2 The World Distribution of MM

The occurrence of MM shows an extreme variation in the different countries [26], with the higher rates in the UK, Australia and Italy [27], which were among the countries with the highest per capita use of asbestos. Odgerel et al. [26] analysed the WHO Mortality Database categorizing 59 countries with good-quality mesothelioma mortality data, 45 countries with poor-quality data and 126 countries with no data. The gender- and age-specific mortality rates of countries with good-quality data were applied to other countries in order to estimate the number of global deaths. The final global estimate was 38,400 mesothelioma deaths per year.

The relation of asbestos exposure and MM occurrence has been investigated by different authors: Park et al. [28] presented the occurrence of MM in 56 world countries with data on mortality and on use of asbestos: mortality showed a log-linear relation to the amount of asbestos used ($R^2 = 0.83$; $p < 0.0001$) (Fig. 1.1). Diandini et al. [29] estimated that in the same countries, the number of PYLL (Potential Years of Life Lost) because of MM totalled 201,000 per year, with an average of 17.0 years per case.

1.3 Surveillance of MM Incidence

Italy is one of the most involved and sensitive countries in asbestos-related diseases' monitoring and control. This is a consequence of the large asbestos consumption until the ban in 1992, with 3,748,550 tons of raw asbestos produced or imported, and a peak between 1976 and 1980 at more than 160,000 tons/year [30]. A permanent surveillance system of MM incidence has been active since 2002, run by the 'National Register of Malignant Mesotheliomas' (Registro Nazionale dei Mesoteliomi)—ReNaM, identifying cases and assessing asbestos exposure [31]. Specific surveillance systems of MM incidence with reliable information completeness, exposure assessment and territorial coverage are scarce [32]. Currently, these systems are ongoing only in Australia [33], France [34], South Korea [35] and Italy [31]. Other countries have MM surveillance systems based on mortality data that are presented later.

The ReNaM acts with a regional structure, based on Regional Operating Centres (COR), that are now active in all the 20 Italian regions. CORs actively search incident MM cases in hospitals and other health care institutions. Diagnostic criteria are coded according to 3 classes of decreasing level of certainty. Occupational history, lifestyle habits and residential history are investigated using a standardized questionnaire, administered by a trained interviewer to the subject or to the next of kin. In each COR, industrial hygienists classify and code the exposure, examining the collected information. Occupational exposure classification is qualitative and coded as definite, probable or possible.[1] Further codes are assigned to indicate environmental (residence near a source of asbestos pollution without work-related exposure), familial (when patients have lived with a cohabitant occupationally exposed) or leisure activities (other nonoccupational exposures such as those due to leisure-time activities) exposures [31].

[1]Definite occupational exposure is assigned to the subjects whose work has involved the use of asbestos or materials containing asbestos. Probable occupational exposure is attributed to the subjects who have worked in a firm where asbestos was certainly used, but whose exposure cannot be documented, and possible occupational exposure to the subjects who have worked in a firm referring to an economic sector where asbestos has been used.

1.4 Incidence of MM in Italy

In the period 1993–2015, a case list of 27,356 incident MM has been collected by ReNaM [31]. In 2014, incidence standardized rate of pleural MM was 3.26 and 0.87 for 100,000 person/years in men and women with 1450 (1081 in men and 369 in women) recorded incident cases; corresponding rates for peritoneal MM were 0.17 and 0.10, based on 59 and 40 cases, respectively [31]. Mean age at diagnosis was around 70 years, and cases younger than 45 years were less than 2%. More than 90% of cases were localized in the pleural cavities, while peritoneal MM cases were 6.5% (5.3% and 9.4% in men and women, respectively), and cases in other body locations were very few (58 in the pericardium and 79 in the tunica vaginalis of the testis). Morphology of more than half of cases was epithelioid. Gender ratio (M/F) was equal to 2.54 overall and 2.64 for pleural cases, constant over time periods. However, it was noticed that gender ratio (M/F) was close or lower than one in towns with relevant environmental exposure and in occupational categories with predominant female occupation [36].

1.5 Occupational and Nonoccupational Exposure to Asbestos in Italy

In the ReNaM data, asbestos exposure has been evaluated for 21,387 MM cases (78.2% of total cases). Among them, occupational exposure has been identified for 69.3% (14,818 cases), while 4.9% were attributed to familial exposure, and 4.4% to environmental exposure.

The distribution of economic sectors involved in occupational asbestos exposure changed over the 1993–2015 observation period. The economic sectors 'asbestos-cement industry', 'shipbuilding and repair' and 'railways maintenance' accounted for 23% of incident cases in the period 1993–1998 and decreased to 9.5% in 2011–2015. Conversely, the 'construction' sector rose from 12.1% in 1993–1998 to 16.8% in 2011–2015 and now is the most frequent occupational sector in MM cases.

In Italy, excess MM risks related to the residence near asbestos-cement plants have been repeatedly documented for the areas of Casale Monferrato [37], Bari [38], Broni [39], and for the shipbuilding in the areas of Leghorn and La Spezia [40]. Casale Monferrato represents an extreme example of the effect of environmental exposure to asbestos, with incidence rates of 90.2/100,000 person year in men and 45.4 in women in 2010–2014, based on 121 incident cases [41]. Nonoccupationally exposed MM cases have been reported also in relation to the chrysotile mine of Balangero [42].

Among MM cases registered between 1993 and 2008, 4.4% showed familial exposure (they lived with an occupationally exposed person), 4.3% environmental exposure (they lived near sources of asbestos pollution and were never occupationally exposed) and 1.6% were exposed during hobby-related or other leisure activities [43].

A spatial cluster analysis was conducted on ReNaM data. It observed clusters of cases also around industries of sectors with no direct use of asbestos, for example, nonasbestos textile, metal engineering and construction [44]. The extent of nonoccupational exposure (mainly environmental and familial exposures) has been estimated in around 10% of cases, mainly due to the residence near asbestos-cement plants and to the cohabitation with occupationally exposed subjects.

In the framework of a collaboration with National Health Institute (Istituto Superiore di Sanità—ISS), an extensive analysis of MM incidence in Italian national priority contaminated sites (NPCSs) has been performed recently, evidencing an overall excess of 1531 cases in those areas [45].

1.6 Epidemiological Surveillance of MM Mortality

MM is a rare and highly fatal neoplasm; therefore, mortality has been used as a proxy of incidence, since cause-specific mortality data are available in most countries, with national coverage. While well aware of the importance of national MM registration systems (characterized by the histological confirmation of diagnosis and the possibility to interview patients or their next of kins about asbestos exposure history), still the analysis of MM mortality can provide relevant information in terms of the disease occurrence and its temporal and spatial distribution.

A study performed in South-Eastern England showed that 87% of ascertained MM cases had mesothelioma correctly mentioned as their cause of death [46].

Epidemiological surveillance of MM mortality is thus performed in several countries, and here we provide only some examples.

The first registry of MM was started in the UK, based on the examination of the causes of death reporting 'mesothelioma' or other causes of interest. The more recent report (period 1968–2016) included about 2500 cases per year in the period 2012–2016, corresponding to the highest rates in the world [47].

In the US, 1999–2015, 45,221 deaths from MM were ascertained [48]. The overall annual number of deaths is still increasing, in particular in older age classes. Although incidence is decreasing in ages younger than 74, over 2500 cases were observed in the age class <55. Maintaining efforts to prevent asbestos exposure and for epidemiological surveillance is warranted.

In Greece, epidemiological surveillance is based on malignant pleural cancer (ICD ninth Revision). Mortality rate increased from 0.047/100,000 in 1983–1993 to 0.156 in 1994–2003 [49].

In Spain, MM mortality surveillance has so far been based on malignant pleural cancer as defined by ICD ninth Revision. There was a higher risk of death due to pleural cancer in areas with asbestos using industries [50]. Rates showed a flattening in 2001–2005 and a decline in women, but forecasts predict that pleural cancer mortality is expected to continue possibly to 2040 [51].

In Brazil, MM mortality was monitored based on national mortality records and an overall mortality rate of 1.1/100,000 was observed in 2003, but the authors underline that these figures may be underestimated [52].

Pasetto et al. presented an analysis of mortality from MM and other asbestos-related cancer in Argentina, Brazil, Colombia and Mexico based on the WHO mortality database and underlined the increasing trend and the possible underestimations [53].

Finally, in Italy, pleural mesothelioma mortality (ICD tenth Revision) has been used since 2003, while previously malignant pleural cancer (ICD ninth Revision) had been used. In the most recent report (2003–2014), mortality is still increasing in men and levelling off in women [54]. The average annual number of deaths was about 1000. Three regions of Northern Italy had mortality rates higher than national average in both genders. Out of 8046 Italian municipalities, 217 showed a statistically significant excess of the number of observed cases versus the regional expected value. These excesses were mainly observed in areas affected by the presence of industries using large amounts of asbestos in the production process or as an insulating material, and also in one Sicilian municipality characterized by the natural occurrence of fluoro-edenite in soil (see paragraph on naturally occurring fibres). These findings contribute to setting priorities for environmental remediation and to developing a communication process with affected communities and associations of victims.

Epidemiological surveillance of MM mortality, besides providing valuable public health information at country level, is also useful in the global environmental health arena.

1.7 Forecast of Temporal Trends in MM Occurrence

The joint analysis of ReNaM data, mortality statistics and asbestos consumption before the ban allowed to forecast MM mortality in Italy, predicting a peak around 2015–2020 [36]. A recent study performing a historical reconstruction of pleural MM mortality since 1970 actually confirmed these predictions [55].

Forecasts of MM incidence or mortality predicted a steady growth of the number of cases in industrialized countries, followed by a plateau or decline in consequence of the restriction in the use of asbestos [56]. Forecasts of MM mortality have been published for Europe [57], Great Britain [58, 59], France [60], Italy [61], The Netherlands [62], Denmark [63], Norway [64], Spain [51] and outside Europe for the US [65], Australia [33], Japan [66] and other Asiatic countries [67]. All predictions have been developed either using national asbestos consumption as proxy of exposure or according to age-period cohort models and provide similar expectations of a reduction in incidence after 30–40 years of reduction of the use of asbestos.

The analysis of the effect of asbestos ban on MM occurrence is methodologically complex given the short time so far elapsed and the long latency after asbestos exposure; however, Jarvholm and Burdorf [68] in Sweden could show a reduction in MM incidence in the more recent birth cohorts that started employment after the reduction of asbestos use.

1.8 The Economical Cost of MM

Based on ReNaM data and econometric analysis, Buresti et al. [69] estimated average medical care costs in 33,000 euro/case, and insurance and compensation costs in 25,000 euro/case, respectively. They also estimated a cost of 200,000 euro per patient for productivity loss, representing most of indirect costs of disease.

1.9 MM and Exposure to Naturally Occurring Fibres

Due to geological reasons, asbestos can be present in soil, where it can occur in outcrops, usually determining relatively low levels of airborne fibres. Anthropic interventions, though, such as those associated with excavations, quarries and agricultural work, can determine localized peaks of fibre concentrations, thus resulting in observable adverse health effects, ranging from pleural plaques to MM [70, 71].

The first report of MM cases associated with the presence of tremolite and chrysotile in soil concerned Turkey [72]. Several studies confirmed these findings in Greece, Cyprus, Turkey, Corsica, Botswana, Afghanistan and New Caledonia; for a review, see Pasetto et al. [73]. Liu et al. [74] and subsequently Luo et al. [75] reported an excess of asbestos-related disease, including MM, in an area of China characterized by the presence of crocidolite in soil. Pan et al. [76] observed a relation of MM risk with proximity to Naturally Occurring Asbestos in California. Considering all the available evidence, tremolite and chrysotile were present in most locations. While mean values of airborne fibres concentrations were low, high concentrations were found in whitewash and materials employed for road paving. In most case series, the sex ratio was close to 1 and the mean age at diagnosis was between 50 and 60, with an appreciable number of cases under 40. These findings point to an aetiologic role of the environmental asbestos exposure in childhood.

Investigations conducted in some contexts were useful in detecting the most important exposure routes and the role of other mineral fibres. Following the initial report of an outbreak of pleural mesothelioma and chronic fibrosing pleurisy in Central Turkey [77], a series of epidemiological studies demonstrated the aetiologic role of erionite, a natural fibrous zeolite found in some volcanic tuffs as an environmental contaminant whose occurrence was observed in the soil, road dust and building stone [78, 79]. Erionite was evaluated by the International Agency for Research on Cancer (IARC) as carcinogenic to humans in 1987, and subsequently this evaluation was confirmed in 2012 [80, 81]. Erionite was recently associated to a cluster of MM in Mexico [82].

In New Caledonia, the initial studies were focused on tremolite in whitewash [18], while subsequent investigations pointed to a major aetiologic role of serpentinite in soil, namely on the roads, and of proximity of serpentinite quarries to the residence of MM cases [83, 84]. In Libby, Montana, the vermiculite ore bed, which was extensively mined, contained up to 26% of amphibole asbestos initially believed to be tremolite, and subsequently shown to be a combination of winchite, richterite and tremolite. MM occurred in excess among vermiculite miners and also in the general population without occupational exposure [83, 84]. A recent study performed in the area of Mount Pollino, in Southern Italy, where natural outcrops of serpentinites and metabasites can contain tremolite, actinolite and chrysotile, showed an excess risk of MM in the villages where the outcrops were close to dwellings and cultivated land [87].

An excess of mortality for malignant pleural cancer[2] was observed in the years 1988–1992 in a municipality in Sicily, in the frame of the epidemiological surveillance of MM mortality in Italy. As no occupational exposure to asbestos was documented, the observation prompted a series of checks. Most cases were histologically confirmed, the sex ratio was close to 1 and exposure to asbestos could be excluded for most of them. On the basis of 26 cases diagnosed between 1998 and 2011 (13 men and 13 women), the incidence of the disease in Biancavilla appeared to be about five-fold the corresponding incidence in Sicily. For subjects diagnosed before 50 or 40 years of age, MM incidence was 20 and 60 times, respectively, the corresponding incidence in Sicily [88]. In the meanwhile, an amphibolic fibre was detected in the material extracted from a quarry located quite close to the town and extensively used in the construction industry and in road paving. The fibre was initially classified as an intermediate phase between tremolite and actinolite [89] and eventually found to be a new mineral, fluoro-edenite [90, 91]. After injection of fluoro-edenite fibres, rats developed MM of pleura and peritoneum [92, 93]. IARC classified fluoro-edenite as carcinogenic to humans in 2014 [94].

1.10 Man-Made Mineral Fibres and MM

Studies have been conducted in relation to different types of man-made mineral fibres. Evidence of carcinogenicity, including the observation of MM, was found in animal studies after exposure to ceramic fibres or slag wool fibres. However, no cases of MM

[2] The indirect estimator of pleural mesothelioma mortality that was used prior the adoption of the tenth Revision of the International Classification of Disease.

have been observed in the large cohort studies on workers in mineral fibres production. No evidence of association with glass fibres was observed in animal or epidemiological studies [95, 96].

Evidence of carcinogenicity was observed for the Silicon Carbide (SiC) whiskers, that were classified as probably carcinogenic to humans (Group 2A), based on evidence of MM in experimental animals [97]. Also different types of Carbon Nanotubes (CNT) were considered, of which only type MWCNT-7 was classified as 'possibly carcinogenic' (group 2B), while the other CNTs were classified in group 3 [97].

1.11 Exposure–Response Relationship Between Asbestos Exposure and MM

Many studies have been conducted to investigate quantitatively the relation between the dose of asbestos exposure and the risk of MM, and results were presented in classical reviews [11]. Here, we present the update of a quantitative review that was first prepared for the II Italian Consensus Conference on Malignant Mesothelioma [98]. We reviewed the reports of absolute or relative MM risk by either quantitative categories or exposure unit published by Medline indexed journals. Potentially relevant articles were searched via Pub-Med and perusal of references in reviews [11, 99–102], and full-text articles from the Pub-Med search. After exclusions based on examination of title, abstract or text, 59 works were retained and divided into two groups: (1) reports based on assessment of exposure to airborne asbestos, or external exposure [4, 8, 19, 57, 103–146], and (2) papers relying on the lung fibre burden or internal exposure [147–155]. Data on study characteristics and MM risk were abstracted according to standard formats adopted in a similar review by the II Italian Consensus Conference on Pleural Mesothelioma [98].

Results from 25 studies were reported by 49 articles with external exposure assessment (Table 1.1). Data from studies with multiple papers were abstracted from the most informative or most recent one. There were 19 cohort and nested case–control studies, mostly on highly exposed asbestos workers plus a cohort of residents in a village of Australian crocidolite miners [114, 138–141] and a general population cohort from the Netherlands [132]. Five population-based case–control studies [16, 115, 116, 119, 143] allowed the exposure–response relationship to be explored at low doses. As effect measure, we estimated the increase in relative risk by unit increase in cumulative exposure in fibre/millilitre year (f/mly), or slope in Table 1.1. Some papers provided this value [103, 109, 112, 146]. When not, we derived it by contrasting the maximum and minimum exposure categories and calculating the ratio between differences in their excess relative risk and in their average or midpoint exposure. Further calculations were needed: (1) to convert incidence rates into rate ratios [105, 123, 138, 142]; (2) to convert million particles per cubic foot into f/mly [123] according to the Hodgson and Darnton coefficient [11]. No slope estimate could be obtained in some cases, due to use of qualitative exposure categories [105, 127], semi-quantitative scores [117, 133], exposure to total dust rather than fibres [146] or lack of results by exposure category [111, 134]. In further two studies [112, 121], only the increase in the proportion of MM deaths over expected total mortality and not the change in relative risk could be calculated.

Some industry-based cohort studies allowed the identification of the type of fibre. The slope was lower for chrysotile-only cohorts (unit relative risk about 1.003) [112, 123, 137] than for mixed or amphibole cohorts (estimates ranging from 1.05 to 1.7).

The slope was higher in case–control studies, corresponding to a nonlinear increase, with steeper increase at low exposure. A particularly high slope was also found among pulp and paper workers [108]. In this cohort, exposure levels were lower than among asbestos workers and close to those found in general population studies. In case–control studies, the unit increase was between 1.5 (in China, where chrysotile had been almost exclusively used) [116] and 4.4 (in France) [119]. A steeper slope at low cumulative exposure had been previously reported [11]. Measurement errors in exposure, perhaps by over-estimation in industry-based and under-

Table 1.1 Exposure–response relationship for mesothelioma

Study # Study (references), main reference	Overall			Exposure assessment	Risk estimator	MM site	Asbestos type	Gender	Lowest		Highest		Slope
		No cases	Relative risk (95% CI)						category	risk	category	risk	
Cohort studies and nested case-control studies													
1 Cape Asbestos, UK ([4, 105, 131]), [105]	Ple Per All	52 46 98		High vs low and <2 years vs ≥ 2 years	Incidence rate per 100,000 years	All	Cro	Men Women	Low and <2 years	38 34	High and ≥2 years	308 133	
2 Turner & Newall, UK ([134, 156]), [134]	Ple Per All	10 0 10		Average level (p/ml), duration (years), CE (p/mly)	Fit of '*cubic residence time*' models[a]	Ple	Mix	Men					
3 UNARCO, USA ([121, 144, 145]), [121]	Ple Per All	7 7 14		CE (f/mly)	Obs. cases/exp. overall mortality	All	Amo	Men	<12	0	24–47	10.2%	0.35%
4 Asbestos-cement, Canada ([8, 113]), [113]	Ple Per All	31 14 45		CE (f/mly)	OR	All	Mix	Men	10	3.3	190	17.5	1.078
5 Rolling stock repairers, Sweden, [133]	All	5		Cumulative index = score × duration	No risk estimate for MMs	All	Mix	Men					
6 Raybestos Manhattan, USA ([112, 124]), [112]	Ple Per All	2 0 2		CE (f/mly)	Obs. cases/exp. overall mortality	Ple	Chr	Men					0.002%
7 Johns Manville, USA, [111]	Ple Per All	6 2 8		CE (mppcfy)	No risk estimate for MMs	All	Mix	Men					
8 Crocidolite miners, Australia ([104, 106, 107, 110, 129, 130, 142]), [142]	Ple Per All	281 48 329		CE (f/mly)	RR[b]	Ple Per	Cro Cro	Men Men	<10 <10	1 1	10–50 10–50	2.23 2.67	1.049 1.067
9 Asbestos-cement workers, Sweden, [103]	Ple	13	7.2 (1.0–54.0)	CE (f/mly)	OR	Ple	Mix	Men					1.7
10 Chrysotile miners, Italy ([135–137]), [137]	Ple Per All	7 1 8	5. 5 (2.2–11.4) 1.1 (0.0–6.1)	CE (f/mly)	SMR	Ple	Chr	Men	<100	5.8	≥400	7.7	1.003

11 Chrysotile miners, Canada ([123, 126]), [123]	Ple	25		CE (f/mly)[c]	RR[d]	Ple	Chr	Men	<300	1	≥900	6.27	1.003
12 Anthophyllite miners, Finland, [127]	Ple Per All	3 1 4	55.8 (11.5–163) 167 (4.2–933)	High/low	SIR	All	Ant	Men	All other workers		Miners and crashing plant workers	67.0	
13 Wittenoom residents, Australia ([114, 138–141]), [138]	Ple Per All	62 3 67		CE (f/mly)	RR[e]	Ple	Cro	Both	<10	1	25–50	5.30	1.132
14 Pulp and paper industry, [108]	Ple	14	2.5 (1.0–6.2)	CE (f/mly)	RR	Ple	Mix	Men	0.01	1	0.10–0.77	1.66	2.535
15 Finnish Asbestos Screening Campaign 1990–1992, [117]	All	13	2.0 (1.0–3.4)	Cumulative index (score × duration)	RR	All	Mix	Men	<40	1	40–89	1.9	
16 Vermiculite miners, USA ([122, 125]), [122]	All	19	94.8 (57.0–148)	CE (f/mly)	HR	All	Lib	Men					1.01
17 Asbestos textiles, France, [109]	Ple Per All	16 8 24		CE (f/mly)	RR	All	Mix	Both	<40	1	≥140	2.3	1.003
18 The Netherlands cohort study, [132]	Ple Per All	145 10 155	3.02 (2.11–4.32)	CE (f/mly)	RR	Ple	Mix	Men					1.08
19 'Amiantus' program, Poland, [146]	All	131		CE (mg/mly)	OR	All	Mix	Both	0	1.0	100	1.53	
Case control studies													
20 Five French regions, 1987–1993 ([115, 120]), [115]	Ple	405	3.6 (2.4–5.3) certain	CE (f/mly)	OR	Ple	Mix	Men	0.001–0.49	1.2	1–9.9	5.2	1.762

(continued)

Table 1.1 (continued)

Study # Study (references), main reference	Overall			Exposure assessment	Risk estimator	MM site	Asbestos type	Gender	Lowest		Highest		Slope
	No cases		Relative risk						category	risk	category	risk	
21 Hamburg, 1988–1991, Germany[f], [143]	Ple	125		CE (f/mly)	OR	Ple	Mix	Men	0–0.15	9.2	1.5–15	32.2	3.813
22 22 departments, 1998–2002, France ([119, 120]), [119]	Ple	437	Men: 11.4 (6.1–21.4) Women: 12.0 (3.5–41.7)	CE (f/mly)	OR	Ple	Mix	Men	0–0.1	4.0	1–10	22.5	4.394
23 Casale Monferrato, 2001–2006, Italy, [16]	Ple	200		CE (f/mly)	OR	Ple	Mix	Both	0–0.1	1	1–10	17.5	3.646
24 Southern China, 1998–2011, [116]	Ple	46		CE (f/mly)	OR	Ple	Chr	Both	0–0.5	28.0	0.5–29	36.0	1.535
Other study designs													
25 Amagasaki population, Japan ([19, 118]), [19]	All	121		Residential distance from industrial source	SMR	All	Mix	Men Women			Closest area Closest area	23.0 47.7	

Abbreviations: *Amo* amosite, *Ant* anthophyllite, *CE* cumulative exposure, *Chr* chrysotile, *Cro* crocidolite, *Exp* expected, *f/mly* fibres per millilitre-year, *HR* hazard ratio, *JEM* job-exposure matrix, *Mix* mixed fibres, *MM* malignant mesothelioma, *mppcfy* million particles per cubic foot-year, *Obs* observed, *OR* odds ratio, *p/mly* particles per millilitre-year, *Per* peritoneum, *Ple* pleura, *RR* rate ratio, *SMR* standardized mortality ratio, *TSFE* time since first exposure, *TSLE* time since last exposure

[a]Where incidence was fitted as a linear function of CE

[b]RR calculated from rates as published

[c]CE reported in mppcfy by the Authors. Conversion factor (1 mppcfy = 3 f/mly) as suggested by Hodgson and Darnton [11]. Mortality rates in Asbestos and Thetford mines calculated from data in Table 9

[d]RR calculated from rates (calculated from data in Table 9)

[e]RR calculated from rates as published

[f]Results from lagged (20 years) analyses

estimation in population-based studies, may have also contributed to such differences.

Results from nine studies were reported by ten articles with lung fibre burden data, providing evidence of monotonically increasing mesothelioma risk by increasing concentration of asbestos fibres or bodies in the lungs [147–155], in agreement with results from studies on external exposure.

1.12 Latency from Asbestos Exposure to MM Occurrence

The interval between the beginning of asbestos exposure and the occurrence of MM is usually very long, with median values exceeding 30 years [147–155].

Incidence of MM after asbestos exposure shows a linear increase with exposure and an exponential increase (with a power of 3 to 4) with time since exposure (usually called latency); therefore, early exposures weight more in the causation, although all exposures do contribute to the increase in MM risk. The relation of MM occurrence with exposure and with latency was investigated since the beginning of investigations on asbestos and MM [147–155]. A detailed summary of the mathematical formulas can be found in reviews [21, 98]. The Health Effects Institute (HEI) review [21] presents the formulas according to different duration of exposure (brief or extended) and type (constant or variable) of exposure. A minimum latency time (lag time) is often adopted, defined as the shortest time assumed for MM occurrence. Contrary to some misinterpretations, the power relation between MM and latency does consider all exposures (except lag time), each with its specific weight depending on the latency time elapsed, as no scientific evidence indicates a threshold.

These power models assume that MM incidence will constantly increase after exposure, with no upper limit. Recent reports, based on longer follow-up, indicate that for pleural MM an attenuation of the risk increase is observed after very long (over 40–50 years) latency, while increase continues for peritoneal MM [106, 159–161].

1.13 Other Risk Factors

1.13.1 Ionizing Radiations

The possible relation between ionizing radiation and MM has been investigated in relation to three categories of exposure: (1) the use of Thorotrast for diagnostic imaging, (2) the external irradiation for cancer treatment and (3) the exposure associated to occupational exposure, in particular in the nuclear industry. Five reports have been identified, reporting on cohort studies of subjects exposed to Thorotrast: two reported an increased frequency of both pleural and peritoneal MM, two an increased frequency of peritoneal MM only, while the fifth did not provide data on MM (review in [162]). The use of Thorotrast occurred in 1930–1955; therefore, the contribution to the present occurrence of MM is likely minimal [24, 98].

An increase in the frequency of MM has been observed in several cohort studies of long-term cancer survivors. The review by Goodman et al. [162] reported Relative Risks (RR) in the range from 6.6 to 25.7 for Hodgkin lymphoma survivors, from 0.8 to 2.24 for non-Hodgkin lymphoma and from 1.29 to 3.74 for breast cancer. Only one study reported on risk after malignancies of the testis, with an RR of 4 for MM. Based on these figures and on the number of incident cases of these malignancies, it was estimated that the number of MM attributable to this exposure in Italy was between 20 and 56 per year [98].

Scientific literature also reported cases of MM in workers exposed to ionizing radiations, but the more frequent source of exposure was the occupational activity in the nuclear industry, where asbestos exposure could not be excluded [162].

1.13.2 Viruses

The possible association of MM with SV40 infection was suggested, and initial studies supported it. However, after a 10-year-long debate with new evidence collected regarding the search of viral DNA in MM and in serum, the more recent studies failed to detect evidence of infection in serum samples collected before the diagnosis, and the conclusions no longer support the hypothesis of a causal association of MM and SV40 viral infection [98].

1.14 Conclusions

MM is a continuing legacy of asbestos exposure, affecting all the countries where asbestos fibres were used, and the also the areas with natural outcrops of mineral fibres.

The extent of asbestos exposure in occupational settings is expected to be decreasing in the countries that adopted exposure reduction measures, while the contribution of different patterns of nonoccupational exposures is likely underestimated, due to their much lower level, although not negligible and possibly sufficient to cause disease.

The relation of MM incidence with dose indicates that risk starts at very low doses, with no threshold, and increases with increasing cumulative exposure. The contribution of other risk factors, different from mineral fibres, is very limited.

Given the clear association with cumulative exposure and the long latency of the disease, asbestos ban is the only real solution to avoid the continuation of MM epidemics.

Conflict of Interest DM and CM acted as expert witnesses for the public prosecutor in court trials on asbestos-related diseases.

References

1. Wagner JC, Sleggs CA, Marchand P. Diffuse pleural mesothelioma and asbestos exposure in the North Western Cape Province. Br J Ind Med. 1960;17:260–71.
2. IARC. Asbestos. In: IARC monographs evaluation of carcinogenic risks to humans, vol. 14. Lyon: International Agency for Research on Cancer; 1977. p. 1–104.
3. IARC. Asbestos. In: Some inorganic and organometallic compounds. IARC monographs evaluation of carcinogenic risks to humans, vol. 2. Lyon: International Agency for Research on Cancer; 1973. p. 17–47.
4. Newhouse ML, Berry G. Predictions of mortality from mesothelial tumours in asbestos factory workers. Br J Ind Med. 1976;33:147–51.
5. Peto J, Seidman H, Selikoff IJ. Mesothelioma mortality in asbestos workers: implications for models of carcinogenesis and risk assessment. Br J Cancer. 1982;45:124–35.
6. Selikoff IJ. Lung cancer and mesothelioma during prospective surveillance of 1249 asbestos insulation workers, 1963-1974. Ann N Y Acad Sci. 1976;271:448–56.
7. McDonald JC, McDonald AD, Gibbs GW, Siemiatycki J, Rossiter CE. Mortality in the chrysotile asbestos mines and mills of Quebec. Arch Environ Health. 1971;22:677.
8. Finkelstein MM. Mortality among employees of an Ontario asbestos-cement factory. Am Rev Resp Dis. 1984;129:754–61.
9. Rubino GF, Piolatto G, Newhouse ML, Scansetti G, Aresini GA, Murray R. Mortality of chrysotile asbestos workers at the Balangero Mine, Northern Italy. Br J Ind Med. 1979;36:187–94.
10. Davis JM. Mineral fibre carcinogenesis: experimental data relating to the importance of fibre type, size, deposition, dissolution and migration. IARC Sci Publ. 1989;90:33–45.
11. Hodgson JT, Darnton A. The quantitative risks of mesothelioma and lung cancer in relation to asbestos exposure. Ann Occup Hyg. 2000;44:565–601.
12. IARC. Asbestos. In: Arsenic, metals, fibres and dusts. IARC monographs evaluation of carcinogenic risks to humans, vol. 100C. Lyon: International Agency for Research on Cancer; 2012. p. 219–310.
13. Landrigan PJ. The third wave of asbestos disease: exposure to asbestos in place. Public health control. Introduction. Ann N Y Acad Sci. 1991;643:xv–xvi.
14. Anderson HA, Lilis R, Daum SM, Fischbein AS, Selikoff IJ. Household-contact asbestos neoplastic risk. Ann N Y Acad Sci. 1976;271:311–23.
15. Ferrante D, Bertolotti M, Todesco A, Mirabelli D, Terracini B, Magnani C. Cancer mortality and incidence of mesothelioma in a cohort of wives of asbestos workers in Casale Monferrato, Italy. Environ Health Perspect. 2007;115:1401–5.
16. Ferrante D, Mirabelli D, Tunesi S, Terracini B, Magnani C. Pleural mesothelioma and occupational and non-occupational asbestos exposure: a case-control study with quantitative risk assessment. Occup Environ Med. 2016;73:147–53.
17. Gardner MJ, Saracci R. Effects on health of non-occupational exposure to airborne mineral fibres. In: Bignon J, Peto J, Saracci R, editors. Non-occupational exposure to mineral fibres, IARC

scientific publications no. 90. Lyon: International Agency for Research on Cancer; 1989. p. 375–97.
18. Goldberg P, Goldberg M, Marne MJ, Hirsch A, Tredaniel J. Incidence of pleural mesothelioma in New Caledonia: a 10-year survey (1978-1987). Arch Environ Health. 1991;46:306–9.
19. Kurumatani N, Kumagai S. Mapping the risk of mesothelioma due to neighborhood asbestos exposure. Am J Respir Crit Care Med. 2008;178:624–9.
20. Magnani C, Agudo A, González CA, Andrion A, Calleja A, Chellini E, Dalmasso P, Escolar A, Hernandez S, Ivaldi C, Mirabelli D, Ramirez J, Turuguet D, Usel M, Terracini B. Multicentric study on malignant pleural mesothelioma and non-occupational exposure to asbestos. Br J Cancer. 2000;83:104–11.
21. HEI Health Effects Institute - Asbestos Research. Asbestos in public and commercial buildings. Cambridge: Health Effects Institute - Asbestos Research; 1991.
22. Magnani C, Bianchi C, Chellini E, Consonni D, Fubini B, Gennaro V, Marinaccio A, Menegozzo M, Mirabelli D, Merler E, Merletti F, Musti M, Oddone E, Romanelli A, Terracini B, Zona A, Zocchetti C, Alessi M, Baldassarre A, Dianzani I, Maule M, Mensi C, Silvestri S. III Italian Consensus Conference on Malignant Mesothelioma of the Pleura. Epidemiology, Public Health and Occupational Medicine related issues. Med Lav. 2015;106:325–32.
23. Novello S, Pinto C, Torri V, Porcu L, Di Maio M, Tiseo M, Ceresoli G, Magnani C, Silvestri S, Veltri A, Papotti M, Rossi G, Ricardi U, Trodella L, Rea F, Facciolo F, Granieri A, Zagonel V, Scagliotti G. The third italian consensus conference for malignant pleural mesothelioma: state of the art and recommendations. Crit Rev Oncol Hematol. 2016;104:9–20.
24. Pinto C, Novello S, Torri V, Ardizzoni A, Betta PG, Bertazzi PA, Casalini GA, Fava C, Fubini B, Magnani C, Mirabelli D, Papotti M, Ricardi U, Rocco G, Pastorino U, Tassi G, Trodella L, Zompatori M, Scagliotti G. Second Italian consensus conference on malignant pleural mesothelioma: state of the art and recommendations. Cancer Treat Rev. 2013;39:328–39.
25. Wolff H, Vehmas T, Oksa P, Rantanen J, Vainio H. Asbestos, asbestosis, and cancer, the Helsinki criteria for diagnosis and attribution 2014: recommendations. Scand J Work Environ Health. 2015;41:5–15.
26. Odgerel CO, Takahashi K, Sorahan T, Driscoll T, Fitzmaurice C, Yoko-O M, Sawanyawisuth K, Furuya S, Tanaka F, Horie S, Zandwijk NV, Takala J. Estimation of the global burden of mesothelioma deaths from incomplete national mortality data. Occup Environ Med. 2017;74:851–8.
27. Delgermaa V, Takahashi K, Park EK, Le GV, Hara T, Sorahan T. Global mesothelioma deaths reported to the World Health Organization between 1994 and 2008. Bull World Health Organ. 2011;89:716–24.
28. Park EK, Takahashi K, Hoshuyama T, Cheng TJ, Delgermaa V, Le GV, Sorahan T. Global magnitude of reported and unreported mesothelioma. Environ Health Perspect. 2011;119:514–8.
29. Diandini R, Takahashi K, Park EK, Jiang Y, Movahed M, Le GV, Lee LJ, Delgermaa V, Kim R. Potential years of life lost (PYLL) caused by asbestos-related diseases in the world. Am J Ind Med. 2013;56:993–1000.
30. Marinaccio A, Binazzi A, Di Marzio D, Scarselli A, Verardo M, Mirabelli D, Gennaro V, Mensi C, Riboldi L, Merler E, Zotti RD, Romanelli A, Chellini E, Silvestri S, Pascucci C, Romeo E, Menegozzo S, Musti M, Cavone D, Cauzillo G, Tumino R, Nicita C, Melis M, Iavicoli S. Pleural malignant mesothelioma epidemic. Incidence, modalities of asbestos exposure and occupations involved from the Italian national register. Int J Cancer. 2012;130:2146–54.
31. Marinaccio A, Binazzi A, Bonafede M, et al. Quinto rapporto. Il Registro Nazionale dei Mesoteliomi. INAIL, Milano. 2015.
32. Ferrante P, Binazzi A, Branchi C, Marinaccio A. National epidemiological surveillance systems of mesothelioma cases. Epidemiol Prev. 2016;40:215–23.
33. Leigh J, Davidson P, Hendrie L, Berry D. Malignant mesothelioma in Australia, 1945-2000. Am J Ind Med. 2002;41:188–201.
34. Goldberg M, Imbernon E, Rolland P, Gilg Soit Ilg A, Savès M, de Quillacq A, Frenay C, Chamming's S, Arveux P, Boutin C, Launoy G, Pairon JC, Astoul P, Galateau-Sallé F, Brochard P. The French national mesothelioma surveillance program. Occup Environ Med. 2006;63:390–5.
35. Jung SH, Kim HR, Koh SB, Yong SJ, Chung MJ, Lee CH, Han J, Eom MS, Oh SS. A decade of malignant mesothelioma surveillance in Korea. Am J Ind Med. 2012;55:869–75.
36. Marinaccio A, Montanaro F, Mastrantonio M, et al. Predictions of mortality from pleural mesothelioma in Italy: a model based on asbestos consumption figures supports results from age-period-cohort models. Int J Cancer. 2005;115:142–7.
37. Magnani C, Dalmasso P, Biggeri A, Ivaldi C, Mirabelli D, Terracini B. Increased risk of malignant mesothelioma of the pleura after residential or domestic exposure to asbestos: a case-control study in Casale Monferrato, Italy. Environ Health Perspect. 2001;109:915–9.
38. Musti M, Pollice A, Cavone D, Dragonieri S, Bilancia M. The relationship between malignant mesothelioma and an asbestos cement plant environmental risk: a spatial case-control study in the city of Bari (Italy). Int Arch Occup Environ Health. 2009;82:489–97.
39. Mensi C, Riboldi L, De Matteis S, Bertazzi PA, Consonni D. Impact of an asbestos cement factory on mesothelioma incidence: global assessment of effects of occupational, familial, and environmental exposure. Environ Int. 2015;74:191–9.

40. Dodoli D, Del Nevo M, Fiumalbi C, Iaia TE, Cristaudo A, Comba P, Viti C, Battista G. Environmental household exposures to asbestos and occurrence of pleural mesothelioma. Am J Ind Med. 1992;21:681–7.
41. Comba P, D'Angelo M, Fazzo L, Magnani C, Marinaccio A, Mirabelli D, Terracini B. Mesothelioma in Italy: the Casale Monferrato model to a national epidemiological surveillance system. Ann Ist Super Sanita. 2018;54:139–48.
42. Mirabelli D, Calisti R, Barone-Adesi F, Fornero E, Merletti F, Magnani C. Excess of mesotheliomas after exposure to chrysotile in Balangero, Italy. Occup Environ Med. 2008;65:815–9.
43. Marinaccio A, Binazzi A, Bonafede M, Corfiati M, Di Marzio D, Scarselli A, Verardo M, Mirabelli D, Gennaro V, Mensi C, Schallemberg G, Merler E, Negro C, Romanelli A, Chellini E, Silvestri S, Cocchioni M, Pascucci C, Stracci F, Ascoli V, Trafficante L, Angelillo I, Musti M, Cavone D, Cauzillo G, Tallarigo F, Tumino R, Melis M. Malignant mesothelioma due to non-occupational asbestos exposure from Italian national surveillance system (ReNaM): epidemiology and public health issues. Occup Environ Med. 2015;72:648–55.
44. Corfiati M, Scarselli A, Binazzi A, et al. Epidemiological patterns of asbestos exposure and spatial clusters of incident cases of malignant mesothelioma from the Italian national registry. BMC Cancer. 2015;15:286.
45. Binazzi A, Marinaccio A, Corfiati M, Bruno C, Fazzo L, Pasetto R, Pirastu R, Biggeri A, Catelan D, Comba P, Zona A. Mesothelioma incidence and asbestos exposure in Italian national priority contaminated sites. Scand J Work Environ Health. 2017;43:550–9.
46. Okello C, Treasure T, Nicholson AG, Peto J, Møller H. Certified causes of death in patients with mesothelioma in South East England. BMC Cancer. 2009;9:28.
47. HSE. www.hse.gov.uk/statistics/causdis/mesothelioma/mesothelioma.pdf. Accessed 28 Sept 2018.
48. Mazurek JM, Syamlal G, Wood JM, Hendricks SA, Weston A. Malignant mesothelioma mortality - United States, 1999-2015. MMWR Morb Mortal Wkly Rep. 2017;66:214–8.
49. Gogou E, Kerenidi T, Chamos V, Zintzaras E, Gourgoulianis KI. Mesothelioma mortality in Greece from 1983 to 2003. Int J Clin Pract. 2009;63:944–8.
50. López-Abente G, Hernández-Barrera V, Pollán M, Aragonés N, Pérez-Gómez B. Municipal pleural cancer mortality in Spain. Occup Environ Med. 2005;62:195–9.
51. López-Abente G, García-Gómez M, Menéndez-Navarro A, Fernández-Navarro P, Ramis R, García-Pérez J, Cervantes M, Ferreras E, Jiménez-Muñoz M, Pastor-Barriuso R. Pleural cancer mortality in Spain: time-trends and updating of predictions up to 2020. BMC Cancer. 2013;13:528.
52. Pedra F, Tambellini AT, Pereira Bde B, da Costa AC, de Castro HA. Mesothelioma mortality in Brazil, 1980-2003. Int J Occup Environ Health. 2008;14(3):170–5. Erratum in: Int J Occup Environ Health. 2009;15:391
53. Pasetto R, Terracini B, Marsili D, Comba P. Occupational burden of asbestos-related cancer in Argentina, Brazil, Colombia, and Mexico. Ann Glob Health. 2014;80:263–8.
54. Fazzo L, Minelli G, De Santis M, Bruno C, Zona A, Conti S, Comba P. Epidemiological surveillance of mesothelioma mortality in Italy. Cancer Epidemiol. 2018;55:184–91.
55. Ferrante P, Mastrantonio M, Uccelli R, Corfiati M, Marinaccio A. Pleural mesothelioma mortality in Italy: time series reconstruction (1970-2009) and comparison with incidence (2003-2008). Epidemiol Prev. 2016;40:205–14.
56. Montanaro F, Bray F, Gennaro V, Merler E, Tyczynski JE, Parkin DM, Strnad M, Jechov'a M, Storm HH, Aareleid T, Hakulinen T, Velten M, Lef'evre H, Danzon A, Buemi A, Daur'es JP, Ménégoz F, Raverdy N, Sauvage M, Ziegler H, Comber H, Paci E, Vercelli M, De Lisi V, Tumino R, Zanetti R, Berrino F, Stanta G, Langmark F, Rachtan J, Mezyk R, Blaszczyk J, Ivan P, Primic-Zakelj M, Martínez AC, Izarzugaza I, Borràs J, Garcia CM, Garau I, Sánchez NC, Aicua A, Barlow L, Torhorst J, Bouchardy C, Levi F, Fisch T, Probst N, Visser O, Quinn M, Gavin A, Brewster D, Mikov M, ENCR Working Group. Pleural mesothelioma incidence in Europe: evidence of some deceleration in the increasing trends. Cancer Causes Control. 2003;14:791–803.
57. Pelucchi C, Malvezzi M, La Vecchia C, Levi F, Decarli A, Negri E. The mesothelioma epidemic in Western Europe: an update. Br J Cancer. 2004;90:1022–4.
58. Hodgson JT, McElvenny DM, Darnton AJ, et al. The expected burden of mesothelioma mortality in Great Britain from 2002 to 2050. Br J Cancer. 2005;92:587–93.
59. Tan E, Warren N, Darnton AJ, Hodgson JT. Projection of mesothelioma mortality in Britain using Bayesian methods. Br J Cancer. 2010;103:430–6.
60. Le Stang N, Belot A, Gilg Soit Ilg A, et al. Evolution of pleural cancers and malignant pleural mesothelioma incidence in France between 1980 and 2005. Int J Cancer. 2010;126:232–8.
61. Marinaccio A, Corfiati M, Binazzi A, Di Marzio D, Scarselli A, Ferrante P, Bonafede M, Verardo M, Mirabelli D, Gennaro V, Mensi C, Schallemberg G, Mazzoleni G, Merler E, Girardi P, Negro C, D'Agostin F, Romanelli A, Chellini E, Silvestri S, Pascucci C, Calisti R, Stracci F, Romeo E, Ascoli V, Trafficante L, Carrozza F, Angelillo IF, Cavone D, Cauzillo G, Tallarigo F, Tumino R, Melis M, Iavicoli S, ReNaM Working Group. The epidemiology of malignant mesothelioma in women: gender differ-

ences and modalities of asbestos exposure. Occup Environ Med. 2018;75:254–62.
62. Segura O, Burdorf A, Looman C. Update of predictions of mortality from pleural mesothelioma in the Netherlands. Occup Environ Med. 2003;60:50–5.
63. Kjaergaard J, Andersson M. Incidence rates of malignant mesothelioma in Denmark and predicted future number of cases among men. Scand J Work Environ Health. 2000;26:112–7.
64. Ulvestad B, Kjaerheim K, Møller B, Andersen A. Incidence trends of mesothelioma in Norway, 1965-1999. Int J Cancer. 2003;107:94–8.
65. Price B, Ware A. Time trend of mesothelioma incidence in the United States and projection of future cases: an update based on SEER data for 1973 through 2005. Crit Rev Toxicol. 2009;39:576–88.
66. Myojin T, Azuma K, Okumura J, Uchiyama I. Future trends of mesothelioma mortality in Japan based on a risk function. Ind Health. 2012;50:197–204.
67. Le GV, Takahashi K, Park EK, et al. Asbestos use and asbestos-related diseases in Asia: past, present and future. Respirology. 2001;16:767–75.
68. Järvholm B, Burdorf A. Emerging evidence that the ban on asbestos use is reducing the occurrence of pleural mesothelioma in Sweden. Scand J Public Health. 2015;43:875–81.
69. Buresti G, Colonna F, Corfiati M, et al. Economic impact of malignant mesothelioma in Italy: an estimate of the public and social costs. Med Lav. 2017;108:358–66.
70. Burlikov T, Michailova L. Asbestos content of the soil and endemic pleural asbestosis. Environ Res. 1970;3:443–51.
71. Hillerdal G. Mesothelioma: cases associated with non-occupational and low dose exposures. Occup Environ Med. 1999;56:505–13.
72. Yazicioglu S, Ilçayto R, Balci K, Sayli BS, Yorulmaz B. Pleural calcification, pleural mesotheliomas, and bronchial cancers caused by tremolite dust. Thorax. 1980;35:564–9.
73. Pasetto R, Comba P, Marconi A. Mesothelioma associated with environmental exposures. Med Lav. 2005;96:330–7.
74. Liu XZ, Luo SQ, Wang ZM, Wang MZ, Zhan CL. An investigation of crocidolite contamination and mesothelioma in a rural area of China. Biomed Environ Sci. 1990;3:156–65.
75. Luo S, Liu X, Mu S, Tsai SP, Wen CP. Asbestos related diseases from environmental exposure to crocidolite in Da-yao, China. I. Review of exposure and epidemiological data. Occup Environ Med. 2003;60:35–41.
76. Pan XL, Day HW, Wang W, Beckett LA, Schenker MB. Residential proximity to naturally occurring asbestos and mesothelioma risk in California. Am J Respir Crit Care Med. 2005;172:1019–25.
77. Baris YI, Sahin AA, Ozesmi M, Kerse I, Ozen E, Kolacan B, Altinörs M, Göktepeli A. An outbreak of pleural mesothelioma and chronic fibrosing pleurisy in the village of Karain/Urgüp in Anatolia. Thorax. 1978;33:181–92.
78. Bariş YI, Grandjean P. Prospective study of mesothelioma mortality in Turkish villages with exposure to fibrous zeolite. J Natl Cancer Inst. 2006;98:414–7.
79. Simonato L, Bariş R, Saracci R, et al. Relation of environmental exposure to erionite fibres to risk of respiratory cancer. IARC Sci Publ. 1989;90:398–405.
80. IARC. Erionite. In: Arsenic, metals, fibres and dusts. IARC monographs evaluation of carcinogenic risks to humans, vol. 100C. Lyon: International Agency for Research on Cancer; 2012. p. 311–6.
81. IARC. Silica and some silicates. IARC monographs evaluation of carcinogenic risks to humans, vol. 42. International Agency for Research on Cancer: Lyon; 1987.
82. Espejo-Herrera N, Gràcia-Lavedan E, Boldo E, Aragonés N, Pérez-Gómez B, Pollán M, Molina AJ, Fernández T, Martín V, La Vecchia C, Bosetti C, Tavani A, Polesel J, Serraino D, Gómez Acebo I, Altzibar JM, Ardanaz E, Burgui R, Pisa F, Fernández-Tardón G, Tardón A, Peiró R, Navarro C, Castaño-Vinyals G, Moreno V, Righi E, Aggazzotti G, Basagaña X, Nieuwenhuijsen M, Kogevinas M, Villanueva CM. Colorectal cancer risk and nitrate exposure through drinking water and diet. Int J Cancer. 2016;139:334–46.
83. Baumann F, Maurizot P, Mangeas M, Ambrosi JP, Douwes J, Robineau B. Pleural mesothelioma in New Caledonia: associations with environmental risk factors. Environ Health Perspect. 2011;119:695–700.
84. Baumann F, Rougier Y, Ambrosi JP, Robineau BP. Pleural mesothelioma in New Caledonia: an acute environmental concern. Cancer Detect Prev. 2007;31:70–6.
85. Naik SL, Lewin M, Young R, Dearwent SM, Lee R. Mortality from asbestos-associated disease in Libby, Montana 1979-2011. J Expo Sci Environ Epidemiol. 2017;27:207–13.
86. Whitehouse AC, Black CB, Heppe MS, Ruckdeschel J, Levin SM. Environmental exposure to Libby asbestos and mesotheliomas. Am J Ind Med. 2008;51:877–80.
87. Caputo A, De Santis M, Manno V, Cauzillo G, Bruni BM, Palumbo L, Conti S, Comba P. Health impact of asbestos fibres naturally occurring in Mount Pollino area (Basilicata Region, Southern Italy). Epidemiol Prev. 2018;42:142–50.
88. Bruno C, Tumino R, Fazzo L, Cascone G, Cernigliaro A, De Santis M, Giurdanella MC, Nicita C, Rollo PC, Scondotto S, Spata E, Zona A, Comba P. Incidence of pleural mesothelioma in a community exposed to fibres with fluoro-edenitic composition in Biancavilla (Sicily, Italy). Ann Ist Super Sanita. 2014;50:111–8.
89. Paoletti L, Batisti D, Bruno C, Di Paola M, Gianfagna A, Mastrantonio M, Nesti M, Comba P. Unusually high incidence of malignant pleural mesothelioma in a town of the eastern Sicily: an epidemiological and

environmental study. Arch Environ Occup Health. 2000;55:392–8.
90. Comba P, Gianfagna A, Paoletti L. The pleural mesothelioma cases in Biancavilla are related to the new fluoro-edenite fibrous amphibole. Arch Environ Occup Health. 2003;58:229–32.
91. Gianfagna A, Oberti R. Fluoro-edenite from Biancavilla (Catania, Sicily, Italy). Crystal chemistry of a new amphibole end-member. Am Mineral. 2001;83:1486–93.
92. Belpoggi F, Tibaldi E, Lauriola M, Bua L, Falcioni L, Chiozzotto D, Manservisi F, Manservigi M, Soffritti M. The efficacy of long-term bioassays in predicting human risks: mesotheliomas induced by fluoro-edenitic fibres present in lava stone from the Etna volcano in Biancavilla, Italy. Eur J Oncol. 2011;16:185–96.
93. Soffritti M, Minardi F, Bua L, Degli Esposti D, Belpoggi F. First experimental evidence of peritoneal and pleural mesotheliomas induced by fluoro-edenite fibres present in Etnean volcanic material from Biancavilla (Sicily, Italy). Eur J Oncol. 2004;9:169–75.
94. IARC. Fluoro-edenite. In: Some nanomaterials and some fibres. IARC monographs on the evaluation of carcinogenic risks to humans, vol. 111. Lyon: International Agency for Research on Cancer; 2017. p. 215–42.
95. IARC. Man-made vitreous fibres. IARC monographs evaluation of carcinogenic risks to humans, vol. 81. International Agency for Research on Cancer: Lyon; 2002.
96. Utell MJ, Maxim LD. Refractory ceramic fiber (RCF) toxicity and epidemiology: a review. Inhal Toxicol. 2010;22:500–21.
97. IARC. Carbon nanotubes. In: Some nanomaterials and some fibres. IARC monographs on the evaluation of carcinogenic risks to humans, vol. 111. Lyon: International Agency for Research on Cancer; 2017. p. 35–214.
98. Magnani C, Fubini B, Mirabelli D, Bertazzi PA, Bianchi C, Chellini E, Gennaro V, Marinaccio A, Menegozzo M, Merler E, Merletti F, Musti M, Pira E, Romanelli A, Terracini B, Zona A. Pleural mesothelioma: epidemiological and public health issues. Report from the Second Italian Consensus Conference on Pleural Mesothelioma. Med Lav. 2013;104:191–202.
99. Berman DW, Crump KS. Update of potency factors for asbestos-related lung cancer and mesothelioma. Crit Rev Toxicol. 2008;38(Suppl 1):1–47.
100. Boffetta P, Stayner LT. Pleural and peritoneal neoplasms. In: Schottenfeld D, Fraumeni JF, editors. Cancer epidemiology and prevention. 3rd ed. New York: Oxford University Press; 2006. p. 659–73.
101. Goodman M, Morgan RW, Ray R, Malloy CD, Zhao K. Cancer in asbestos-exposed occupational cohorts: a meta-analysis. Cancer Causes Control. 1999;10:453–65.
102. Lash TL, Crouch EA, Green LC. A meta-analysis of the relation between cumulative exposure to asbestos and relative risk of lung cancer. Occup Environ Med. 1997;54:254–63.
103. Albin M, Jakobsson K, Attewell R, et al. Mortality and cancer morbidity in cohorts of asbestos cement workers and referents. Br J Ind Med. 1990;47:602–10.
104. Berry G, de Klerk NH, Reid A, et al. Malignant pleural and peritoneal mesotheliomas in former miners and millers of crocidolite at Wittenoom, Western Australia. Occup Environ Med. 2004;61:e14.
105. Berry G, Newhouse ML, Wagner JC. Mortality from all cancers of asbestos factory workers in East London 1933-80. Occup Environ Med. 2000;57:782–5.
106. Berry G, Reid A, Aboagye-Sarfo P, de Klerk NH, Olsen NJ, Merler E, Franklin P, Musk AW. Malignant mesotheliomas in former miners and millers of crocidolite at Wittenoom (Western Australia) after more than 50 years follow-up. Br J Cancer. 2012;106:1016–20.
107. Berry G. Prediction of mesothelioma, lung cancer, and asbestosis in former Wittenoon asbestos workers. Br J Ind Med. 1991;48:793–802.
108. Carel R, Boffetta P, Kauppinen T, Teschke K, Andersen A, Jäppinen P, Pearce N, Rix BA, Bergeret A, Coggon D, Persson B, Szadkowska-Stanczyk I, Kielkowski D, Henneberger P, Kishi R, Facchini LA, Sala M, Colin D, Kogevinas M. Exposure to asbestos and lung and pleural cancer mortality among pulp and paper industry workers. J Occup Environ Med. 2002;44:579–84.
109. Clin B, Morlais F, Launoy G, Guizard AV, Dubois B, Bouvier V, Desoubeaux N, Marquignon MF, Raffaelli C, Paris C, Galateau-Salle F, Guittet L, Letourneux M. Cancer incidence within a cohort occupationally exposed to asbestos: a study of dose—response relationships. Occup Environ Med. 2011;68:832–6.
110. de Klerk NH, Armstrong BK, Musk AW, Hobbs MS. Cancer mortality in relation to measures of occupational exposure to crocidolite at Wittenoom Gorge in Western Australia. Br J Ind Med. 1989;46:529–36.
111. Enterline PE, Hartley J, Henderson V. Asbestos and cancer: a cohort followed up to death. Br J Ind Med. 1987;44:396–401.
112. Finkelstein MM, Meisenkothen C. Malignant mesothelioma among employees of a Connecticut factory that manufactured friction materials using chrysotile asbestos. Ann Occup Hyg. 2010;54:692–6.
113. Finkelstein MM. Analysis of the exposure-response relationship for mesothelioma among asbestos-cement factory workers. Ann N Y Acad Sci. 1991;643:85–9.
114. Hansen J, de Klerk NH, Musk AW, Hobbs MS. Environmental exposure to crocidolite and mesothelioma: exposure-response relationships. Am J Respir Crit Care Med. 1998;157:69–75.

115. Iwatsubo Y, Pairon JC, Boutin C, Ménard O, Massin N, Caillaud D, Orlowski E, Galateau-Salle F, Bignon J, Brochard P. Pleural mesothelioma: dose-response relation at low levels of asbestos exposure in a French population-based case-control study. Am J Epidemiol. 1998;148:133–42.
116. Jiang Z, Chen T, Chen J, Ying S, Gao Z, He X, Miao C, Yu M, Feng L, Xia H, Wu W, Chen R, Morinaga K, Lou J, Zhang X. Hand-spinning chrysotile exposure and risk of malignant mesothelioma: a case-control study in Southeastern China. Int J Cancer. 2018;142:514–23.
117. Koskinen K, Pukkala E, Martikainen R, Reijula R, Karjalainen A. Different measures of asbestos exposure in estimating risk of lung cancer and mesothelioma among construction workers. J Occup Environ Med. 2002;44:1190–6.
118. Kumagai S, Kurumatani N. Asbestos fiber concentration in the area surrounding a former asbestos cement plant and excess mesothelioma deaths in residents. Am J Ind Med. 2009;52:790–8.
119. Lacourt A, Gramond C, Rolland P, Ducamp S, Audignon S, Astoul P, Chamming's S, Gilg Soit Ilg A, Rinaldo M, Raherison C, Galateau-Salle F, Imbernon E, Pairon JC, Goldberg M, Brochard P. Occupational and non-occupational attributable risk of asbestos exposure for malignant pleural mesothelioma. Thorax. 2014;69:532–9.
120. Lacourt A, Leffondré K, Gramond C, Ducamp S, Rolland P, Gilg Soit Ilg A, Houot M, Imbernon E, Févotte J, Goldberg M, Brochard P. Temporal patterns of occupational asbestos exposure and risk of pleural mesothelioma. Eur Respir J. 2012;39:1304–12.
121. Langer AM. Health experience of some US and Canadian workers exposed to asbestos: foundation for risk assessment. In: Nolan RP, Langer AM, Ross M, Wicks FJ, Martin RF, editors. The health effects of chrysotile, Canadian mineralogist special publication 5. Ottawa: Mineralogical Association of Canada; 2001. p. 9–20.
122. Larson TC, Antao VC, Bove FJ. Vermiculite worker mortality: estimated effects of occupational exposure to Libby amphibole. J Occup Environ Med. 2010;52:555–60.
123. Liddell FD, McDonald AD, McDonald JC. The 1891–1920 birth cohort of Quebec chrysotile miners and millers: development from 1904 and mortality to 1992. Ann Occup Hyg. 1997;41:13–36.
124. McDonald AD, Fry JS, Woolley AJ, McDonald JC. Dust exposure and mortality in an American chrysotile asbestos friction products plant. Br J Ind Med. 1984;41:151–7.
125. McDonald JC, Harris J, Armstrong B. Mortality in a cohort of vermiculite miners exposed to fibrous amphibole in Libby, Montana. Occup Environ Med. 2004;61:363–6.
126. McDonald JC, Liddell FD, Dufresne A, McDonald AD. The 1891-1920 birth cohort of Quebec chrysotile miners and millers: mortality 1976-88. Br J Ind Med. 1993;50:1073–81.
127. Meurman LO, Pukkala E, Hakama M. Incidence of cancer among antophyllite asbestos miners in Finland. Occup Environ Med. 1994;51:421–5.
128. Mowé G, Gylseth B, Hartveit F, Skaug V. Fiber concentration in lung tissue of patients with malignant mesothelioma: a case-control study. Cancer. 1985;56:1089–93.
129. Musk AW, de Klerk NH, Olsen N, et al. Mortality in miners and millers of crocidolite in Western Australia: follow-up to 1999. Ann Occup Hyg. 2002;46(Suppl 1):90–2.
130. Musk AW, de Klerk NH, Reid A, et al. Mortality of former crocidolite (blue asbestos) miners and millers at Wittenoom. Occup Environ Med. 2008;65:541–3.
131. Newhouse ML, Berry G, Wagner JC. Mortality of factory workers in East London 1933-80. Br J Ind Med. 1985;42:4–11.
132. Offermans NS, Vermeulen R, Burdorf A, Goldbohm RA, Kauppinen T, Kromhout H, van den Brandt PA. Occupational asbestos exposure and risk of pleural mesothelioma, lung cancer, and laryngeal cancer in the Prospective Netherlands Cohort Study. J Occup Environ Med. 2014;56:6–19.
133. Ohlson CG, Klaesson B, Hogstedt C. Mortality among asbestos-exposed workers in a railroad workshop. Scand J Work Environ Health. 1984;10:283–91.
134. Peto J. The hygiene standard for chrysotile asbestos. Lancet. 1978;1:484–9.
135. Piolatto G, Negri E, La Vecchia C, Pira E, De Carli A, Peto J. An update on cancer mortality among chrysotile asbestos miners in Balangero, northern Italy. Br J Ind Med. 1990;47:810–4.
136. Pira E, Pelucchi C, Piolatto PG, et al. Mortality from cancer and other causes in the Balangero cohort of chrysotile asbestos miners. Occup Environ Med. 2009;66:805–9.
137. Pira E, Romano C, Donato F, Pelucchi C, Vecchia C, Boffetta P. Mortality from cancer and other causes among Italian chrysotile asbestos miners. Occup Environ Med. 2017;74:558–63.
138. Reid A, Berry G, de Klerk N, Hansen J, Heyworth J, Ambrosini G, Fritschi L, Olsen N, Merler E, Musk AW. Age and sex differences in malignant mesothelioma after residential exposure to blue asbestos (crocidolite). Chest. 2007;131:376–82.
139. Reid A, Berry G, Heyworth J, et al. Predicted mortality from malignant mesothelioma among women exposed to blue asbestos at Wittenoom, Western Australia. Occup Environ Med. 2009;66:169–74.
140. Reid A, Franklin P, Olsen N, Sleith J, Samuel L, Aboagye-Sarfo P, de Klerk N, Musk AW. All-cause mortality and cancer incidence among adults exposed to blue asbestos during childhood. Am J Ind Med. 2013;56:133–45.
141. Reid A, Heyworth J, de Klerk N, Musk AW. The mortality of women exposed environmentally and domestically to blue asbestos at Wittenoom, Western Australia. Occup Environ Med. 2008;65:743–9.

142. Reid A, Merler E, Peters S, Jayasinghe N, Bressan V, Franklin P, Brims F, de Klerk NH, Musk AW. Migration and work in postwar Australia: mortality profile comparisons between Australian and Italian workers exposed to blue asbestos at Wittenoom. Occup Environ Med. 2018;75:29–36.
143. Rödelsperger K, Jöckel KH, Pohlabeln H, et al. Asbestos and man-made vitreous fibers as risk factors for diffuse malignant mesothelioma: results from a German hospital based case-control study. Am J Ind Med. 2001;39:262–75.
144. Seidman H, Selikoff IJ, Gelb SK. Mortality experience of amosite asbestos factory workers: dose-response relationships 5 to 40 years after onset of short-term work exposure. Am J Ind Med. 1986;10:479–514.
145. Seidman H, Selikoff IJ, Hammond EC. Short-term asbestos work exposure and long-term observation. Ann N Y Acad Sci. 1979;330:61–89.
146. Świątkowska B, Szeszenia-Dąbrowska N. Mesothelioma continues to increase even 40 years after exposure - evidence from long-term epidemiological observation. Lung Cancer. 2017;108:121–5.
147. Albin M, Johanssen L, Pooley FD, et al. Mineral fibres, fibrosis, and asbestos bodies in lung tissue from deceased asbestos cement workers. Br J Ind Med. 1990;47:767–74.
148. Gilham C, Rake C, Burdett G, Nicholson AG, Davison L, Franchini A, Carpenter J, Hodgson J, Darnton A, Peto J. Pleural mesothelioma and lung cancer risks in relation to occupational history and asbestos lung burden. Occup Environ Med. 2016;73:290–9.
149. Howel D, Gibbs A, Arblaster L, et al. Mineral fibre analysis and routes of exposure to asbestos in the development of mesothelioma in an English region. Occup Environ Med. 1999;56:51–8.
150. Johansson LG, Albin MP, Jakobsson KM, Welinder HEC, Ranstam PJ, Attewell RG. Ferruginous bodies and pulmonary fibrosis in dead low to moderately exposed asbestos cement workers: histological examination. Br J Ind Med. 1987;44:550–8.
151. McDonald JC, Armstrong B, Case B, et al. Mesothelioma and asbestos fiber type. Evidence from lung tissue analyses. Cancer. 1989;63:1544–7.
152. McDonald JC, Armstrong BG, Edwards CW, et al. Casereferent survey of young adults with mesothelioma: I. Lung fibre analyses. Ann Occup Hyg. 2001;45:513–8.
153. Rödelsperger K, Woitowitz HJ, Brückel B, et al. Dose-response relationship between amphibole fiber lung burden and mesothelioma. Cancer Detect Prev. 1999;23:183–93.
154. Rogers AJ, Leigh J, Berry G, et al. Relationship between lung asbestos fiber type and concentration and relative risk of mesothelioma. A case-control study. Cancer. 1991;67:1912–20.
155. Tuomi T, Huuskonen MS, Virtamo M, et al. Relative risk of mesothelioma associated with different levels of exposure to asbestos. Scand J Work Environ Health. 1991;17:404–8.
156. Peto J, Doll R, Hermon C, et al. Relationship of mortality to measures of environmental asbestos pollution in an asbestos textile factory. Ann Occup Hyg. 1985;29:305–55.
157. Lanphear BP, Buncher CR. Latent period for malignant mesothelioma of occupational origin. J Occup Med. 1992;34:718–21.
158. Marinaccio A, Binazzi A, Cauzillo G, Cavone D, Zotti RD, Ferrante P, Gennaro V, Gorini G, Menegozzo M, Mensi C, Merler E, Mirabelli D, Montanaro F, Musti M, Pannelli F, Romanelli A, Scarselli A, Tumino R, Italian Mesothelioma Register (ReNaM) Working Group. Analysis of latency time and its determinants in asbestos related malignant mesothelioma cases of the Italian register. Eur J Cancer. 2007;43:2722–8.
159. Barone Adesi F, Ferrante D, Bertolotti M, et al. Long-term mortality from pleural and peritoneal cancer after exposure to asbestos. Possible role of asbestos clearance. Int J Cancer. 2008;123:912–6.
160. Ferrante D, Chellini E, Merler E, Pavone V, Silvestri S, Miligi L, Gorini G, Bressan V, Girardi P, Ancona L, Romeo E, Luberto F, Sala O, Scarnato C, Menegozzo S, Oddone E, Tunesi S, Perticaroli P, Pettinari A, Cuccaro F, Mattioli S, Baldassarre A, Barone-Adesi F, Cena T, Legittimo P, Marinaccio A, Mirabelli D, Musti M, Pirastu R, Ranucci A, Magnani C, The Working Group. Italian pool of asbestos workers cohorts: mortality trends of asbestos-related neoplasms after long time since first exposure. Occup Environ Med. 2017;74:887–98.
161. Reid A, de Klerk NH, Magnani C, Ferrante D, Berry G, Musk AW, Merler E. Mesothelioma risk after 40 years since first exposure to asbestos: a pooled analysis. Thorax. 2014;69:843–50.
162. Goodman JE, Nascarella MA, Valberg PA. Ionizing radiation: a risk factor for mesothelioma. Cancer Causes Control. 2009;20:1237–54.

Asbestos and the Pathophysiology of Mesothelioma

2

Nico van Zandwijk and Glen Reid

2.1 Introduction

Malignant mesothelioma, or simply mesothelioma, originates from the mesothelial lining of the pleural cavity, the pericardium and the abdominal cavity including the tunica vaginalis. Christopher Wagner was among the first to recognize the relation between asbestos exposure and mesothelioma [1]. More than half a century later, an abundant body of evidence has accumulated confirming that occupational and environmental asbestos exposure has a causative role in the majority of cases of this highly malignant condition. Exposure to erionite, an asbestos-like fibre, ionizing irradiation and chronic inflammation of the pleura have also been recognized as additional causes [2]. Despite the prominent carcinogenic potential of asbestos fibres, it usually takes more than 20 years from the date of first asbestos exposure until manifestation of disease. Latency periods range from around 20 to more than 50 years explaining why mesothelioma is often diagnosed in patients with advanced age [3] and why asbestos is referred to as a 'Time Bomb with a Long Fuse' [4]. Lung cancer, ovarian cancer (and probably cancers in other organ sites), pulmonary fibrosis (asbestosis), pleural plaques and pleural effusions are the malignant and non-malignant pathologies occurring after asbestos exposure [5–8]. Whereas lung cancer studies revealed a clear synergism between (occupational) asbestos exposure and cigarette smoking [9], smoking alone doesn't seem to contribute to the development of mesothelioma.

2.2 History of Asbestos

The history of asbestos dates back at least 4000 years. Asbestos was found to be an important ingredient of Finnish pottery that was produced around 2500 BC, and also featured as a magical (i.e. fire-resistant) material (stone) in ancient Greek and Roman writings [10, 11]. The term asbestos is derived from the ancient Greek term for *inextinguishable* and covers a collection of minerals (hydrated silicates) naturally occurring in a fibrous form. Asbestos fibres are traditionally divided into serpentine and amphibole forms, and the shape (length and aspect ratio) of these fibres is thought to play an important role in carcinogenicity. While in the

N. van Zandwijk (✉)
Faculty of Medicine, The University of Sydney, Camperdown, NSW, Australia

Specialist Sydney Local Health District, Concord Repatriation General Hospital, Concord, NSW, Australia
e-mail: nico.vanzandwijk@sydney.edu.au

G. Reid
Faculty of Medicine, The University of Sydney, Camperdown, NSW, Australia

Department of Pathology, Dunedin School of Medicine, University of Otago, Dunedin, New Zealand
e-mail: glen.reid@otago.ac.nz

G. L. Ceresoli et al. (eds.), *Mesothelioma*, https://doi.org/10.1007/978-3-030-16884-1_2

past, evidence pointed mainly to long asbestos fibres, a recent review has focused more attention on short asbestos fibres [12]. Amphibole fibres are straight, stiff and particularly strong, and include amosite (brown asbestos), crocidolite (blue asbestos), anthophyllite, tremolite and actinolite. Amphiboles have been used for the production of asbestos cement, insulation materials, tiles and numerous other products. Chrysotile (white asbestos) is the sole serpentine form of asbestos with curly, pliable fibres suitable for building materials, insulation products and fabrics.

Asbestos use surged in the late nineteenth century in Europe (Italy and Russia) and Canada, with commercial (mechanized) mining of these minerals driven by increasing applications during the industrial revolution. Commercial amphibole mining began with amosite in South Africa and crocidolite in Australia in the beginning of the 1900s. Boosted by its fire-retarding properties, asbestos was increasingly used after WWII in building materials as well as in a wide range of products for everyday life [13].

2.3 Exposure to Asbestos in the Occupational Setting

The association between asbestos and lung fibrosis provided the first indication that asbestos exposure in an occupational setting could be dangerous. Scattered reports on asbestos-induced fibrosis had appeared in the 1920s [14, 15] and contributed to the establishment of workplace (dust) regulations in the UK [16]. The neoplastic consequences of asbestos exposure were discovered 20 years later by the renowned study of Sir Richard Doll, revealing the causal association between occupational asbestos exposure and lung cancer [17]. Ten years later, a similar path was followed and mesothelioma was linked to asbestos exposure. The landmark publication of Wagner appeared shortly after a number of isolated case reports describing mesothelioma in patients after occupational asbestos exposure [18, 19]. The rapidly rising asbestos consumption in the second half of the previous century was followed, around 20 years later, by a major increase in mesothelioma incidence [20, 21]. In this context, it is important to underline that preventive measures including workplace regulations and asbestos bans did not become effective before the 1980s. However, when these regulations were eventually introduced in Europe and Australia, an acceleration in asbestos consumption was noted in most Asian countries to the extent that it is estimated that currently 60% of the world's chrysotile production is consumed in Asia.

Over the last 50 years, a number of case–control studies have further analysed the relationship between occupational asbestos exposure and mesothelioma and have confirmed the causal link identified by Wagner [22–28]. A recent example of a national survey from France—which estimated asbestos exposures of individuals who worked in the construction and shipbuilding industries or who were involved in the manufacture of asbestos cement, metal-working industry or the manufacture/repair of motor vehicles—once more confirmed a clear dose relationship between asbestos exposure and occurrence of mesothelioma [29]. Additionally, this study provided attributable risk data and an estimation of the risk of non-occupational asbestos exposures in females. The commercial use of asbestos in France was predominantly chrysotile; therefore, these data cannot be generalized to other (developing) countries with a different pattern of industrialization and using different types of asbestos.

2.4 Environmental Asbestos Exposure

In the past, mesothelioma was mostly attributed to exposure of asbestos in the occupational environment. Today, it is recognized that there are multiple non-occupational pathways for exposure to asbestos, generally referred to as environmental asbestos exposure (Fig. 2.1) [30].

2.4.1 Para-Occupational Exposure

Para-occupational asbestos exposure is defined as the exposure of family members of asbestos-

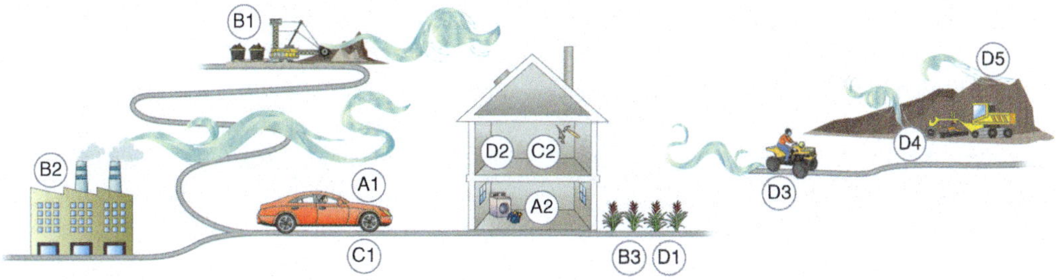

Fig. 2.1 Potential pathways for environmental exposure to asbestos. (**a**) Para-occupational exposure occurs when asbestos-exposed workers function as vectors for transporting fibres. Household contacts can be exposed in worker vehicles (*a1*) or through contact with worker clothes or other dust deposits in the home (*a2*). (**b**) Environmental exposure from industrial operations. Airborne contamination to communities can be attributed to emissions from nearby mining operations (*b1*) or asbestos industry (*b2*). Communities can also be exposed to railings or asbestos-laden industrial waste materials when used in roadways or soils (*b3*). (**c**) Exposure to commercial asbestos-containing products. Asbestos is in numerous products, including automotive brakes (*c1*) and several housing materials that can be readily disturbed during home maintenance or renovation projects (*c2*). (**d**) Naturally occurring asbestos (NOA). In several parts of the world, humans have been exposed to asbestos through local use of NOA materials for roads and soil amendments (*d1*) and as a component in whitewash, stucco or other building materials (*d2*). Human contact with locations of exposed NOA can result in fibre release through recreational interaction (*d3*) and development projects (*d4*). NOA materials can also be released through natural erosion and wind (*d5*). Adapted from C. W. Noonan. Ann Transl Med;5(11):234 with permission of the author

exposed workers, who serve as a vector for the transport of asbestos fibres into the household setting. The most common activity attributed to para-occupational asbestos exposure is laundering of asbestos-contaminated clothes. Interestingly, the asbestos lung fibre burden among para-occupationally exposed women with mesothelioma was found to be in the same range as in male mesothelioma cases with moderate occupational exposure [13]. Over the past decades, several hundred mesothelioma cases have been reported among family members of workers in industries with asbestos exposure including mining, shipbuilding and cement manufacturing [31]. An impressive report on para-occupational exposures came from the crocidolite mine in Wittenoom, Western Australia, where between 1943 and 1992, 40 cases of mesothelioma were detected in women not involved in asbestos mining or milling [32]. It is assumed that environmental (airborne) exposures and exposure to tailings from the mine will have contributed to the cause of mesothelioma in these cases. A recent meta-analysis of para-occupational exposure and mesothelioma found an odds ratio of 5.0 (2.5–10 CI) for domestic asbestos exposure [33].

2.4.2 Environmental Exposure

Environmental asbestos exposures typically take place in the vicinity of industrial operations and asbestos mines, and there are reports showing decreasing mesothelioma risk with increasing distance from industrial asbestos activities [34, 35]. Thus, the outdoor environment provides an important source of asbestos exposure. However, in recent years, it has become apparent that the indoor environment may also pose a serious risk factor. Living in a house with loose-fill (amosite) roof insulation confers an increased risk of cancer (in particular mesothelioma) [36], and it is clear that renovation of asbestos-contaminated homes and buildings is contributing to the mesothelioma epidemic [37]. Victims' groups and lawyers involved in the claims of asbestos victims were the first to point to the 'changing face of mesothelioma' and demanded attention for the role of non-occupational asbestos exposure in causing disease. The early assessment of cancer outcomes in New York City firefighters, who were massively exposed to asbestos and multiple other carcinogens after the attacks on the World Trade Centre on 11 September 2001, reveals an increased cancer incidence and a high prevalence of disease conditions thought to be the consequence of chronic inflammation [38]. It is difficult to judge these early findings, but considering the fact that lung and mesothelioma carcinogenesis are estimated to take at least 20 years, much more time is needed to reliably estimate the consequences of an unprecedented intense exposure to toxic, asbestos-containing dust.

Mesothelioma registry data from Australia confirm that the number of mesothelioma cases with exposure to asbestos during home renovation has increased in recent years [21], underlining the importance of awareness campaigns to warn people not to disturb asbestos-containing materials. The ongoing excessive consumption of asbestos in developing countries urgently calls for action, but it is doubtful if the mesothelioma epidemic that is currently building up in these countries can be effectively prevented [39]. In this respect, it should be underlined that the pathological diagnosis of mesothelioma is notoriously difficult and frequently requires an expert pathologist [40, 41]. Apart from the difficulties in making a correct mesothelioma diagnosis, underreporting of mesothelioma in developing nations has been noticed [39, 42, 43]. Underreporting may have contributed to an attitude of 'mesothelioma is not a problem here' and explain the lack of attention for the dangers of (occupational and environmental) asbestos in many countries worldwide.

2.4.3 Naturally Occurring Asbestos

Apart from occupational, para-occupational and environmental asbestos and related mineral exposures, we may have unintended contact with 'natural' asbestos in rocks and soils. Naturally occurring asbestos (NOA) is a term used to describe fibrous minerals that constitute a natural component of rocks and soil, although they may or may not meet the regulatory definitions of asbestos [44]. Several geographic areas with deposits of natural occurring asbestos have been identified: tremolite and chrysotile are found in villages in Turkey, Greece, Corsica, Cyprus and New Caledonia; erionite is present in Cappadocia; and crocidolite in commonly found in rural southwestern China [45–50]. In some of these places, the naturally occurring asbestos was used for whitewashing and stucco and in others for the pavement of roads. The mesothelioma incidence rates among people living around these typically rural sites were elevated when compared with global background rates and, similar to studies of asbestos plants, the mesothelioma risk was inversely correlated with the distance from the asbestos deposit. The male-to-female ratios were lower than for mesotheliomas in the occupational setting and frequently approach 1:1 [51]. Our understanding of the risks of naturally occurring asbestos has increased in recent years, and studies from New Caledonia, Turkey and the US have identified the most likely sources of environmental asbestos exposures (roads, soils, whitewash and stucco), underlining that not every natural environment is safe.

2.5 The Chrysotile Controversy

Ninety to 95% of all asbestos mined and utilized worldwide was chrysotile [52]. On the basis of historical asbestos consumption data and age-adjusted mortality rates, an evident (ecological) association between the increasing mortality from mesothelioma and increasing asbestos consumption was established in 2007 [53]. This worldwide association study underlines that the consensus among scientists, who reviewed the asbestos literature and concluded that all forms of asbestos are carcinogenic, is correct [54]. The term 'safe use of chrysotile asbestos' propagated by Chrysotile Association, a Canada-based lobby group of chrysotile producers, has been used to avoid expansion of trading bans for all forms of asbestos [55–57]. The debate about the 'safety' of chrysotile came to a head in 1997 following the blanket ban on asbestos usage by France. A dispute with Canada ensued, with claims of damaged economic interests and impedance of free trade in view of the alleged safety of chrysotile. After much discussion, the World Trade Organization ruled that chrysotile was dangerous, and in the subsequent years, it became a requirement for all countries wishing to enter the European Union to ban all forms of asbestos. The anti-chrysotile position has also been adopted by the United Nations, United States Environmental Protection Agency (though not the US government) and the International Labour Organization (WHO. Elimination of asbestos related diseases. WHO; 2006). It is important to note that the Canadian support for Chrysotile was not unanimous. The Canadian Cancer Society (2010), the Canadian Medical association (2009) and the Canadian Public Health Association (2010) opposed the exportation of chrysotile to developing countries. After the Quebec provincial election in 2012, the winning party (Parti Québécois) followed through with the election promise to halt asbestos mining and to cancel a multimillion dollar loan promised by the Canadian government to reopen the mines that were closed in 2011. Since this time, the International Chrysotile Association (ICA), funded and controlled by foreign asbestos interests, continues to defend the 'safe use of chrysotile' despite a plethora of scientific evidence showing the opposite. The Directors of the ICA represent asbestos interests in Russia, Kazakhstan, Brazil, India, Mexico and Zimbabwe and lobby governments not to ban asbestos [58, 59]. It is assumed that the 'safe use of chrysotile' campaigns together with the accelerated economic developments in Asia have contributed to the dramatic shift of the world's asbestos consumption to Asian countries [60].

The complexity of establishing the relation between asbestos (chrysotile) exposure and mesothelioma should not be underestimated. The long latency between (first) asbestos exposure and cancer (mesothelioma) is a confounding factor, and deaths from cardiovascular disease and cancers other than mesothelioma partly obscure the link between asbestos and mesothelioma [61]. Moreover, observational studies usually are not designed to cover periods of 50 years or more, and studies with a follow up of 10–20 years are unable to establish a reliable association between chrysotile exposure and mesothelioma. The importance of continued observations is underlined by data from the Australian Mesothelioma Registry revealing a marked increase over time of the age-specific mesothelioma incidence rates for individuals aged 75 years or older [21]. Taking into consideration the complexity of making a correct mesothelioma diagnosis [62], it is understandable why it has taken so many years to confirm the association between chrysotile exposure and the occurrence of mesothelioma [63, 64].

Proponents of chrysotile hypothesize that this form of asbestos is unable to cause significant toxicity due to the ability of chrysotile fibres to undergo rapid, longitudinal splitting into smaller fibrils. The splitting into smaller fragments was thought to lead to a more rapid clearance from the lung (decreased half-life) and less carcinogenicity [65]. Animal studies had also suggested a relationship between fibre dimensions and carcinogenic potential (Stanton hypothesis), with longer fibres being more carcinogenic [66]. Moreover, pathological studies with fibre counts in lung tissue and fibre classification revealed significant amounts of amphibole fibres (tremolite) in the lungs of chrysotile workers [67, 68]. These amphiboles rather than chrysotile were suspected to constitute the real cause of mesothelioma. Similar studies in autopsy cases of mesothelioma patients revealed a high prevalence of amphibole fibres [69]. In addition, the relationship between lung asbestos fibre type/burden and relative risk of mesothelioma was supported by the outcomes of a case–control study [70]. However, in an analysis of 186 human lung and mesothelioma samples by high-resolution analytical electron microscopy, long thin asbestos fibres comprised only 2.3% of the fibres present; 89.4% were ≤5 μm and 92.7% were ≤0.25 μm in width, suggesting a contribution of these shorter fibres to the pathogenesis of mesothelioma [71]. In 2017, the first longitudinal intraindividual asbestos fibre quantitation data became available [72]. Sequential biopsies of 12 patients with asbestos-related disease had been collected at a median interval of 8 years (range 4–21). Over time, the fibre burden seemed to have increased, and chrysotile was found to be the main fibre present in the tissue samples (66.7%). Considering the theory of 'rapid clearance' of chrysotile from the lungs, the high biopersistence of chrysotile fibres in the lungs of patients with asbestos-related disease came as a genuine surprise. This study also underlined the complexity of fibre analyses and added a new dimension to the chrysotile debate. Previous studies measuring asbestos fibres in the lungs of patients have taken the fibre burden as a surrogate for asbestos carcinogenesis and potentially overlooked the most important steps of mesothelioma carcinogenesis that are assumed to take place in the parietal pleura [10].

The potency of amphibole asbestos fibres to induce mesothelioma has been re-evaluated recently. While amphiboles appear to have a greater link to mesothelioma, it is suspected that chrysotile may have a similar potential as amphiboles, when lung cancer is concerned [73]. The high lung cancer rates in a prospective study of 37 years in smoking and non-smoking chrysotile miners in China provide a good example supporting this idea [74]. Finally, it is important to mention that researchers with a conflict of interest (due to financial support from the asbestos industry) have influenced the chrysotile debate. As such they are responsible for a black page in the history of research into asbestos-related diseases [75].

2.6 Non-Asbestos Causes of Mesothelioma

2.6.1 Erionite

Not every mesothelioma is elicited by minerals categorized under the name asbestos. Exposure to erionite, a fibrous zeolite but resembling asbestos [76] and present in volcanic regions around the world, is associated with mesothelioma. Environmental exposure to erionite present in volcanic deposits in the Cappadocia region of Turkey, where it is used to whitewash houses, has been established as the origin of an unusually high incidence of mesothelioma [77, 78]. Subsequent experimental studies confirmed the carcinogenic potential of this mineral [79]. Interestingly, there is also a high incidence of lung cancers noted among the inhabitants of this region [80], and similar observations have been made in other parts of the world [81, 82]. As a consequence of the very high (>50%) incidence of erionite-associated mesothelioma, genetic predisposition studies have been undertaken. These suggest that the mesothelioma epidemic must result from an interaction between genetics and erionite exposure [83, 84].

2.6.2 Ionizing Irradiation

The association between mesothelioma and radiation exposure comes from case reports, case series and retrospective cohort studies. The total number of radiation-exposed individuals studied is much smaller than in studies of asbestos exposure. Evidence for an elevated risk of developing mesothelioma following radiotherapy for Hodgkin and non-Hodgkin lymphoma, childhood tumours or breast cancer has been provided in a number of studies [85–88]. Similar observations were made in patients exposed to radioactive contrast (Thorotrast) and in individuals exposed to radiation in nuclear plants [89, 90]. Experiments with intraperitoneal injection of plutonium dioxide in rats confirmed that a variety of tumours including mesothelioma were induced in a high percentage (30%) of the exposed animals [91].

2.6.3 Chronic Inflammation

Scattered reports of mesothelioma following chronic inflammation of the pleura (or peritoneum) have appeared since the 1980s. Chronic empyema and tuberculosis, chronic diverticulitis and recurrent peritonitis (Crohn's disease) were among the preconditions [92–95]. These case reports do not allow more than speculation about the carcinogenic pathways and inflammatory mediators involved, although continuous overproduction of certain cytokines has been suspected to play an important role [96].

2.6.4 Carbon Nanotubes

A variety of man-made fibres have been studied for their potential etiological role in inducing mesothelioma. Systematic reviews of vitreous fibres conclude that that there is insufficient support for an increased risk of mesothelioma following exposure to rock wool and glass fibres [97]. Carbon nanotubes, applied in a variety of products and—as with asbestos in the past—rapidly gaining popularity, are likely to behave as biopersistent fibres with a carcinogenic potential [98]. Similar to asbestos fibres, carbon nanotubes will lodge in the lungs after inhalation and migrate to the pleura and give rise to a (chronic) inflammatory reaction [99]. Notwithstanding the fact that the literature on the health effects of carbon nanotubes and mesothelioma is scarce, the asbestos tragedy teaches us that our awareness of the potential dangers of man-made mineral fibres should be high. In other words, these nanomaterials should only be released into the environment if extensive carcinogenic testing has confirmed their safety [10].

2.6.5 Simian Virus 40

In 1996, a potential causative role of simian virus 40 (SV40)—an oncogenic polyomavirus endemic in rhesus monkeys and a contaminant of the poliovirus vaccine of the 1950s—in the development of mesothelioma was proposed by UK investigators [100]. It was theorized that 30–100 million individuals in the US and many more worldwide might have received SV40-contaminated polio vaccine, thereby increasing their future risk of mesothelioma [101]. Initially, a few reports seemed to support this theory, but none of the larger epidemiological studies that followed have been able to confirm this association [102–104]. Within this context, it is appropriate to mention experimental studies revealing that mice became more susceptible to asbestos carcinogenesis after being infected with SV40 or transfected with SV40 large T-antigen (Tag) [105] and that transgenic mice in which expression of the SV40 large T antigen is limited to the mesothelium are particularly susceptible to asbestos carcinogenesis [106]. Interestingly, these experimental tumours don't have the same mutations as human mesothelioma.

2.7 Mesothelioma Carcinogenesis

Until recently, it has been assumed that the mesothelial cell represented the progenitor cell for mesothelioma. However, when mesothelial cells are damaged, sub-mesothelial (multipotent) stem cells may contribute to repair/regeneration [10, 107, 108]. Therefore, it is unclear whether the mesothelioma progenitor cell is derived from a sub-mesothelial (multipotent) cell, from the differentiated mesothelial cell or both [10]. Another point that needs our attention is the hypothesis that mesothelioma primarily originates in the parietal pleura and thereafter involves the visceral pleura. The carcinogenic (initiating) role of asbestos fibres that accumulated near the parietal pleura seems likely, but since pathological studies have primarily focused on asbestos fibres in lung parenchyma, our understanding of mesothelioma carcinogenesis is far from complete. Taking clinical and experimental evidence together, it seems likely that inhaled asbestos fibres will end up in the pleura, induce a chronic inflammatory reaction and lead to 'frustrated phagocytosis' followed by genetic and epigenetic changes in the mesothelium [109, 110]. In addition, fibre-induced changes in signalling pathways [111], iron-catalysed generation of free radicals [112] and the release of alarmins such as HMGB1 [113] have been postulated to play a role in carcinogenesis.

Cytogenetic studies have revealed that instead of being associated with oncogene mutations, mesothelioma is primarily caused by a lack of tumour-suppressing mechanisms. More recent studies employing next-generation sequencing have reinforced this notion [114–116]. The cyclin-dependent kinase inhibitor 2A (*CDKN2A*), neurofibromatosis type 2 (*NF2*) and BRCA1-associated protein (*BAP1*) are the most frequently mutated tumour-suppressor genes [114]. *CDKN2A* deletions are found in about 70%, inactivating NF2 mutations in 35–40% and *BAP1* alterations in 60% of mesothelioma cases. *NF2*, *CDKN2A* and *BAP1* deletions also contribute to mesothelioma development in mouse models [117–120]. There is increasing evidence that in certain individuals there might have been a genetic basis for more susceptibility to asbestos carcinogenesis [121–123], and *BAP1* mutation carriers found a high incidence of malignancies in contrast to family members who did not carry a mutation. As *BAP1* mutations were found less frequent in patients with sporadic mesothelioma, it is hoped that additional gene-disease correlation studies will further elucidate susceptibility factors [124]. Functional studies have demonstrated the feasibility of targeting BAP1 protein partners as well as genes up- and downstream of BAP1 functions. For example, the molecular targeting of EZH2 overexpression in mesothelioma tumour cells lacking BAP1 activity has been postulated as an approach to treatment [125] and has reached the clinical trial stage [126].

In addition to the frequent loss of tumour-suppressor genes, array-based investigations have reported gene expression changes that distinguish mesothelioma from mesothelium [127], provide a prognostic signature [128], identify potential therapeutic targets [129] and define molecular sub-groups [130]. Many of these changes result in growth promoting upregulation of genes involved metabolism [131], cell cycle and mitosis [129], signalling pathways [127] and epithelial–mesenchymal transition [130]. More recent next-generation sequencing has confirmed many of these transcriptomic changes [114, 132]. As well as changes between mesothelioma and normal tissue, gene expression changes in mesothelial and lung epithelial cells induced by asbestos exposure have been explored, both in vitro [133–135] and in various animal models [136, 137]. Changes induced by asbestos include alterations to cell signalling, apoptosis, inflammatory response and fibrogenesis. However, the specific contribution of many of these changes to mesothelioma remains to be determined.

More recently, non-coding RNA genes have also been implicated in mesothelioma pathogenesis, with the microRNA family of non-coding of gene regulators gaining increasing attention in recent years. These short (21–23 nucleotides) posttranscriptional repressors of mRNA translation are predominantly downregulated in cancer contributing to upregulation of growth-promoting genes [138], with a growing number of reports implicating roles for microRNAs in mesothelioma carcinogenesis and biology [139]. Compared to the effects of asbestos exposure on protein coding gene expression, there is limited information concerning asbestos-induced changes in microRNA levels. While expression profiling in asbestos-exposed mesothelial cells and animal models is needed to clarify the role of microRNAs in mesothelioma carcinogenesis, several studies suggest they may appear at an early stage. For example, silencing the tumour-suppressor miR-34 family imparts malignant characteristics to mesothelial cells [140], and mice genetically engineered to have LOH in *Nf2* and *Cdkn2a* develop aggressive tumours with reduced p53 and miR-34a expression [141]. In addition, the inflammatory effects of asbestos fibres are associated with altered methylation patterns in mesothelioma [142, 143], and epigenetic silencing has been found to suppress levels of miR-34b/c [144], miR-145 [145] and miR-126 [146]. Other mechanisms are responsible for the reduced expression of additional microRNAs: miR-31 is frequently co-deleted with *CDKN2A* [147], while gene dosage also affects expression of miR-137 [148]. Intriguingly, while the latter display tumour-suppressor properties in mesothelioma cells, they are also found at elevated levels in the tumours of patients with shorter survival [148, 149] suggesting different roles during tumour progression.

Accumulating evidence suggests that changes in microRNA expression contribute to the increased migration and invasion characteristic of mesothelioma cells. Increasing the levels of miR-29c-3p [150], miR-31 [147], miR-34b/c [144], miR-137 [148] and miR-145 [145] all inhibit invasion. Changes in miR-205 were associated with increased epithelial–mesenchymal transition, with expression lower in non-epithelioid tumours and cell lines [151]. Other microRNAs including members of the miR-15 [152] and miR-34 [144] families, miR-193a-3p [153] and miR-302b [154], regulate expression of cell cycle and apoptosis-related genes and proliferation. However, while the list of dysregulated microRNAs with tumour-suppressor activity in mesothelioma continues to grow, only a handful have shown therapeutic potential by inhibiting tumour growth in vivo [139]. Of these, miR-16 has developed furthest clinically. It is significantly downregulated in mesothelioma tumours and cell lines, and restoring levels using a mimic inhibited mesothelioma growth in vitro and in vivo [152]; these results supported a phase I trial which yielded promising results [155]. The contribution of miR-16 family members to chemoresistance [152], PD-L1 [156] and mesothelin expression [157] suggests that microRNAs may have the potential to contribute to combination therapy.

2.8 Conclusion

The relationship between occupational and non-occupational asbestos exposure and development of mesothelioma is well established. In occupational studies, the number of males diagnosed with mesothelioma was definitely higher than that of females. However, when studies with non-occupational asbestos exposure are taken into account, this gender difference seems to disappear. In recent years, the risk of environmental asbestos has been more accurately defined, while non-asbestos risk factors such as irradiation have been added. Special attention is warranted for the potential risk of carbon nanotubes, bearing structural similarities with asbestos fibres. Despite the acceptance by global health organizations more than 40 years ago of the evidence that all forms of asbestos are carcinogenic, asbestos manufacturers worldwide have continued their lobby for so-called 'safe chrysotile use'. This lobby, closely resembling that of the tobacco industry, contributes to the continuing (massive) environmental pollution in developing countries and the creation of the health problems of tomorrow. The disclosure that certain asbestos researchers, paid (directly or indirectly) by the asbestos industry, participated in the 'chrysotile debate' constitutes a black page in the history of research of asbestos-related diseases and underlines the crucial role of 'conflict-of-interest' statements.

Progress has been made in our understanding of the biology of mesothelioma and the molecular changes occurring in mesothelioma cells. Overall, the number of genes with recurrent mutations in mesothelioma is relatively limited, and mostly comprises tumour-suppressor genes. A role of BAP1 mutations in familial mesothelioma is very likely. Mutations in BAP1 are also common in sporadic mesothelioma, and additional studies may provide new approaches for the treatment of tumours exhibiting loss of BAP1 or other tumour-suppressor genes. Similarly, microRNAs are also frequently dysregulated in mesothelioma, and their roles in carcinogenesis and tumour progression are slowly becoming clear. The continued investigation into mesothelioma biology is essential to identify new preventive and therapeutic strategies and to provide hope for patients suffering from this devastating predominantly man-made cancer.

Acknowledgements/Conflict of Interest Statement Professor Nico van Zandwijk would like to express his gratitude for the support given by Sydney Local Health District while writing this chapter. Associate Professor Glen Reid changed position—from the University of Sydney to the University of Otago—while contributing to this chapter. Both authors declare to be unaware of any conflict of interest.

References

1. Wagner JC, Sleggs CA, Marchand P. Diffuse pleural mesothelioma and asbestos exposure in the North Western Cape Province. Br J Ind Med. 1960;17:260–71.
2. Attanoos RL, Churg A, Galateau-Salle F, Gibbs AR, Roggli VL. Malignant mesothelioma and its non-Asbestos causes. Arch Pathol Lab Med. 2018;142(6):753–60.
3. Bianchi C, Giarelli L, Grandi G, Brollo A, Ramani L, Zuch C. Latency periods in asbestos-related mesothelioma of the pleura. Eur J Cancer Prev. 1997;6(2):162–6.
4. Linton A, Vardy J, Clarke S, van Zandwijk N. The ticking time-bomb of asbestos: its insidious role in the development of malignant mesothelioma. Crit Rev Oncol Hematol. 2012;84(2):200–12.

5. Ferrante D, Mirabelli D, Tunesi S, Terracini B, Magnani C. Pleural mesothelioma and asbestos exposure: a case-control study with quantitative risk assessment-response to Marsh and Benson's letter. Occup Environ Med. 2017;74(2):157–8.
6. Pira E, Romano C, Violante FS, Farioli A, Spatari G, La Vecchia C, et al. Updated mortality study of a cohort of asbestos textile workers. Cancer Med. 2016;5(9):2623–8.
7. Ndlovu N, Rees D, Murray J, Vorajee N, Richards G, teWaterNaude J. Asbestos-related diseases in mineworkers: a clinicopathological study. ERJ Open Res. 2017;3(3):00022-2017.
8. Pairon JC, Andujar P, Rinaldo M, Ameille J, Brochard P, Chamming's S, et al. Asbestos exposure, pleural plaques, and the risk of death from lung cancer. Am J Respir Crit Care Med. 2014;190(12):1413–20.
9. Ngamwong Y, Tangamornsuksan W, Lohitnavy O, Chaiyakunapruk N, Scholfield CN, Reisfeld B, et al. Additive synergism between asbestos and smoking in lung cancer risk: a systematic review and meta-analysis. PLoS One. 2015;10(8):e0135798.
10. Roe OD, Stella GM. Malignant pleural mesothelioma: history, controversy and future of a manmade epidemic. Eur Respir Rev. 2015;24(135):115–31.
11. Pira E, Donato F, Maida L, Discalzi G. Exposure to asbestos: past, present and future. J Thorac Dis. 2018;10(Suppl 2):S237–S45.
12. Boulanger G, Andujar P, Pairon JC, Billon-Galland MA, Dion C, Dumortier P, et al. Quantification of short and long asbestos fibers to assess asbestos exposure: a review of fiber size toxicity. Environ Health. 2014;13:59.
13. Roggli VL, Sharma A, Butnor KJ, Sporn T, Vollmer RT. Malignant mesothelioma and occupational exposure to asbestos: a clinicopathological correlation of 1445 cases. Ultrastruct Pathol. 2002;26(2):55–65.
14. Cooke WE. Fibrosis of the lungs due to the inhalation of asbestos dust. Br Med J. 1924;2(3317):140–2, 147.
15. Cooke WE. Pulmonary asbestosis. Br Med J. 1927;2(3491):1024–5.
16. Gloyne SR, Merewether ER. Asbestos. In: Occupation and health: encyclopedia of hygiene, pathology, and social welfare. Geneva: International Labour Office; 1938. p. S1–15.
17. Doll R. Mortality from lung cancer in asbestos workers. Br J Ind Med. 1955;12(2):81–6.
18. Van Der Schoot HC. [Asbestosis & pleural tumors]. Ned Tijdschr Geneeskd. 1958;102(23):1125–6.
19. Weiss A. [Cancer of pleura in pulmonary asbestosis determined morphologically in vivo]. Medizinische. 1953;6(3):93–4.
20. Lehnert M, Kraywinkel K, Heinze E, Wiethege T, Johnen G, Fiebig J, et al. Incidence of malignant mesothelioma in Germany 2009-2013. Cancer Causes Control. 2017;28(2):97–105.
21. Soeberg MJ, Leigh J, van Zandwijk N. Malignant mesothelioma in Australia 2015: current incidence and asbestos exposure trends. J Toxicol Environ Health B Crit Rev. 2016;19(5–6):173–89.
22. Agudo A, Gonzalez CA, Bleda MJ, Ramirez J, Hernandez S, Lopez F, et al. Occupation and risk of malignant pleural mesothelioma: a case-control study in Spain. Am J Ind Med. 2000;37(2):159–68.
23. Aguilar-Madrid G, Robles-Perez E, Juarez-Perez CA, Alvarado-Cabrero I, Rico-Mendez FG, Javier KG. Case-control study of pleural mesothelioma in workers with social security in Mexico. Am J Ind Med. 2010;53(3):241–51.
24. Howel D, Arblaster L, Swinburne L, Schweiger M, Renvoize E, Hatton P. Routes of asbestos exposure and the development of mesothelioma in an English region. Occup Environ Med. 1997;54(6):403–9.
25. Iwatsubo Y, Pairon JC, Boutin C, Menard O, Massin N, Caillaud D, et al. Pleural mesothelioma: dose-response relation at low levels of asbestos exposure in a French population-based case-control study. Am J Epidemiol. 1998;148(2):133–42.
26. Rees D, Goodman K, Fourie E, Chapman R, Blignaut C, Bachmann MO, et al. Asbestos exposure and mesothelioma in South Africa. S Afr Med J. 1999;89(6):627–34.
27. Rodelsperger K, Jockel KH, Pohlabeln H, Romer W, Woitowitz HJ. Asbestos and man-made vitreous fibers as risk factors for diffuse malignant mesothelioma: results from a German hospital-based case-control study. Am J Ind Med. 2001;39(3):262–75.
28. Pintos J, Parent ME, Case BW, Rousseau MC, Siemiatycki J. Risk of mesothelioma and occupational exposure to asbestos and man-made vitreous fibers: evidence from two case-control studies in Montreal, Canada. J Occup Environ Med. 2009;51(10):1177–84.
29. Lacourt A, Gramond C, Rolland P, Ducamp S, Audignon S, Astoul P, et al. Occupational and non-occupational attributable risk of asbestos exposure for malignant pleural mesothelioma. Thorax. 2014;69(6):532–9.
30. Noonan CW. Environmental asbestos exposure and risk of mesothelioma. Ann Transl Med. 2017;5(11):234.
31. Donovan EP, Donovan BL, McKinley MA, Cowan DM, Paustenbach DJ. Evaluation of take home (para-occupational) exposure to asbestos and disease: a review of the literature. Crit Rev Toxicol. 2012;42(9):703–31.
32. Reid A, Berry G, Heyworth J, de Klerk NH, Musk AW. Predicted mortality from malignant mesothelioma among women exposed to blue asbestos at Wittenoom, Western Australia. Occup Environ Med. 2009;66(3):169–74.
33. Goswami E, Craven V, Dahlstrom DL, Alexander D, Mowat F. Domestic asbestos exposure: a review of epidemiologic and exposure data. Int J Environ Res Public Health. 2013;10(11):5629–70.
34. Tarres J, Alberti C, Martinez-Artes X, Abos-Herrandiz R, Rosell-Murphy M, Garcia-Allas I, et al. Pleural mesothelioma in relation to meteorological conditions and residential distance from an industrial source of asbestos. Occup Environ Med. 2013;70(8):588–90.

35. Kurumatani N, Kumagai S. Mapping the risk of mesothelioma due to neighborhood asbestos exposure. Am J Respir Crit Care Med. 2008;178(6):624–9.
36. Korda RJ, Clements MS, Armstrong BK, Law HD, Guiver T, Anderson PR, et al. Risk of cancer associated with residential exposure to asbestos insulation: a whole-population cohort study. Lancet Public Health. 2017;2(11):e522–e8.
37. Olsen NJ, Franklin PJ, Reid A, de Klerk NH, Threlfall TJ, Shilkin K, et al. Increasing incidence of malignant mesothelioma after exposure to asbestos during home maintenance and renovation. Med J Aust. 2011;195(5):271–4.
38. Zeig-Owens R, Webber MP, Hall CB, Schwartz T, Jaber N, Weakley J, et al. Early assessment of cancer outcomes in New York City firefighters after the 9/11 attacks: an observational cohort study. Lancet. 2011;378(9794):898–905.
39. Bianchi C, Bianchi T. Global mesothelioma epidemic: trend and features. Indian J Occup Environ Med. 2014;18(2):82–8.
40. Henderson DW, Reid G, Kao SC, van Zandwijk N, Klebe S. Challenges and controversies in the diagnosis of mesothelioma: part 1. Cytology-only diagnosis, biopsies, immunohistochemistry, discrimination between mesothelioma and reactive mesothelial hyperplasia, and biomarkers. J Clin Pathol. 2013;66(10):847–53.
41. Henderson DW, Reid G, Kao SC, van Zandwijk N, Klebe S. Challenges and controversies in the diagnosis of malignant mesothelioma: part 2. Malignant mesothelioma subtypes, pleural synovial sarcoma, molecular and prognostic aspects of mesothelioma, BAP1, aquaporin-1 and microRNA. J Clin Pathol. 2013;66(10):854–61.
42. Soeberg MJ, Luong MA, Tran VT, Tran AT, Nguyen TT, Bui D, et al. Estimating the incidence of malignant mesothelioma in Vietnam: a pilot descriptive cancer registration study. Int J Occup Environ Health. 2016;22(2):167–72.
43. Park EK, Takahashi K, Hoshuyama T, Cheng TJ, Delgermaa V, Le GV, et al. Global magnitude of reported and unreported mesothelioma. Environ Health Perspect. 2011;119(4):514–8.
44. Harper M. 10th Anniversary critical review: naturally occurring asbestos. J Environ Monit. 2008;10(12):1394–408.
45. Bayram M, Bakan ND. Environmental exposure to asbestos: from geology to mesothelioma. Curr Opin Pulm Med. 2014;20(3):301–7.
46. Constantopoulos SH. Environmental mesothelioma associated with tremolite asbestos: lessons from the experiences of Turkey, Greece, Corsica, New Caledonia and Cyprus. Regul Toxicol Pharmacol. 2008;52(1 Suppl):S110–5.
47. McConnochie K, Simonato L, Mavrides P, Christofides P, Mitha R, Griffiths DM, et al. Mesothelioma in cyprus. IARC Sci Publ. 1989;90:411–9.
48. Luce D, Brochard P, Quenel P, Salomon-Nekiriai C, Goldberg P, Billon-Galland MA, et al. Malignant pleural mesothelioma associated with exposure to tremolite. Lancet. 1994;344(8939–8940):1777.
49. Luo S, Liu X, Mu S, Tsai SP, Wen CP. Asbestos related diseases from environmental exposure to crocidolite in Da-yao, China. I. Review of exposure and epidemiological data. Occup Environ Med. 2003;60(1):35–41; discussion-2.
50. Baumann F, Maurizot P, Mangeas M, Ambrosi JP, Douwes J, Robineau B. Pleural mesothelioma in New Caledonia: associations with environmental risk factors. Environ Health Perspect. 2011;119(5):695–700.
51. Baumann F, Buck BJ, Metcalf RV, McLaurin BT, Merkler DJ, Carbone M. The presence of asbestos in the natural environment is likely related to mesothelioma in young individuals and women from Southern Nevada. J Thorac Oncol. 2015;10(5):731–7.
52. Frank AL, Joshi TK. The global spread of asbestos. Ann Glob Health. 2014;80(4):257–62.
53. Lin RT, Takahashi K, Karjalainen A, Hoshuyama T, Wilson D, Kameda T, et al. Ecological association between asbestos-related diseases and historical asbestos consumption: an international analysis. Lancet. 2007;369(9564):844–9.
54. Allen TC, Cagle PT, Churg AM, Colby TV, Gibbs AR, Hammar SP, et al. Localized malignant mesothelioma. Am J Surg Pathol. 2005;29(7):866–73.
55. Kazan-Allen L. The debate on banning asbestos. CMAJ. 2001;165(9):1189; author reply 91-3.
56. Kazan-Allen L. Asbestos poisons World Trade Organization atmosphere. Int J Health Serv. 2001;31(3):481–93.
57. Greenberg M. The defence of chrysotile, 1912-2007. Int J Occup Environ Health. 2008;14(1):57–66.
58. Ruff K. How Canada changed from exporting asbestos to banning asbestos: the challenges that had to be overcome. Int J Environ Res Public Health. 2017;14(10):E1135.
59. Ruff K. How Canada's asbestos industry was defeated in Quebec. New Solut. 2017;26(4):543–56.
60. Courtice MN, Lin S, Wang X. An updated review on asbestos and related diseases in China. Int J Occup Environ Health. 2012;18(3):247–53.
61. Andersen PK, Geskus RB, de Witte T, Putter H. Competing risks in epidemiology: possibilities and pitfalls. Int J Epidemiol. 2012;41(3):861–70.
62. Guo Z, Carbone M, Zhang X, Su D, Sun W, Lou J, et al. Improving the accuracy of mesothelioma diagnosis in China. J Thorac Oncol. 2017;12(4):714–23.
63. Jiang Z, Chen T, Chen J, Ying S, Gao Z, He X, et al. Hand-spinning chrysotile exposure and risk of malignant mesothelioma: a case-control study in Southeastern China. Int J Cancer. 2018;142(3):514–23.
64. Gao Z, Hiroshima K, Wu X, Zhang J, Shao D, Shao H, et al. Asbestos textile production linked to malignant peritoneal and pleural mesothelioma in women: analysis of 28 cases in Southeast China. Am J Ind Med. 2015;58(10):1040–9.
65. Mossman BT, Churg A. Mechanisms in the pathogenesis of asbestosis and silicosis. Am J Respir Crit Care Med. 1998;157(5 Pt 1):1666–80.

66. Harington JS. Fiber carcinogenesis: epidemiologic observations and the Stanton hypothesis. J Natl Cancer Inst. 1981;67(5):977–89.
67. Gaudichet A, Sebastien P, Clark NJ, Pooley FD. Identification and quantification of asbestos fibres in human tissues. IARC Sci Publ. 1980;30:61–8.
68. Rowlands N, Gibbs GW, McDonald AD. Asbestos fibres in the lungs of chrysotile miners and millers—a preliminary report. Ann Occup Hyg. 1982;26(1–4):411–5.
69. Rogers AJ, Leigh J, Berry G, Ferguson DA, Mulder HB, Ackad M. Relationship between lung asbestos fiber type and concentration and relative risk of mesothelioma. A case-control study. Cancer. 1991;67(7):1912–20.
70. Dufresne A, Harrigan M, Masse S, Begin R. Fibers in lung tissues of mesothelioma cases among miners and millers of the township of Asbestos, Quebec. Am J Ind Med. 1995;27(4):581–92.
71. Suzuki Y, Yuen SR, Ashley R. Short, thin asbestos fibers contribute to the development of human malignant mesothelioma: pathological evidence. Int J Hyg Environ Health. 2005;208(3):201–10.
72. Feder IS, Tischoff I, Theile A, Schmitz I, Merget R, Tannapfel A. The asbestos fibre burden in human lungs: new insights into the chrysotile debate. Eur Respir J. 2017;49(6):1602534.
73. Berman DW, Crump KS. Update of potency factors for asbestos-related lung cancer and mesothelioma. Crit Rev Toxicol. 2008;38(Suppl 1):1–47.
74. Wang X, Yano E, Qiu H, Yu I, Courtice MN, Tse LA, et al. A 37-year observation of mortality in Chinese chrysotile asbestos workers. Thorax. 2012;67(2):106–10.
75. Pezerat H. Chrysotile biopersistence: the misuse of biased studies. Int J Occup Environ Health. 2009;15(1):102–6.
76. Dogan AU, Dogan M, Hoskins JA. Erionite series minerals: mineralogical and carcinogenic properties. Environ Geochem Health. 2008;30(4):367–81.
77. Baris YI, Sahin AA, Ozesmi M, Kerse I, Ozen E, Kolacan B, et al. Outbreak of pleural mesothelioma and chronic fibrosing pleurisy in village of Karain-Urgup in Anatolia. Thorax. 1978;33(2):181–92.
78. Baris YI, Grandjean P. Prospective study of mesothelioma mortality in Turkish villages with exposure to fibrous zeolite. J Natl Cancer Inst. 2006;98(6):414–7.
79. Wagner JC, Skidmore JW, Hill RJ, Griffiths DM. Erionite exposure and mesotheliomas in rats. Br J Cancer. 1985;51(5):727–30.
80. Baris B, Demir AU, Shehu V, Karakoca Y, Kisacik G, Baris YI. Environmental fibrous zeolite (erionite) exposure and malignant tumors other than mesothelioma. J Environ Pathol Toxicol Oncol. 1996;15(2–4):183–9.
81. Ortega-Guerrero MA, Carrasco-Nunez G, Barragan-Campos H, Ortega MR. High incidence of lung cancer and malignant mesothelioma linked to erionite fibre exposure in a rural community in Central Mexico. Occup Environ Med. 2015;72(3):216–8.
82. Carbone M, Baris YI, Bertino P, Brass B, Comertpay S, Dogan AU, et al. Erionite exposure in North Dakota and Turkish villages with mesothelioma. Proc Natl Acad Sci U S A. 2011;108(33):13618–23.
83. Roushdy-Hammady I, Siegel J, Emri S, Testa JR, Carbone M. Genetic-susceptibility factor and malignant mesothelioma in the Cappadocian region of Turkey. Lancet. 2001;357(9254):444–5.
84. Dogan AU, Baris YI, Dogan M, Emri S, Steele I, Elmishad AG, et al. Genetic predisposition to fiber carcinogenesis causes a mesothelioma epidemic in Turkey. Cancer Res. 2006;66(10):5063–8.
85. De Bruin ML, Burgers JA, Baas P, van 't Veer MB, Noordijk EM, Louwman MW, et al. Malignant mesothelioma after radiation treatment for Hodgkin lymphoma. Blood. 2009;113(16):3679–81.
86. Travis LB, Fossa SD, Schonfeld SJ, McMaster ML, Lynch CF, Storm H, et al. Second cancers among 40,576 testicular cancer patients: focus on long-term survivors. J Natl Cancer Inst. 2005;97(18):1354–65.
87. Peterson JT Jr, Greenberg SD, Buffler PA. Non-asbestos-related malignant mesothelioma. A review. Cancer. 1984;54(5):951–60.
88. Farioli A, Ottone M, Morganti AG, Compagnone G, Romani F, Cammelli S, et al. Radiation-induced mesothelioma among long-term solid cancer survivors: a longitudinal analysis of SEER database. Cancer Med. 2016;5(5):950–9.
89. Stey C, Landolt-Weber U, Vetter W, Sauter C, Marincek B. Malignant peritoneal mesothelioma after Thorotrast exposure. Am J Clin Oncol. 1995;18(4):313–7.
90. Goodman JE, Nascarella MA, Valberg PA. Ionizing radiation: a risk factor for mesothelioma. Cancer Causes Control. 2009;20(8):1237–54.
91. Sanders CL, Jackson TA. Induction of mesotheliomas and sarcomas from "hot spots" of 239 PuO 2 activity. Health Phys. 1972;22(6):755–9.
92. Hillerdal G, Berg J. Malignant mesothelioma secondary to chronic inflammation and old scars. Two new cases and review of the literature. Cancer. 1985;55(9):1968–72.
93. Roviaro GC, Sartori F, Calabro F, Varoli F. The association of pleural mesothelioma and tuberculosis. Am Rev Respir Dis. 1982;126(3):569–71.
94. Riddell RH, Goodman MJ, Moossa AR. Peritoneal malignant mesothelioma in a patient with recurrent peritonitis. Cancer. 1981;48(1):134–9.
95. Butnor KJ, Pavlisko EN, Sporn TA, Roggli VL. Malignant peritoneal mesothelioma and Crohn disease. J Clin Pathol. 2017;70(3):228–32.
96. Landskron G, De la Fuente M, Thuwajit P, Thuwajit C, Hermoso MA. Chronic inflammation and cytokines in the tumor microenvironment. J Immunol Res. 2014;2014:149185.
97. Boffetta P, Donaldson K, Moolgavkar S, Mandel JS. A systematic review of occupational exposure to synthetic vitreous fibers and mesothelioma. Crit Rev Toxicol. 2014;44(5):436–49.

98. Moller P, Jacobsen NR. Weight of evidence analysis for assessing the genotoxic potential of carbon nanotubes. Crit Rev Toxicol. 2017;47(10):867–84.
99. Ryman-Rasmussen JP, Cesta MF, Brody AR, Shipley-Phillips JK, Everitt JI, Tewksbury EW, et al. Inhaled carbon nanotubes reach the subpleural tissue in mice. Nat Nanotechnol. 2009;4(11):747–51.
100. Pepper C, Jasani B, Navabi H, Wynford-Thomas D, Gibbs AR. Simian virus 40 large T antigen (SV40LTAg) primer specific DNA amplification in human pleural mesothelioma tissue. Thorax. 1996;51(11):1074–6.
101. Poulin DL, DeCaprio JA. Is there a role for SV40 in human cancer? J Clin Oncol. 2006;24(26):4356–65.
102. Cristaudo A, Foddis R, Vivaldi A, Buselli R, Gattini V, Guglielmi G, et al. SV40 enhances the risk of malignant mesothelioma among people exposed to asbestos: a molecular epidemiologic case-control study. Cancer Res. 2005;65(8):3049–52.
103. Strickler HD, International SVWG. A multicenter evaluation of assays for detection of SV40 DNA and results in masked mesothelioma specimens. Cancer Epidemiol Biomark Prev. 2001;10(5):523–32.
104. Strickler HD, Goedert JJ, Devesa SS, Lahey J, Fraumeni JF Jr, Rosenberg PS. Trends in U.S. pleural mesothelioma incidence rates following simian virus 40 contamination of early poliovirus vaccines. J Natl Cancer Inst. 2003;95(1):38–45.
105. Kane AB. Animal models of malignant mesothelioma. Inhal Toxicol. 2006;18(12):1001–4.
106. Robinson C, Dick IM, Wise MJ, Holloway A, Diyagama D, Robinson BW, et al. Consistent gene expression profiles in MexTAg transgenic mouse and wild type mouse asbestos-induced mesothelioma. BMC Cancer. 2015;15:983.
107. Herrick SE, Mutsaers SE. Mesothelial progenitor cells and their potential in tissue engineering. Int J Biochem Cell Biol. 2004;36(4):621–42.
108. Bolen JW, Hammar SP, McNutt MA. Reactive and neoplastic serosal tissue. A light-microscopic, ultrastructural, and immunocytochemical study. Am J Surg Pathol. 1986;10(1):34–47.
109. Jaurand MC, Fleury-Feith J. Pathogenesis of malignant pleural mesothelioma. Respirology. 2005;10(1):2–8.
110. Roe OD, Anderssen E, Helge E, Pettersen CH, Olsen KS, Sandeck H, et al. Genome-wide profile of pleural mesothelioma versus parietal and visceral pleura: the emerging gene portrait of the mesothelioma phenotype. PLoS One. 2009;4(8):e6554.
111. Heintz NH, Janssen-Heininger YM, Mossman BT. Asbestos, lung cancers, and mesotheliomas: from molecular approaches to targeting tumor survival pathways. Am J Respir Cell Mol Biol. 2010;42(2):133–9.
112. Chew SH, Toyokuni S. Malignant mesothelioma as an oxidative stress-induced cancer: an update. Free Radic Biol Med. 2015;86:166–78.
113. Yang H, Rivera Z, Jube S, Nasu M, Bertino P, Goparaju C, et al. Programmed necrosis induced by asbestos in human mesothelial cells causes high-mobility group box 1 protein release and resultant inflammation. Proc Natl Acad Sci U S A. 2010;107(28):12611–6.
114. Bueno R, Stawiski EW, Goldstein LD, Durinck S, De Rienzo A, Modrusan Z, et al. Comprehensive genomic analysis of malignant pleural mesothelioma identifies recurrent mutations, gene fusions and splicing alterations. Nat Genet. 2016;48(4):407–16.
115. Guo G, Chmielecki J, Goparaju C, Heguy A, Dolgalev I, Carbone M, et al. Whole-exome sequencing reveals frequent genetic alterations in BAP1, NF2, CDKN2A, and CUL1 in malignant pleural mesothelioma. Cancer Res. 2015;75(2):264–9.
116. Lo Iacono M, Monica V, Righi L, Grosso F, Libener R, Vatrano S, et al. Targeted next-generation sequencing of cancer genes in advanced stage malignant pleural mesothelioma: a retrospective study. J Thorac Oncol. 2015;10(3):492–9.
117. Altomare DA, Menges CW, Xu J, Pei J, Zhang L, Tadevosyan A, et al. Losses of both products of the Cdkn2a/Arf locus contribute to asbestos-induced mesothelioma development and cooperate to accelerate tumorigenesis. PLoS One. 2011;6(4):e18828.
118. Altomare DA, Vaslet CA, Skele KL, De Rienzo A, Devarajan K, Jhanwar SC, et al. A mouse model recapitulating molecular features of human mesothelioma. Cancer Res. 2005;65(18):8090–5.
119. Jongsma J, van Montfort E, Vooijs M, Zevenhoven J, Krimpenfort P, van der Valk M, et al. A conditional mouse model for malignant mesothelioma. Cancer Cell. 2008;13(3):261–71.
120. Xu J, Kadariya Y, Cheung M, Pei J, Talarchek J, Sementino E, et al. Germline mutation of Bap1 accelerates development of asbestos-induced malignant mesothelioma. Cancer Res. 2014;74(16):4388–97.
121. Ascoli V, Romeo E, Carnovale Scalzo C, Cozzi I, Ancona L, Cavariani F, et al. Familial malignant mesothelioma: a population-based study in central Italy (1980-2012). Cancer Epidemiol. 2014;38(3):273–8.
122. Matullo G, Guarrera S, Betti M, Fiorito G, Ferrante D, Voglino F, et al. Genetic variants associated with increased risk of malignant pleural mesothelioma: a genome-wide association study. PLoS One. 2013;8(4):e61253.
123. Testa JR, Cheung M, Pei J, Below JE, Tan Y, Sementino E, et al. Germline BAP1 mutations predispose to malignant mesothelioma. Nat Genet. 2011;43(10):1022–5.
124. Ascoli V, Cozzi I, Vatrano S, Izzo S, Giorcelli J, Romeo E, et al. Mesothelioma families without inheritance of a BAP1 predisposing mutation. Cancer Genet. 2016;209(9):381–7.
125. LaFave LM, Beguelin W, Koche R, Teater M, Spitzer B, Chramiec A, et al. Loss of BAP1 function leads to EZH2-dependent transformation. Nat Med. 2015;21(11):1344–9.
126. Zauderer MG, Szlosarek P, Le Moulec S, Popat S, Taylor P, Planchard D, et al. Phase 2,

multicenter study of the EZH2 inhibitor tazemetostat as monotherapy in adults with relapsed or refractory (R/R) malignant mesothelioma (MM) with BAP1 inactivation. J Clin Oncol. 2018;36(15_suppl; abstr):8515.

127. Gordon GJ, Rockwell GN, Jensen RV, Rheinwald JG, Glickman JN, Aronson JP, et al. Identification of novel candidate oncogenes and tumor suppressors in malignant pleural mesothelioma using large-scale transcriptional profiling. Am J Pathol. 2005;166(6):1827–40.
128. Pass HI, Liu Z, Wali A, Bueno R, Land S, Lott D, et al. Gene expression profiles predict survival and progression of pleural mesothelioma. Clin Cancer Res. 2004;10(3):849–59.
129. Lopez-Rios F, Chuai S, Flores R, Shimizu S, Ohno T, Wakahara K, et al. Global gene expression profiling of pleural mesotheliomas: overexpression of aurora kinases and P16/CDKN2A deletion as prognostic factors and critical evaluation of microarray-based prognostic prediction. Cancer Res. 2006;66(6):2970–9.
130. de Reynies A, Jaurand MC, Renier A, Couchy G, Hysi I, Elarouci N, et al. Molecular classification of malignant pleural mesothelioma: identification of a poor prognosis subgroup linked to the epithelial-to-mesenchymal transition. Clin Cancer Res. 2014;20(5):1323–34.
131. Singhal S, Wiewrodt R, Malden LD, Amin KM, Matzie K, Friedberg J, et al. Gene expression profiling of malignant mesothelioma. Clin Cancer Res. 2003;9(8):3080–97.
132. Sugarbaker DJ, Richards WG, Gordon GJ, Dong L, De Rienzo A, Maulik G, et al. Transcriptome sequencing of malignant pleural mesothelioma tumors. Proc Natl Acad Sci U S A. 2008;105(9):3521–6.
133. Nymark P, Lindholm PM, Korpela MV, Lahti L, Ruosaari S, Kaski S, et al. Gene expression profiles in asbestos-exposed epithelial and mesothelial lung cell lines. BMC Genomics. 2007;8:62.
134. Ramos-Nino ME, Heintz N, Scappoli L, Martinelli M, Land S, Nowak N, et al. Gene profiling and kinase screening in asbestos-exposed epithelial cells and lungs. Am J Respir Cell Mol Biol. 2003;29(3 Suppl):S51–8.
135. Shukla A, MacPherson MB, Hillegass J, Ramos-Nino ME, Alexeeva V, Vacek PM, et al. Alterations in gene expression in human mesothelial cells correlate with mineral pathogenicity. Am J Respir Cell Mol Biol. 2009;41(1):114–23.
136. Putnam EA, Smartt A, Groves A, Schwanke C, Brezinski M, Pershouse MA. Gene expression changes after exposure to six-mix in a mouse model. J Immunotoxicol. 2008;5(2):139–44.
137. Sabo-Attwood T, Ramos-Nino M, Bond J, Butnor KJ, Heintz N, Gruber AD, et al. Gene expression profiles reveal increased mClca3 (Gob5) expression and mucin production in a murine model of asbestos-induced fibrogenesis. Am J Pathol. 2005;167(5):1243–56.
138. Garzon R, Calin GA, Croce CM. MicroRNAs in Cancer. Annu Rev Med. 2009;60:167–79.
139. Reid G. MicroRNAs in mesothelioma: from tumour suppressors and biomarkers to therapeutic targets. J Thorac Dis. 2015;7(6):1031–40.
140. Tanaka N, Toyooka S, Soh J, Tsukuda K, Shien K, Furukawa M, et al. Downregulation of microRNA-34 induces cell proliferation and invasion of human mesothelial cells. Oncol Rep. 2013;29(6):2169–74.
141. Menges CW, Kadariya Y, Altomare D, Talarchek J, Neumann-Domer E, Wu Y, et al. Tumor suppressor alterations cooperate to drive aggressive mesotheliomas with enriched cancer stem cells via a p53-miR-34a-c-Met axis. Cancer Res. 2014;74(4):1261–71.
142. Christensen BC, Houseman EA, Godleski JJ, Marsit CJ, Longacker JL, Roelofs CR, et al. Epigenetic profiles distinguish pleural mesothelioma from normal pleura and predict lung asbestos burden and clinical outcome. Cancer Res. 2009;69(1):227–34.
143. Christensen BC, Godleski JJ, Roelofs CR, Longacker JL, Bueno R, Sugarbaker DJ, et al. Asbestos burden predicts survival in pleural mesothelioma. Environ Health Perspect. 2008;116(6):723–6.
144. Kubo T, Toyooka S, Tsukuda K, Sakaguchi M, Fukazawa T, Soh J, et al. Epigenetic silencing of microRNA-34b/c plays an important role in the pathogenesis of malignant pleural mesothelioma. Clin Cancer Res. 2011;17(15):4965–74.
145. Cioce M, Ganci F, Canu V, Sacconi A, Mori F, Canino C, et al. Protumorigenic effects of mir-145 loss in malignant pleural mesothelioma. Oncogene. 2014;33(46):5319–31.
146. Andersen M, Trapani D, Ravn J, Sorensen JB, Andersen CB, Grauslund M, et al. Methylation-associated silencing of microRNA-126 and its host gene EGFL7 in malignant pleural mesothelioma. Anticancer Res. 2015;35(11):6223–9.
147. Ivanov SV, Goparaju CM, Lopez P, Zavadil J, Toren-Haritan G, Rosenwald S, et al. Pro-tumorigenic effects of miR-31 loss in mesothelioma. J Biol Chem. 2010;285(30):22809–17.
148. Johnson TG, Schelch K, Cheng YY, Williams M, Sarun KH, Kirschner MB, et al. Dysregulated expression of the microRNA miR-137 and its target YBX1 contribute to the invasive characteristics of malignant pleural mesothelioma. J Thorac Oncol. 2018;13(2):258–72.
149. Matsumoto S, Nabeshima K, Hamasaki M, Shibuta T, Umemura T. Upregulation of microRNA-31 associates with a poor prognosis of malignant pleural mesothelioma with sarcomatoid component. Med Oncol. 2014;31(12):303.
150. Pass HI, Goparaju C, Ivanov S, Donington J, Carbone M, Hoshen M, et al. hsa-miR-29c* is linked to the prognosis of malignant pleural mesothelioma. Cancer Res. 2010;70(5):1916–24.
151. Fassina A, Cappellesso R, Guzzardo V, Dalla Via L, Piccolo S, Ventura L, et al. Epithelial-mesenchymal transition in malignant mesothelioma. Mod Pathol. 2012;25(1):86–99.

152. Reid G, Pel ME, Kirschner MB, Cheng YY, Mugridge N, Weiss J, et al. Restoring expression of miR-16: a novel approach to therapy for malignant pleural mesothelioma. Ann Oncol. 2013;24(12):3128–35.
153. Williams M, Kirschner MB, Cheng YY, Hanh J, Weiss J, Mugridge N, et al. miR-193a-3p is a potential tumor suppressor in malignant pleural mesothelioma. Oncotarget. 2015;6(27):23480–95.
154. Khodayari N, Mohammed KA, Lee H, Kaye F, Nasreen N. MicroRNA-302b targets Mcl-1 and inhibits cell proliferation and induces apoptosis in malignant pleural mesothelioma cells. Am J Cancer Res. 2016;6(9):1996–2009.
155. van Zandwijk N, Pavlakis N, Kao SC, Linton A, Boyer MJ, Clarke S, et al. Safety and activity of microRNA-loaded minicells in patients with recurrent malignant pleural mesothelioma: a first-in-man, phase 1, open-label, dose-escalation study. Lancet Oncol. 2017;18(10):1386–96.
156. Kao SC, Cheng YY, Williams M, Kirschner MB, Madore J, Lum T, et al. Tumor suppressor microRNAs contribute to the regulation of PD-L1 expression in malignant pleural mesothelioma. J Thorac Oncol. 2017;12(9):1421–33.
157. De Santi C, Vencken S, Blake J, Haase B, Benes V, Gemignani F, et al. Identification of MiR-21-5p as a functional regulator of mesothelin expression using MicroRNA capture affinity coupled with next generation sequencing. PLoS One. 2017;12(1):e0170999.

3 Screening Issues in Exposed Subjects and Early Diagnosis

Manlio Mencoboni, Paola Taveggia, Claudio Francesco Simonassi, and Rosa Angela Filiberti

3.1 Introduction

Asbestos is a natural fibrous mineral. It has been increasingly used for a variety of applications around the world, especially heavy industry and construction activities. WHO estimates that 125 million workers are exposed to asbestos [1]. Many domestic tools or products are responsible for a nonoccupational exposure as well.

So hundreds of millions of people are at risk of developing an asbestos-caused disease because of occupational, environmental, or domestic exposure. Malignant mesothelioma (MM), pleural, peritoneal, testicular, and pericardial is the most lethal one. The WHO estimates that asbestos may be responsible for more than 100,000 deaths yearly. MM develops with a latency of 20–60 years from asbestos exposure [2]. Malignant pleural mesothelioma (MPM) is the most common.

M. Mencoboni (✉) · P. Taveggia
Oncology Department, ASL 3 Villa Scassi Hospital, Genoa, Italy
e-mail: Manlio.mencoboni@fastwebnet.it; Paola.taveggia@asl3.liguria.it

C. F. Simonassi
Pneumology Department, ASL 3 Villa Scassi Hospital, Genoa, Italy
e-mail: Claudiofrancesco.simonassi@asl3.liguria.it

R. A. Filiberti
Clinical Epidemiology Unit, Ospedale Policlinico San Martino, Genoa, Italy
e-mail: Rosa.filiberti@hasanmartino.it

Exposure to asbestos fibers is considered as the main cause of MM [2, 3] even if additional factors including SV40 infection [4–6] and exposure to radiation, especially high-dose radiotherapy of lymphoma and other chest malignancies [2], may also cause mesothelioma, possibly in concert with asbestos [7].

Recently, germline heterozygous inactivating mutations of the BRCA1-associated protein-1 (BAP1) gene have been identified as the cause of the high penetrance hereditary BAP1 cancer syndrome [8, 9]. BAP1 syndrome includes multiple cancers. Mesothelioma, even if not exposed to asbestos, is one of these cancers.

MM is divided into three histology categories: epithelioid, sarcomatoid, and biphasic. Epithelioid histology accounts for about 70% of all MMs and is less aggressive, sarcomatoid histology is the most aggressive one, and biphasic subtype has intermediate features. But all these histologies share ominous prognosis.

Differential diagnosis of mesothelioma is sometimes very difficult. Epithelioid MM looks like renal or non-small cell lung cancer. Sarcomatoid histotype is similar to carcinosarcoma or to other sarcomas. Immunohistochemical tissue markers (such as calretinin or WT-1) are very useful to diagnose MM [10].

These tissue markers, however, will not be the focus of this chapter. We will focus on soluble biomarkers potentially useful for preventive or clinical screening purposes. Only soluble biomarkers are manageable for mass screening, and

G. L. Ceresoli et al. (eds.), *Mesothelioma*, https://doi.org/10.1007/978-3-030-16884-1_3

Table 3.1 Main Mesothelioma biomarkers

Marker	Collection	Use	Pros	Cons
HMGB1	Serum-plasma	Exposure/diagnosis	Promising	Difficult determination
MicroRNA	Serum-plasma	Exposure/diagnosis	Promising	Difficult determination/variability
Proteomic signature	Serum-plasma	Exposure/diagnosis/prognosis	Promising	Few patients studied
Mesothelin and SMRP	Serum-plasma	Exposure/diagnosis/prognosis	Easy to test	Not reliable by itself (low sensitivity and specificity)
MPF	Serum-plasma	Exposure/diagnosis/prognosis	Easy to test	Not reliable by itself
Osteopontin	Serum-plasma	Exposure/diagnosis/prognosis	Easy to test	Reliable only for exposure
Fibulin-3	Serum-plasma	Exposure/diagnosis	Easy to test	Low sensitivity and specificity

most screening studies have used them. Actually new effective biomarkers are needed for MM screening and detection at earlier stages and to develop tailored therapies.

Low-dose computed tomography screening studies for MM have been conducted by several investigators, but CT scans resulted in low cases of true malignancies detected together with a certain number of benign diseases requiring follow-up. As a matter of fact, radiologic screening studies have not proven effective for detecting early-stage MPM among asbestos-exposed subjects.

So soluble biomarkers are crucial: biomarkers are cellular, biochemical, or molecular alterations that are measurable in cells, in tissues, or in biological media [11]. Biomarkers refer to a biological condition, including tumors. Biomarkers can be divided into two categories:

- Prevention (biomarkers of exposure, risk prediction)
- Clinical and diagnostic biomarkers (biomarkers of diagnosis, prognosis, treatment response)

Early MM detection could allow therapeutic interventions at a potentially treatable stage, but when monitoring high-risk subjects, it is necessary to have a sensitive and highly specific test in order to avoid false-positive results. Asbestos-exposed workers may represent an ideal cohort to be followed, because of the higher risk of developing MM and since there is an increased probability that the studied marker be raised in this group, compared to unexposed populations. Over the past decades, advances in molecular biology have led to the identification of several potential biomarkers in blood for early MM detection; nevertheless, at present there are no validated biomarkers proved to have sufficient specificity and sensitivity to be used. We will review the state of the art of soluble biomarkers that are more suitable for prevention and screening and might be useful to evaluate the response to therapy (Table 3.1).

3.2 High-Mobility Group Box 1

High-mobility group box 1 (HMGB1) is a pro-inflammatory cytokine but has several different functions, as well. It is usually found in the nucleus, where it stabilizes nucleosomes and contributes to DNA transcription, replication, and recombination. In case of inflammation, HMGB1 can translocate from the nucleus to the cytosol and then be secreted into the extracellular environment and from this to systemic circulation [12–14]. Inflammatory cells, such as granulocytes and macrophages, can produce HMGB1 as well and diffuse it from the cytosol in the extracellular milieu, where it displays pro-inflammatory activity-producing TNF alpha [15,

16]. In case of inflammation, HMGB1 is acetylated, and this prevents from nuclear translocation. Asbestos fibers cause chronic inflammation, and HMGB1 increases in extracellular matrix and inside the mesothelial cells. HMGB1, due to asbestos exposure, triggers the process of cell transformation in mesothelial cells that is usually associated with acetylated form [17]. So it has been demonstrated that HMGB1 levels in the sera from patients with malignant peritoneal mesothelioma were significantly higher than those of non-mesothelioma subjects with a history of exposure to asbestos [18, 19]. In Japanese patients with malignant pleural mesothelioma (MPM) serum, HMGB1 was also a prognostic marker [19]. The role of HMGB1 in exposed subjects (ES) or in patients affected by benign diseases caused by asbestos exposure (ABD) is still unknown. Recently, it has been published that the level of HMGB1 was significantly elevated in ES and ABD subjects. For clinical diagnosis, these results indicated that serum HMGB1 is a sensitive and specific biomarker to discriminate asbestosis and MM from healthy or ES [20, 21]. Moreover, a recent paper has shown in cellular and murine level that salicylates inhibit the activities of extracellular HMGB1 and that at least part of the anticancer effects of aspirin are due to inhibition of HMGB1's activities and are COX-2 independent [22]. So the role and the importance of HMGB1 are increasing, and further interesting investigations are warranted. This is one of the most promising new markers.

3.3 miRNA

miRNAs (microRNAs) are small sequences of RNA involved in regulation of gene expression. They are circulating and regulate many cellular activities: proliferation, apoptosis, metabolism, and angiogenesis. They are characterized by high stability under different conditions [23] and play important roles in several processes such as cell growth, differentiation, proliferation, angiogenesis, stress response, tissue remodeling, disease, and malignancy [24–29]. A multitude of miRNAs are differentially expressed in specimens from MM, asbestos-exposed, and healthy subjects. Some miRNA seems to be most significant. Actually tumors generate a characteristic miRNA fingerprint in the cellular fraction of peripheral blood [30]. miR-103 levels were able to discriminate MM patients from asbestos-exposed subjects and healthy controls [31]. Moreover, miR-625-3p levels showed the ability in differentiating MM from asbestosis patients [32]. Another study has identified two different serum miRNA signatures (with several miRNAs) correlating with MM histological subtype and clinical outcome [33]. Investigation of miR-34b/c activity has demonstrated that downregulation of miR-34 family members induces proliferation of mesothelial cells, playing an important role in carcinogenesis [34]. Adenovirus-mediated miR34b/c gene therapy has shown promise in the treatment of malignant pleural mesothelioma (MPM) [35]. Many studies have been performed about miRNA and MM. But differences in miRNA profiling methods and the technological approaches adopted are a real problem in comparing results from different papers. Therefore, the identification of minimally invasive, inexpensive diagnostic/prognostic tests with miRNA for MM is still negative.

3.4 Proteomics

Myriad of proteins are expressed by an organism or a system under defined conditions. The study of some of these proteins might be a useful tool for early diagnosis in MM.

Actually a serum-based 13-protein classifier with an AUC of 0.95 and an overall accuracy of 92% for detection of MM in the asbestos-exposed population using the SOMAscan™ proteomic assay has been developed [36].

Another seven glycopeptide signature has been identified by selected reaction monitoring (SRM) assay technology in MM cells and used to investigate surfaceome-derived serum candidate biomarker panels for MM [37]. This panel accurately discriminated MM from healthy subjects.

Moreover, in combination with mesothelin ELISA, it significantly improved the diagnostic accuracy of mesothelin in differentiating MM from non-small-cell lung cancer (NSCLC) [37]. Therefore, the proteomic approach seems to be a very promising approach.

3.5 Mesothelin and Soluble Mesothelin-Related Peptides (SMRPs)

Soluble mesothelin-related peptides (SMRPs) are found in normal mesothelial cells and are overexpressed in various cancers. They are membrane-bound peptides that can be processed to yield megakaryocyte-potentiating factor (MPF) and mesothelin, which remains attached to the cell membrane via glycophosphatidylinositol linkage [38, 39].

SMRPs are found in human serum and in pleural fluid and have been proposed as marker for the diagnosis of MM and for differentiating MM among asbestos-exposed individuals and patients with benign pleural diseases or with pleural metastases from carcinomas [40, 41] as well as a prognostic marker [42, 43]. Moreover, the evidence of increased serum SMRP concentrations in individuals with past exposure to asbestos compared to nonexposed, and in subjects with pleural asbestos-related diseases (i.e., pleural plaques and fibrosis), has suggested a possible role of SMRP for detecting the disease in early stages [44, 45]. Robinson et al. first hypothesized the possibility to use SMRP in surveillance of asbestos-exposed individuals as an early marker of MM in a retrospective study. The authors found increased serum SMRP values in 7 samples from a random pool of 40 healthy, asbestos-exposed individuals. Three out of the seven subjects were diagnosed with MM at 15, 26, and 69 months after blood drawing, while one subject was diagnosed with non-small cell lung cancer 4 years after sampling. In addition, two of other eight patients with MM had increased levels at 12–48 months before diagnosis. No MMs were seen in subjects with normal mesothelin levels during an 8-year follow-up [40]. Creaney et al. [45] determined serial serum SMRP levels in a large retrospective study of prospectively collected samples of healthy asbestos-exposed individuals. 106 out of 118 mesotheliomas diagnosed over a period of 12 years had serum samples available before diagnosis. Mesothelin levels were higher than the cutoff value of 2.5 nmol/L in last serum sample before the diagnosis in 17 of them. Generally, median SMRP concentration was higher in premorbid samples of subjects with MM, compared with individuals with no subsequent malignant disease. Positivity for SMRP was found in 7 out of 43 individuals with a serum sample available within 6 months of diagnosis. The authors showed that the percentage of mesothelin-positive samples increases to 40% when considering a progressive raise in serial samplings, rather than an absolute increase. A study from Felten et al. [46] on blood samples from formerly asbestos-exposed and nonexposed controls showed that SMRP concentration may increase between 6 and 18 months before the onset of MM symptoms. Nevertheless, the authors could not find an adequate cutoff value for abnormality. Although retrospective studies have been encouraging, the possible use of mesothelin as a MM screening tool in healthy asbestos-exposed populations has been investigated with contradicting results and is still objective of scientific debate [41, 44, 47–49]. Generally, prospective studies have shown that the marker has a low sensitivity. The poor cancer diagnostic value of SMRP might partially be explained by the large time interval between sample collection and MM diagnosis [47, 50, 51], but the efficacy of SMRP is also hampered by its lower concentration in sarcomatous or mixed mesotheliomas and by a high rate of false-positive cases that could lead to unnecessary procedures and anxiety in exposed subjects [41, 44]. In fact, a meta-analysis evaluating SMRP in MPM and in symptomatic or high-risk controls showed that SMRP better discriminated controls from patients with advanced epithelioid or biphasic MM compared to those with early stage or sarcomatoid type and had low sensitivity (32%) for early disease at 95% specificity [43].

So SMRP and mesothelin have been extensively studied. By themselves they have high specificity but unfortunately low sensitivity, so they cannot play a role in the early diagnosis of

MM. In the future, it is likely that they can be associated to other biomarkers to ameliorate their sensitivity.

In addition, several pathological conditions, such as renal impairment, can elevate serum mesothelin levels, so it is necessary to take care of these conditions [52]. Moreover these levels are also affected by some individual characteristics such as age, body mass index, and current smoking that should be taken into account when evaluating SMRP in non-mesothelioma subjects as they could increase the percentage of false MM positives [53, 54].

3.6 Megakaryocyte-Potentiating Factor (MPF)

MPF is a cytokine sharing with mesothelin the same coding gene and has been measured by different ELISA assays in blood of MM patients and different control subjects to test its ability to diagnose MM [55–57]. Higher serum MPF levels were detected in MM patients, compared to healthy subjects, individuals with benign asbestos-related diseases, or lung cancer patients [58, 59], but, generally, it has been shown that MPF diagnostic performance is similar to SMRP, while the combination of the two biomarkers has given inconsistent results [55, 57, 60].

3.7 Osteopontin

Osteopontin (OPN) is a glycoprotein that mediates cell-matrix interaction and cell signaling and is overexpressed in several human neoplasms such as lung, breast, and colon cancer [61]. Pass and colleagues found that serum osteopontin levels were significantly higher in patients with pleural mesothelioma than in those with exposure to asbestos. In addition, high sensitivity and specificity were found comparing patients with stage I mesothelioma and patients with exposure to asbestos. These results suggested the potential use of OPN as a diagnostic marker for MM patients [62]. The diagnostic performance of OPN for MM was investigated in other studies that validated these results [63], but, conversely, other authors did not confirm the utility of OPN as a diagnostic marker [64–67]. A more recent systematic review and meta-analysis showed that pooled sensitivity for serum OPN measurement for diagnosing MM was 57% and specificity 81% [68], so the role of OPN in mesothelioma screening is limited. On the other side, OPN might be used as a marker of extent of asbestos exposure [69].

3.8 Fibulin

Fibulin-3 is a conserved member of the extracellular glycoprotein fibulin family encoded by the gene epidermal growth factor, containing fibulin-like extracellular matrix protein 1 (EFEMP1, [70]) involved in the regulation of MM cell proliferation and migration [71]. Analyzing plasma fibulin-3, pleural effusion fibulin-3, and tumor tissue fibulin, Pass et al. showed that fibulin-3 preferentially stained MM tumor cells, with a sensitivity of 97% and a specificity of 95%, suggesting that fibulin-3 was a potential diagnostic marker for MM [72]. However, other research did not replicate these data and reported a much lower sensitivity of fibulin-3 for MM diagnosis [73, 74] and suggested a better association of fibulin-3 with prognosis rather than diagnosis [74]. A comprehensive meta-analysis in MPM cases including 6 studies, 468 MPM patients, and 664 controls evaluated the clinical diagnostic value of fibulin-3 for MPM finding a sensitivity and specificity of 62% and 82%, respectively [71].

3.9 Conclusions

Early MM detection could allow therapeutic interventions at a potentially treatable stage, but when monitoring high-risk subjects, it is necessary to have a sensitive and highly specific test in order to avoid false-positive results.

Over the past decades, advances in molecular biology have led to the identification of several potential biomarkers in blood for early MM detection in high-risk subjects such as workers exposed to asbestos. It is likely that only asbestos-exposed workers may represent an ideal cohort to be followed, because of the higher risk of developing MM and since there is an increased probability that the studied marker be raised in this group, compared to unexposed populations. Actually, screening is only worthwhile in a population with a very high probability of disease as MM is still a rare disease even in high-risk subjects. Furthermore, exposed subjects can be closely followed and are motivated to be included in follow-up studies and give the possibility to test early therapeutic intervention. Surveillance currently includes health history, chest X-ray, and spirometry, but so far these tools have poor power in predicting the disease. There is a great interest in blood biomarkers on their potential use in screening for the early detection of MM; nevertheless, thus far, the studies on this topic have led to variable results. There are no satisfactory results, and no marker seems to be eligible in the surveillance of subjects at risk of MM when used alone. Some potential explanations for different results include the different assays used for markers and different control populations used, which may not be reflective of high-risk screening populations. In the future, the combination of different markers might help to distinguish mesothelioma from benign asbestos-related diseases and asbestos-exposed subjects. But we must keep in mind that improvements in other fields of research regarding MM are wanted such as early-stage treatment. Actually, for screening to be justifiable, treatment of early-stage disease should improve outcome, and it is still uncertain whether this is the case for mesothelioma at the moment.

References

1. Marsili D, Terracini B, Santana VS, et al. Prevention of asbestos-related disease in countries currently using asbestos. Int J Environ Res Public Health. 2016;13:494. https://doi.org/10.3390/ijerph13050494.
2. Carbone M, Ly BH, Dodson RF, et al. Malignant mesothelioma: facts, myths, and hypotheses. J Cell Physiol. 2012;227:44–58. https://doi.org/10.1002/jcp.22724.
3. Qi F, Okimoto G, Jube S, et al. Continuous exposure to chrysotile asbestos can cause transformation of human mesothelial cells via HMGB1 and TNF-alpha signaling. Am J Pathol. 2013;183:1654–66. https://doi.org/10.1016/j.ajpath.2013.07.029.
4. Gazdar AF, Carbone M. Molecular pathogenesis of malignant mesothelioma and its relationship to simian virus 40. Clin Lung Cancer. 2003;5:177–81. https://doi.org/10.3816/CLC.2003.n.031.
5. Carbone M, Rizzo P, Pass H. Simian virus 40: the link with human malignant mesothelioma is well established. Anticancer Res. 2000;20:875–7.
6. Carbone M. Simian virus 40 and human tumors: it is time to study mechanisms. J Cell Biochem. 1999;76:189–93. https://doi.org/10.1002/(SICI)1097-4644(20000201)76:2<189::AID-JCB3>3.0.CO;2-J.
7. Baumann F, Ambrosi JP, Carbone M. Asbestos is not just asbestos: an unrecognised health hazard. Lancet Oncol. 2013;14:576–8. https://doi.org/10.1016/S1470-2045(13)70257-2.
8. Testa JR, Cheung M, Pei J, et al. Germline BAP1 mutations predispose to malignant mesothelioma. Nat Genet. 2011;43:1022–5. https://doi.org/10.1038/ng.912.
9. Carbone M, Yang H, Pass HI, et al. BAP1 and cancer. Nat Rev Cancer. 2013;13:153–9. https://doi.org/10.1038/nrc3459.
10. Pass HI, Carbone M, Krug LM, et al. Benign and malignant mesothelioma. In: De Vita VT, Hellmann S, Rosemberg SA, editors. Cancer, principles & practice of oncology. 10th ed. Baltimore: Lippincott Williams & Wilkins; 2014. p. 1738–60.
11. Hulka BS, Wilcosky TC, Griffith JD. Biological markers in epidemiology. New York: Oxford University Press; 1990.
12. Naglova H, Bucova M. HMGB1and its physiologicaland pathological roles. Bratisl Lek Listy. 2012;113(3):163–71.
13. Kang R, Zhang Q, Zeh HJ III, Lotze MT, Tang D. HMGB1 in cancer: good, bad, or both? Clin Cancer Res. 2013;19(15):4046–57.
14. Sims GP, Rowe DC, Rietdijk ST, Herbst R, Coyle AJ. HMGB1 and RAGE in inflammation and cancer. Annu Rev Immunol. 2010;28:367–88.
15. Lu B, Antoine DJ, Kwan K, et al. JAK/STAT1 signaling promotes HMGB1 hyperacetylation and nuclear translocation. Proc Natl Acad Sci U S A. 2014;111:3068–73. https://doi.org/10.1073/pnas.1316925111.
16. Carneiro VC, de Moraes Maciel R, de Abreu da Silva IC, et al. The extracellular release of *Schistosoma mansoni* HMGB1 nuclear protein is mediated by acetylation. Biochem Biophys Res Commun. 2009;390:1245–9. https://doi.org/10.1016/j.bbrc.2009.10.129.
17. Jube S, Rivera ZS, Bianchi ME, et al. Cancer cell secretion of the DAMP protein HMGB1 supports progression in malignant mesothelioma. Cancer Res. 2012;72:3290–301. https://doi.org/10.1158/0008-5472.CAN11-3481.

18. Tabata C, Kanemura S, Tabata R, et al. Serum HMGB1 as a diagnostic marker for malignant peritoneal mesothelioma. J Clin Gastroenterol. 2013;47(8):684–8.
19. Tabata C, Shibata E, Tabata R, et al. Serum HMGB1 as a prognostic marker for malignant pleural mesothelioma. BMC Cancer. 2013;13:205.
20. Ying S, Jiang Z, He X, Yu M, Chen R, Chen J, Ru G, Chen Y, Chen W, Zhu L, Li T, Zhang Y, Guo X, Yin X, Zhang X, Lou J. Serum HMGB1 as a potential biomarker for patients with asbestos-related diseases. Dis Markers. 2017;2017:5756102. https://doi.org/10.1155/2017/5756102.
21. Chen Z, Gaudino G, Pass HI, Carbone M, Yan H. Diagnostic and prognostic biomarkers for malignant mesothelioma: an update. Transl Lung Cancer Res. 2017;6(3):259–69. https://doi.org/10.21037/tlcr.2017.05.06.
22. Yang H, Pellegrini L, Napolitano A, Giorgi C, Jube S, Preti A, Jennings CJ, De Marchis F, Flores EG, Larson D, Pagano I, Tanji M, Powers A, Kanodia S, Gaudino G, Pastorino S, Pass HI, Pinton P, Bianchi ME, Carbone M. Aspirin delays mesothelioma growth by inhibiting HMGB1-mediated tumor progression. Cell Death Dis. 2015;6:e1786. https://doi.org/10.1038/cddis.2015.153.
23. Micolucci L, Akhtar MM, Olivieri F, Rippo MR, Procopio AD. Diagnostic value of microRNAs in asbestos exposure and malignant mesothelioma: systematic review and qualitative meta-analysis. Oncotarget. 2016;7(36):58606–37.
24. Carrington JC, Ambros V. Role of microRNAs in plant and animal development. Science. 2003;301:336–8.
25. Kumar MS, Lu J, Mercer KL, Golub TR, Jacks T. Impaired microRNA processing enhances cellular transformation and tumorigenesis. Nat Genet. 2007;39:673–7.
26. Suárez Y, Sessa WC. MicroRNAs as novel regulators of angiogenesis. Circ Res. 2009;104:442–54.
27. Olivieri F, Rippo MR, Prattichizzo F, Babini L, Graciotti L, Recchioni R, Procopio AD. Toll like receptor signaling in "inflammaging": microRNA as new players. Immun Ageing. 2013;10:11.
28. Olivieri F, Rippo MR, Procopio AD, Fazioli F. Circulating inflamma-miRs in aging and age-related diseases. Front Genet. 2013;4:121.
29. Rippo MR, Olivieri F, Monsurrò V, Prattichizzo F, Albertini MC, Procopio AD. MitomiRs in human inflamm-aging: a hypothesis involving miR-181a, miR-34a and miR-146a. Exp Gerontol. 2014;56:154–63.
30. Häusler SFM, Keller A, Chandran PA, Ziegler K, Zipp K, Heuer S, Krockenberger M, Engel JB, Hönig A, Scheffler M, Dietl J, Wischhusen J. Whole blood-derived miRNA profiles as potential new tools for ovarian cancer screening. Br J Cancer. 2010;103:693–700.
31. Weber DG, Johnen G, Bryk O, Jöckel K-H, Brüning T. Identification of miRNA-103 in the cellular fraction of human peripheral blood as a potential biomarker for malignant mesothelioma—a pilot study. PLoS One. 2012;7:e30221.
32. Kirschner MB, Cheng YY, Badrian B, Kao SC, Creaney J, Edelman JJB, Armstrong NJ, Vallely MP, Musk AW, Robinson BWS, McCaughan BC, Klebe S, Mutsaers SE, et al. Increased circulating miR-625-3p: a potential biomarker for patients with malignant pleural mesothelioma. J Thorac Oncol. 2012;7:1184–91.
33. Lamberti M, Capasso R, Lombardi A, Di Domenico M, Fiorelli A, Feola A, Perna AF, Santini M, Caraglia M, Ingrosso D. Two different serum MiRNA signatures correlate with the clinical outcome and histological subtype in pleural malignant mesothelioma patients. PLoS One. 2015;10:e0135331.
34. Tanaka N, Toyooka S, Soh J, Tsukuda K, Shien K, Furukawa M, Muraoka T, Maki Y, Ueno T, Yamamoto H, Asano H, Otsuki T, Miyoshi S. Downregulation of microRNA-34 induces cell proliferation and invasion of human mesothelial cells. Oncol Rep. 2013;29:2169–74.
35. Ueno T, Toyooka S, Fukazawa T, Kubo T, Soh J, Asano H, Muraoka T, Tanaka N, Maki Y, Shien K, Furukawa M, Sakaguchi M, Yamamoto H, et al. Preclinical evaluation of microRNA-34b/c delivery for malignant pleural mesothelioma. Acta Med Okayama. 2014;68:23–6.
36. Ostroff RM, Mehan MR, Stewart A, Ayers D, Brody EN, Williams SA, Levin S, Black B, Harbut M, Carbone M, Goparaju C, Pass HI. Early detection of malignant pleural mesothelioma in asbestos-exposed individuals with a noninvasive proteomics-based surveillance tool. PLoS One. 2012;7(10):e46091.
37. Cerciello F, Choi M, Nicastri A, et al. Identification of a seven glycopeptide signature for malignant pleural mesothelioma in human serum by selected reaction monitoring. Clin Proteomics. 2013;10:16. https://doi.org/10.1186/1559-0275-10-16.
38. Hassan R, Bera T, Pastan I. Mesothelin: a new target for immunotherapy. Clin Cancer Res. 2004;10:3937–42.
39. Chang K, Pastan I. Molecular cloning of mesothelin, a differentiation antigen present on mesothelium, mesotheliomas, and ovarian cancers. Proc Natl Acad Sci U S A. 1996;93:136–40.
40. Robinson BWS, Creaney J, Lake R, Nowak A, Musk AW, de Klerk N, Winzell P, Hellstrom KE, Hellstrom I. Mesothelin-family proteins and diagnosis of mesothelioma. Lancet. 2003;362:1612–6.
41. Scherpereel A, Grigoriu B, Conti M, Gey T, Grégoire M, Copin MC, Devos P, Chahine B, Porte H, Lassalle P. Soluble mesothelin-related peptides in the diagnosis of malignant pleural mesothelioma. Am J Respir Crit Care Med. 2006;173:1155–60.
42. Weber DG, Taeger D, Pesch B, Kraus T, Brüning T, Johnen G. Soluble mesothelin-related peptides (SMRP) - high stability of a potential tumor marker for mesothelioma. Cancer Biomark. 2007;3:287–2927.
43. Hollevoet K, Reitsma JB, Creaney J, Grigoriu BD, Robinson BW, Scherpereel A, Cristaudo A, Pass HI, Nackaerts K, Rodríguez Portal JA, Schneider J,

Muley T, Di Serio F, Baas P, Tomasetti M, Rai AJ, van Meerbeeck JP. Serum mesothelin for diagnosing malignant pleural mesothelioma: an individual patient data meta-analysis. J Clin Oncol. 2012;30:1541–9.
44. Park EK, Sandrini A, Yates DH, Creaney J, Robinson BW, Thomas PS, Johnson AR. Soluble mesothelin-related protein in an asbestos-exposed population: the dust diseases board cohort study. Am J Respir Crit Care Med. 2008;178:832–7.
45. Creaney J, Olsen NJ, Brims F, Dick IM, Musk AW, de Klerk NH, Skates SJ, Robinson BW. Serum mesothelin for early detection of asbestos-induced cancer malignant mesothelioma. Cancer Epidemiol Biomark Prev. 2010;19:2238–46.
46. Felten MK, Khatab K, Knoll L, Schettgen T, Muller-Berndorff H, Kraus T. Changes of mesothelin and osteopontin levels over time in formerly asbestos-exposed power industry workers. Int Arch Occup Environ Health. 2014;87(2):195–204.
47. Filiberti R, Marroni P, Spigno F, Merlo DF, Mortara V, Caruso P, Cioè A, Michelazzi L, Bruzzone A, Bobbio B, Simonassi C, Del Corso L, Galli R, Racchi O, Dini G, Linares R, Mencoboni M. Is soluble mesothelin-related protein an upfront predictive marker of pleural mesothelioma? A prospective study on Italian workers exposed to asbestos. Oncology. 2014;86:33–43.
48. Beyer HL, Geschwindt RD, Glover CL, Tran L, Hellstrom I, Hellstrom KE, Miller MC, Verch T, Allard WJ, Pass HI, Sardesai NY. MESOMARK: a potential test for malignant pleural mesothelioma. Clin Chem. 2007;53:666–72.
49. Gube M, Taeger D, Weber DG, Pesch B, Brand P, Johnen G, Müller-Lux A, Gross IM, Wiethege T, Weber A, Raithel HJ, Kraus T, Brüning T. Performance of biomarkers SMRP, CA125, and CYFRA 21-1 as potential tumor markers for malignant mesothelioma and lung cancer in a cohort of workers formerly exposed to asbestos. Arch Toxicol. 2011;85:185–92.
50. Gube M, Taeger D, Weber DG, et al. Performance of biomarkers SMRP, CA125, and CYFRA 21-1 as potential tumor markers for malignant mesothelioma and lung cancer in a cohort of workers formerly exposed to asbestos. Arch Toxicol. 2011;85:185–92.
51. Roe OD, Creaney J, Lundgren S, Larsson E, Sandeck H, Boffetta P, Nilsen TI, Robinson B, Kjaerheim K. Mesothelin-related predictive and prognostic factors in malignant mesothelioma: a nested case-control study. Lung Cancer. 2008;61:235–43.
52. Boudville N, Paul R, Robinson BW, et al. Mesothelin and kidney function—analysis of relationship and implications for mesothelioma screening. Lung Cancer. 2011;73:320–4.
53. Filiberti R, Marroni P, Mencoboni M, Mortara V, Caruso P, Cioè A, Michelazzi L, Merlo DF, Bruzzone A, Bobbio B, Delcorso L, Galli R, Taveggia P, Dini G, Spigno F. Individual predictors of increased serum mesothelin in asbestos-exposed workers. Med Oncol. 2013;30:422.
54. Hollevoet K, Van Cleemput J, Thimpont J, De Vuyst P, Bosquée L, Nackaerts K, Germonpré P, Vansteelandt S, Kishi Y, Delanghe JR, van Meerbeeck JP. Serial measurements of mesothelioma serum biomarkers in asbestos-exposed individuals: a prospective longitudinal cohort study. J Thorac Oncol. 2011;6:889–95.
55. Hollevoet K, Nackaerts K, Thimpont J, et al. Diagnostic performance of soluble mesothelin and megakaryocyte potentiating factor in mesothelioma. Am J Respir Crit Care Med. 2010;181:620–514.
56. Sato T, Suzuki Y, Mori T, et al. Newly established ELISA for N-ERC/mesothelin improves diagnostic accuracy in patients with suspected pleural mesothelioma. Cancer Med. 2014;3:1377–84.
57. Creaney J, Sneddon S, Dick IM, et al. Comparison of the diagnostic accuracy of the MSLN gene products, mesothelin and megakaryocyte potentiating factor, as biomarkers for mesothelioma in pleural effusions and serum. Dis Markers. 2013;35:119–27.
58. Shiomi K, Miyamoto H, Segawa T, et al. Novel ELISA system for detection of N-ERC/mesothelin in the sera of mesothelioma patients. Cancer Sci. 2006;97:928–32.
59. Onda M, Nagata S, Ho M, et al. Megakaryocyte potentiation factor cleaved from mesothelin precursor is a useful tumor marker in the serum of patients with mesothelioma. Clin Cancer Res. 2006;12:4225–31.
60. Creaney J, Yeoman D, Demelker Y, et al. Comparison of osteopontin, megakaryocyte potentiating factor, and mesothelin proteins as markers in the serum of patients with malignant mesothelioma. J Thorac Oncol. 2008;3:851–7.
61. Coppola D, Szabo M, Boulware D, et al. Correlation of osteopontin protein expression and pathological stage across a wide variety of tumor histologies. Clin Cancer Res. 2004;10:184–9024.
62. Pass HI, Lott D, Lonardo F, et al. Asbestos exposure, pleural mesothelioma, and serum osteopontin levels. N Engl J Med. 2005;353:1564–73.
63. Cristaudo A, Bonotti A, Simonini S, et al. Combined serum mesothelin and plasma osteopontin measurements in malignant pleural mesothelioma. J Thorac Oncol. 2011;6:1587–93.
64. Cristaudo A, Foddis R, Bonotti A, et al. Comparison between plasma and serum osteopontin levels: usefulness in diagnosis of epithelial malignant pleural mesothelioma. Int J Biol Markers. 2010;25:164–70.
65. Rai AJ, Flores RM, Mathew A, et al. Soluble mesothelin related peptides (SMRP) and osteopontin as protein biomarkers for malignant mesothelioma: analytical validation of ELISA based assays and characterization at mRNA and protein levels. Clin Chem Lab Med. 2010;48:271–825.
66. Grigoriu BD, Scherpereel A, Devos P, et al. Utility of osteopontin and serum mesothelin in malignant pleural mesothelioma diagnosis and prognosis assessment. Clin Cancer Res. 2007;13:2928–35.

67. Paleari L, Rotolo N, Imperatori A, et al. Osteopontin is not a specific marker in malignant pleural mesothelioma. Int J Biol Markers. 2009;24:112–710.
68. Hu ZD, Liu XF, Liu XC, et al. Diagnostic accuracy of osteopontin for malignant pleural mesothelioma: a systematic review and meta-analysis. Clin Chim Acta. 2014;433:44–8.
69. Park EK, Thomas PS, Johnson AR, Yates DH. Osteopontin levels in an asbestos-exposed population. Clin Cancer Res. 2009;15(15):1362–9.
70. Zhang Y, Marmorstein LY. Focus on molecules: fibulin-3 (EFEMP1). Exp Eye Res. 2010;90:374–5.
71. Pei D, Li Y, Liu X, et al. Diagnostic and prognostic utilities of humoral fibulin-3 in malignant pleural mesothelioma: evidence from a meta-analysis. Oncotarget. 2017;8:13030–8.
72. Pass HI, Levin SM, Harbut MR, et al. Fibulin-3 as a blood and effusion biomarker for pleural mesothelioma. N Engl J Med. 2012;367:1417–27.
73. Creaney J, Dick IM, Meniawy TM, et al. Comparison of fibulin-3 and mesothelin as markers in malignant mesothelioma. Thorax. 2014;69:895–902.
74. Kirschner MB, Pulford E, Hoda MA, et al. Fibulin-3 levels in malignant pleural mesothelioma are associated with prognosis but not diagnosis. Br J Cancer. 2015;113:963–9.

Genetics and Epigenetics of Mesothelioma

4

Anna Aspesi, Marika Sculco, Simonetta Guarrera, Elisabetta Casalone, Laura Moro, Corrado Magnani, Giuseppe Matullo, and Irma Dianzani

4.1 Introduction

The definition of the malignant mesothelioma (MM) genome may have important endpoints, both in terms of pathobiology and translation to clinical practice. Generally, the identification of DNA changes within a tumor genome is useful to identify the molecular events that lead to carcinogenesis or tumor progression, i.e., the driver mutations. Early studies focused on the analysis of single genes, especially *TP53*. Looking at melanoma and lung cancer genomes, these studies achieved the important milestone of deciphering the mutational profile (signature) generated by two carcinogens, i.e., UV radiation and smoke carcinogens, respectively [1, 2]. The advent of next generation sequencing (NGS) and novel bioinformatic approaches allowed to explore systematically a large number of tumor types. The seminal studies by Stratton and co-workers allowed to identify several signatures, each associated with exposure to a specific carcinogen or due to key events in carcinogenesis, such as inactivation of specific DNA repair mechanisms or activation of deamination enzymes [2].

The identification of abnormalities in specific pathways shed light on shared carcinogenetic pathways in tumors with or without the same histological origin, paving the road to the creation of pathway-specific targeted drugs. In addition, tumor classification may be supported by looking at the tumor genome and transcriptome.

Furthermore, it is important to consider that the individual germline genome can modulate the response to carcinogens and hence transformation. Genetic risk factors are well known for several tumors and may have important translational output. For example, individuals carrying such risk factors may benefit from the implementation of screening programs aimed at early diagnosis of tumors. Additionally, the same risk factor may modify specific carcinogenic pathways and response to specific therapies.

Finally, it is well known that tumor suppressor genes may also be inactivated by epigenetic mechanisms. The term "epigenetic" refers to

A. Aspesi · M. Sculco · I. Dianzani (✉)
Department of Health Sciences, University of Piemonte Orientale, Novara, Italy
e-mail: anna.aspesi@med.uniupo.it; marika.sculco@uniupo.it; irma.dianzani@med.uniupo.it

S. Guarrera · E. Casalone · G. Matullo
Department of Medical Sciences, University of Turin, Turin, Italy

Italian Institute for Genomic Medicine, Turin, Italy
e-mail: simonetta.guarrera@iigm.it; elisabetta.casalone@iigm.it; giuseppe.matullo@unito.it

L. Moro
Department of Pharmaceutical Sciences, University of Piemonte Orientale, Novara, Italy
e-mail: laura.moro@uniupo.it

C. Magnani
Unit of Cancer Epidemiology, CPO-Piemonte, Department of Translational Medicine, University of Piemonte Orientale, Novara, Italy
e-mail: corrado.magnani@uniupo.it

G. L. Ceresoli et al. (eds.), *Mesothelioma*, https://doi.org/10.1007/978-3-030-16884-1_4

heritable and reversible changes in the mechanisms that regulate gene activity without altering the genomic sequence. In recent years, there is increasing evidence of the major role of epigenetic mechanisms in tumorigenesis, as well as in drug-response. Much attention is also devoted to epigenetic changes as biomarkers of early disease detection, prognosis, and response to therapy.

In this review, different patterns of genetic and epigenetic signatures of the malignant pleural mesothelioma (MPM) genomes will be discussed, together with peculiar aspects of genetic predisposition and gene/environment interactions. The potential use of these genetic/epigenetic signatures for the development of future therapeutics will also be addressed.

4.2 Genetic Risk Factors of Mesothelioma

MPM carcinogenesis is caused in the large majority of cases by asbestos or asbestos-like fibers exposure. It is well known that the level of asbestos exposure directly correlates with the risk of MM ([3], more details are given in a different chapter of this book), but several epidemiological studies suggested that different individuals may respond differently to this carcinogen. An important observation is that only about 10% of the workers heavily exposed to asbestos develop MPM [4]. Additionally, several papers reported familial aggregations of MPM [5]. These observations suggested the hypothesis of an inherited predisposition that modifies the carcinogenic effect of asbestos.

Generally, inherited predisposition factors are DNA variants that occur in the germline genome and modify the function of a specific gene. They are divided into three classes, depending on the relative risk (RR) they carry: low-, moderate-, and high-risk factors.

Low-risk factors are DNA variants that subtly modify the function of a gene or a biochemical pathway. In this case, a single DNA variant does not have any substantial effect on human phenotypes, but many DNA variants affecting the same biochemical pathway may alter its functions, favoring disease development. Therefore, the disease risk does not follow the rules of Mendelian heredity, because each variant is inherited independently from the others.

Risk factors are identified using genome wide association studies (GWAS) on thousands of patients and controls [6]. Large numbers are required to obtain statistically significant results, because each variant confers a low risk. The aim of these studies is to identify DNA variants that are differently represented in patients versus controls. These studies are expected to increase the knowledge of asbestos carcinogenesis and improve risk evaluation.

So far, only two GWAS on MPM have been performed, both including several hundreds of patients and controls, but not enough to obtain statistically significant results [7, 8]. However, both studies identified a region associated with the MPM status, that included *FOXK1*, encoding for an interactor of BAP1 (BRCA1-associated protein 1), a well-known high-risk factor for MPM.

BAP1 codes for a tumor suppressor that is frequently deleted in the genomes of several tumors, including cutaneous melanoma, uveal melanoma, mesothelioma, and others [9].

Germline variants in *BAP1* characterize the *BAP1*-tumor predisposition syndrome (*BAP1*-TPDS, MIM#614327) [10]. Tumor predisposition syndromes are due to germline mutations in tumor suppressor genes and are inherited with an autosomal dominant pattern. The patients with these syndromes show a high or moderate risk for specific tumors during their whole life. Often they develop several independent tumors.

Individuals with *BAP1*-TPDS show a high risk of developing mesothelioma, cutaneous and uveal melanoma, clear cell renal carcinoma, and basal cell carcinoma [10]. Moreover, they develop peculiar nonmalignant skin tumors, called atypical Spitz tumors or MBAITs (BAP1-mutated atypical intradermal tumors) or bapomas [10, 11].

Patients with *BAP1*-TPDS and uveal melanoma have a poor prognosis [10, 12], whereas those with mesothelioma seem to have a longer survival than those without *BAP1*-TPDS [13].

Ninety-seven families with *BAP1*-TPDS have been identified so far, 48 of them included patients with MM; thus, this syndrome is indeed very rare [11, 14–38]. Age at onset of mesothelioma in patients with *BAP1*-TPDS is earlier than that in patients without this syndrome [13, 26]. Most of the MM are MPM and show an epithelioid histotype, while peritoneal mesothelioma (PM) has been rarely reported [10]. The prevalence of *BAP1*-TPDS among patients with familial MPM varied between 6% (9/153) and 7.7% (3/39) [26, 31] and was higher than the prevalence observed in sporadic cases [23, 39, 40].

Other tumors have been reported in patients with *BAP1*-TPDS, i.e., breast cancer [12, 14, 21, 22], cholangiocarcinoma [12, 22, 41], meningioma [18, 25, 38, 41], neuroendocrine tumors [18, 19], non-small cell lung cancer (NSCLC) [12, 18, 19, 42], thyroid carcinoma [21, 43], and mucoepidermoid carcinoma of the tongue [23].

BAP1 (#MIM 603089) is located on 3p21.1 and encodes for a ubiquitin carboxy-terminal hydrolase, a nuclear enzyme that catalyzes the cleavage of a ubiquitin residue from its target proteins. The product of the gene, BAP1, has three domains: the ubiquitin C-terminal hydrolase domain and two nuclear localization sequences. The BAP1 protein together with FOXK1, HCFC1, ASXL1/2, and OGT [44] forms a multiprotein complex.

BAP1 has been implicated in DNA repair, chromatin modulation, transcriptional regulation, cell proliferation, cell death, and glucidic metabolism [45–49]. The mechanism of BAP1-dependent carcinogenesis is not known, but these functions are not mutually exclusive. *BAP1* is involved in DNA repair by the HRR (homologous recombination repair) pathway [49].

Bap1 (+/−) mice are more sensitive to asbestos compared with wild-type mice [50, 51]. Quantification of asbestos exposure has been reported only for four individuals with MPM and *BAP1*-TPDS: all showed very low exposure [31, 52].

BAP1 germline mutations cause loss of function, and only ten of the different mutations have been identified in patients within apparently nonconsanguineous families [24]. Recurrent mutations could be due to mutable hot spots, such as CpG dinucleotides.

Eleven other genes were reported to confer predisposition to MPM: *CDKN2A*, *PALB2*, *BRCA1*, *FANCI*, *ATM*, *SLX4*, *BRCA2*, *FANCC*, *FANCF*, *PMS1*, and *XPC* [32, 53] (Table 4.1). All these genes but *PMS1* are tumor suppressors, responsible for cancer predisposition syndromes with specific tumor spectra. In particular, *BRCA1*, *BRCA2*, *ATM*, *SLX4*, and *PALB2* can predispose women to breast and ovarian cancer whereas *BRCA1* and *BRCA2* also to prostate and pancreatic carcinomas [61]; *CDKN2A* to melanoma and pancreatic cancer [54]; and *XPC* to basal cell carcinoma, squamous cell carcinoma, and melanoma [62]. *PMS1* is involved in MMR (DNA mismatch repair) and possibly in cancer predisposition [63, 64].

Homozygous germline variants in *BRCA1* (also called *FANCS*); *BRCA2* (*FANCD1*); *FANCC*,

Table 4.1 High- or moderate-risk predisposition genes

Gene	Function	Reference
BAP1	Deubiquitination enzyme, cell proliferation, DNA repair pathway (HRR)	[11, 12, 14–39, 41–43, 54–60]
CDKN2A	Cell cycle regulation	[32]
ATM	Cell cycle regulation, DNA repair pathway (HRR)	[53]
BRCA1	DNA repair pathway (HRR)	[53]
BRCA2	DNA repair pathway (HRR)	[53]
FANCC	DNA repair pathway (HRR)	[53]
FANCF	DNA repair pathway (HRR)	[53]
FANCI	DNA repair pathway (HRR)	[53]
PALB2	DNA repair pathway (HRR)	[53]
SLX4	DNA repair pathway (HRR)	[53]
XPC	DNA repair pathway (NER)	[53]

Only genes harboring germline PTVs in MM patients are included. *HRR* homologous recombination repair, *NER* nucleotide excision repair

FANCI, *FANCF*, and *SLX4* (*FANCP*); and *PALB2* (*FANCN*) are found in patients with Fanconi anemia, a recessive disease that predisposes to a variety of hematological and solid tumors. This disorder can be caused by at least 20 different genes [65], all acting in a specific signaling pathway activated in response to cross-linking agents.

Mutations in *XPC* cause the recessive disease xeroderma pigmentosum (MIM# 278720). *XPC* is involved in the NER (nucleotide excision repair) pathway, a DNA repair system that removes the pyrimidine dimers induced by exposure to ultraviolet radiation.

In most cases, the loss of the wild-type allele, due to a further acquired mutation, induces carcinogenesis in the target tissues of patients with a germline variant. Except for *CDKN2A*, which is involved in the control of cell proliferation, all these genes have a role in DNA repair.

Anecdotal studies allow to include two more genes involved in cancer predisposition syndromes, *NF2* and *TP53*, because MPM was reported in patients with neurofibromatosis Type 2 or Li-Fraumeni syndrome, due to germline variants in *NF2* or *TP53* [66, 67], respectively.

Interestingly, some of these genes are often somatically mutated in MPM, i.e., *BAP1*, *CDKN2A*, *NF2*, and *TP53* [55, 68, 69].

The involvement of DNA repair genes in MPM risk has been confirmed by others [70] and is in accordance with the observation that 12% of patients with different types of metastatic tumors were reported to carry germline variants, 75% of which in DNA repair genes [71].

Most probably, the development of a specific tumor type in patients with these germline mutations depends on the carcinogen to which they are exposed. If the carcinogen is asbestos, the tumor is likely MPM. Analysis of the genomic signature of the different cancers affecting these patients may confirm this hypothesis.

4.3 The Mesothelioma Genome

Deciphering tumor genomes is important both to gather information about the processes that induce carcinogenesis and to identify druggable pathways in the landscape of precision oncology.

Different methodologies are required to identify point mutations or large rearrangements and copy number variants (CNVs). Ideally, rearrangements and CNVs are studied on the whole genome by using CGH (comparative genomic hybridization) arrays, SNP (single nucleotide polymorphism) arrays, or whole genome sequencing. These methods simultaneously identify all copy gains and copy losses in a genome. Point mutations (also called single nucleotide variants, SNVs) are detected by NGS. Different approaches may be used. Targeted resequencing screens hundreds of known cancer genes that are usually analyzed in the regions corresponding to exons (panel NGS analysis). Exome analysis has the advantage of studying all the genes of the human genome, with a focus on exons. Using appropriate bioinformatic tools, CNVs and rearrangements may be identified in exomes, but not those affecting noncoding regions.

Whole genome analysis addresses the entire genome and could theoretically identify all variants, but management of big data may be time-consuming. In addition, the role of the majority of the genome noncoding regions is not known, so the functional interpretation of variants is difficult.

Usually the cancer and the blood cell genomes are sequenced at the same time to distinguish somatic from germline variants. It should be considered that a very large amount of mutations are generated in each tumor cell at every cell division because of its genetic instability. Therefore, most of these variants are passenger (neutral) variants; only a small number are driver mutations, those that confer a selective advantage to the cell. It has been calculated that only half of the driver mutations in tumors are located in known cancer genes, whereas the others reside in genes or regions whose effect on carcinogenesis is still unknown [72].

The first studies reporting copy gains and copy losses in the mesothelioma genome were published 20 years ago (Table 4.2) [9, 55, 56, 69, 73–80], but point mutations in mesothelioma have been addressed only after the implementation of NGS strategies (Table 4.3) [9, 55–59, 68, 69, 74, 76, 78, 79, 81–85]. Most studies are focused on

Table 4.2 Mesothelioma genome: genes harboring somatic CNVs

#	Gene	Aberration	Function	Reference
1	***NF2***	Loss, Chr rearrangements, fusion	Cell shape, cell growth, cell adhesion	[55, 56, 69, 73–77]
2	***BAP1***	Loss, Chr rearrangements, fusion	Deubiquitinating enzyme, cell proliferation, DNA repair pathway (HRR)	[9, 69, 74, 76, 77]
3	***CDKN2A***[c]	Loss, Chr rearrangements	Cell cycle regulation	[55, 56, 69, 73, 75, 77, 78], [79][a]
4	***TRAF7***	Loss	Ubiquitin-protein transferase activity	[76]
5	***LATS2***	Loss	Mitosis, cytoskeleton damage response	[69, 74, 76]
6	***CDKN2B***[c]	Loss	Cell cycle regulation	[55, 69, 78], [79][a]
7	***SETD2***	Loss, fusion	Regulation of chromatin	[69, 75–77]
8	***FGFR3***	Loss	Cell shape, cell growth, cell adhesion	[76]
9	*PBRM1*	Loss, fusion	Regulation of chromatin, DNA replication	[69, 75, 77]
10	***HUWE1***	Loss	Ubiquitination	[76]
11	*GRM8*	Loss	Transcription regulation	[76]
12	*PTEN*	Loss, fusion	Phosphatase activity	[69, 74]
13	***TP53***	Loss	Cell division, DNA repair pathway, senescence, apoptosis	[55, 69, 74, 76]
14	***LATS1***	Loss	Cell cycle regulation	[69, 74]
15	***STK11***	Fusion	Protein tyrosine kinase	[69, 74], [75][b]
16	*CDH5*	Loss	Cell adhesion, cytoskeleton organization	[74]
17	*ERRFI1*	Loss	Cell growth, cell stress, cell signaling	[74]
18	*SDHB*	Loss	Citric acid cycle regulation, respiratory chain regulation	[74]
19	*RAP1*	Loss	Signal transduction, cell adhesion, cell junction formation	[74]
20	***RASSF1***[c]	Loss	Cell cycle regulation, apoptosis, DNA repair pathway	[74]
21	*DUSP7*	Loss	MAPK pathway	[74]
22	*PTPN13*	Loss	Apoptosis, cell growth, differentiation, mitotic cycle	[74, 77]
23	*PTPRD*	Loss	Cell growth, differentiation, mitotic cycle	[74]
24	*RB1*	Loss	Cell cycle regulation	[74, 77]
25	*ING1*	Loss	Cell growth arrest, apoptosis	[74]
26	*SPRY2*	Loss	Protein translocation	[74]
27	*CDKN3*	Loss	Cell cycle regulation	[74]
28	***SMARCB1***	Loss	Regulator of chromatin	[74, 75, 77]
29	*CHEK2*	Loss	DNA repair pathway, cell cycle arrest, apoptosis	[74, 75, 77]
30	*DMC1*	Loss	Meiotic homologous recombination	[74]
31	*RICTOR*	Gain	Cell growth, cell proliferation	[74]
32	*TRIO*	Gain	Actin remodeling, cell migration, cell growth	[74]
33	*RHEB*	Gain	Cell cycle regulation, cell growth	[74]
34	*DPP10*	Chrom break	Potassium channels regulation	[80]
35	*EPHA6*	Chrom break	Transferase activity	[80]
36	*EYS/PRIM2*	Chrom break	Integrity of photoreceptor cells	[80]
37	*NRG3*	Chrom break	Neuroblast proliferation, migration, and differentiation	[80]

(continued)

Table 4.2 (continued)

#	Gene	Aberration	Function	Reference
38	*NOS2A*	Chrom break	Oxidoreductase activity, neurotransmission, antimicrobial activity	[80]
39	*RAB11FIP4*	Chrom break	Regulation of endocytic traffic	[80]
40	*CA10*	Chrom break	Brain development	[80]
41	*MAP2K6/ CA10*	Chrom break	Activating protein kinase	[80]
42	*ARSG*	Chrom break	Hormone biosynthesis, modulation of cell signaling, degradation of macromolecules	[80]
43	*CCDC123 (CEP89)*	Chrom break	Organelle biogenesis and maintenance, cell cycle progression	[80]
44	*CHODL*	Chrom break	Neurogenesis, motor axon growth, and guidance	[80]
45	*DLG2*	Chrom break	Regulation of synaptic stability	[80]
46	*GRK5/ KCNJ12*	Chrom break	Apoptosis, cell proliferation, cell cycle regulation/controlling the resting membrane potential	[80]
47	*CCDC46 (CEP112)*	Chrom break	Cell division, centrosome	[80]
48	*TANC2*	Chrom break	Morphogenesis of the optic cup	[80]
49	***TERT***	Gain	Telomerase maintenance	[77, 81]
50	***CUL1***	Loss	Ubiquitination, protein degradation	[55]
51	*NOSIP*	Fusion	Ubiquitination	[69]
52	*LIFR*	Fusion	Cell differentiation, cell proliferation, cell survival	[69, 77]
53	*CLTC*	Fusion	Intracellular trafficking	[69, 77]
54	*RRBP1*	Fusion	Protein transport, translocation, transport	[69]
55	*DTD1*	Fusion	DNA replication	[69]
56	*RPTOR*	Gain	Cell growth	[69]
57	*BRD4*	Gain	Regulation of chromatin, DNA repair pathway, DNA replication	[69]
58	*TNFRSF14*	Gain	Host-virus interaction	[75]
59	*DVL1*	Gain	Developmental protein, cell proliferation	[75]
60	*ACSL6*	Gain	Fatty acid metabolism	[75]
61	*RECQL4*	Gain	Chromosome segregation, DNA repair	[75, 77]
62	*MYC*	Gain	Cell cycle progression, apoptosis, cellular transformation	[75]
63	*KDM5A*	Gain	Regulation of chromatin	[75]
64	*HOXC11*	Gain	Morphogenesis, cell growth	[75]
65	*HOXC13*	Gain	Morphogenesis, cell growth	[75]
66	*TRIM33*	Loss	Transcription regulation, ubiquitination	[75, 77]
67	*UBE4B*	Loss	Ubiquitination	[75]
68	*MLL3 (KMT2C)*	Loss	Methylation, transcription regulation	[75]
69	*WRN*	Loss	DNA repair, replication, transcription, telomere maintenance	[75]
70	*BMPR1A*	Loss	Cell differentiation	[75]
71	*SUFU*	Loss	Developmental protein, cell proliferation	[75]
72	*PTPN11*	Loss	Cell growth, differentiation, mitotic cycle	[75]
73	*CASC5 (KNL1)*	Loss	Chromosome segregation, spindle elongation	[75]
74	*RABEP1*	Loss	Endocytosis, protein transport, apoptosis	[75]
75	*SUZ12*	Loss	Chromatin regulation, methylation	[75]

Table 4.2 (continued)

#	Gene	Aberration	Function	Reference
76	***ASXL1***	Loss	Chromatin regulation, transcription	[75]
77	*PDGFB*	Loss	Embryonic development, cell proliferation, cell migration, cell survival, chemotaxis	[75, 77]
78	*MKL1*	Loss	Smooth muscle cell differentiation	[75, 77]
79	*EP300*	Loss	Chromatin regulation, cell growth, cell division, cell differentiation	[75, 77]
80	*PATZ1*	Loss	Chromatin regulation	[75, 77]
81	***MYH9***	Loss	Cytokinesis, cell shape, cytoskeleton reorganization	[56, 75, 77]
82	*CLTCL1*	Loss	Chromatin modeling, transcription regulation	[75, 77]
83	*BCR*	Loss	Chemical signaling, migration	[75, 77]
84	*RAF1*	Gain	Cell proliferation, cell differentiation, apoptosis, survival	[75][b]
85	***KIT***	Gain	Cell growth, cell division, cell survival, cell migration	[75][b]
86	*CCND3*	Gain	Cell cycle regulation	[75][b]
87	*TFEB*	Gain	Transcription regulation	[75][b]
88	*ELN*	Gain	Extracellular matrix structural constituent	[75][b]
89	*HIP1*	Gain	Structural constituent of cytoskeleton	[75][b]
90	*RUNX1T1*	Gain	DNA-binding transcription factor activity	[75][b]
91	*NOTCH1*	Gain	DNA-binding transcription factor activity	[75][b]
92	*RALGDS*	Gain	GTPase regulator activity	[75][b]
93	*FGFR2*	Gain	Cell shape, cell growth	[75][b]
95	*CCDN1*	Gain	Cell cycle regulation	[75][b]
96	*KRAS*	Gain	Cell proliferation, cell differentiation, apoptosis, survival	[75][b]
97	*FUS*	Gain	Regulation of gene expression	[75][b]
98	*HERPUD1*	Gain	Protein processing in endoplasmic reticulum, unfolded protein response	[75][b]
99	*BRCA1*	Gain	DNA repair pathway (HRR)	[75][b]
100	*RARA*	Gain	Regulation of development, differentiation, apoptosis, transcription	[75][b]
101	*CANT1*	Gain	Pyrimidine metabolism	[75][b]
102	*ELL*	Gain	Transcription	[75][b]
103	*AKT2*	Gain	Metabolism, cell proliferation, cell survival, cell growth, angiogenesis	[75][b]
104	*APOBEC3B*	Loss	Deoxycytidine deaminase activity	[77]
105	*MN1*	Loss	Transcription regulator	[77]
106	*EWSR1*	Loss	Gene expression, cell signaling, RNA processing, and transport	[77]
107	*MAPK1*	Loss	Cell proliferation, differentiation, transcription regulation, development	[77]
108	*SEPT5*	Loss	Cell division, cytoskeletal organization	[77]
109	*LZTR1*	Loss	Transcriptional regulator	[77]
110	*NCKIPSD*	Loss	Signal transduction, stress fiber formation	[77]
111	*SDHA*	Gain	Complex of the mitochondrial respiratory chain	[77]
112	*DROSHA*	Gain	miRNA synthesis	[77]
113	*ILR7*	Gain	VDJ recombination (lymphocyte)	[77]
114	*FCGR2B*	Gain	Phagocytosis, regulation of antibody production	[77]

(continued)

Table 4.2 (continued)

#	Gene	Aberration	Function	Reference
115	*CDC73*	Gain	Cell division, cell cycle	[77]
116	*PTPRC*	Gain	Cell growth, differentiation, mitosis	[77]
117	*MDM4*	Gain	p53 regulator	[77]
118	*ELK4*	Gain	Chromatin regulation, transcription	[77]
119	*SLC45A3*	Gain	Transmembrane transport	[77]
120	*HLF*	Gain	Transcription regulation	[77]
121	*MSI2*	Gain	Transcription regulation	[77]
122	***RNF43***	Gain	Ubiquitination	[77]
123	*PPM1D*	Gain	Cell stress response	[77]
124	***BRIP1***	Gain	DNA repair pathway (HRR)	[77]
125	*CD79B*	Gain	Transmembrane signaling receptor activity	[77]
126	*DDX5*	Gain	Coregulator of transcription, regulator of splicing, processing of small noncoding RNAs	[77]
127	*AXIN2*	Gain	DNA repair pathway (MMR), cell proliferation, cell death, ubiquitination	[77]
128	*PRKAR1A*	Gain	Ubiquitination	[77]
129	*ROS1*	Loss	Cell growth, differentiation	[77]
130	*CACNA1D*	Loss	Muscle contraction, hormone, or neurotransmitter release	[77]
131	*FLT3*	Loss	Hematopoiesis	[75, 77]
132	*FOXO1*	Loss	Myogenic growth, differentiation	[77]
133	*EPS15*	Loss	Cell growth	[77]
134	*WHSC1*	Loss	Transcriptional regulation, developmental transcription factors	[77]
135	*RAP1GDS1*	Loss	Proton-transporting ATPase activity	[77]
136	***FBXW7***	Loss	Cell cycle regulation, ubiquitination	[77]
137	*FAT1*	Loss	Cell proliferation	[77]
138	*NFIB*	Loss	Transcriptional activator	[77]
139	*MLLT3*	Loss	Chromatin regulation, transcription	[77]
140	*BRCA2*	Loss	DNA repair pathway (HRR)	[77]
141	*LHFP*	Loss	Transmembrane protein	[77]
142	*LCP1*	Loss	Actin-binding protein	[77]
143	*PMS2*	Gain	DNA repair pathway (MMR)	[77]
144	*EIF4A2*	Gain	Translation regulation	[77]
145	*HNRNPA2B1*	Gain	mRNA metabolism and transport	[77]
146	***EGFR***	Gain	Cell growth	[75, 77]
147	***MET***[c]	Gain	Cell survival, cell migration, embryogenesis, invasion	[77]
148	*RAD21*	Gain	DNA double-strand breaks pathway	[77]
149	*KLF6*	Gain	Transcriptional activator	[75][b], [77]
150	*NAB2*	Gain	Transcriptional regulator	[77]
151	*MLLT6*	Gain	Histone-binding protein	[77]
152	*CIC*	Gain	Transcriptional regulator	[77]
153	*FAM131B*	Gain	Cell proliferation, differentiation	[77]
154	*PLAG1*	Gain	Transcriptional activator	[77]
155	*CHCHD7*	Gain	Metabolism of proteins, mitochondrial protein import	[77]
156	*NUTM2B*	Gain	Intracellular protein	[77]
157	*NUTM2A*	Gain	Intracellular protein	[77]
158	*ETNK1*	Gain	Transferase activity	[77]
159	*DICER1*	Gain	Metabolism of RNA	[77]

Table 4.2 (continued)

#	Gene	Aberration	Function	Reference
160	***ZNF521***	Gain	Protein domain-specific binding	[77]
161	*ABL1*	Gain	Cell differentiation, cell division, cell adhesion, stress response	[79][a]
162	*COL1A1*	Gain	Member of group I collagen	[79][a]
163	*PITCH1*	Loss	Embryonic development	[78]

HRR homologous recombination repair, *MMR* mismatch repair
Genes underscored and in bold also harbor PTVs
[a]Gene that can also be lost by epigenetic mechanisms
[b]Tumor type not specified
[c]Peritoneal mesothelioma

Table 4.3 Mesothelioma genome: genes harboring somatic point mutations or small indels

#	Gene	Function	Reference
1	***BAP1***	Deubiquitinating enzyme, cell proliferation, DNA repair pathway (HRR)	[9, 55–57, 59, 68, 69, 74, 76, 78, 81–85], [79][a]
2	***NF2***	Cell shape, cell growth, cell adhesion	[55, 56, 68, 69, 74, 76, 81, 84], [78][d], [58][c]
3	***TP53***	Cell division, DNA repair pathway, senescence, apoptosis	[55, 56, 68, 69, 76, 81, 84, 85], [79][a], [58][c]
4	***LATS2***	Mitosis, cytoskeleton damage response	[76, 84]
5	***TERT***[b]	Telomerase maintenance, senescence	[81]
6	*RIF1*	DNA repair pathway, regulation of chromatin, regulation of replication timing	[76]
7	***CUL1***	Ubiquitination, protein degradation	[55]
8	*RDX*	Cytoskeleton	[55]
9	*TAOK1*	Transferase activity	[55]
10	*PIK3C2B*	Cell proliferation, cell survival, cell migration, and intracellular protein trafficking	[55]
11	***EGFR***	Cell proliferation, apoptosis, angiogenesis, cell migration, cell adhesion, invasion	[68], [79][a]
12	***LATS1***	Cell cycle regulation	[55, 84]
13	***SMARCB1***	Regulator of chromatin	[68, 74]
14	***CDKN2A***[e]	Cell cycle regulation	[69, 78, 81, 84], [58][c]
15	***CDKN2B***[e]	Cell cycle regulation	[78, 81, 84]
16	*PIK3C2A*	Cell proliferation, cell survival, cell migration, and intracellular protein trafficking	[68]
17	*PDGFRA*	Growth factors receptor	[68]
18	*HRAS*	Cell transduction, cell growth, cell division	[68]
19	***KIT***	Cell growth, cell division, cell survival, cell migration	[68]
20	*KDR*	Transferase activity	[68]
21	***STK11***	Protein tyrosine kinase	[68, 78]
22	***MET***[e]	Cell survival, cell migration, embryogenesis, invasion	[68]
23	***FBXW7***	Cell cycle regulation, ubiquitination	[68]
24	*SMAD4*	Cell proliferation	[68]
25	*ERBB4*	Cell growth	[68]
26	*CSF1R*	Cytokine involved in production, differentiation, and function of macrophages	[68]
27	*APC*[e]	Cell division, cell adhesion, cell polarization	[68]
28	*RET*	Cell proliferation	[68]

(continued)

Table 4.3 (continued)

#	Gene	Function	Reference
29	***FGFR3***	Cell shape, cell growth, cell adhesion	[68, 76]
30	***TRAF7***	Ubiquitin-protein transferase activity	[78]
31	*DDX3X*	ATP-dependent RNA helicase activity	[78]
32	*RYR2*	Calcium regulation	[78]
33	*CFAP45*	Cell migration	[78]
34	*SETDB1*	Methyltransferase activity	[69], [58][c]
35	*SETD5*	Methyltransferase activity	[69]
36	*ULK2*	Axonal elongation	[69]
37	*DDX51*	Nucleic acid binding and hydrolase activity	[69]
38	***SETD2***	Regulation of chromatin	[69], [78][d], [57][c]
39	*APOBEC2*	Cytidine deaminase, RNA editing	[56]
40	***MYH9***	Cytokinesis, cell shape, cytoskeleton reorganization	[56]
41	*PTPRT*	Signal transduction, cellular adhesion	[56]
42	***RNF43***	Ubiquitination	[56]
43	*SCRN2*	Dipeptidase activity	[56]
44	*CENPE*	Chromosome movement, spindle elongation	[56]
45	*RHOA*	Signal transduction pathway, cell adhesion	[56]
46	*SAV1*	Protein degradation, transcription, RNA splicing	[84], [58][c]
47	***RASSF1***[e]	Cell cycle regulation, apoptosis, DNA repair pathway	[84]
48	*STK3 (MST2)*	Apoptosis	[84]
49	*MST1*	Ciliary motility (lung cells), cell signaling	[84]
50	***HUWE1***	Ubiquitination	[76]
51	*NF1*	MAPK pathway	[79][a]
52	*PREX2*	GTPase activator	[79][a]
53	*KDM5C*	Chromatin remodeling	[79][a]
54	*KDM6A*	Demethylation	[78][c]
55	***ASXL1***	Chromatin regulation, transcription	[78][c]
56	***BRIP1***	DNA repair pathway (HRR)	[78][c]
57	*SMPD4*	Response to DNA damage, cellular stress, and tumor necrosis factor	[58][c]
58	*ARPC1A*	Actin filament binding	[58][c]
59	*PLA2G5*	Inflammatory response	[58][c]
60	*INTS4*	Transcription	[58][c]
61	*PIBF1*	Steroid hormone progesterone	[58][c]
62	*ATP1B2*	Electrochemical gradient establishing and maintaining	[58][c]
63	*PMSD3*	Embryonic development, growth control, homeostasis	[58][c]
64	*TTYH*	Ion transport	[58][c]
65	*LACE1*	Mitochondrial protein homeostasis	[58][c]
66	*ORM1*	Acute inflammation	[58][c]
67	*RHBDF1*	Cell survival, cell proliferation, cell migration	[58][c]
68	*KCNJ2*	Potassium channel	[58][c]
69	*P2RY12*	Platelet aggregation, blood coagulation	[58][c]
70	*ANKRD65*	Intracellular protein	[58][c]
71	*OIT3*	Liver development and function	[58][c]
72	*EED*	Histone methyltransferase activity, cellular senescence, embryonic development	[58][c]
73	*FOXM1*	Transcriptional activator, cell proliferation	[58][c]
74	*ICAM2*	Intercellular adhesion molecule	[58][c]
75	*KNCJ2*	Chondrocyte differentiation	[58][c]

Table 4.3 (continued)

#	Gene	Function	Reference
76	***ZNF521***	Protein domain-specific binding	[58][c]
77	*NLRP9*	Innate immune response	[58][c]
78	*PLXNB2*	Axon guidance, cell migration	[58][c]
79	*MSH5*	DNA repair pathway (MMR)	[58][c]
80	*EPBH2*	Developmental processes in the nervous system	[59][c]
81	*GTPBP3*	Mitochondrial tRNA modification	[59][c]
82	*STYK1*	Transferase activity	[59][c]
83	*TMEM18*	Transmembrane protein	[59][c]

HRR homologous recombination repair, *MMR* mismatch repair
Genes underscored and in bold also harbor CNVs
[a]Tumor type not specified
[b]Both in peritoneal and pleural mesothelioma
[c]Peritoneal mesothelioma
[d]GOF (gain of function)
[e]Gene that can also be lost by epigenetic mechanisms

MPM and show that MPM genomes include a large number of chromosomal abnormalities, such as CNVs and chromosomal translocations often leading to gene fusion, but a relatively low number of protein altering mutations compared with most tumors [60]. These alterations involve mostly tumor suppressor genes. A great inter-individual heterogeneity is also typical.

A recent study on CNVs in MPM was performed by Hylebos et al. [77]. They used information obtained using CGH arrays on 85 MPM patients and stored within The Cancer Genome Atlas (TCGA). Data were validated on a panel of 21 patients using low-pass whole genome sequencing. Both datasets showed losses on chromosomes 1, 3, 4, 6, 9, 13, and 22 in 25% of tumors. These losses included *CDKN2A*, *NF2*, *BAP1*, *EP300*, *SETD2*, and *PBRM1*. Copy number gains were less represented compared to losses. They were located on chromosomes 1, 5, 7, and 17 and occurred in 15% of tumors. Genes affected by these gains were *TERT*, *FCGR2B*, *CD79B*, and *PRKAR1A*. In conclusion, recurrent CNVs were detected in both datasets, occurring in regions harboring known MPM-associated genes and genes not previously linked to MPM.

The first studies addressing the MPM mutational landscape were reported by Lo Iacono et al. and Guo et al., independently in 2015, using different NGS approaches [55, 68]. A limit of both studies is that they included patients who had been subjected to chemotherapy; thus, it is possible that a portion of the mutations was due to the mutagenic effect of the drugs [60]. Lo Iacono et al. investigated 52 cancer genes in FFPE (formalin-fixed, paraffin-embedded) tumor samples of 123 MPM patients [68]. Mutated genes included *TP53*, *SMARCB1*, *BAP1*, *PDGFRA*, *KIT*, *KDR*, *HRAS*, *PIK3CA*, *STK11*, and *NF2*. The most represented pathways were the p53/DNA repair and the phosphatidylinositol 3-kinase-AKT. Guo et al. performed whole exome sequencing in fresh tumor samples from 22 patients [55]. These samples showed frequent genetic alterations in *BAP1*, *NF2*, *CDKN2A*, and *CUL1*. The MAPK and the Wnt signaling pathway frequently carried alterations.

Bueno et al. reported data on 216 MPM genomes, 99 of which were studied by whole exome and 103 by panel sequencing (344 genes) [69]. These data were paralleled by RNAseq, an approach that investigates all the RNA species transcribed and allows to validate the functional effect of genetic anomalies. They identified the following genes that are often mutated or lost in MPM: *BAP1*, *NF2*, *TP53*, *SETD2*, *DDX3X*, *ULK2*, *RYR2*, *CFAP45*, *SETDB1*, *DDX51*, *TRAF7*, and *SF3B1*. The pathways that were more frequently affected were Hippo, mTOR, histone methylation, RNA helicase, and p53 signaling [69].

De Rienzo et al. performed whole genome sequencing of 10 MPM patients [56]. The identified mutations and copy number aberrations were validated by targeted resequencing of 9 genes in 147 additional samples (*BAP1*, *NF2*, *TP53*, *MYH9*, *MYH6*, *MYH10*, *PIK3C2A*, *RHOA*, *TNFRSF1A*). A further 136 patients were analyzed for *TP53*, *BAP1*, *NF2*, and *CDKN2A*, which were the most frequently mutated genes. *TP53* variants were more often found in women. Interestingly, three patients showed germline PTVs (protein-truncating variants) in *BAP1* [56].

Exome NGS was also performed on cells from pleural effusions from 27 patients with MPM. Mutations in *BAP1*, *CDKN2A*, and *NF2* and loss of *TRAF7*, *LATS2*, *SETD2*, and *TP53* were identified [76], suggesting that analysis of pleural effusions might be used to monitor the MPM molecular evolution.

Looking at 61 primary mesothelioma cultures, Tranchant et al. identified a subgroup of tumors harboring both *LATS2* and *NF2* mutations [84]. Co-occurring mutations in these genes were associated with a poor prognosis. These cell lines showed abnormalities both in the Hippo signaling pathway and mTOR protein expression suggesting specific therapeutic strategies.

FFPE portions from 11 patients (7 MPM and 4 PM) were studied by Ugurluer et al. using a NGS panel including 236 cancer genes [78]. In MPM samples the mutations most commonly found were in *BAP1*, *CDKN2A/B*, and *NF2*. Other PTVs were found in *PTCH1*, *SETD2*, *STK11*, *KDM6A*, *ASXL1*, and *BRIP1*.

Two PM reported by Ugurluer et al. showed mutations in *BAP1* or *NF2*, whereas the other two did not show PTVs. The whole genome of two PM was reported by Sheffield et al. in 2015 [58]. The two patients reported different histology and different response to chemotherapy. The first had an epithelioid histology, a high disease burden, and did not respond to chemotherapy, whereas the second showed minimal clinical symptoms; histology was poor-prognosis sarcomatoid MM but responded well to treatment. The two tumors shared PTVs in *NF2* but were elsewhere very different. The first had only 18 variants, whereas the second had more than 260 variants in each of the 2 samples that were studied, corresponding to a status called somatic hypermutation. Another study focused on 12 patients with PM [59]. They used copy number analysis and exome sequencing and targeted sequencing and found a low number of CNVs (mostly losses) and SNVs. The gene that was more frequently affected was *BAP1*, whereas *NF2* and *CDKN2A* were not affected. One of the patients carried a nonsense germline variant paired to gene loss in the tumor; thus, he had *BAP1*-TPDS.

Overall, PM seems to have a mutation rate lower than MPM, but driver mutations in PM seem to affect the same genes that are often involved in MPM.

A limit of these studies is that they do not generally consider the hypothesis of intra-tumor heterogeneity, which may be an important issue in mesothelioma considering that there are hints of a polyclonal origin of carcinogenesis [86]. The paper by Zhang et al. focused on testicular MM is a good example of intra-tumor heterogeneity and rapid molecular evolution [87]. They performed whole genome sequencing using DNA obtained from FFPE samples of four successive tumors from a single patient. The first sample was obtained from the primary tumor, whereas the other samples were from a local recurrent tumor, an inguinal lymph node metastasis and a recurrent tumor from the same localization. This study evaluated the tumor progression looking at molecular events. The signature of molecular lesions and also the mutated genes were different from those reported for MPM. Other patients should be studied to evaluate whether this testicular MM is different from the other MM [87].

Tumor exome sequencing may give important information about carcinogenesis in individuals who develop multiple independent tumors. This approach was followed in the case of a 73-year-old male who developed two independent lung cancers (adenocarcinoma and squamous cell carcinoma) and a malignant PM with an epithelioid histology. The patient was a heavy smoker and did not report asbestos exposure. The somatic mutational signatures of the two lung tumors were in agreement with the smoking carcinogen effect, and the mutated genes corresponded to those reported for the tumor types. Conversely, the PM showed a very low number of somatic events, including one PTV in *BAP1* and one in *SETD2*. Several low-risk variants in DNA repair genes could account for the PM predisposition in this patient.

The mutation types prevalent in the tumor genome may be identified in large studies [69]. In particular, Bueno et al. analyzed the mesothelioma exome for transitions (C > T, T > C) and transversions (C > A, C > G, T > A, T > G), taking into account the flanking base immediately 5′ and 3′ of the somatic base (so-called triplets). They identified five distinct signatures (S1, S2, S4, S5, and S6) that are operative in MPMs, two of them being the most represented (S1 and S2). The patterns of contribution of these signatures were different between MPM and lung cancers, in agreement with epidemiological studies that revealed that MPM is not related to smoking like lung cancer. For example, signature S3, characterized by C > A transversions, caused by bulky adducts, is not shown by MPM but is typical of cigarette smoking, an exposure that is not epidemiologically associated with MPM.

The S1 signature is characterized by no predominant transition or transversion and is considered indicative of a base-agnostic mutagen such as reactive oxygen species (ROS) [88, 89]. The S2 signature is represented by C > T transitions at NpCpG trinucleotides and is attributed to an endogenous mechanism, the deamination of 5-methylcytosine to thymine in CpG dinucleotides. The S4 signature is characterized by C > T transitions and is typical of repair errors at UV-induced pyrimidine dimer sites observed in melanoma. Signature S5 shows C > T transitions or C > G transversions at TpCpN nucleotides, considered as indicative of the function of APOBEC enzymes responsible for cytidine deamination and frequently activated in cancer [88, 89].

In conclusion, the study of Bueno et al. identified a mutational pattern concordant with the effect of asbestos exposure (i.e., S1 signature) [69]. The authors did not observe a significant difference of this signature in samples with (n = 69) or without (17) asbestos exposure, but this may depend on the fact that asbestos fiber quantification in the lung was available only for 64/217 patients, whereas asbestos exposure of the other patients was reported, but not quantified.

Overall it is expected that asbestos causes DNA damage in two ways, first by inducing chromosomal breaks by interfering with spindle fibers during cell division and second by inducing inflammation and ROS production. The first mechanism may explain some of the chromosomal rearrangements whereas the second some of the point mutations.

4.4 Translation to the Clinics: Druggable Targets

The identification of driver mutations in mesothelioma is expected to pave the way to precision oncology. In general, this task may be particularly difficult in MPM, considering the wide inter-individual and possibly intra-tumor heterogeneity. Moreover, MPM driver mutations in protein-coding genes are rarer than in other tumors [72]. On the other hand, it is important to note that all these studies reported a frequent involvement of *BAP1*, *NF2*, *CDKN2A*, and *SETD2*.

A thorough evaluation of possible translational steps is beyond the scope of this review, and we refer to other chapters of this book and specific literature [90, 91]. We only mention that PARP or EZH2 inhibitor drugs have been considered for tumors characterized by *BAP1* loss, CDK4/6 or PRMT5 inhibitors for tumors with *CDKN2A* mutations, FAK inhibitors for tumors with *NF2* mutations, and PI3K-AKT inhibitors for tumors with *PI3K-AKT* abnormalities [90]. More in detail, a phase II clinical trial in *BAP1*-deficient patients with the EZH2 inhibitor, tazemetostat, was recently opened to accrual (NCTO02860286); a phase II clinical trial to evaluate the CDK4/6 inhibitor, ribociclib, in solid tumors carrying relevant CDK4/6, cyclinD1/3, or p16^{INK4A} aberrations, including MPMs, has been designed (NCT02187783); while after a randomized switch maintenance, clinical trial (NCT01870609) with the FAK inhibitor defactinib (VS-6063) versus placebo was discontinued in late 2015, in 2016 a new single-center clinical trial tested defactinib before surgery for MPM (NCT02004028); at last, the modest response obtained in a phase I study of apitolisib (GDC-0980), dual phosphatidylinositol-3-kinase, and mammalian target of rapamycin kinase inhibitor (NCT00854152) indicated that combination regimens must be explored.

Conversely, predisposing factors may also give some therapeutic opportunities to the patients that carry them. Patients with ovarian cancer and germline variants in *BRCA1* or *BRCA2* respond to PARP1 inhibitors drugs, through a mechanism called synthetic lethality [92, 93]. This mechanism is induced when two (or more) variants are not lethal singularly but are lethal when both are present in a cell [94]. PARP1 is a nuclear enzyme that functions in three DNA repair systems, i.e., SSBs (single-strand breaks), BER (base excision repair), and alt-NHEJ (alternative nonhomologous end joining) [95]. PARP1 binds to SSBs and causes the formation of polymers of ADP-ribose (PAR) on its target proteins (this phenomenon is called PARylation). PARs are required for the recruitment of SSBs repair scaffolding proteins. PARP1 auto-PARylation is followed by its release from DNA and inactivation [94]. PARP1inhibitors traps PARP1 to the site of DNA damage and interfere with the progression of the replication fork causing the accumulation of SSBs that evolve to DSBs (double-strand breaks), following replication fork collapse. Both HRR and NHEJ (nonhomologous end joining) are used to repair DSBs and restart replication forks stalled by PARP1 inhibitors. When HRR is deficient, because of loss of *BRCA1* or *BRCA2*, the damage cannot be repaired by alt-NHEJ, because this system requires PARP1. If these systems are not functional, cells can only use classical NHEJ, which causes chromosomal anomalies, genomic instability, and cell death [96].

PARP1 inhibitors could inhibit growth of cells that have lost both *BAP1* alleles either because of a germline and a somatic variant or because of two somatic variants. Tumor cells in patients with a germline variant in *BAP1* have a very high likelihood of a second somatic variant on the wild-type allele. Thus, theoretically, in patients with a germline variant in *BAP1* MPM, tumor tissue could have a more homogeneous *BAP1* loss than in sporadic patients and may better respond to this treatment. Patients with germline mutations in other HRR genes may also show such behavior.

4.5 Tumor Epigenetics

The mechanisms underlying tumor initiation and progression involve also epigenome aberrations that share an intricate relationship with genetic instability in the tumor evolution process.

Epigenetic includes three main regulatory mechanisms: histone modifications, DNA methylation, and microRNA (miRNA)-mediated gene regulation.

Histones are members of a highly conserved family of proteins that associate with DNA to organize chromatin in the nucleus. Several post-translational modifications may occur at N-terminal histone tails, including the addition or removal of methyl and acetyl residues. Histone modification is associated with the transcriptional regulation of genes, promoting the transition between open and close chromatin conformation.

DNA methylation consists in the addition of a methyl residue (–CH3) to the cytosine residues within the dinucleotide CpG. DNA methylation mainly occurs at the carbon-5 position of the cytosine ring [97], even though a small fraction (~2%) may occur at cytosines in any context of the genome, or also in a non-CpG context in embryonic stem cells [98]. CpGs DNA methylation may occur in gene promoters, where a high concentration of CpGs dinucleotides can be seen in the so-called CpG islands. Promoter DNA methylation is a well-known mechanism to repress gene transcription, leading to gene silencing through inhibition of transcription factor binding to DNA [99]. Deregulation of the DNA methylation levels may result in cell transformation. Diffuse genome-wide hypomethylation is frequently seen in cancer cells, together with site-specific hypermethylation [100, 101].

miRNAs are a class of small noncoding RNAs involved in gene silencing through a posttranscriptional mechanism that requires miRNA binding to 3′-UTR regions of mRNAs and leads to translation inhibition or mRNA degradation [102]. Dysregulation of miRNAs has been associated to cancer development [103–105], and they have been proposed as tools for cancer diagnosis, classification, prognosis, and treatment [106–109].

Epigenetic alterations may be critical determinants of malignant transformation of pleural mesothelial cells following asbestos exposure. The relationship between DNA methylation modifications and *in vitro* asbestos exposure in MeT5A mesothelial cell lines was recently described [110]. The authors report slight DNA methylation in MeT5A cells after both crocidolite and chrysotile treatments, mainly in genes involved in the regulation of cellular matrix and adhesion, which are mechanisms for mesothelial infiltration and injury, facilitating epithelial-to-mesenchymal transition (EMT) in MPM. This finding may suggest an involvement of methylation changes as potential modulators of asbestos-induced pleural injury.

Evidence of relationship between asbestos burden and promoter methylation of selected tumor suppressor genes (*APC*, *CCND2*, *CDKN2A*, *CDKN2B*, *HPPBP1*, and *RASSF1*) was also reported in lung tissue from MPM patients. Moreover, the increase in methylation of these genes correlates with asbestos body counts [111]. Inactivation of *CDKN2A* by methylation was also reported by Kobayashi et al. [112].

The examination of over 6000 CpG islands in MPM and lung adenocarcinomas showed that 387 genes (6.3%) and 544 genes (8.8%) were hypermethylated in MPM and adenocarcinoma, respectively, and that the two malignancies have characteristic DNA methylation patterns, likely a result of different pathologic processes [113]. Moreover, Goto et al. suggest that *KAZALD1*, *MAPK13*, and *TMEM30B* genes, which were specifically methylated only in MPM, could serve as potential diagnostic markers.

In a larger study of 158 mesothelioma specimens and 18 normal pleura samples, Christensen et al. reported that the DNA methylation profile of 803 cancer-associated genes was able to discriminate normal pleura from mesothelioma and was a predictor of shorter survival [114].

Aberrant promoter methylation of *WIF-1* and *SFRP1*, *2*, *4* genes was found in MPM tissue and mesothelioma cell lines [115]. The analysis of 52 MPM samples and 38 histologically non-tumor lung samples identified higher methylation levels of *ESR1*, *SLC6A20*, and *SYK* genes in MPM [116]. The combination of *SLC6A20*, *SYK*, and *APC* yielded a sensitivity of 92% and a specificity of 73% as positive markers for MPM. The inclusion of *ESR1* methylation as a third positive marker increased sensitivity but reduced specificity.

Cheng et al. [117] reported downregulation of the *ZIC1* gene via promoter methylation in MPM. This gene acts as a tumor suppressor, targeting apoptosis-related miRNAs. In particular, miR-23a and miR-27a are expressed at higher levels in epithelioid MPM patients with shorter survival. These studies highlight that epigenetic silencing through promoter hypermethylation is a frequent event in MPM.

Other studies looked for miRNAs involved in MPM development. Guled et al. [118] identified a number of miRNAs that were differentially expressed between MPM tissue and normal pericardium.

With an *in vitro* study, Pass et al. reported that miR-29c-5p may be a tumor suppressor in MPM and thus a potential therapeutic target [119].

Several miRNA-targeted therapeutics have reached clinical testing. For example, miR-16 is involved in a phase I clinical trial, MesomiR 1. The trial is based on the work by Reid et al. who reported the downregulation of miR-15-16 in MPM tissue and cell lines associated with increased levels of the target oncogenes *CCND1* and *Bcl-2* [120]. Restoring miRNA expression, cell growth is inhibited, and cells acquire sensitivity to gemcitabine and pemetrexed. miR-16 is also a regulator of programmed death ligand 1 (*PD-L1*) in MPM and may therefore contribute to immune system evasion [120].

In MPM, miR-34b/c and miR-126 are regulated by methylation and oxidative stress [121, 122]. Several studies showed that miR-34b/c is a regulator of C-*MET* and *BCL*-2 oncogenes, and its downregulation promotes transformation of mesothelial cells [122–124]. *In vivo* studies showed that during oxidative stress, miR-126 compromises mitochondrial function, induces autophagy by altering cell metabolism, and inhibits cell growth and tumor formation, showing that increased autophagy has a protective role in MPM [121, 125].

The identification of miRNA target genes is of paramount importance for understanding how these small noncoding RNAs regulate MPM cell function. A recent approach [126] identified miR-21-5p as a candidate regulator of *MSLN* (mesothelin). The increased expression of miR-21-5p reduced MSLN expression and inhibited MPM cell proliferation, uncovering a potential tumor suppressing miRNA in MPM.

A single miRNA can regulate many genes, and one gene may be targeted by many miRNAs. *MCL-1* is overexpressed in MPM and is associated with the resistance to apoptosis and chemotherapy [127]. Khodayari et al. reported that the transfection of MPM cells with miR-302b reduced MCL-1 expression, decreasing cell and tumor growth and inducing apoptosis [128]. The same antitumor activity has been observed for miR-193a-3p, suggesting that miRNA replacement therapy to target *MCL-1* may provide an effective treatment for MPM [129].

4.6 Epigenetic as a Potential Diagnostic Biomarker

Epigenetic markers are considered potential biomarkers for early diagnosis and prognosis in cancer research [130].

DNA methylation is rather stable but may change across time [131], and it can be modified by several factors during lifetime [132], such as lifestyle, environmental exposures, aging, and diseases [133, 134]. The DNA methylation asset of each individual is thus considered as an adaptive phenomenon potentially linking environmental factors and development of disease phenotypes [135]. Aberrant DNA methylation is found as an early event in tumor development and has been suggested as a tool for early cancer detection and prognosis [136, 137], including MPM [138].

Whereas tumor tissue DNA methylation is widely investigated in MPM, only few studies addressed the relationship between DNA methylation in blood-derived specimens and MPM.

With a targeted study focused on free serum DNA of mesothelioma patients, Fischer et al. [139] investigated the methylation status of the promoter region of nine candidate genes that were previously shown to be epigenetically altered in MPM tissue and cell lines. The authors reported hypermethylation in the promoter region of *FHIT* and the gene encoding for E-cadherin and to a lower extent *ACP1A*, *RASSF1A*, and *DARK* genes. Intermediate values were observed for *CDKN2A*, *APC1*, *ARF*, and *RARβ* [139]. The same study reported a correlation of the methylation levels of *DAPK*, *RASSF1A*, and *RARβ* genes with overall survival, though the effect was only seen in combination.

A recent study [140] investigated for the first time the whole genome DNA methylation levels in peripheral blood cells to assess the potentiality of DNA methylation profiles in blood to discriminate MPM cases from asbestos-exposed controls without MPM. The authors report significant case/control differential DNA methylation (>800 CpG sites) with consistent hypomethylation in MPM cases with respect to controls. Moreover, a small panel of seven differentially methylated CpGs was able to significantly increase discrimination between cases and controls (AUC = 0.81 vs AUC = 0.89) when considering DNA methylation together with asbestos exposure vs asbestos exposure alone.

miRNAs have been also suggested as promising candidates for the development of noninvasive techniques for early cancer detection and as therapeutic targets [141, 142]. Specific miRNA profiles have been suggested as diagnostic/prognostic biomarkers also for MPM [143–146]. Aberrant miRNA profiles have been already described in MPM tissue and biological fluids [145, 146]. Weber at al. [147], in a pilot study, identified miR-103a-3p in peripheral blood cells as a potential marker for the discrimination of mesothelioma patients from both asbestos-exposed controls and general population. The use of miR-103a-3p improved the discrimination power of serum mesothelin, reaching a sensitivity of 95% and a specificity of 81% when the two biomarkers were combined [147].

More recently, Cavalleri et al. further validated the suitability of miR-103a-3p as a MPM biomarker. A miR-103a-3p/miR-30e-3p signature of plasma-derived extracellular vesicles distinguished MPM patients from subjects reporting a past asbestos exposure with a sensitivity of 95.5% and a specificity of 80.0% [148]. While miR-103a-3p is a potential biomarker, several other studies that investigated miRNA deregulation in plasma/serum yielded heterogeneous and inconclusive results.

miR-200 family members have been suggested as potential candidates for discriminating MPM from lung cancer [144, 145, 149, 150]. Gee et al. reported downregulated miRNAs as potential biomarkers to distinguish MPM and lung adenocarcinoma [149]. Also Benjamin et al. identified a panel of three deregulated miRNAs (miR-193-3p, miR-200c, miR-192) reaching a sensitivity of 100% and a specificity of 94% to discriminate MPM from carcinoma of epithelial origin that may invade the pleura [145, 150]. High diagnostic accuracy was also reached by using a panel of four miRNAs (miR-126, miR-143, miR-145, and miR-652) that were significantly downregulated in MPM compared with nonneoplastic pleura [151]. Santarelli et al. quantified the levels of 88 miRNAs reported to be associated with cancer in 10 samples of MPM and 1 sample of healthy mesothelial tissue using a customized PCR Array [146]. The study identified three miRNAs (miR-335, miR-126, and miR-32), but only miR-126 replicated in 27 FFPE MPM samples and 27 adjacent healthy pleural tissues. Limits of these studies were the small number of miRNA investigated and the different methods used to preserve samples (RNA later in discovery and FFPE in replication phase).

The downregulation of miR-126 is also a significant prognostic factor associated with poor survival [152]. Andersen et al. showed an epigenetic downregulation of miR-126 and its host gene *EGFL7*. Silencing of *EGFL7* is associated with a poor clinical outcome in epithelioid subtype [152]. Understanding DNA hypermethylation of *EGFL7* and miR-126 may provide potential avenue for therapeutic intervention.

The first study suggesting that miRNA can be used to predict survival outcomes identified miR-29c-5p as an independent prognostic factor for time to disease progression [119]. Pass et al. identified a signature as a potential tool for predicting survival, based on the expression of let-7c-5p and miR-151a-5p in 52 MPM tumors [153].

4.7 Conclusions and Future Developments

The identification of driver mutations in MPM is a prerequisite for precision medicine, and the results are expected in the long run. The presence of germline predisposing mutations in tumor suppressor genes may be useful to identify the driver genes in cancers and address their specific therapy. miRNAs are also attractive therapeutic targets because of their powerful regulatory functions.

Additionally, different epigenetic profiles, which include miRNA and DNA methylation, in peripheral blood might be a useful tool to monitor exposed subjects.

References

1. Pfeifer GP. Environmental exposures and mutational patterns of cancer genomes. Genome Med. 2010;2:54.
2. Alexandrov LB, Nik-Zainal S, Wedge DC, Aparicio SAJR, Behjati S, Biankin AV, et al. Signatures of mutational processes in human cancer. Nature. 2013;500:415–21.
3. Ferrante D, Mirabelli D, Tunesi S, Terracini B, Magnani C. Pleural mesothelioma and occupational and non-occupational asbestos exposure: a case-control study with quantitative risk assessment. Occup Environ Med. 2016;73:147–53.
4. Hodgson JT, Darnton A. The quantitative risks of mesothelioma and lung cancer in relation to asbestos exposure. Ann Occup Hyg. 2000;44:565–601.
5. Ugolini D, Neri M, Ceppi M, Cesario A, Dianzani I, Filiberti R, et al. Genetic susceptibility to malignant mesothelioma and exposure to asbestos: the influence of the familial factor. Mutat Res. 2008;658:162–71.

6. Sud A, Kinnersley B, Houlston RS. Genome-wide association studies of cancer: current insights and future perspectives. Nat Rev Cancer. 2017;17:692–704.
7. Matullo G, Guarrera S, Betti M, Fiorito G, Ferrante D, Voglino F, et al. Genetic variants associated with increased risk of malignant pleural mesothelioma: a genome-wide association study. PLoS One. 2013;8:e61253.
8. Cadby G, Mukherjee S, Musk AWB, Reid A, Garlepp M, Dick I, et al. A genome-wide association study for malignant mesothelioma risk. Lung Cancer. 2013;82:1–8.
9. Nasu M, Emi M, Pastorino S, Tanji M, Powers A, Luk H, et al. High incidence of somatic BAP1 alterations in sporadic malignant mesothelioma. J Thorac Oncol. 2015;10:565–76.
10. Pilarski R, Rai K, Cebulla C, Abdel-Rahman M. BAP1 tumor predisposition syndrome. Seattle: University of Washington; 2016.
11. Carbone M, Ferris LK, Baumann F, Napolitano A, Lum CA, Flores EG, et al. BAP1 cancer syndrome: malignant mesothelioma, uveal and cutaneous melanoma, and MBAITs. J Transl Med. 2012;10:179.
12. Njauw C-NJ, Kim I, Piris A, Gabree M, Taylor M, Lane AM, et al. Germline BAP1 inactivation is preferentially associated with metastatic ocular melanoma and cutaneous-ocular melanoma families. PLoS One. 2012;7:e35295.
13. Baumann F, Flores E, Napolitano A, Kanodia S, Taioli E, Pass H, et al. Mesothelioma patients with germline BAP1 mutations have 7-fold improved long-term survival. Carcinogenesis. 2015;36:76–81.
14. Testa JR, Cheung M, Pei J, Below JE, Tan Y, Sementino E, et al. Germline BAP1 mutations predispose to malignant mesothelioma. Nat Genet. 2011;43:1022–5.
15. Haugh AM, Njauw C-N, Bubley JA, Verzì AE, Zhang B, Kudalkar E, et al. Genotypic and phenotypic features of BAP1 Cancer syndrome: a report of 8 new families and review of cases in the literature. JAMA Dermatol. 2017;153:999–1006.
16. Rai K, Pilarski R, Boru G, Rehman M, Saqr AH, Massengill JB, et al. Germline BAP1 alterations in familial uveal melanoma. Genes Chromosomes Cancer. 2017;56:168–74.
17. O'Shea SJ, Robles-Espinoza CD, McLellan L, Harrigan J, Jacq X, Hewinson J, et al. A population-based analysis of germline BAP1 mutations in melanoma. Hum Mol Genet. 2017;26:717–28.
18. Abdel-Rahman MH, Pilarski R, Cebulla CM, Massengill JB, Christopher BN, Boru G, et al. Germline BAP1 mutation predisposes to uveal melanoma, lung adenocarcinoma, meningioma, and other cancers. J Med Genet. 2011;48:856–9.
19. Wadt K, Choi J, Chung J-Y, Kiilgaard J, Heegaard S, Drzewiecki KT, et al. A cryptic BAP1 splice mutation in a family with uveal and cutaneous melanoma, and paraganglioma. Pigment Cell Melanoma Res. 2012;25:815–8.
20. Wiesner T, Fried I, Ulz P, Stacher E, Popper H, Murali R, et al. Toward an improved definition of the tumor spectrum associated with BAP1 germline mutations. J Clin Oncol. 2012;30:e337–40.
21. Popova T, Hebert L, Jacquemin V, Gad S, Caux-Moncoutier V, Dubois-d'Enghien C, et al. Germline BAP1 mutations predispose to renal cell carcinomas. Am J Hum Genet. 2013;92:974–80.
22. Pilarski R, Cebulla CM, Massengill JB, Rai K, Rich T, Strong L, et al. Expanding the clinical phenotype of hereditary BAP1 cancer predisposition syndrome, reporting three new cases. Genes Chromosomes Cancer. 2014;53:177–82.
23. Betti M, Casalone E, Ferrante D, Romanelli A, Grosso F, Guarrera S, et al. Inference on germline BAP1 mutations and asbestos exposure from the analysis of familial and sporadic mesothelioma in a high-risk area. Genes Chromosomes Cancer. 2015;54:51–62.
24. Rai K, Pilarski R, Cebulla CM, Abdel-Rahman MH. Comprehensive review of BAP1 tumor predisposition syndrome with report of two new cases. Clin Genet. 2016;89:285–94.
25. Cheung M, Kadariya Y, Talarchek J, Pei J, Ohar JA, Kayaleh OR, et al. Germline BAP1 mutation in a family with high incidence of multiple primary cancers and a potential gene-environment interaction. Cancer Lett. 2015;369:261–5.
26. Ohar JA, Cheung M, Talarchek J, Howard SE, Howard TD, Hesdorffer M, et al. Germline BAP1 mutational landscape of Asbestos-exposed malignant mesothelioma patients with family history of Cancer. Cancer Res. 2016;76:206–15.
27. Abdel-Rahman MH, Rai K, Pilarski R, Davidorf FH, Cebulla CM. Germline BAP1 mutations misreported as somatic based on tumor-only testing. Familial Cancer. 2016;15:327–30.
28. Ribeiro C, Campelos S, Moura CS, Machado JC, Justino A, Parente B. Well-differentiated papillary mesothelioma: clustering in a Portuguese family with a germline BAP1 mutation. Ann Oncol. 2013;24:2147–50.
29. Cheung M, Talarchek J, Schindeler K, Saraiva E, Penney LS, Ludman M, et al. Further evidence for germline BAP1 mutations predisposing to melanoma and malignant mesothelioma. Cancer Genet. 2013;206:206–10.
30. Turunen JA, Markkinen S, Wilska R, Saarinen S, Raivio V, Täll M, et al. BAP1 germline mutations in finnish patients with uveal melanoma. Ophthalmology. 2016;123:1112–7.
31. Betti M, Aspesi A, Ferrante D, Sculco M, Righi L, Mirabelli D, et al. Sensitivity to asbestos is increased in patients with mesothelioma and pathogenic germline variants in BAP1 or other DNA repair genes. Genes Chromosomes Cancer. 2018;57(11):573–83.
32. Betti M, Aspesi A, Biasi A, Casalone E, Ferrante D, Ogliara P, et al. CDKN2A and BAP1 germline mutations predispose to melanoma and mesothelioma. Cancer Lett. 2016;378:120–30.

33. Harbour JW, Onken MD, Roberson EDO, Duan S, Cao L, Worley LA, et al. Frequent mutation of BAP1 in metastasizing uveal melanomas. Science. 2010;330:1410–3.
34. Höiom V, Edsgärd D, Helgadottir H, Eriksson H, All-Ericsson C, Tuominen R, et al. Hereditary uveal melanoma: a report of a germline mutation in BAP1. Genes Chromosomes Cancer. 2013;52:378–84.
35. Busam KJ, Wanna M, Wiesner T. Multiple epithelioid spitz nevi or tumors with loss of BAP1 expression. JAMA Dermatol. 2013;149:335.
36. Gupta MP, Lane AM, DeAngelis MM, Mayne K, Crabtree M, Gragoudas ES, et al. Clinical characteristics of uveal melanoma in patients with germline BAP1 mutations. JAMA Ophthalmol. 2015;133:881–7.
37. Gerami P, Yélamos O, Lee CY, Obregon R, Yazdan P, Sholl LM, et al. Multiple cutaneous melanomas and clinically atypical moles in a patient with a novel germline BAP1 mutation. JAMA Dermatol. 2015;151:1235–9.
38. de la Fouchardière A, Cabaret O, Savin L, Combemale P, Schvartz H, Penet C, et al. Germline BAP1 mutations predispose also to multiple basal cell carcinomas. Clin Genet. 2015;88:273–7.
39. Rusch A, Ziltener G, Nackaerts K, Weder W, Stahel RA, Felley-Bosco E. Prevalence of BRCA-1 associated protein 1 germline mutation in sporadic malignant pleural mesothelioma cases. Lung Cancer. 2015;87:77–9.
40. Sneddon S, Leon JS, Dick IM, Cadby G, Olsen N, Brims F, et al. Absence of germline mutations in BAP1 in sporadic cases of malignant mesothelioma. Gene. 2015;563:103–5.
41. Wadt KAW, Aoude LG, Johansson P, Solinas A, Pritchard A, Crainic O, et al. A recurrent germline BAP1 mutation and extension of the BAP1 tumor predisposition spectrum to include basal cell carcinoma. Clin Genet. 2015;88:267–72.
42. Aoude LG, Wadt K, Bojesen A, Crüger D, Borg A, Trent JM, et al. A BAP1 mutation in a Danish family predisposes to uveal melanoma and other cancers. PLoS One. 2013;8:e72144.
43. McDonnell KJ, Gallanis GT, Heller KA, Melas M, Idos GE, Culver JO, et al. A novel BAP1 mutation is associated with melanocytic neoplasms and thyroid cancer. Cancer Genet. 2016;209:75–81.
44. White AE, Harper JW. Cancer. Emerging anatomy of the BAP1 tumor suppressor system. Science. 2012;337:1463–4.
45. Daou S, Hammond-Martel I, Mashtalir N, Barbour H, Gagnon J, Iannantuono NVG, et al. The BAP1/ASXL2 histone H2A deubiquitinase complex regulates cell proliferation and is disrupted in cancer. J Biol Chem. 2015;290:28643–63.
46. Yu H, Pak H, Hammond-Martel I, Ghram M, Rodrigue A, Daou S, et al. Tumor suppressor and deubiquitinase BAP1 promotes DNA double-strand break repair. Proc Natl Acad Sci U S A. 2014;111:285–90.
47. Ji Z, Mohammed H, Webber A, Ridsdale J, Han N, Carroll JS, et al. The forkhead transcription factor FOXK2 acts as a chromatin targeting factor for the BAP1-containing histone deubiquitinase complex. Nucleic Acids Res. 2014;42:6232–42.
48. Bononi A, Yang H, Giorgi C, Patergnani S, Pellegrini L, Su M, et al. Germline BAP1 mutations induce a Warburg effect. Cell Death Differ. 2017;24:1694–704.
49. Ismail IH, Davidson R, Gagné J-P, Xu ZZ, Poirier GG, Hendzel MJ. Germline mutations in BAP1 impair its function in DNA double-strand break repair. Cancer Res. 2014;74:4282–94.
50. Napolitano A, Pellegrini L, Dey A, Larson D, Tanji M, Flores EG, et al. Minimal asbestos exposure in germline BAP1 heterozygous mice is associated with deregulated inflammatory response and increased risk of mesothelioma. Oncogene. 2016;35:1996–2002.
51. Xu J, Kadariya Y, Cheung M, Pei J, Talarchek J, Sementino E, et al. Germline mutation of Bap1 accelerates development of asbestos-induced malignant mesothelioma. Cancer Res. 2014;74:4388–97.
52. Betti M, Aspesi A, Sculco M, Matullo G, Magnani C, Dianzani I. Genetic predisposition for malignant mesothelioma: a concise review. Mutat Res. 2019;781:1–10.
53. Betti M, Casalone E, Ferrante D, Aspesi A, Morleo G, Biasi A, et al. Germline mutations in DNA repair genes predispose asbestos-exposed patients to malignant pleural mesothelioma. Cancer Lett. 2017;405:38–45.
54. Aoude LG, Wadt KAW, Pritchard AL, Hayward NK. Genetics of familial melanoma: 20 years after *CDKN2A*. Pigment Cell Melanoma Res. 2015;28:148–60.
55. Guo G, Chmielecki J, Goparaju C, Heguy A, Dolgalev I, Carbone M, et al. Whole-exome sequencing reveals frequent genetic alterations in BAP1, NF2, CDKN2A, and CUL1 in malignant pleural mesothelioma. Cancer Res. 2015;75:264–9.
56. De Rienzo A, Archer MA, Yeap BY, Dao N, Sciaranghella D, Sideris AC, et al. Gender-specific molecular and clinical features underlie malignant pleural mesothelioma. Cancer Res. 2016;76:319–28.
57. Vanni I, Coco S, Bonfiglio S, Cittaro D, Genova C, Biello F, et al. Whole exome sequencing of independent lung adenocarcinoma, lung squamous cell carcinoma, and malignant peritoneal mesothelioma. Medicine (Baltimore). 2016;95:e5447.
58. Sheffield BS, Tinker AV, Shen Y, Hwang H, Li-Chang HH, Pleasance E, et al. Personalized oncogenomics: clinical experience with malignant peritoneal mesothelioma using whole genome sequencing. PLoS One. 2015;10:e0119689.
59. Alakus H, Yost SE, Woo B, French R, Lin GY, Jepsen K, et al. BAP1 mutation is a frequent somatic event in peritoneal malignant mesothelioma. J Transl Med. 2015;13:122.
60. Carbone M, Gaudino G, Yang H. Recent insights emerging from malignant mesothelioma genome sequencing. J Thorac Oncol. 2015;10:409–11.
61. Petrucelli N, Daly MB, Pal T. BRCA1- and BRCA2-associated hereditary breast and ovarian cancer. Seattle: University of Washington; 2016.
62. Kraemer KH, DiGiovanna JJ. Xeroderma pigmentosum. Seattle: University of Washington; 2016.

63. Peltomäki P. Lynch syndrome genes. Familial Cancer. 2005;4:227–32.
64. Wang Y, Zhou X, Song Y, Ji X, Zhang A, Zhang G, et al. The mismatch repair gene hPMS1 (human postmeiotic segregation 1) is down regulated in oral squamous cell carcinoma. Gene. 2013;524:28–34.
65. Mehta PA, Tolar J. Fanconi Anemia. Seattle: University of Washington; 2018.
66. Ceelen WP, Van Dalen T, Van Bockstal M, Libbrecht L, Sijmons RH. Malignant peritoneal mesothelioma in a patient with Li-Fraumeni syndrome. J Clin Oncol. 2011;29:e503–5.
67. Baser ME, Rai H, Wallace AJ, Evans DGR. Neurofibromatosis 2 (NF2) and malignant mesothelioma in a man with a constitutional NF2 missense mutation. Familial Cancer. 2005;4:321–2.
68. Lo Iacono M, Monica V, Righi L, Grosso F, Libener R, Vatrano S, et al. Targeted next-generation sequencing of cancer genes in advanced stage malignant pleural mesothelioma: a retrospective study. J Thorac Oncol. 2015;10:492–9.
69. Bueno R, Stawiski EW, Goldstein LD, Durinck S, De Rienzo A, Modrusan Z, et al. Comprehensive genomic analysis of malignant pleural mesothelioma identifies recurrent mutations, gene fusions and splicing alterations. Nat Genet. 2016;48:407–16.
70. Panou V, Gadiraju M, Wolin A, Weipert CM, Skarda E, Husain AN, et al. Frequency of germline mutations in cancer susceptibility genes in malignant mesothelioma. J Clin Oncol. 2018;36:2863–71.
71. Robinson DR, Wu Y-M, Lonigro RJ, Vats P, Cobain E, Everett J, et al. Integrative clinical genomics of metastatic cancer. Nature. 2017;548:297–303.
72. Martincorena I, Raine KM, Gerstung M, Dawson KJ, Haase K, Van Loo P, et al. Universal Patterns of Selection in Cancer and Somatic Tissues. Cell. 2017;171:1029–1041.e21.
73. Lee WC, Testa JR. Somatic genetic alterations in human malignant mesothelioma (review). Int J Oncol. 1999;14:181–8.
74. Bott M, Brevet M, Taylor BS, Shimizu S, Ito T, Wang L, et al. The nuclear deubiquitinase BAP1 is commonly inactivated by somatic mutations and 3p21.1 losses in malignant pleural mesothelioma. Nat Genet. 2011;43:668–72.
75. Borczuk AC, Pei J, Taub RN, Levy B, Nahum O, Chen J, et al. Genome-wide analysis of abdominal and pleural malignant mesothelioma with DNA arrays reveals both common and distinct regions of copy number alteration. Cancer Biol Ther. 2016;17:328–35.
76. Sneddon S, Dick I, Lee YCG, Musk AWB, Patch A-M, Pearson JV, et al. Malignant cells from pleural fluids in malignant mesothelioma patients reveal novel mutations. Lung Cancer. 2018;119:64–70.
77. Hylebos M, Van Camp G, Vandeweyer G, Fransen E, Beyens M, Cornelissen R, et al. Large-scale copy number analysis reveals variations in genes not previously associated with malignant pleural mesothelioma. Oncotarget. 2017;8:113673–86.
78. Ugurluer G, Chang K, Gamez ME, Arnett AL, Jayakrishnan R, Miller RC, et al. Genome-based mutational analysis by next generation sequencing in patients with malignant pleural and peritoneal mesothelioma. Anticancer Res. 2016;36:2331–8.
79. Kim JE, Kim D, Hong YS, Kim K-P, Yoon YK, Lee DH, et al. Mutational profiling of malignant mesothelioma revealed potential therapeutic targets in EGFR and NRAS. Transl Oncol. 2018;11:268–74.
80. Bueno R, De Rienzo A, Dong L, Gordon GJ, Hercus CF, Richards WG, et al. Second generation sequencing of the mesothelioma tumor genome. PLoS One. 2010;5:e10612.
81. Tallet A, Nault J-C, Renier A, Hysi I, Galateau-Sallé F, Cazes A, et al. Overexpression and promoter mutation of the TERT gene in malignant pleural mesothelioma. Oncogene. 2014;33:3748–52.
82. Yoshikawa Y, Sato A, Tsujimura T, Emi M, Morinaga T, Fukuoka K, et al. Frequent inactivation of the BAP1 gene in epithelioid-type malignant mesothelioma. Cancer Sci. 2012;103:868–74.
83. Zauderer MG, Bott M, McMillan R, Sima CS, Rusch V, Krug LM, et al. Clinical characteristics of patients with malignant pleural mesothelioma harboring somatic BAP1 mutations. J Thorac Oncol. 2013;8:1430–3.
84. Tranchant R, Quetel L, Tallet A, Meiller C, Renier A, de Koning L, et al. Co-occurring mutations of tumor suppressor genes, LATS2 and NF2, in malignant pleural mesothelioma. Clin Cancer Res. 2017;23:3191–202.
85. Kiyotani K, Park J-H, Inoue H, Husain A, Olugbile S, Zewde M, et al. Integrated analysis of somatic mutations and immune microenvironment in malignant pleural mesothelioma. Oncoimmunology. 2017;6:e1278330.
86. Comertpay S, Pastorino S, Tanji M, Mezzapelle R, Strianese O, Napolitano A, et al. Evaluation of clonal origin of malignant mesothelioma. J Transl Med. 2014;12:301.
87. Zhang S, Zhang Q, Sun Q, Tang J, Chen J, Ji N, et al. Genome evolution analysis of recurrent testicular malignant mesothelioma by whole-genome sequencing. Cell Physiol Biochem. 2018;45:163–74.
88. Alexandrov LB, Nik-Zainal S, Wedge DC, Campbell PJ, Stratton MR. Deciphering signatures of mutational processes operative in human cancer. Cell Rep. 2013;3:246–59.
89. Nik-Zainal S, Alexandrov LB, Wedge DC, Van Loo P, Greenman CD, Raine K, et al. Mutational processes molding the genomes of 21 breast cancers. Cell. 2012;149:979–93.
90. Yap TA, Aerts JG, Popat S, Fennell DA. Novel insights into mesothelioma biology and implications for therapy. Nat Rev Cancer. 2017;17:475–88.
91. McCambridge AJ, Napolitano A, Mansfield AS, Fennell DA, Sekido Y, Nowak AK, et al. Progress in the management of malignant pleural mesothelioma in 2017. J Thorac Oncol. 2018;13:606–23.

92. Fong PC, Boss DS, Yap TA, Tutt A, Wu P, Mergui-Roelvink M, et al. Inhibition of poly(ADP-ribose) polymerase in tumors from BRCA mutation carriers. N Engl J Med. 2009;361:123–34.
93. Swisher EM, Lin KK, Oza AM, Scott CL, Giordano H, Sun J, et al. Rucaparib in relapsed, platinum-sensitive high-grade ovarian carcinoma (ARIEL2 part 1): an international, multicentre, open-label, phase 2 trial. Lancet Oncol. 2017;18:75–87.
94. Lord CJ, Ashworth A. PARP inhibitors: synthetic lethality in the clinic. Science. 2017;355:1152–8.
95. Brown JS, O'Carrigan B, Jackson SP, Yap TA. Targeting DNA repair in cancer: beyond PARP inhibitors. Cancer Discov. 2017;7:20–37.
96. Ohmoto A, Yachida S. Current status of poly(ADP-ribose) polymerase inhibitors and future directions. Onco Targets Ther. 2017;10:5195–208.
97. Jin B, Li Y, Robertson KD. DNA methylation: superior or subordinate in the epigenetic hierarchy? Genes Cancer. 2011;2:607–17.
98. Lister R, Pelizzola M, Dowen RH, Hawkins RD, Hon G, Tonti-Filippini J, et al. Human DNA methylomes at base resolution show widespread epigenomic differences. Nature. 2009;462:315–22.
99. Deaton AM, Bird A. CpG islands and the regulation of transcription. Genes Dev. 2011;25:1010–22.
100. Esteller M. Aberrant DNA methylation as a cancer-inducing mechanism. Annu Rev Pharmacol Toxicol. 2005;45:629–56.
101. Portela A, Esteller M. Epigenetic modifications and human disease. Nat Biotechnol. 2010;28:1057–68.
102. Macfarlane L-A, Murphy PR. MicroRNA: biogenesis, function and role in cancer. Curr Genomics. 2010;11:537–61.
103. Romero-Cordoba SL, Salido-Guadarrama I, Rodriguez-Dorantes M. Hidalgo-Miranda A: miRNA biogenesis: biological impact in the development of cancer. Cancer Biol Ther. 2014;15:1444–55.
104. Hata A, Kashima R. Dysregulation of microRNA biogenesis machinery in cancer. Crit Rev Biochem Mol Biol. 2016;51:121–34.
105. Melo SA, Esteller M. Disruption of microRNA nuclear transport in human cancer. Semin Cancer Biol. 2014;27:46–51.
106. Steer CJ, Subramanian S. Circulating microRNAs as biomarkers: a new frontier in diagnostics. Liver Transpl. 2012;18:265–9.
107. Allegra A, Alonci A, Campo S, Penna G, Petrungaro A, Gerace D, et al. Circulating microRNAs: new biomarkers in diagnosis, prognosis and treatment of cancer (review). Int J Oncol. 2012;41:1897–912.
108. Wu W, Sun M, Zou G-M, Chen J. MicroRNA and cancer: current status and prospective. Int J Cancer. 2007;120:953–60.
109. Tutar L, Tutar E, Özgür A, Tutar Y. Therapeutic targeting of microRNAs in cancer: future perspectives. Drug Dev Res. 2015;76:382–8.
110. Casalone E, Allione A, Viberti C, Pardini B, Guarrera S, Betti M, et al. DNA methylation profiling of asbestos-treated MeT5A cell line reveals novel pathways implicated in asbestos response. Arch Toxicol. 2018;92(5):1785–95.
111. Christensen BC, Godleski JJ, Marsit CJ, Houseman EA, Lopez-Fagundo CY, Longacker JL, et al. Asbestos exposure predicts cell cycle control gene promoter methylation in pleural mesothelioma. Carcinogenesis. 2008;29:1555–9.
112. Kobayashi N, Toyooka S, Yanai H, Soh J, Fujimoto N, Yamamoto H, et al. Frequent p16 inactivation by homozygous deletion or methylation is associated with a poor prognosis in Japanese patients with pleural mesothelioma. Lung Cancer. 2008;62:120–5.
113. Goto Y, Shinjo K, Kondo Y, Shen L, Toyota M, Suzuki H, et al. Epigenetic profiles distinguish malignant pleural mesothelioma from lung adenocarcinoma. Cancer Res. 2009;69:9073–82.
114. Christensen BC, Houseman EA, Godleski JJ, Marsit CJ, Longacker JL, Roelofs CR, et al. Epigenetic profiles distinguish pleural mesothelioma from normal pleura and predict lung asbestos burden and clinical outcome. Cancer Res. 2009;69:227–34.
115. Kohno H, Amatya VJ, Takeshima Y, Kushitani K, Hattori N, Kohno N, et al. Aberrant promoter methylation of WIF-1 and SFRP1, 2, 4 genes in mesothelioma. Oncol Rep. 2010;24:423–31.
116. Tsou JA, Galler JS, Wali A, Ye W, Siegmund KD, Groshen S, et al. DNA methylation profile of 28 potential marker loci in malignant mesothelioma. Lung Cancer. 2007;58:220–30.
117. Cheng YY, Kirschner MB, Cheng NC, Gattani S, Klebe S, Edelman JJB, et al. ZIC1 is silenced and has tumor suppressor function in malignant pleural mesothelioma. J Thorac Oncol. 2013;8:1317–28.
118. Guled M, Lahti L, Lindholm PM, Salmenkivi K, Bagwan I, Nicholson AG, et al. CDKN2A, NF2, and JUN are dysregulated among other genes by miRNAs in malignant mesothelioma -A miRNA microarray analysis. Genes Chromosomes Cancer. 2009;48:615–23.
119. Pass HI, Goparaju C, Ivanov S, Donington J, Carbone M, Hoshen M, et al. hsa-miR-29c* is linked to the prognosis of malignant pleural mesothelioma. Cancer Res. 2010;70:1916–24.
120. Reid G, Pel ME, Kirschner MB, Cheng YY, Mugridge N, Weiss J, et al. Restoring expression of miR-16: a novel approach to therapy for malignant pleural mesothelioma. Ann Oncol. 2013;24:3128–35.
121. Tomasetti M, Nocchi L, Staffolani S, Manzella N, Amati M, Goodwin J, et al. MicroRNA-126 suppresses mesothelioma malignancy by targeting IRS1 and interfering with the mitochondrial function. Antioxid Redox Signal. 2014;21:2109–25.
122. Kubo T, Toyooka S, Tsukuda K, Sakaguchi M, Fukazawa T, Soh J, et al. Epigenetic silencing of microRNA-34b/c plays an important role in the pathogenesis of malignant pleural mesothelioma. Clin Cancer Res. 2011;17:4965–74.
123. Tanaka N, Toyooka S, Soh J, Tsukuda K, Shien K, Furukawa M, et al. Downregulation of microRNA-34 induces cell proliferation and invasion of human mesothelial cells. Oncol Rep. 2013;29:2169–74.

124. Maki Y, Asano H, Toyooka S, Soh J, Kubo T, Katsui K, et al. MicroRNA miR-34b/c enhances cellular radiosensitivity of malignant pleural mesothelioma cells. Anticancer Res. 2012;32:4871–5.
125. Tomasetti M, Monaco F, Manzella N, Rohlena J, Rohlenova K, Staffolani S, et al. MicroRNA-126 induces autophagy by altering cell metabolism in malignant mesothelioma. Oncotarget. 2016;7:36338–52.
126. Vencken S, Hassan T, McElvaney NG, Smith SGJ. Greene CM: miR-CATCH: microRNA capture affinity technology. Methods Mol Biol. 2015;1218:365–73.
127. Soini Y, Kinnula V, Kaarteenaho-Wiik R, Kurttila E, Linnainmaa K, Pääkkö P. Apoptosis and expression of apoptosis regulating proteins bcl-2, mcl-1, bcl-X, and bax in malignant mesothelioma. Clin Cancer Res. 1999;5:3508–15.
128. Khodayari N, Mohammed KA, Lee H, Kaye F, Nasreen N. MicroRNA-302b targets Mcl-1 and inhibits cell proliferation and induces apoptosis in malignant pleural mesothelioma cells. Am J Cancer Res. 2016;6:1996–2009.
129. Williams M, Kirschner MB, Cheng YY, Hanh J, Weiss J, Mugridge N, et al. miR-193a-3p is a potential tumor suppressor in malignant pleural mesothelioma. Oncotarget. 2015;6:23480–95.
130. Yang X, Dai W, Kwong DL, Szeto CYY, Wong EH, Ng WT, et al. Epigenetic markers for noninvasive early detection of nasopharyngeal carcinoma by methylation-sensitive high resolution melting. Int J Cancer. 2015;136:E127–35.
131. Bjornsson HT, Sigurdsson MI, Fallin MD, Irizarry RA, Aspelund T, Cui H, et al. Intra-individual change over time in DNA methylation with familial clustering. JAMA. 2008;299:2877–83.
132. Christensen BC, Houseman EA, Marsit CJ, Zheng S, Wrensch MR, Wiemels JL, et al. Aging and environmental exposures alter tissue-specific DNA methylation dependent upon CpG island context. PLoS Genet. 2009;5:e1000602.
133. Kanherkar RR, Bhatia-Dey N, Csoka AB. Epigenetics across the human lifespan. Front Cell Dev Biol. 2014;2:49.
134. Bell CG, Beck S. The epigenomic interface between genome and environment in common complex diseases. Brief Funct Genomics. 2010;9:477–85.
135. Marsit CJ. Influence of environmental exposure on human epigenetic regulation. J Exp Biol. 2015;218:71–9.
136. Shivapurkar N, Gazdar AF. DNA methylation based biomarkers in non-invasive cancer screening. Curr Mol Med. 2010;10:123–32.
137. Dong Y, Zhao H, Li H, Li X, Yang S. DNA methylation as an early diagnostic marker of cancer (review). Biomed Rep. 2014;2:326–30.
138. Vandermeers F, Neelature Sriramareddy S, Costa C, Hubaux R, Cosse J-P, Willems L. The role of epigenetics in malignant pleural mesothelioma. Lung Cancer. 2013;81:311–8.
139. Fischer JR, Ohnmacht U, Rieger N, Zemaitis M, Stoffregen C, Kostrzewa M, et al. Promoter methylation of RASSF1A, RARbeta and DAPK predict poor prognosis of patients with malignant mesothelioma. Lung Cancer. 2006;54:109–16.
140. Guarrera S, Viberti C, Cugliari G, Allione A, Casalone E, Betti M, et al. Peripheral blood DNA methylation as potential biomarker of malignant pleural mesothelioma in asbestos-exposed subjects. J Thorac Oncol. 2019;14:527–39.
141. Bolha L, Ravnik-Glavač M, Glavač D. Circular RNAs: biogenesis, function, and a role as possible cancer biomarkers. Int J Genomics. 2017;2017:6218353.
142. Di Leva G, Garofalo M, Croce CM. MicroRNAs in cancer. Annu Rev Pathol. 2014;9:287–314.
143. Ramírez-Salazar EG, Salinas-Silva LC, Vázquez-Manríquez ME, Gayosso-Gómez LV, Negrete-Garcia MC, Ramírez-Rodriguez SL, et al. Analysis of microRNA expression signatures in malignant pleural mesothelioma, pleural inflammation, and atypical mesothelial hyperplasia reveals common predictive tumorigenesis-related targets. Exp Mol Pathol. 2014;97:375–85.
144. Birnie KA, Prêle CM, Thompson PJ, Badrian B, Mutsaers SE. Targeting microRNA to improve diagnostic and therapeutic approaches for malignant mesothelioma. Oncotarget. 2017;8:78193–207.
145. Kirschner MB, Cheng YY, Badrian B, Kao SC, Creaney J, Edelman JJB, et al. Increased circulating miR-625-3p: a potential biomarker for patients with malignant pleural mesothelioma. J Thorac Oncol. 2012;7:1184–91.
146. Santarelli L, Strafella E, Staffolani S, Amati M, Emanuelli M, Sartini D, et al. Association of MiR-126 with soluble mesothelin-related peptides, a marker for malignant mesothelioma. PLoS One. 2011;6:e18232.
147. Weber DG, Casjens S, Johnen G, Bryk O, Raiko I, Pesch B, et al. Combination of MiR-103a-3p and mesothelin improves the biomarker performance of malignant mesothelioma diagnosis. PLoS One. 2014;9:e114483.
148. Cavalleri T, Angelici L, Favero C, Dioni L, Mensi C, Bareggi C, et al. Plasmatic extracellular vesicle microRNAs in malignant pleural mesothelioma and asbestos-exposed subjects suggest a 2-miRNA signature as potential biomarker of disease. PLoS One. 2017;12:e0176680.
149. Gee GV, Koestler DC, Christensen BC, Sugarbaker DJ, Ugolini D, Ivaldi GP, et al. Downregulated microRNAs in the differential diagnosis of malignant pleural mesothelioma. Int J Cancer. 2010;127:2859–69.
150. Benjamin H, Lebanony D, Rosenwald S, Cohen L, Gibori H, Barabash N, et al. A diagnostic assay based on microRNA expression accurately identifies malignant pleural mesothelioma. J Mol Diagn. 2010;12:771–9.
151. Andersen M, Grauslund M, Ravn J, Sørensen JB, Andersen CB, Santoni-Rugiu E. Diagnostic potential of miR-126, miR-143, miR-145, and miR-652 in malignant pleural mesothelioma. J Mol Diagn. 2014;16:418–30.

152. Andersen M, Trapani D, Ravn J, Sørensen JB, Andersen CB, Grauslund M, et al. Methylation-associated silencing of microRNA-126 and its host gene EGFL7 in malignant pleural mesothelioma. Anticancer Res. 2015;35:6223–9.

153. De Santi C, Melaiu O, Bonotti A, Cascione L, Di Leva G, Foddis R, et al. Deregulation of miRNAs in malignant pleural mesothelioma is associated with prognosis and suggests an alteration of cell metabolism. Sci Rep. 2017;7:3140.

5 Microenvironment and Immunology of the Human Pleural Malignant Mesothelioma

Elisabeth Digifico, Cristina Belgiovine, Alberto Mantovani, and Paola Allavena

5.1 Introduction

A state of chronic non-resolving inflammation is the hallmark of malignant pleural mesothelioma (MPM), a very aggressive neoplastic disease whose pathogenesis has been strongly associated with occupational exposure to airborne asbestos fibers and long-term tissue damage [1, 2].

Upon inhalation of asbestos in the lungs, macrophages are locally recruited and activated for phagocytosis in an attempt to clear the fibers away but are eventually unable to eliminate them, due to their nondegradable nature. Epithelial cells in the lungs and pleura and especially local and newly recruited immune cells participate in the inflammatory process triggered by asbestos, through the production of several cytokines and reactive chemical species. This "frustrated phagocytosis" of asbestos fibers leads to a state of chronic non-resolving inflammation and to a fibrogenic response, both contributing—in the long run—to transformation of normal pleural cells into neoplastic cells [2–4].

In this context, cells of the local immunological network, especially inflammatory cells of the innate immunity, play a major role in tumor onset and development by fueling a state of chronic inflammation.

Cancer-related inflammation is an established hallmark of cancer [5]. Epidemiological, genetic, and experimental evidence demonstrated that chronic inflammation can increase cancer risk and promotes tumor progression and metastatic spread [6, 7].

A number of studies have characterized the local infiltration of inflammatory leukocytes in human malignant mesothelioma and the expression of several reactive/inflammatory mediators [2–4, 8–10].

In most studies, however, conclusive results are hampered by the difficulty to have large cohorts of samples from this relatively rare tumor, especially considering that not all the patients undergo surgical resection and provide an adequate sample for immunohistochemical investigation.

Of the different histotypes of MPM, epithelioid, sarcomatoid, and biphasic, much less information is available on the latter two, due to their lower incidence.

In this chapter we present an organized characterization of each immune cell subset that populates the tumor microenvironment and of the major mediators of the inflammatory milieu.

E. Digifico · C. Belgiovine
Humanitas University, Milan, Italy

A. Mantovani (✉)
Humanitas University, Milan, Italy

IRCCS Humanitas Clinical and Research Center, Milan, Italy
e-mail: alberto.mantovani@humanitasresearch.it

P. Allavena
IRCCS Humanitas Clinical and Research Center, Milan, Italy

G. L. Ceresoli et al. (eds.), *Mesothelioma*, https://doi.org/10.1007/978-3-030-16884-1_5

5.2 Immune Cells in the Tumor Microenvironment of Malignant Pleural Mesothelioma

The stroma of solid tumors is typically a disorganized and heterogeneous mixture of different cell types, mostly fibroblasts and immune cells, and an aberrant matrix where new vessels have grown. The composition of the tumor microenvironment (TME) is subject to individual changes among patients and specific histological subtypes but also to dynamic modifications, for instance, after exposure to antitumor therapies; moreover, it can evolve over time following complex interactions between the tumor and the host [11, 12].

All pathological studies on tissues from MPM patients report a rich immune infiltrate predominantly composed of macrophages and T lymphocytes. Other immune cells such as B lymphocytes, regulatory T cells (Tregs), dendritic cells (DCs), myeloid-derived suppressor cells (MDSCs), and natural killer (NK), neutrophils, and mast cells have also been reported (Fig. 5.1).

NK cells, cytotoxic and helper T cells, and DCs may contribute to sustain a protective antitumor immune response, while Tregs and myeloid

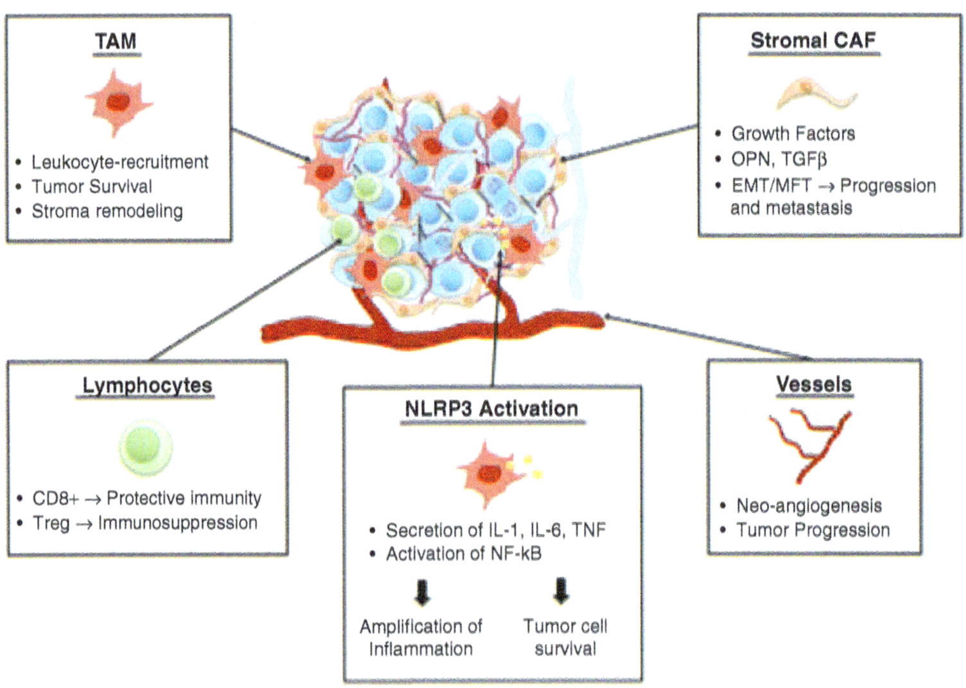

Fig. 5.1 Human malignant pleural mesothelioma MPM tissues have a complex microenvironment highly infiltrated by inflammatory cells. Mostly represented are tumor-associated macrophages (TAMs), specialized phagocytic cells of the innate immunity that engulf the nondegradable asbestos fibers in the lungs and produce several inflammatory mediators and support tumor cell survival. Among cells of the adaptive immunity are T lymphocytes, including cytotoxic effector CD8+ cells, with antitumor functions, and Tregs, which suppress antitumor responses. In MPM tumors, asbestos fibers (danger signal) trigger the activation of the inflammasome platform (e.g., NLRP3) with secretion of the inflammatory cytokine IL-1β which activates the transcription factor NF-kB and initiates the inflammatory cascade. Released cytokines and chemokines amplify the inflammatory reaction with enhanced leukocyte recruitment; production of growth factors that support neo-angiogenesis and tumor cell proliferation. Stromal cancer-associated fibroblasts (CAF) produce growth factors, matrix proteins (e.g., osteopontin, OPN) and TGFβ, which induce epithelial to mesenchymal transition (EMT) and mesothelial to fibroblastic transition (MFT)

cells (macrophages and MDSCs) are usually associated with an immunosuppressive milieu that favors tumor progression.

5.2.1 Macrophages and Myeloid Suppressor Cells

Macrophages are specialized phagocytic cells of the innate immunity; they are present in all phases of the mesothelioma pathological process. Since the early exposure to airborne asbestos, the nondegradable fibers in the lungs and along pleural lining provide a "danger signal" that triggers the release of inflammatory cytokines and chemokines which stimulate the recruitment of new phagocytic leukocytes (neutrophils and monocytes) [13, 14]. Neutrophils are relatively short-living cells and die in few days, but monocytes differentiate into long-lasting macrophages and become major producers of reactive oxygen and nitrogen species and of inflammatory cytokines. Thus, macrophages, in their attempt to clear the fibers away, are likely the most responsible for the chronic non-resolving inflammation that characterizes the pleural premalignant sites [1, 3].

Once the tumor has established, the presence of tumor-associated macrophages (TAMs), like in other solid tumors, is regulated by the production of monocyte attractants, such as the chemokine CCL2, produced by cancer and stromal cells [15–17]. Tumor cells attract monocytes to their own advantage, as macrophages differentiated under the influence of tumor-secreted products acquire an immunosuppressive phenotype and tumor-promoting functions (e.g., production of growth factors for cancer cells and neo-vessels) [15]. Indeed, it is now established that TAM density in tumors is usually associated with tumor progression and poor patient prognosis [15, 18].

The inflammatory macrophages at premalignant sites and the pro-tumoral TAMs in established mesothelioma tissues display different phenotypes and functions. This "plasticity" is a hallmark of macrophages and is regulated by the different nature of the local stimuli encountered by differentiating monocytes. In a simplified scheme, their broad spectrum of activation has two polarized extremes: the M1 (or classically activated) macrophages and the M2 (or alternatively activated). The former (M1) represents the immune-competent cells acting against bacterial infections and producing pro-inflammatory cytokines, such as IL-1β, TNFα, and IL-12, promoting protective Th1 responses. M2 macrophages, instead, suppress Th1 immunity and promote tumor proliferation and neo-angiogenesis. Thus, although it is now recognized that the full spectrum of TAM activation is more complex than previously perceived, there is a general consensus that macrophages in tumors acquire phenotype and functions typical of the M2-like polarization [15, 19]. This notion is useful for the use of specific M2 markers in MPM tissue, possibly predicting their tumor-promoting and immunosuppressive functions. All the published studies investigating the presence of TAMs in MPM tissues with the pan-macrophage marker CD68, agree that both epithelial and non-epithelial MPM contain a large proportion of CD68+ TAMs, whose proportion can reach up to 40–50% of all cells.

In a series of 52 surgical patients, Burt et al. found that high levels of CD68+ macrophages were associated with worst patient prognosis only in sarcomatoid MPM and not in tumors with epithelial features [20]. These TAMs expressed also typical M2-like markers such as CD163, CD206, and the IL-4 receptor α. Similar results were later reported by two groups who found that single immune cell counts for CD163+ cells did not correlate with clinical outcome, but the ratio of CD163+/CD68+ macrophages was a significant prognostic marker for overall survival in epithelioid mesothelioma patients [21, 22].

The interplay between MPM cells and macrophages has a crucial role in shifting TAMs toward immunosuppressive and pro-tumorigenic cells [23]. This shift is promoted also by tumor-infiltrating lymphocytes (TILs) that produce IL-4, IL-13, and IL-10, typical stimuli inducing the M2 phenotype of myeloid cells [24, 25]. In vitro studies showed that macrophages co-cultured with MPM tumor cells or their pleural effusions acquire an M2-like phenotype [26] and release significant amounts of prostaglandins (e.g., PGE2) which have immunosuppressive effects in the TME by stimulating the development of Tregs [23, 27]. Indeed, the number of CD68+ macrophages was found to be correlated with the density of Tregs in patient tumors [28]. In a recent study the authors investigated the immunoscore of 302 MPM samples with a tissue microarray and correlated the density of each leukocyte population with patient survival. In line with the above findings, low numbers of macrophages (CD68+), Tregs (FOXP3+), and neutrophils (NP57+) were associated with longer survival in epithelioid MPM patients [29]. Neutrophils are less represented than macrophages in tumor tissues; nevertheless, their presence has been investigated in some studies. Besides the above-mentioned report, Awad et al. found an inverse correlation between neutrophil infiltration and T cell density [30].

In line with these findings, in murine tumor models of MPM, depletion of macrophages with zoledronic acid, prior to tumor cell injection, strongly reduced tumor take and growth [31].

Monocytes, the circulating precursors of TAMs, have been studied as prognostic marker in MPM patients. In a large series of 667 cases, higher preoperative monocyte counts negatively correlated with overall survival in both epithelioid and sarcomatoid mesothelioma [20]. Another study reported that a decreased lymphocyte/monocyte ratio (i.e., many monocytes) was associated with poor survival [32]. Finally, a high neutrophil-to-lymphocyte ratio was also as independent poor prognostic factors [33]. Overall, the high representation of macrophages within tumor tissues, or of myeloid circulating cells, constantly appears to be associated with faster tumor progression.

Other myeloid immune cells with suppressive function are the so-called myeloid-derived suppressor cells (MDSCs), a phenotypically heterogeneous population related to monocytes and neutrophils [34, 35].

MDSCs inhibit the proliferation and functional activity of CD4+ and CD8+ T cells by producing arginase (ARG1), inducible nitric oxide synthase (iNOS), indoleamine 2,3-dioxygenase 1 (IDO1), and PGE2. In cancer, MDSCs increase in response to tumor-derived factors, such as GM-CSF and prostaglandins, and by inhibiting adaptive immunity they favor tumor growth and disease progression. In a murine mesothelioma model, treatment with celecoxib, a COX-2 inhibitor, reduced the production of PGE2 and the numbers of MDSCs, leading to improved antitumor response to dendritic cell-based immunotherapy [36].

In another study, the authors aimed to target bromodomain proteins BRD2, BRD4, and BRD9 which are highly expressed in the malignant pleura. In a preclinical MPM model, bromodomain inhibitors not only reduced cancer cell proliferation but also induced immunogenic cell death and modified the composition of the TME. The results indicated the antitumor efficacy of Bromodomain inhibitors was largely due to a decrease of MDSC and an increase of CD8+ T lymphocytes [37].

5.2.2 Lymphocytes

T and B lymphocytes belong to the adaptive immune system. In the tumor context, tumor-infiltrating lymphocytes (TILs) play a pivotal role in antitumor responses. CD8+ T cells are able, upon recognition of a specific tumor-antigen on the Major Histocompatibility Complex, to directly kill tumor cells through the production of cytotoxic factors such as perforins and granzymes. T helper CD4+ cells can activate antigen-presenting cells (APCs) and support the action of CD8+ T lymphocytes and natural killer (NK) cells by producing IFNγ, overall favoring the antitumor immune response against cancer [38, 39].

The presence in tumors of CD8+ T lymphocytes is usually taken as a sign of antigen-specific antitumor immune response. In many solid tumors, high levels of T cells, in particular of cytotoxic CD8+ T cells, confer a survival benefit [40–42]. Several studies have reported that MPM tissues harbor variable numbers of T lymphocytes. Already in 1982 it was recognized that lymphoid infiltration correlated with a significantly longer patient survival, although at the time it was not possible to identify the different lymphoid subsets [43]. In more recent years, a better characterization has been performed; there is an overall concordance that the presence at high density of CD8+ in MPM can be a marker of active antitumor responses, associated with improved survival [22, 44, 45].

CD4+ T lymphocytes also correlate with better response to cisplatin-/pemetrexed-based chemotherapy [46] and in a large series of epithelioid tumors, with better prognosis when considered together with CD20+ B lymphocytes [29].

A recent study investigated leukocyte infiltration in diagnostic biopsies of MPM patients. The results demonstrated that the more aggressive histotype (sarcomatoid/biphasic) had higher CD8+ T lymphocytes and PD-L1 expression on tumor cells, while epithelioid tumors had higher CD4+ T and CD20+ B lymphocytes. At variance with the other studies, high density of CD8+ T cells correlated with lower response to chemotherapy and worse survival [47]. This different finding may be explained by the fact that higher CD8+ T cells were also associated with higher amount of CD68+ macrophages.

In MPM, as in many other tumors, the cytotoxic function of CD8+ T cell is inhibited by the molecule programmed cell death 1 (PD-L1) or PD-L2 (checkpoints of the immune response), expressed by tumor cells or by immunosuppressive cells in the stroma, such as TAMs and MDSCs [48]. Their counter-receptor (PD-1) is expressed on activated CD4+ and CD8+ T cells. The interaction between PD-1+ T cells and PD-L1+ cancer/stromal cells inhibits the function of T lymphocytes and leads to tumor immune evasion [47, 49, 50]. With the advent of immunotherapy with checkpoint inhibitors that achieved remarkable tumor regressions in some patients [51–53], it is indispensable to understand whether the lymphoid infiltrate expresses the PD-1 molecule, taken as a marker of immune exhaustion. Between 16% and 65% of the investigated MPM express PD-L1, with the highest immunoreactivity found in non-epithelioid mesothelioma [28, 54–59]. The presence of the PD-1/PD-L1 axis leads to inhibition of the endogenous antitumor immune response and to faster disease progression; PD-L1 levels in MPM is an independent prognostic marker of worse overall survival [46, 55–60]. In a study with 43 MPM patients, the authors investigated by flow cytometry, on disaggregated tumor samples, the phenotype of infiltrating leukocytes. Their results demonstrated that PD-L1-positive tumors had significantly more CD45+ leukocytes and in particular more CD3+ CD8+ T cells with PD-1 expression and also higher CD4+/FOXP3+ Tregs [30]. A similar analysis was performed on fine needle aspirate samples that did not require enzymatic dissociation for flow cytometry [61]. The authors were able to immunophenotype the infiltrating leukocytes and to determine the status of PD-1 expression by CD4+ and CD8+ lymphocytes, as well as the presence of myeloid cells (CD33+ monocytes and CD66b+ granulocytes). This methodology is of interest because it can be performed immediately on fresh diagnostic material and may be more representative of the tumor microenvironment than the analysis performed on the dissociated samples [61].

A recent study from Lee et al. [62] characterized the immune infiltrate and the PD-1/PD-1 L status of MPM using CyTOF analysis. Two tumor subtypes with distinct immune phenotypes were identified: TiME-I and TiME-II. The first contained significantly greater numbers of exhausted CD8+ T cells (PD-1+CTLA-4+CD8+ T cells) with the ability to produce IFNγ and of plasmacytoid DC (pDC) expressing high levels of CD40 and CD86. In contrast, TiME-II tumors contained more Tregs expressing high ICOS and CTLA-4 markers, CXCR4+CD38- (naive) CD8+ T cells, as well as neutrophils, conventional DCs (cDC), and TAMs with high PD-L1 and producing IL-10. Further in-depth studies demonstrated that TiME-I tumors had more neo-antigen abundance and elevated levels of MHC class I and II proteins, compared with TiME-II tumors. Of interest, these signatures had prognostic significance in that patients with TiME-I tumors had a more favorable survival [62]. The results of this study point out that the presence of PD-1 by T cell effectors is not always a sign of immune exhaustion, but—instead—may testify that these T lymphocytes are, or have been, antigen-primed, and therefore the tumor is immunogenic. On the same line, PD-1L upregulation (which is mainly induced by IFNγ) by cancer or stromal cells may be taken as a sign of antitumor immune response. The issue if this immune response is still active or has been completely abrogated by PD-1L remains to be determined.

Other immune checkpoints have now been recognized: lymphocyte activity can be inhibited also by the molecules TIM-3 and LAG-3; their presence has been described on CD4+, CD8+ T cells, and NK cells in the effusions of mesothelioma patients [46] as well as on diagnostic biopsies [61].

B lymphocytes are able to act as APCs, to stimulate T cells and to differentiate into antibody-secreting plasma cells. B cells are usually non abundant in solid tumors and frequently are located in aggregates with some T cells, called tertiary lymphoid structures (TLS). In some tumors, B cells in TLS are associated with better prognosis [63, 64], while sparse B cells in the stroma are not, or correlate with worse survival, as in pancreatic cancer [65]. Low numbers of CD20+ B cells are usually found in MPM, although some patients with higher B cell infiltration (up to 50% of CD45+ cells) have been reported [44, 66, 67]. Of the few studies performed, an association between B lymphocyte counts and better patient outcome has been reported [22]. In another study, the authors reported that high numbers of CD20+ B lymphocytes correlated with better prognosis when considered together with low numbers of CD163+ macrophages [22]. The exact role of B cells in MPM is, however, still controversial. With their antibody response, these cells can also sustain and potentiate the chronic inflammation which favors tumor growth and progression.

As mentioned above, the subset of CD4+FOXP3+ T cells is endowed with potent immunosuppressive activity: Tregs have a pivotal role in physiology to maintain self-tolerance and avoid autoimmune diseases. In tumors their presence is usually associated with poor prognosis, since they are able to suppress activation and proliferation of cytotoxic T cells [12, 22, 66]. Conversely, low Tregs are associated with longer survival in epithelioid MPM patients [29]. Moreover, it has been shown that the number of Tregs decreased in patients pretreated with cisplatin and pemetrexed [28].

NK cells are lymphocytes displaying natural cytotoxicity against tumor cells in an antigen-independent manner. Few NK cells infiltrate the solid masses of MPM, but some are found in the malignant pleural effusions, where they can constitute up to 10–15% of total cells. These NK cells have little cytotoxic potential, and also blood NK cells from patients have lower cytotoxicity than healthy individuals [68]. In vitro exposure to asbestos seems to impair NK cytotoxicity and to decrease the expression of the activating receptor NKp46 [68]. These cells, however, are not anergic and can be rescued by activating cytokines such as IL-2 [69].

5.3 The Inflammatory Microenvironment of MPM

5.3.1 Reactive Oxygen and Nitrogen Species

It is known that asbestos fibers give rise to cellular damage and generation of reactive oxygen and nitrogen species (ROS/RNS) which cause oxidation and nitrosylation of DNA and proteins [70, 71].

Oxidants play important roles in the initiation of numerous signal transduction pathways that are linked to proliferation/apoptosis and inflammation [72]. RNS are molecules with antimicrobial activity, derived from nitric oxide and superoxide (O_2^-) which are induced during inflammation in macrophages in response to LPS or IFNγ [73]. ROS are chemically reactive molecules containing oxygen, such as peroxides, superoxide, hydroxyl radical, and singlet oxygen. Under homeostasis, low levels of ROS production exert several important roles in cell signaling and immune; in contrast, during environmental or cellular injury, increased ROS/RNS levels cause oxidative stress, with implications in DNA and cellular damage. In the context of MPM, ROS/RNS are induced by asbestos fibers both through a direct effect on mesothelial cells and an indirect effect on the recruited inflammatory cells. ROS/RNS overproduction and chronic non-resolving inflammation are the major factors responsible for the processes of cell transformation and malignant evolution [74].

These highly reactive molecules can induce DNA damage and genomic instability (DNA strand breaks and base modifications) and protein alterations (e.g., in DNA repair enzymes) [75]. It has been demonstrated that occupational exposure to asbestos causes increased DNA double-strand breaks in comparison to non-exposed workers [76]. Aberrant inflammatory cytokine expression and NF-kB activation also predispose cells to carcinogenesis by a variety of mechanisms, for instance, by increasing cell survival, proliferation, and angiogenesis. The direct toxic effect of asbestos on pleural cells was strongly inhibited by the concomitant production of TNF, which supported cell survival via the NF-kB pathway; thus, an increased number of surviving pleural cells are susceptible to malignant transformation [77].

A possible scenario in the asbestos-induced oncogenesis process is that pleural cells which survive the direct injury are continuously exposed to inflammatory mediators and reactive ROS/RNS. Initially, DNA damage is successfully repaired, but over time, if DNA damage is no more fixed, and if random mutations have ablated tumor suppressor genes or cell cycle checkpoint genes, pleural cells proliferate and enter the carcinogenesis process [78–81] (Fig. 5.2).

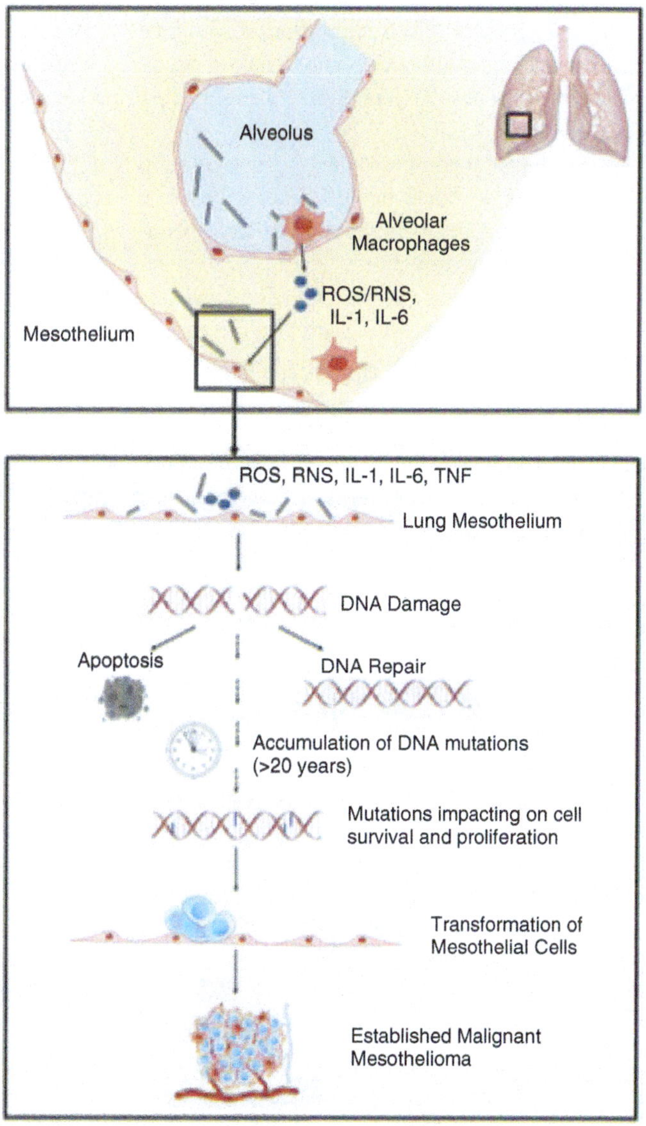

Fig. 5.2 Upon introduction of asbestos fibers in the lung alveoli, local macrophages are activated in an attempt to clear the fibers away, a process of "frustrated phagocytosis" to their nondegradable nature. Asbestos-induced inflammatory reaction leads to a state of chronic non-resolving inflammation. Reactive oxygen and nitrogen species (ROS/RNS) and inflammatory cytokines (IL-1β, IL-6, TNF) cause in mesothelial cells DNA damage and genetic alterations (e.g., in tumor suppressor genes) and inhibition of DNA repair mechanisms. This process of inflammation-induced carcinogenesis may require several years, being in fact the results of a balance between continuous random mutations and successful DNA repair, mesothelial cell death or cell proliferation, recognition by the immune system or escape from it

5.3.2 NLRP3 Inflammasome Activation and IL-1

Asbestos fibers in the lungs are able to directly activate the NOD-like receptor NLRP3, a component of the inflammasome, in innate immunity cells, leading to the production and secretion of active IL-1β and IL-18 in the microenvironment [13, 82]. IL-1 is the first member of a complex family of structurally related cytokines that are central mediators of innate immunity and inflammation [83]. The family includes several ligand isoforms (most known are IL-1α, IL-β, and IL-33) and other ligands that serve as receptor antagonists, such as IL-1Ra. The receptor family is also complex and is composed of an active signaling receptor (IL-1RI), non-signaling decoy receptors (e.g., IL-1RII), and receptor regulators (e.g., IL-1R8).

This structural complexity and tight regulation are necessary to fine-tune the balance between amplification of defensive immunity and uncontrolled inflammation [83].

IL-1β signals via the MyD88-IRAK-NF-κB pathway and stimulates the secretion of secondary inflammatory mediators, including TNF and IL-6, several chemokines, growth factors, and enzymes of the inflammatory cascade.

IL-1β, together with other inflammatory cytokines, is produced in vitro by cultured human mesothelial cells and alveolar macrophages treated with asbestos or other similar fibers [82, 84]. In a mouse xenograft model with human MPM cells, the release of several cytokines was impaired upon treatment with IL-1Ra (Anakinra), confirming the primary role of IL-1 in triggering the downstream amplification of the inflammatory cascade [82]. In the last decade, inflammasome activation and IL-1 secretion have been considered key components of the tumor-promoting inflammation [85]. IL-1-triggered responses amplify the recruitment of inflammatory cells, promote neo-angiogenesis, and lead to suppression of antitumor immunity [85]. Furthermore, chronic NLRP3 activation and IL-1β/IL-18 production induce a mesothelial to fibroblastic transition (MFT) that is considered the initial step of MPM tumorigenesis, with a gain of mesenchymal markers (vimentin, N-cadherin) and loss of epithelial markers (e.g., E-cadherin) [86]. Among the factors responsible for MFT are the cytokines IL-6 and CXCL8, as well as the fibroblast growth factor (FGF), also triggered by asbestos [86].

Of interest, treatment with chemotherapeutic drugs and consequent cell death may also activate the inflammasome and increase the levels of IL-1β and of other pro-inflammatory mediators. In SCID mice bearing a human MPM cell line, inhibition of IL-1R signaling (Anakinra) combined with cisplatin resulted in greater antitumor effect compared to cisplatin alone [87]. These data confirm that IL-1β signaling has a significant role in the progression of MPM. Indeed, the interest of IL-1 blocking agents in oncology has dramatically increased in the last years; of note IL-1β inhibition with a specific antibody could significantly reduce incident lung cancer and related mortality in a large cohort of high-risk patients [88]. These findings constitute a rationale to use inflammation-targeting therapies in human MPM and to consider chemopreventing strategies against inflammation-related IL-1β/IL1R signaling in high-risk individuals who have been chronically exposed to asbestos [89].

5.3.3 Other Inflammatory Cytokines and Chemokines

As mentioned above, IL-1-mediated activation of the transcription factor NF-kB results in the transcription of several inflammatory genes. In MPM tissues, and especially in pleural effusions, several soluble inflammatory mediators are present, such as TNF, IL-6, and the chemokines CXCL8 and CCL2; in addition, a number of growth factors are expressed for epithelial cells, vessels, and stromal cells, including vascular endothelial growth factor (VEGF), hepatocyte growth factor (HGF), transforming growth factor beta (TGF-β), platelet-derived growth factor (PDGF), and insulin-like growth factor (IGF) and FGF [90–93].

TNF is a pro-inflammatory cytokine able to activate several cellular processes; by stimulating

NF-kB it induces the production of chemokines and adhesion molecules, important for the arrival of inflammatory leukocytes. In addition, low levels of TNF stimulate angiogenesis and the activation of quiescent fibroblasts in the stroma [16]. As a matter of fact, at concentrations usually found in the microenvironment, TNF sustains cancer progression; on the other hand, very high levels of TNF potently induce necrotic cell death in various cancer types [16].

IL-6 is a pleiotropic cytokine acting on immune cells and also on epithelial cells and the microenvironment. It is a major cytokine of the acute phase response but also importantly involved in the chronic process of inflammation. In the tumor microenvironment its role is strictly correlated with the activation of several pathways, such as STAT3, Ras/MAPK/ERK, AP1/JNK, Cox2, PI3K/AKT, Wnt, and Notch3/Jagged1. These pathways, especially STAT3, stimulate cancer cell survival [94] and may be involved in the acquisition of chemoresistance during therapy, while activation of STAT3 in immune cells (e.g., by IL-6 and IL-10) leads to immunosuppression [95].

Pleural effusions of mesothelioma patients contain substantial levels of IL-6 [96–99]. Its involvement in this disease has been studied as potential autocrine growth factor and angiogenesis promoter [96, 100]; of note, IL-6 receptor inhibition abrogated VEGF expression in cultured mesothelial cells [101]. IL-6 is also involved in the acquisition of chemoresistance, although this aspect is controversial in mesothelioma tumors [100]. Unlike other solid tumors where serum levels of IL-6 correlate with poor prognosis (e.g., NSCLC, pancreatic and breast adenocarcinoma), its prognostic significance is less clear in MPM, but its presence is linked with other factors predicting poor prognosis, such as CRP and high numbers of platelet [98, 102, 103].

IL-1, TNF, and IL-6 strongly stimulate the expression of several genes coding for chemokines. A major factor in monocyte recruitment inside tumor tissues is CCL2, also known as monocyte chemoattractant protein-1 (MCP1) [6, 17]. Both MPM tumor cells and macrophages are able to produce CCL2, and its release is the main mechanism for monocyte recruitment from the blood [26]. Higher levels of CCL2 are present in the pleural effusion of MPM patients, compared to benign pleural effusions [104, 105].

IL-8, also known as CXCL8, is produced by macrophages, endothelial and epithelial cells upon infection or tissue injury, and stimulates the migration of granulocytes to the affected site [106]; in that context, CXCL8 also promotes the resolution of the pathological processes [107]. In the tumor context, this chemokine is responsible for the recruitment of neutrophils and also MDSCs, prompting the formation of an immunosuppressive microenvironment. CXCL8 is also a potent angiogenic factor and inducer of the epithelial-mesenchymal transition (EMT) [108, 109]. In mice exposed to asbestos, CXCL8, IL-6, and IL-1β were overexpressed and fueled the inflammation preceding tumor formation [110, 111]. In a xenograft mouse model, CXCL8 inhibition decreased tumor growth, confirming the important role of this chemokine in tumor progression [112, 113].

Pleural effusion from human mesothelioma patients contains substantial levels of CXCL8. In addition to its pro-angiogenic and chemoattractant role, in vitro studies on cultured mesothelioma cells reported an autocrine proliferative effect of CXCL8 on cancer cells [113–115].

Previous studies demonstrated that chemotherapy-treated mesothelioma cells may survive the apoptotic insult and enter a state of senescence, which is characterized by a senescence-associated secretory phenotype (SASP); CXCL8 and IL-6 were among the most secreted cytokines [116]. A recent study reported that an inhibitor to the chaperon molecule HSP90 (known to sensitize tumor cells to some chemotherapeutics) blunted chemokine secretion and the correlated CXCL8-mediated survival of mesothelioma cells [113].

5.3.4 Stromal Cells and Matrix-Related Factors

Stromal cells are a major determinant of solid tumors, and recent evidence has highlighted their complex interaction with cancer cells and locally infiltrating leukocytes. Cancer-associated fibroblasts (CAFs) typically display a non-quiescent phenotype, as instead occurs in normal tissues, and are indeed an important source of soluble or matrix-bound biological mediators, such as growth factors for cancer and endothelial cells. CAFs and the vessel network are thus importantly involved during tumor development and sustain cancer cell proliferation and their ability to invade the surrounding tissues [117, 118].

In malignant mesothelioma, CAFs acquire an activated phenotype due to the local expression of FGF-2, PDGF-AA (platelet-derived growth factor-AA), and TGFβ produced by cancer and stromal cells [119]. In turn, they secrete abundant matrix components and proteolytic enzymes which eventually lead to the construction of an aberrant extracellular matrix with continuous remodeling. CAFs also produce other growth factors such as VEGF, thereby stimulating the angiogenic network, tumor development, and resistance to therapy [82, 119–125]. In mouse model it is demonstrated that their inhibition reduces mesothelioma cell growth in vitro [122].

As in many other tumors, human MPM tissues contain many vessels, and the histological evaluation of angiogenesis is an independent factor of poor prognosis [126]. There is evidence in a rat model of mesothelioma that targeting CAFs with an inhibitor of the Hedgehog signaling pathway decreased tumor volume and growth rate. Histological evaluations determined that target genes of this pathway (e.g., fibronectin and VEGF) were predominantly down-modulated in the stromal compartment [127, 128].

Transforming growth factor β (TGFβ) is a master regulator of stromal cells. TGFβ is a secreted cytokine produced by tumor cells with the ability to induce oncogenic transformation of non-cancerous cells in vitro [129]. The TGFβ family comprises different members involved in various physiological processes, for instance, in the regulation of embryonic development, and also in pathological conditions such as cancer [130]. TGFβ has been implicated in tumor progression through its regulation of cell growth, differentiation, and migration and has been also implicated in cell apoptosis, epithelial to mesenchymal transition (EMT), and matrix regulation. In normal cells such as fibroblasts, TGFβ is a potent activator of their matrix-producing function; by contrast, in immune cells, TGFβ is potently suppressive: it inhibits Th1-mediated T cell responses, expands Tregs, and polarizes macrophages toward pro-tumor [130, 131]. In the pleural effusions of mesothelioma patients, TGFβ is present at high levels and likely exerts two complementary functions: the creation of a suppressive environment and the development of tumor cells with EMT phenotype and invasive ability [26, 48, 131, 132].

The canonical Smad-mediated TGFβ signaling upregulates the ERK and AKT pathways in target cells. In a recent study, using a mouse model of mesothelioma xenografts, the authors showed that treatment with pirfenidone (an antifibrotic drug) blocked the TGFβ-induced upregulation of ERK and AKT and modified the tumor microenvironment. The most important modifications were a reduction in the expression of matrix-associated genes, such as several types of collagens, matrix glycoproteins, and gremlin1 (an antagonist to bone morphogenetic proteins); these molecules are implicated in driving cancer cells to a migratory and invasive phenotype [133]. Having such complex roles, TGFβ has always been considered a difficult target molecule in cancer. Nevertheless some approaches have been attempted. A clinical study was performed in a small number of advanced mesothelioma patients to evaluate the effect of a neutralizing anti-TGFβ antibody. No clinical responses were observed, but 5 patients out of 13 treated had immunoregulatory effects and produced enhanced levels of antibodies against tumor cell lysates; these patients had an increased median overall survival (15 vs 7.5 months) compared to patients not producing antibodies [134]. These results suggest that TGFβ-blockade may be worth pursuing and that effective compounds directed to this cytokine or its receptors may be useful to normalize the tumor microenvironment [131].

Mesothelin and Osteopontin are two matricellular glycoproteins that are overexpressed in mesothelioma and were found to be associated with tumor progression in some studies. Osteopontin is produced by various cell types, including macrophages, and is frequently overexpressed in tumors. It is able to promote oncogenic features such as cell proliferation, survival, migration, and neo-angiogenesis [135–137]. Serum levels of Osteopontin are usually high in MPM, and this protein has been proposed as diagnostic marker or as marker for therapy response [138]. Similarly, Mesothelin levels in blood were assessed in MPM patients along the course of chemotherapy. A rise of 10% in serum mesothelin could predict disease progression with a sensitivity of 96% and specificity of 74% [139].

5.4 Conclusions

The tumor microenvironment of human MPM is characterized by the presence of an abundant leukocyte infiltrate, a fingerprint of the inflammatory origin of this tumor. The myeloid lineage (macrophages, MDSCs) usually predominates and exerts strong immunosuppressive effects on adaptive T cell-mediated antitumor immune responses. Macrophages also promote disease progression by directly supporting tumor cell survival and proliferation and by stimulating neo-angiogenesis. In this scenario, several components of the inflammatory cascade (reactive chemical species, IL-1-orchestrated cytokines and chemokines) are expressed in the tumor stroma or accumulate in pleural effusions. Several cytokines have been investigated also in the plasma of MPM patients, with the intent to define biomarkers for early diagnosis or response to treatments. These studies, so far, have not provided reproducible and clinically useful assays.

Tumor-induced immune dysfunction and the intrinsic resistance of mesothelioma cells to anti-proliferative chemotherapy suggest to test alternative therapeutic approaches. Antibody-based immunotherapy against checkpoint inhibitors is currently being pursued in mesothelioma patients. Due to its inflammatory nature, it would be reasonable also to investigate novel strategies targeting specific inflammatory circuits, such as depletion or re-programming of the tumor-promoting macrophages, as well as inhibition of specific cytokines, especially IL-1β, at the summit of the inflammatory cascade. The recent availability of several target-specific drugs and the increasing clinical knowledge in therapy combinations justify the hope that this tumor might be treated in the future with more success than previously achieved.

Acknowledgments Cristina Belgiovine is supported by a fellowship form Fondazione Veronesi, Milan, Italy.

References

1. Liu G, Cheresh P, Kamp DW. Molecular basis of asbestos-induced lung disease. Annu Rev Pathol. 2013;8:161–87.
2. Mossman BT, Churg A. Mechanisms in the pathogenesis of asbestosis and silicosis. Am J Respir Crit Care Med. 1998;157(5 Pt 1):1666–80.
3. Mossman BT, Lippmann M, Hesterberg TW, Kelsey KT, Barchowsky A, Bonner JC. Pulmonary endpoints (lung carcinomas and asbestosis) following inhalation exposure to asbestos. J Toxicol Environ Health B Crit Rev. 2011;14(1–4):76–121.
4. Bograd AJ, Suzuki K, Vertes E, Colovos C, Morales EA, Sadelain M, et al. Immune responses and immunotherapeutic interventions in malignant pleural mesothelioma. Cancer Immunol Immunother. 2011;60(11):1509–27.
5. Hanahan D, Weinberg RA. Hallmarks of cancer: the next generation. Cell. 2011;144(5):646–74.
6. Mantovani A, Allavena P, Sica A, Balkwill F. Cancer-related inflammation. Nature. 2008;454(7203):436–44.
7. Aggarwal BB, Gehlot P. Inflammation and cancer: how friendly is the relationship for cancer patients? Curr Opin Pharmacol. 2009;9(4):351–69.
8. Thompson JK, Westbom CM, Shukla A. Malignant mesothelioma: development to therapy. J Cell Biochem. 2014;115(1):1–7.
9. Izzi V, Masuelli L, Tresoldi I, Foti C, Modesti A, Bei R. Immunity and malignant mesothelioma: from mesothelial cell damage to tumor development and immune response-based therapies. Cancer Lett. 2012;322(1):18–34.
10. Solbes E, Harper RW. Biological responses to asbestos inhalation and pathogenesis of asbestos-related benign and malignant disease. J Investig Med. 2018;66(4):721–7.
11. Yap TA, Aerts JG, Popat S, Fennell DA. Novel insights into mesothelioma biology and implications for therapy. Nat Rev Cancer. 2017;17(8):475–88.
12. Minnema-Luiting J, Vroman H, Aerts J, Cornelissen R. Heterogeneity in immune cell content in malignant pleural mesothelioma. Int J Mol Sci. 2018;19(4):1041.

13. Dostert C, Petrilli V, Van Bruggen R, Steele C, Mossman BT, Tschopp J. Innate immune activation through Nalp3 inflammasome sensing of asbestos and silica. Science. 2008;320(5876):674–7.
14. Sekido Y. Molecular pathogenesis of malignant mesothelioma. Carcinogenesis. 2013;34(7):1413–9.
15. Mantovani A, Marchesi F, Malesci A, Laghi L, Allavena P. Tumour-associated macrophages as treatment targets in oncology. Nat Rev Clin Oncol. 2017;14(7):399–416.
16. Balkwill F. TNF-alpha in promotion and progression of cancer. Cancer Metastasis Rev. 2006;25(3):409–16.
17. Conti I, Rollins BJ. CCL2 (monocyte chemoattractant protein-1) and cancer. Semin Cancer Biol. 2004;14(3):149–54.
18. Kitamura T, Qian BZ, Pollard JW. Immune cell promotion of metastasis. Nat Rev Immunol. 2015;15(2):73–86.
19. Murray PJ, Allen JE, Biswas SK, Fisher EA, Gilroy DW, Goerdt S, et al. Macrophage activation and polarization: nomenclature and experimental guidelines. Immunity. 2014;41(1):14–20.
20. Burt BM, Rodig SJ, Tilleman TR, Elbardissi AW, Bueno R, Sugarbaker DJ. Circulating and tumor-infiltrating myeloid cells predict survival in human pleural mesothelioma. Cancer. 2011;117(22):5234–44.
21. Cornelissen R, Lievense LA, Maat AP, Hendriks RW, Hoogsteden HC, Bogers AJ, et al. Ratio of intratumoral macrophage phenotypes is a prognostic factor in epithelioid malignant pleural mesothelioma. PLoS One. 2014;9(9):e106742.
22. Ujiie H, Kadota K, Nitadori JI, Aerts JG, Woo KM, Sima CS, et al. The tumoral and stromal immune microenvironment in malignant pleural mesothelioma: a comprehensive analysis reveals prognostic immune markers. Oncoimmunology. 2015;4(6):e1009285.
23. Izzi V, Chiurchiu V, D'Aquilio F, Palumbo C, Tresoldi I, Modesti A, et al. Differential effects of malignant mesothelioma cells on THP-1 monocytes and macrophages. Int J Oncol. 2009;34(2):543–50.
24. Mantovani A, Sozzani S, Locati M, Allavena P, Sica A. Macrophage polarization: tumor-associated macrophages as a paradigm for polarized M2 mononuclear phagocytes. Trends Immunol. 2002;23(11):549–55.
25. Hanahan D, Coussens LM. Accessories to the crime: functions of cells recruited to the tumor microenvironment. Cancer Cell. 2012;21(3):309–22.
26. Chene AL, d'Almeida S, Blondy T, Tabiasco J, Deshayes S, Fonteneau JF, et al. Pleural effusions from patients with mesothelioma induce recruitment of monocytes and their differentiation into M2 macrophages. J Thorac Oncol. 2016;11(10):1765–73.
27. Baratelli F, Lin Y, Zhu L, Yang SC, Heuze-Vourc'h N, Zeng G, et al. Prostaglandin E2 induces FOXP3 gene expression and T regulatory cell function in human CD4+ T cells. J Immunol. 2005;175(3):1483–90.
28. Marcq E, Siozopoulou V, De Waele J, van Audenaerde J, Zwaenepoel K, Santermans E, et al. Prognostic and predictive aspects of the tumor immune microenvironment and immune checkpoints in malignant pleural mesothelioma. Oncoimmunology. 2017;6(1):e1261241.
29. Chee SJ, Lopez M, Mellows T, Gankande S, Moutasim KA, Harris S, et al. Evaluating the effect of immune cells on the outcome of patients with mesothelioma. Br J Cancer. 2017;117(9):1341–8.
30. Awad MM, Jones RE, Liu H, Lizotte PH, Ivanova EV, Kulkarni M, et al. Cytotoxic T cells in PD-L1-positive malignant pleural mesotheliomas are counterbalanced by distinct immunosuppressive factors. Cancer Immunol Res. 2016;4(12):1038–48.
31. Veltman JD, Lambers ME, van Nimwegen M, Hendriks RW, Hoogsteden HC, Hegmans JP, et al. Zoledronic acid impairs myeloid differentiation to tumour-associated macrophages in mesothelioma. Br J Cancer. 2010;103(5):629–41.
32. Tanrikulu AC, Abakay A, Komek H, Abakay O. Prognostic value of the lymphocyte-to-monocyte ratio and other inflammatory markers in malignant pleural mesothelioma. Environ Health Prev Med. 2016;21(5):304–11.
33. Kao SC, Klebe S, Henderson DW, Reid G, Chatfield M, Armstrong NJ, et al. Low calretinin expression and high neutrophil-to-lymphocyte ratio are poor prognostic factors in patients with malignant mesothelioma undergoing extrapleural pneumonectomy. J Thorac Oncol. 2011;6(11):1923–9.
34. Mondanelli G, Bianchi R, Pallotta MT, Orabona C, Albini E, Iacono A, et al. A relay pathway between arginine and tryptophan metabolism confers immunosuppressive properties on dendritic cells. Immunity. 2017;46(2):233–44.
35. Sica A, Strauss L, Consonni FM, Travelli C, Genazzani A, Porta C. Metabolic regulation of suppressive myeloid cells in cancer. Cytokine Growth Factor Rev. 2017;35:27–35.
36. Veltman JD, Lambers ME, van Nimwegen M, Hendriks RW, Hoogsteden HC, Aerts JG, et al. COX-2 inhibition improves immunotherapy and is associated with decreased numbers of myeloid-derived suppressor cells in mesothelioma. Celecoxib influences MDSC function. BMC Cancer. 2010;10:464.
37. Riganti C, Lingua MF, Salaroglio IC, Falcomata C, Righi L, Morena D, et al. Bromodomain inhibition exerts its therapeutic potential in malignant pleural mesothelioma by promoting immunogenic cell death and changing the tumor immune-environment. Oncoimmunology. 2018;7(3):e1398874.
38. Friedman KM, Prieto PA, Devillier LE, Gross CA, Yang JC, Wunderlich JR, et al. Tumor-specific CD4+ melanoma tumor-infiltrating lymphocytes. J Immunother. 2012;35(5):400–8.
39. Van Acker HH, Capsomidis A, Smits EL, Van Tendeloo VF. CD56 in the immune system: more than a marker for cytotoxicity? Front Immunol. 2017;8:892.
40. Schreiber RD, Old LJ, Smyth MJ. Cancer immunoediting: integrating immunity's roles in cancer suppression and promotion. Science. 2011;331(6024):1565–70.
41. Galon J, Costes A, Sanchez-Cabo F, Kirilovsky A, Mlecnik B, Lagorce-Pages C, et al. Type, density, and location of immune cells within human

colorectal tumors predict clinical outcome. Science. 2006;313(5795):1960–4.
42. Gentles AJ, Newman AM, Liu CL, Bratman SV, Feng W, Kim D, et al. The prognostic landscape of genes and infiltrating immune cells across human cancers. Nat Med. 2015;21(8):938–45.
43. Leigh RA, Webster I. Lymphocytic infiltration of pleural mesothelioma and its significance for survival. S Afr Med J. 1982;61(26):1007–9.
44. Anraku M, Cunningham KS, Yun Z, Tsao MS, Zhang L, Keshavjee S, et al. Impact of tumor-infiltrating T cells on survival in patients with malignant pleural mesothelioma. J Thorac Cardiovasc Surg. 2008;135(4):823–9.
45. Yamada N, Oizumi S, Kikuchi E, Shinagawa N, Konishi-Sakakibara J, Ishimine A, et al. CD8+ tumor-infiltrating lymphocytes predict favorable prognosis in malignant pleural mesothelioma after resection. Cancer Immunol Immunother. 2010;59(10):1543–9.
46. Marcq E, Waele J, Audenaerde JV, Lion E, Santermans E, Hens N, et al. Abundant expression of TIM-3, LAG-3, PD-1 and PD-L1 as immunotherapy checkpoint targets in effusions of mesothelioma patients. Oncotarget. 2017;8(52):89722–35.
47. Pasello G, Zago G, Lunardi F, Urso L, Kern I, Vlacic G, et al. Malignant pleural mesothelioma immune microenvironment and checkpoint expression: correlation with clinical-pathological features and intratumor heterogeneity over time. Ann Oncol. 2018;29(5):1258–65.
48. Lievense LA, Cornelissen R, Bezemer K, Kaijen-Lambers ME, Hegmans JP, Aerts JG. Pleural effusion of patients with malignant mesothelioma induces macrophage-mediated T cell suppression. J Thorac Oncol. 2016;11(10):1755–64.
49. Ishida Y, Agata Y, Shibahara K, Honjo T. Induced expression of PD-1, a novel member of the immunoglobulin gene superfamily, upon programmed cell death. EMBO J. 1992;11(11):3887–95.
50. Thompson RH, Gillett MD, Cheville JC, Lohse CM, Dong H, Webster WS, et al. Costimulatory B7-H1 in renal cell carcinoma patients: indicator of tumor aggressiveness and potential therapeutic target. Proc Natl Acad Sci U S A. 2004;101(49):17174–9.
51. Ribas A, Kirkwood JM, Flaherty KT. Anti-PD-1 antibody treatment for melanoma. Lancet Oncol. 2018;19(5):e219.
52. Allison JP. Checkpoints. Cell. 2015;162(6):1202–5.
53. Ceresoli GL, Mantovani A. Immune checkpoint inhibitors in malignant pleural mesothelioma. Lancet Oncol. 2017;18(5):559–61.
54. Patil NS, Righi L, Koeppen H, Zou W, Izzo S, Grosso F, et al. Molecular and histopathological characterization of the tumor immune microenvironment in advanced stage of malignant pleural mesothelioma. J Thorac Oncol. 2018;13(1):124–33.
55. Combaz-Lair C, Galateau-Salle F, McLeer-Florin A, Le Stang N, David-Boudet L, Duruisseaux M, et al. Immune biomarkers PD-1/PD-L1 and TLR3 in malignant pleural mesotheliomas. Hum Pathol. 2016;52:9–18.
56. Cedres S, Ponce-Aix S, Zugazagoitia J, Sansano I, Enguita A, Navarro-Mendivil A, et al. Analysis of expression of programmed cell death 1 ligand 1 (PD-L1) in malignant pleural mesothelioma (MPM). PLoS One. 2015;10(3):e0121071.
57. Inaguma S, Lasota J, Wang Z, Czapiewski P, Langfort R, Rys J, et al. Expression of ALCAM (CD166) and PD-L1 (CD274) independently predicts shorter survival in malignant pleural mesothelioma. Hum Pathol. 2018;71:1–7.
58. Mansfield AS, Roden AC, Peikert T, Sheinin YM, Harrington SM, Krco CJ, et al. B7-H1 expression in malignant pleural mesothelioma is associated with sarcomatoid histology and poor prognosis. J Thorac Oncol. 2014;9(7):1036–40.
59. Khanna S, Thomas A, Abate-Daga D, Zhang J, Morrow B, Steinberg SM, et al. Malignant mesothelioma effusions are infiltrated by CD3(+) T cells highly expressing PD-L1 and the PD-L1(+) tumor cells within these effusions are susceptible to ADCC by the anti-PD-L1 antibody avelumab. J Thorac Oncol. 2016;11(11):1993–2005.
60. Cedres S, Ponce-Aix S, Pardo-Aranda N, Navarro-Mendivil A, Martinez-Marti A, Zugazagoitia J, et al. Analysis of expression of PTEN/PI3K pathway and programmed cell death ligand 1 (PD-L1) in malignant pleural mesothelioma (MPM). Lung Cancer. 2016;96:1–6.
61. Lizotte PH, Jones RE, Keogh L, Ivanova E, Liu H, Awad MM, et al. Fine needle aspirate flow cytometric phenotyping characterizes immunosuppressive nature of the mesothelioma microenvironment. Sci Rep. 2016;6:31745.
62. Lee HS, Jang HJ, Choi JM, Zhang J, de Rosen VL, Wheeler TM, et al. Comprehensive immunoproteogenomic analyses of malignant pleural mesothelioma. JCI insight. 2018;3(7):98575.
63. Fridman WH, Pages F, Sautes-Fridman C, Galon J. The immune contexture in human tumours: impact on clinical outcome. Nat Rev Cancer. 2012;12(4):298–306.
64. Di Caro G, Bergomas F, Grizzi F, Doni A, Bianchi P, Malesci A, et al. Occurrence of tertiary lymphoid tissue is associated with T-cell infiltration and predicts better prognosis in early-stage colorectal cancers. Clin Cancer Res. 2014;20(8):2147–58.
65. Castino GF, Cortese N, Capretti G, Serio S, Di Caro G, Mineri R, et al. Spatial distribution of B cells predicts prognosis in human pancreatic adenocarcinoma. Oncoimmunology. 2016;5(4):e1085147.
66. Hegmans JP, Hemmes A, Hammad H, Boon L, Hoogsteden HC, Lambrecht BN. Mesothelioma environment comprises cytokines and T-regulatory cells that suppress immune responses. Eur Respir J. 2006;27(6):1086–95.
67. Zhang L, Conejo-Garcia JR, Katsaros D, Gimotty PA, Massobrio M, Regnani G, et al. Intratumoral T cells, recurrence, and survival in epithelial ovarian cancer. N Engl J Med. 2003;348(3):203–13.
68. Nishimura Y, Kumagai-Takei N, Matsuzaki H, Lee S, Maeda M, Kishimoto T, et al. Functional alteration of

natural killer cells and cytotoxic T lymphocytes upon asbestos exposure and in malignant mesothelioma patients. Biomed Res Int. 2015;2015:238431.
69. Vacca P, Martini S, Garelli V, Passalacqua G, Moretta L, Mingari MC. NK cells from malignant pleural effusions are not anergic but produce cytokines and display strong antitumor activity on short-term IL-2 activation. Eur J Immunol. 2013;43(2):550–61.
70. Manning CB, Vallyathan V, Mossman BT. Diseases caused by asbestos: mechanisms of injury and disease development. Int Immunopharmacol. 2002;2(2–3):191–200.
71. Matsuzaki H, Maeda M, Lee S, Nishimura Y, Kumagai-Takei N, Hayashi H, et al. Asbestos-induced cellular and molecular alteration of immunocompetent cells and their relationship with chronic inflammation and carcinogenesis. J Biomed Biotechnol. 2012;2012:492608.
72. Shukla A, Gulumian M, Hei TK, Kamp D, Rahman Q, Mossman BT. Multiple roles of oxidants in the pathogenesis of asbestos-induced diseases. Free Radic Biol Med. 2003;34(9):1117–29.
73. Iovine NM, Pursnani S, Voldman A, Wasserman G, Blaser MJ, Weinrauch Y. Reactive nitrogen species contribute to innate host defense against Campylobacter jejuni. Infect Immun. 2008;76(3):986–93.
74. Benedetti S, Nuvoli B, Catalani S, Galati R. Reactive oxygen species a double-edged sword for mesothelioma. Oncotarget. 2015;6(19):16848–65.
75. Colotta F, Allavena P, Sica A, Garlanda C, Mantovani A. Cancer-related inflammation, the seventh hallmark of cancer: links to genetic instability. Carcinogenesis. 2009;30(7):1073–81.
76. Marczynski B, Czuppon AB, Marek W, Reichel G, Baur X. Increased incidence of DNA double-strand breaks and anti-ds DNA antibodies in blood of workers occupationally exposed to asbestos. Hum Exp Toxicol. 1994;13(1):3–9.
77. Yang H, Bocchetta M, Kroczynska B, Elmishad AG, Chen Y, Liu Z, et al. TNF-alpha inhibits asbestos-induced cytotoxicity via a NF-kappaB-dependent pathway, a possible mechanism for asbestos-induced oncogenesis. Proc Natl Acad Sci U S A. 2006;103(27):10397–402.
78. Kamp DW, Graceffa P, Pryor WA, Weitzman SA. The role of free radicals in asbestos-induced diseases. Free Radic Biol Med. 1992;12(4):293–315.
79. Maples KR, Johnson NF. Fiber-induced hydroxyl radical formation: correlation with mesothelioma induction in rats and humans. Carcinogenesis. 1992;13(11):2035–9.
80. Hardy JA, Aust AE. The effect of iron binding on the ability of crocidolite asbestos to catalyze DNA single-strand breaks. Carcinogenesis. 1995;16(2):319–25.
81. Chew SH, Toyokuni S. Malignant mesothelioma as an oxidative stress-induced cancer: an update. Free Radic Biol Med. 2015;86:166–78.
82. Hillegass JM, Miller JM, MacPherson MB, Westbom CM, Sayan M, Thompson JK, et al. Asbestos and erionite prime and activate the NLRP3 inflammasome that stimulates autocrine cytokine release in human mesothelial cells. Part Fibre Toxicol. 2013;10:39.
83. Garlanda C, Dinarello CA, Mantovani A. The interleukin-1 family: back to the future. Immunity. 2013;39(6):1003–18.
84. Murphy FA, Poland CA, Duffin R, Donaldson K. Length-dependent pleural inflammation and parietal pleural responses after deposition of carbon nanotubes in the pulmonary airspaces of mice. Nanotoxicology. 2013;7(6):1157–67.
85. Mantovani A, Barajon I, Garlanda C. IL-1 and IL-1 regulatory pathways in cancer progression and therapy. Immunol Rev. 2018;281(1):57–61.
86. Thompson JK, MacPherson MB, Beuschel SL, Shukla A. Asbestos-induced mesothelial to fibroblastic transition is modulated by the inflammasome. Am J Pathol. 2017;187(3):665–78.
87. Westbom C, Thompson JK, Leggett A, MacPherson M, Beuschel S, Pass H, et al. Inflammasome modulation by chemotherapeutics in malignant mesothelioma. PLoS One. 2015;10(12):e0145404.
88. Ridker PM, MacFadyen JG, Thuren T, Everett BM, Libby P, Glynn RJ. Effect of interleukin-1beta inhibition with canakinumab on incident lung cancer in patients with atherosclerosis: exploratory results from a randomised, double-blind, placebo-controlled trial. Lancet. 2017;390(10105):1833–42.
89. Kadariya Y, Menges CW, Talarchek J, Cai KQ, Klein-Szanto AJ, Pietrofesa RA, et al. Inflammation-related IL1beta/IL1R signaling promotes the development of asbestos-induced malignant mesothelioma. Cancer Prev Res (Phila). 2016;9(5):406–14.
90. Judge S, Thomas P, Govindarajan V, Sharma P, Loggie B. Malignant peritoneal mesothelioma: characterization of the inflammatory response in the tumor microenvironment. Ann Surg Oncol. 2016;23(5):1496–500.
91. Gavett SH, Parkinson CU, Willson GA, Wood CE, Jarabek AM, Roberts KC, et al. Persistent effects of Libby amphibole and amosite asbestos following subchronic inhalation in rats. Part Fibre Toxicol. 2016;13:17.
92. Fukagawa NK, Li M, Sabo-Attwood T, Timblin CR, Butnor KJ, Gagne J, et al. Inhaled asbestos exacerbates atherosclerosis in apolipoprotein E-deficient mice via CD4+ T cells. Environ Health Perspect. 2008;116(9):1218–25.
93. Dragon J, Thompson J, MacPherson M, Shukla A. Differential susceptibility of human pleural and peritoneal mesothelial cells to asbestos exposure. J Cell Biochem. 2015;116(8):1540–52.
94. Guo Y, Xu F, Lu T, Duan Z, Zhang Z. Interleukin-6 signaling pathway in targeted therapy for cancer. Cancer Treat Rev. 2012;38(7):904–10.
95. Yu H, Pardoll D, Jove R. STATs in cancer inflammation and immunity: a leading role for STAT3. Nat Rev Cancer. 2009;9(11):798–809.
96. Bielefeldt-Ohmann H, Marzo AL, Himbeck RP, Jarnicki AG, Robinson BW, Fitzpatrick DR. Interleukin-6 involvement in mesothelioma pathobiology: inhibition by interferon alpha immunotherapy. Cancer Immunol Immunother. 1995;40(4):241–50.

97. Monti G, Jaurand MC, Monnet I, Chretien P, Saint-Etienne L, Zeng L, et al. Intrapleural production of interleukin 6 during mesothelioma and its modulation by gamma-interferon treatment. Cancer Res. 1994;54(16):4419–23.
98. Nakano T, Chahinian AP, Shinjo M, Tonomura A, Miyake M, Togawa N, et al. Interleukin 6 and its relationship to clinical parameters in patients with malignant pleural mesothelioma. Br J Cancer. 1998;77(6):907–12.
99. Schmitter D, Lauber B, Fagg B, Stahel RA. Hematopoietic growth factors secreted by seven human pleural mesothelioma cell lines: interleukin-6 production as a common feature. Int J Cancer. 1992;51(2):296–301.
100. Adachi Y, Aoki C, Yoshio-Hoshino N, Takayama K, Curiel DT, Nishimoto N. Interleukin-6 induces both cell growth and VEGF production in malignant mesotheliomas. Int J Cancer. 2006;119(6):1303–11.
101. Adachi Y, Yoshio-Hoshino N, Aoki C, Nishimoto N. VEGF targeting in mesotheliomas using an interleukin-6 signal inhibitor based on adenovirus gene delivery. Anticancer Res. 2010;30(6):1947–52.
102. Kao SC-H, Harvie R, Paturi F, Taylor R, Davey R, Abraham R, et al. The predictive role of serum VEGF in an advanced malignant mesothelioma patient cohort treated with thalidomide alone or combined with cisplatin/gemcitabine. Lung Cancer. 2012;75(2):248–54.
103. Abdul Rahim SN, Ho GY, Coward JI. The role of interleukin-6 in malignant mesothelioma. Transl Lung Cancer Res. 2015;4(1):55–66.
104. Gueugnon F, Leclercq S, Blanquart C, Sagan C, Cellerin L, Padieu M, et al. Identification of novel markers for the diagnosis of malignant pleural mesothelioma. Am J Pathol. 2011;178(3):1033–42.
105. Thomas R, Cheah HM, Creaney J, Turlach BA, Lee YC. Longitudinal measurement of pleural fluid biochemistry and cytokines in malignant pleural effusions. Chest. 2016;149(6):1494–500.
106. Mantovani A, Savino B, Locati M, Zammataro L, Allavena P, Bonecchi R. The chemokine system in cancer biology and therapy. Cytokine Growth Factor Rev. 2010;21(1):27–39.
107. Brinkmann V, Reichard U, Goosmann C, Fauler B, Uhlemann Y, Weiss DS, et al. Neutrophil extracellular traps kill bacteria. Science. 2004;303(5663):1532–5.
108. Ostrand-Rosenberg S. Immune surveillance: a balance between protumor and antitumor immunity. Curr Opin Genet Dev. 2008;18(1):11–8.
109. Fridlender ZG, Sun J, Mishalian I, Singhal S, Cheng G, Kapoor V, et al. Transcriptomic analysis comparing tumor-associated neutrophils with granulocytic myeloid-derived suppressor cells and normal neutrophils. PLoS One. 2012;7(2):e31524.
110. Haegens A, Barrett TF, Gell J, Shukla A, Macpherson M, Vacek P, et al. Airway epithelial NF-kappaB activation modulates asbestos-induced inflammation and mucin production in vivo. J Immunol. 2007;178(3):1800–8.
111. Hillegass JM, Shukla A, Lathrop SA, MacPherson MB, Beuschel SL, Butnor KJ, et al. Inflammation precedes the development of human malignant mesotheliomas in a SCID mouse xenograft model. Ann N Y Acad Sci. 2010;1203:7–14.
112. Galffy G, Mohammed KA, Nasreen N, Ward MJ, Antony VB. Inhibition of interleukin-8 reduces human malignant pleural mesothelioma propagation in nude mouse model. Oncol Res. 1999;11(4):187–94.
113. di Martino S, Amoreo CA, Nuvoli B, Galati R, Strano S, Facciolo F, et al. HSP90 inhibition alters the chemotherapy-driven rearrangement of the oncogenic secretome. Oncogene. 2018;37(10):1369–85.
114. Antony VB, Hott JW, Godbey SW, Holm K. Angiogenesis in mesotheliomas: role of mesothelial cell derived IL-8. Chest. 1996;109(3, Supplement):21S–2S.
115. Galffy G, Mohammed KA, Dowling PA, Nasreen N, Ward MJ, Antony VB. Interleukin 8: an autocrine growth factor for malignant mesothelioma. Cancer Res. 1999;59(2):367–71.
116. Canino C, Mori F, Cambria A, Diamantini A, Germoni S, Alessandrini G, et al. SASP mediates chemoresistance and tumor-initiating-activity of mesothelioma cells. Oncogene. 2012;31(26):3148–63.
117. Wiseman BS, Werb Z. Stromal effects on mammary gland development and breast cancer. Science. 2002;296(5570):1046–9.
118. Kalluri R. The biology and function of fibroblasts in cancer. Nat Rev Cancer. 2016;16(9):582–98.
119. Li Q, Wang W, Yamada T, Matsumoto K, Sakai K, Bando Y, et al. Pleural mesothelioma instigates tumor-associated fibroblasts to promote progression via a malignant cytokine network. Am J Pathol. 2011;179(3):1483–93.
120. Lo A, Wang LS, Scholler J, Monslow J, Avery D, Newick K, et al. Tumor-promoting desmoplasia is disrupted by depleting FAP-expressing stromal cells. Cancer Res. 2015;75(14):2800–10.
121. Comar M, Zanotta N, Zanconati F, Cortale M, Bonotti A, Cristaudo A, et al. Chemokines involved in the early inflammatory response and in pro-tumoral activity in asbestos-exposed workers from an Italian coastal area with territorial clusters of pleural malignant mesothelioma. Lung Cancer. 2016;94:61–7.
122. Rizwan M, Ajay K, SuTao Z, Guangbin X, Pierluigi S, Lynne SD, et al. Malignant mesothelioma growth inhibition by agents that target the VEGF and VEGF-C autocrine loops. Int J Cancer. 2003;104(5):603–10.
123. Strizzi L, Catalano A, Vianale G, Orecchia S, Casalini A, Tassi G, et al. Vascular endothelial growth factor is an autocrine growth factor in human malignant mesothelioma. J Pathol. 2001;193(4):468–75.
124. Van TT, Hanibuchi M, Goto H, Kuramoto T, Yukishige S, Kakiuchi S, et al. SU6668, a multiple tyrosine kinase inhibitor, inhibits progression of

human malignant pleural mesothelioma in an orthotopic model. Respirology. 2012;17(6):984–90.
125. Safi A, Sadmi M, Martinet N, Menard O, Vaillant P, Gallati H, et al. Presence of elevated levels of platelet-derived growth factor (PDGF) in lung adenocarcinoma pleural effusions. Chest. 1992;102(1):204–7.
126. Edwards JG, Cox G, Andi A, Jones JL, Walker RA, Waller DA, et al. Angiogenesis is an independent prognostic factor in malignant mesothelioma. Br J Cancer. 2001;85(6):863–8.
127. Wang LC, Lo A, Scholler J, Sun J, Majumdar RS, Kapoor V, et al. Targeting fibroblast activation protein in tumor stroma with chimeric antigen receptor T cells can inhibit tumor growth and augment host immunity without severe toxicity. Cancer Immunol Res. 2014;2(2):154–66.
128. Meerang M, Berard K, Felley-Bosco E, Lauk O, Vrugt B, Boss A, et al. Antagonizing the hedgehog pathway with vismodegib impairs malignant pleural mesothelioma growth in vivo by affecting stroma. Mol Cancer Ther. 2016;15(5):1095–105.
129. Moses HL, Roberts AB, Derynck R. The discovery and early days of TGF-beta: a historical perspective. Cold Spring Harb Perspect Biol. 2016;8(7):a021865.
130. Akhurst RJ, Hata A. Targeting the TGFbeta signalling pathway in disease. Nat Rev Drug Discov. 2012;11(10):790–811.
131. Pickup M, Novitskiy S, Moses HL. The roles of TGFbeta in the tumour microenvironment. Nat Rev Cancer. 2013;13(11):788–99.
132. Nishimura Y, Maeda M, Kumagai-Takei N, Lee S, Matsuzaki H, Wada Y, et al. Altered functions of alveolar macrophages and NK cells involved in asbestos-related diseases. Environ Health Prev Med. 2013;18(3):198–204.
133. Li C, Rezov V, Joensuu E, Vartiainen V, Ronty M, Yin M, et al. Pirfenidone decreases mesothelioma cell proliferation and migration via inhibition of ERK and AKT and regulates mesothelioma tumor microenvironment in vivo. Sci Rep. 2018;8(1):10070.
134. Stevenson JP, Kindler HL, Papasavvas E, Sun J, Jacobs-Small M, Hull J, et al. Immunological effects of the TGFbeta-blocking antibody GC1008 in malignant pleural mesothelioma patients. Oncoimmunology. 2013;2(8):e26218.
135. Fedarko NS, Jain A, Karadag A, Van Eman MR, Fisher LW. Elevated serum bone sialoprotein and osteopontin in colon, breast, prostate, and lung cancer. Clin Cancer Res. 2001;7(12):4060–6.
136. Shevde LA, Samant RS. Role of osteopontin in the pathophysiology of cancer. Matrix Biol. 2014;37:131–41.
137. Robinson BW, Creaney J, Lake R, Nowak A, Musk AW, de Klerk N, et al. Soluble mesothelin-related protein--a blood test for mesothelioma. Lung Cancer. 2005;49(Suppl 1):S109–11.
138. Pass HI, Lott D, Lonardo F, Harbut M, Liu Z, Tang N, et al. Asbestos exposure, pleural mesothelioma, and serum osteopontin levels. N Engl J Med. 2005;353(15):1564–73.
139. Arnold DT, De Fonseka D, Hamilton FW, Rahman NM, Maskell NA. Prognostication and monitoring of mesothelioma using biomarkers: a systematic review. Br J Cancer. 2017;116(6):731–41.

Preclinical Models in Mesothelioma

6

Ilaria Fuso Nerini and Roberta Frapolli

6.1 Introduction

Malignant mesothelioma (MM) is a highly aggressive cancer whose pathogenesis is related to asbestos exposure. The combination of cisplatin and pemetrexed is the frontline therapy, but in most cases it gives only short-term responses, and there are few second-line options. Consequently, MM has a poor prognosis, and the median survival time is around 12–16 months. Increased knowledge of the molecular mechanisms of its development has prompted the design of different clinical studies addressing specific targets, but the impact on patients' long-term survival is minimal. Only the addition of bevacizumab to the first-line regimen has given a slight but significant survival gain of 2–3 months [1]. The benefits with immunotherapy have been disappointing, and although immune checkpoint inhibitors are considered an option for second-line therapy, their efficacy remains unproven [2]. There is therefore a pressing need for novel treatments for MM.

Studies in MM patients present some difficulties, for the following main reasons:

1. MM is a rare tumor, so few patients can be enrolled in randomized clinical trials.
2. Invasive procedures are required for sampling neoplastic lesions, limiting the possibility of collecting specimens during tumor evolution and/or drug response.
3. The peculiar growth pattern of MM, together with the presence of fibrosis, pleural thickening, and pleural effusion, makes evaluation of the clinical response a challenge because of the difficulties in quantifying the tumor burden.

Preclinical studies are therefore needed to deepen our understanding of the disease. Despite some intrinsic limitations, experimental models can reproduce the main features of MM and thus give us the possibility to fill some gaps of knowledge related to its pathogenesis, molecular lesions, and microenvironment complexity. They can also be useful to identify prognostic/predictive biomarkers and test new therapeutic strategies.

Here we present an overview of the reported *in vitro* and *in vivo* preclinical models of MM with particular focus on their advantages and challenges. We give our critical view of the potential applications and limitations of each model when extrapolations to the clinic are made, since the choice of the best models for each experiment is crucial to obtain reliable data. Additional material on this topic can be found in the reviews published by Singh [3] and Robinson [4].

I. Fuso Nerini · R. Frapolli (✉)
Department of Oncology, Istituto di Ricerche Farmacologiche Mario Negri IRCCS, Milan, Italy
e-mail: ilaria.fusonerini@marionegri.it; roberta.frapolli@marionegri.it

G. L. Ceresoli et al. (eds.), *Mesothelioma*, https://doi.org/10.1007/978-3-030-16884-1_6

6.2 *In Vitro* Models of Malignant Mesothelioma

6.2.1 2D Cell Cultures

Cellosaurus (http://web.expasy.org/cgi-bin/cellosaurus/search) lists 473 MM cell lines (433 of human origin, 31 mouse, 8 rat, 1 rainbow trout) on April 2019. Many other cell lines have been generated and are probably owned exclusively by the laboratory where they were developed.

6.2.1.1 Human Primary Cell Cultures

Primary cultures derive from cells taken directly from living tissue, such as surgical tumor tissue or pleural fluid. The procedure for developing primary MM cultures generally involves a few steps: (1) blending the tumor into small pieces of 1–3 mm^2, (2) optional incubation with collagenase or dispase, (3) filtering through a cell sieve, and (4) adding the single-cell suspension to culture medium with special supplements (e.g., hydrocortisone, epidermal growth factor, heparin, insulin, transferrin, selenium, and beta-mercaptoethanol, besides fetal calf serum). Subculturing is allowed only for a limited number of times (generally to expand cell numbers and remove fibroblast contamination) for about 15 population doublings, with a culture life-span of approximately 1 month. Other preparation methods involve the isolation of cells with epithelial-like morphology from the tumor mass by mechanical scraping and their selection by differential attachment [5].

Spontaneous immortalization of MM primary cultures is very frequent, even more than other tumor types. Stable cell lines have an almost unlimited growth potential. They are one of the tools of choice for preclinical research due to the easy handling and high-throughput capacity and are useful for studying the mechanisms of tumor progression, aggressiveness, and drug response.

Characterizing these cell lines is necessary to confirm maintenance of the original tumor subtype, which must be monitored over time. The characterization generally comprises the analysis of immunoreactivity to typical MM markers (e.g., mesothelin, calretinin, 5T4, podoplanin, cytokeratins, and HBME1), karyotyping, and/or short tandem repeat/single-nucleotide polymorphism analysis. Further characterization includes human leucocyte antigen typing, scanning electron microscopy, or whole exome sequencing.

Important efforts have been made to develop large collections of stable MM cell cultures. They have often been run in parallel with the establishment of tissue biobanks (bioresources of MM tissue and blood, linked to a detailed clinical database), given the availability of biopsy samples. The UK MesobanK is the result of a national effort in the UK that has led to the collection of 26 primary MM cultures (http://www.mesobank.com) [6]. Oehl et al. have established 159 primary cultures from human MM samples [7].

6.2.1.2 Human Cell Lines Induced by *In Vitro* Transformation

The main challenge in the development of new MM *in vitro* models is selecting the most suitable starting biological material. Although this is a common problem for many other tumor types, it is even more difficult for MM, since its cell of origin is still uncertain. The majority of studies assume that MM originates from the pleural mesothelial cell, while some researchers believe that other cell types (e.g., mesothelial progenitor cells) are responsible for MM occurrence. The lack of general agreement on the definition of cell transformation adds difficulties in the interpretation of results.

In vitro cell transformation can be prompted by exposure to asbestos. However, the efficiency of transformation is low, because human mesothelial cells are highly sensitive and their exposure to asbestos fibers causes extensive death. Unlike asbestos, erionite is poorly cytotoxic and frequently induces transformation with long-term exposure. Other studies report that inflammatory cytokines, such as IL-1β and TNF-α, are necessary to trigger *in vitro* transformation. Co-culturing of mesothelial cells with macrophages protects them from asbestos-induced cell death and triggers the formation of 3D foci [3].

Other *in vitro* models have been developed by inducing the expression of specific oncogenes in human mesothelial cells. Current genetic engineering technologies easily allow to introduce an unlimited range of mutations. However, choosing the proper mutations that trigger cell transformation remains a big challenge because of our scant knowledge of the exact steps of MM pathogenesis.

- MeT-5A cells have been obtained by transfection of mesothelial cells from pleural fluids of non-cancerous individuals with a plasmid containing simian virus 40 (SV40) large T antigen [8]. The SV40 protein directly inhibits p53 and Rb tumor suppressor pathways. The viral gene can accelerate the cell cycle of mesothelial cells, but is not sufficient to transform them. MeT-5A cells can undergo 60–70 population doublings before senescence, with a culture life-span of approximately 5–6 months. They are sensitive to the cytotoxic effects of asbestos fibers and are non-tumorigenic in mice.
- Some models of MM oncogenesis involve introducing additional mutations in MeT-5A cells, thus supporting the hypothesis that multiple, instead of single, molecular steps are required to produce a malignant phenotype. EJ-ras cells have been generated by introduction of a constitutively activated isoform of p21 ras oncogene in MeT-5A and can form tumors in nude mice. MeT-5A cells also become tumorigenic by transfection with the growth factor PDGFA, whose autocrine signaling has an important role in the malignancy of MM. A chimeric protein disrupting a DNA methyltransferase complex DNMT1/PCNA/ubiquitin-like could induce a tumorigenic phenotype in MeT-5A cells, probably as a consequence of global DNA hypomethylation [3].
- LP-9 cells are peritoneal normal mesothelial cells and have been extensively characterized [9]. They have been used as starting material to prepare novel MM models by introducing or overexpressing oncogenes (e.g., *TERT1*, the catalytic component of telomerase). Some omental mesothelial cell lines have been established by retroviral transduction with both human papillomavirus 16 E6/E7 and *TERT* genes [5].

6.2.1.3 Murine Cell Lines

Similarly to human cell lines, immortalized murine mesothelial cells include cells isolated from spontaneous MM or generated by *in vitro* transformation of mouse primary mesothelial cells [10]. These cell lines present the phenotypical and functional features of MM and have been used for *in vitro* assays or implanted in immunocompetent mice of the same genotype for *in vivo* studies. AB1, AB12, AB22, 40, 40L, AE17, and AK7 cells were derived from spontaneously arising MM in wild-type mice injected intraperitoneally with asbestos [11–13]. TGM cell series (e.g., TGM299h, TGM304i, TGM270i, TGM266i) originated from SV40 TAg transgenic mice [14]. iMESO are SV40-immortalized cell lines derived from wild-type and NF2-mutated mice that showed anchorage-independent growth but that are not tumorigenic in mice. RN5 cells originate from an Nf2+/− mouse exposed repeatedly to crocidolite. They have persistent growth *in vitro* and are highly tumorigenic *in vivo* [15].

Sheddon et al. recently characterized the mutational landscape of 15 murine MM cell lines derived from different murine strains using whole exome sequencing. They analyzed somatic mutations and copy number variations and concluded that murine MM has a similar mutation rate to human MM [16].

6.2.2 3D Cell Cultures

3D cell cultures offer an evolution of *in vitro* cancer modeling and originate from the effort to develop a more accurate system to reproduce the *in vivo* features of MM better. Spheroids are used to model more realistic cellular junctions between epithelial cells and interactions between tumor cells and extracellular matrix. From the exterior to the center of spheroids, gradients of nutrient concentration and cell proliferation form spontaneously. Central necrosis and regions of hypoxia often develop, thus naturally mimicking small avascular tumors. Even drug diffusion kinetics can be partially reproduced within spheroids.

Different 3D models have been developed:

- *Spheroids* have been developed by seeding cell suspensions on 3D structures made of artificial matrix (e.g., polyHEMA). Cells are immortalized cell lines or primary cultures. Mazzocchi et al. recently obtained a collection of MM organoids incorporating patient-derived tumor cells that showed high cellular heterogeneity and variable responses to chemotherapy, in line with the clinical evolution of the original tumors [17].
- *Tumor fragment spheroids* (TFS) are an *ex vivo* model of living tumor. Small fragments of the original tumor tissue are allowed to grow into 3D structures. Tumor cells can form spheroids without an artificial matrix, exploiting the cells' ability to produce and self-organize complex ECM structures and cell-cell interactions. Similarly to the original tumor, cells in TFS are highly genetically or epigenetically heterogeneous. In some cases, the TFS contain viable tumor cells for weeks to months, while the cells disaggregated from the same tumors failed to proliferate [18, 19]. Large global gene expression profiling on 2D and 3D cultures of the same MM cell line served to identify the genes (mainly related to Warburg effect) that are specific to the 3D biological structure of tumors [20].
- *Organ-on-a-chip* is an innovative technology based on the integration of bioengineering with microfluidics to mimic *in vivo* conditions better. Besides 3D architecture and cell-cell/cell-matrix interactions, these platforms can combine complex parameters, such as circulation. Multiple tissues can be seeded within one platform thus allowing to investigate the interactions between cancer cells and different host tissues [17, 21].

6.2.3 Applications for *In Vitro* Malignant Mesothelioma Models

In vitro models are fast, reproducible, economical and can be easily genetically manipulated. Therefore they are used in numerous applications of basic and translational research. For example, different *in vitro* assays are used to investigate the role of specific genes or pathways in MM pathogenesis and aggressiveness. Thus a mutated protein with driver activity in MM could be investigated as a possible target for novel pharmacological therapies. Cell cultures are also used for high-throughput drug screening, to assess the efficacy of experimental compounds or combinations. Similarly, mechanisms of action of drugs can be deeply investigated. Another application of *in vitro* MM models is the identification of novel prognostic/predictive biomarkers. In this case, molecules that confer sensitivity or resistance to drugs can only be definitely validated correlating their levels in tumor biopsies with clinical outcome. However, *in vitro* studies serve to screen the response of tumor cells to multiple drug treatments, which is not feasible in the clinical setting. Potentially, co-clinical *in vitro* models (primary 2D or 3D cell cultures) for each patient can be developed, to help predict the individual response to anticancer drugs. Cell lines from the same patient at different stages during disease progression can be useful to study the mechanisms of pharmacological resistance.

Advantages and challenges of the different models are summarized in Table 6.1. *In vitro* studies reduce the need for animal experiments, in keeping with the 3R policy first described by

Table 6.1 Summary of the main pros and cons of *in vitro* MM models and their main applications in preclinical research

		Advantages	Disadvantages	Main applications
2D cell cultures	Primary cell cultures	• Cost-effective • Easy downstream processing • Same genotype as the parent tissue; not "dedifferentiated" • Absolute control of physical environment	• Relatively short life-span in culture • Very susceptible to contamination • Low reproducibility; considerable variation in population and between preparations • Homogeneous distribution of nutrients, waste, and drugs • Lack of 3D structure; reduced cell-to-cell interactions; unnatural substrate	Investigation of the role of genes in MM progression Testing novel therapeutic options against MM Study of the mechanisms of action of specific drugs against MM Identification and/or validation of novel prognostic/predictive biomarkers
	Cell lines induced by *in vitro* transformation	• Cost-effective • Easy to maintain • Easy downstream processing • High-throughput capacity • Absolute control of physical environment • Easy genetic manipulation	• Cells change over time in culture (genotypic and phenotypic drifting) • Lack of cellular heterogeneity/complexity similar to the original tumor; less biologically relevant models • Lack of 3D structure; reduced cell-to-cell interactions; unnatural substrate • Complex mechanisms of cancer biology (e.g., angiogenesis, metastasis, interstitial fluid pressure, interactions with mesothelial lining, immune infiltration) cannot be reproduced • Homogeneous distribution of nutrients, waste, and drugs • Co-culture unable to establish a microenvironment	
3D cell cultures	Spheroids from cell lines, tumor fragment spheroids, organ-on-a-chip	• More accurate representation of the *in vivo* scenario; better reflects cell differentiation, polarization, cell behavior • Gene expression profile more similar to *in vivo* tumors • Increased cell-to-cell and cell-to-extracellular matrix signaling • Co-culture of multiple cells mimics microenvironment better • Heterogeneous distribution of nutrients, waste, and drug • More predictive drug response than 2D cell cultures	• Added expense • Complex culture system • Complex downstream processing	Analysis of gene function in cancer progression Study of cell-to-cell and cell-to-matrix interactions Study of therapeutic efficacy of anticancer drugs and combinations Identification and/or validation of novel prognostic/predictive biomarkers

Russell and Burch in 1959 [22]. They can be considered complementary approaches to animal testing, although not true alternatives. A major problem is that many of the existing immortalized lines were generated a number of years ago and no longer represent original tumors. Cell lines maintained *in vitro* may suffer selective stress due to the necessity for growth without the tumor microenvironment. As a consequence they lose the typical heterogeneity of the human cancer and may experience a genetic drift different from the primary tumors. This is an important hindrance to *in vitro* studies using cell cultures and, together with the absence of proper tumor-stroma interactions, limits the predictivity of clinical trial results.

6.3 *In Vivo* Models of Malignant Mesothelioma

6.3.1 Asbestos-Induced Models

The first epidemiological studies suggesting a relationship between the risk of MM and asbestos exposure date back to the 1960s [23, 24]. Since then a number of preclinical studies have been done to unravel the pathogenic mechanisms behind MM. Various animal species were exposed to asbestos fibers by inhalation [25–27] or by intrapleural/intratracheal/intraperitoneal injections [28–32]. Inhalation is the most representative route since human exposure mainly occurs through breathing. However, the experimental procedures are expensive and potentially hazardous for researchers and the environment. Moreover, the efficiency in inducing MM is low compared to the other routes (about 5% vs 25–98%, respectively). On the other hand, intrapleural, intratracheal, and intraperitoneal injections introduce asbestos through an unnatural route, exposing mesothelial cells to local concentrations of fibers higher than those reached with human exposure. Despite this disadvantage, the intraperitoneal route allows the easiest delivery and has been widely used to test the carcinogenic potential of different asbestos fibers. Peritoneal MM accounts for about 10% of MM and shares the same pathogenesis and poor drug sensitivity with the more common pleural MM. Studies in rats indicated that the length of the fibers is directly related to their tumorigenicity [11, 33–35]. MM occurs in 56–97.5% of exposed rats, depending on the dose and type of fiber, with all the possible morphological patterns (i.e., tubular, papillary, solid, and spindle cell) observed in humans [35, 36].

Studies in mice after intraperitoneal injection of asbestos substantially confirm the relationship between fiber length and the carcinogenic effect. In this species the incidence of MM after asbestos exposure ranged between 25% and 45%, with a latency of about 7 months [37, 38]. In BALB/c and CBA mice, Davis et al. reported the formation of thick, hemorrhagic ascites and in some cases solid masses in the peritoneum. The cytological and ultrastructural characterization of the serous effusions identified all three histological subtypes of MM (epithelioid, biphasic, and sarcomatoid) with a relatively high frequency of epithelioid. The malignant cells were also cultured *in vitro* and established as continuous cell lines that were tumorigenic when reinoculated in syngeneic mice [38].

Asbestos-induced models use the same carcinogen as in humans resulting in a similar development process, anatomical localization, and morphology, thus reproducing the human disease well. Nevertheless, the low penetrance and the long lag time make these models hard to use for pharmacological studies.

6.3.2 Xenograft Models

MM xenografts were obtained by injecting human MM cells into immunocompromised mice, such as nude, SCID, or NOD/SCID mice, to avoid the rejection of the foreign tissue. Cells can be injected subcutis or orthotopically into the pleural or peritoneal cavity. These models produce MM in a higher percentage of mice than asbestos-induced models, and the tumors maintain most of the molecular and histological features of the human disease.

The establishment of xenograft models of human MM was first described by Chahinian et al. [39]. They obtained fresh tumor specimens from three MM patients and transplanted them in BALB/c nude mice, subcutaneously or intraperitoneally. No tumor growth was seen in the peritoneum, whereas a 65% success rate was reached with the subcutaneous graft. Histological examinations of the transplanted tumors revealed similar characteristics to those of the original tumors.

In 1991 the first human MM cell lines were established from pleural effusions [40], laying the foundations for a number of transplantable xenograft models. However, the subcutaneous tissues do not adequately reproduce the serous cavities, so more suitable models were obtained inoculating MM cells intraperitoneally [41–43]. The possibility to perform orthotopic implantation of human-derived specimens through a thoracotomy was then described [44, 45]. The tumors reproduced the clinical behavior of MM in humans well, with extensive spread in the ipsilateral and contralateral pleural cavities and mediastinal lymph nodes. However, surgical implantation of the tumor may cause inflammation, tissue repair processes, and fibrosis, possibly interfering with the graft due to the production of cytokines and growth factors. To avoid these problems, less invasive transthoracic injections of MM cells were done in nude rats [46] and mice [47, 48]. Both models maintained the pathological and clinical features of human MM.

Overall, xenografts are good tools for preclinical pharmacological screening, but these models have to be selected bearing in mind the following aspects:

- Long-term passaging of cell lines reduces heterogeneity and leads to genetic drift caused by genomic instability, hampering the ability of the preclinical models to accurately mimic clinical MM. Patient-derived xenografts, in which human tumor specimens were engrafted directly in immunocompromised mice, address this problem [49].
- The lack of a fully proficient immune system may lead to an altered tumor microenvironment. Tumor-infiltrating immune cells produce cytokines, chemokines, proteases, and other bioactive molecules (reactive oxygen species, histamine, nitric oxide) that can influence tissue remodeling and new vessel formation, affecting tumor growth, metastasis, and response to chemotherapy [50]. This last point is the main drawback of the xenograft approach, especially considering the growing importance of immunotherapy in oncology.

6.3.3 Syngeneic Models

Syngeneic models of MM were obtained by subcutaneous or orthotopic injection of murine MM cell lines into host mice with the same genetic background (same inbred mouse strain). The establishment of MM cell lines from murine MM was first described in 1992. They were obtained from ascites of asbestos-exposed BALB/c (i.e., AB1, AB2, AB12, AB13, and AB22 cell lines) and CBA (i.e., AC14, AC16, AC28, AC29, AC31, AC32, and AC34 cell lines) mice. All three histotypes (epithelial, biphasic, and sarcomatoid) were observed with a prevalence of the epithelioid form, as in human patients [38]. These cell lines were tumorigenic when injected in mice, giving highly reproducible models growing in immunocompetent mice [38]. Additional models (40, 40L, AE17, and AK7) were described in C57BL/6 mice [12, 51, 52].

Extensive characterization of the AB, AC, and AE cell series *in vitro* and *in vivo* supports the use of these models for preclinical pharmacological studies [13, 16].

The ability of these preclinical models to reproduce the human disease in the context of a fully proficient immune system offers a way to investigate therapeutic strategies targeting not only the neoplastic cells but also the complex microenvironment. Using syngeneic models of peritoneal MM, Miselis and colleagues clearly demonstrated the contribution of tumor-associated macrophages (TAMs) to tumor growth, invasion, and metastasis [53]. Dynamic mechanisms too have been proposed, by which progressive accumulation of host immune and stromal cells and expression of inflammatory mediators support tumor progression [54, 55].

6.3.4 Genetically Engineered Models

Less than 10% of people exposed to asbestos develop MM, suggesting that additional factors are needed for its pathogenesis. Genetically this neoplasm is characterized by frequent somatic lesions, mainly in the *NF2*, *CDKN2a/ARF*, and *BAP-1* loci which are recognized as the main drivers of tumorigenesis [56]. Introducing genetic alterations in the mouse genome has led to the development of transgenic mice as animal models for MM studies.

Mutations of the *p53* tumor suppressor gene are rarely reported in MM; nevertheless, *p53*-deficient mice showed a higher incidence and faster tumor progression than wild-type mice [57, 58].

Altomare et al. described a mouse model obtained by exposing heterozygous *Nf2*$^{(+/-)}$ mice to repeated asbestos treatments. They observed higher susceptibility to MM, with an incidence of 85% in *Nf2*$^{(+/-)}$ and 59% in *Nf2*$^{(+/+)}$ mice and mean survival time of 44 and 56 weeks, respectively. The tumors recapitulated the main molecular features of the human disease including activation of Akt; homozygous deletion of the tumor suppressor genes *p16(Ink4A)*, *p14 (ARF)/p19(Arf)*, and *p15(Ink4B)*; and loss of the *Nf2* protein/Merlin [59].

Ink4a$^{(+/-)}$, *Arf*$^{(+/-)}$, and *Ink4a;Arf*$^{(+/-)}$ genetically modified mice were used to examine the impact of these mutations on MM development after asbestos exposure, showing that the inactivation of *Arf* but not of *Ink4a* may be required for the pathogenesis of MM. In heterozygous *Ink4a;Arf*$^{(+/-)}$ mice, biallelic inactivation of the two tumor suppressor genes after asbestos exposure was observed, together with accelerated tumorigenesis, in accordance with the data obtained in a conditional mouse model of MM in which the adeno-Cre-mediated homozygous loss of *Ink4a* and *Arf* caused MM without asbestos exposure [60].

BAP1 somatic mutations were first reported in MM in 2011 [61]. The same year germline mutations of *BAP1* were discovered in two US families with a high incidence of MM after modest levels of asbestos exposure [62]. Germline mutations of *BAP1* were observed also in a European family with four cases of MM without any known exposure to asbestos [63], thus leading to the idea that *BAP1* mutation may drive MM development even without exposure to the carcinogen. Three different heterozygous *Bap1* mouse models were generated (a *Bap1*-null model and two knock-in models carrying mutations analogous to those reported in the two US families). Overall, these mutants shared an increased susceptibility to MM after peritoneal injection of asbestos. The incidence of MM was double and the median survival time shorter in *Bap1*-mutants than wild-type mice. Without asbestos exposure, spontaneous tumors were observed in about two-thirds of *Bap1* mice, but only two developed MM, supporting the fundamental role of the interaction between genes and environment in MM pathogenesis [64].

These genetically modified models have given further knowledge of the MM pathogenesis, development, and molecular biology, but they are not suitable for pharmacological studies because of the high incidence of spontaneous unrelated tumors and the incomplete penetrance of MM that does not occur in all the animals. To overcome these problems, Robinson et al. generated the MexTAg mice, specifically expressing the large T antigen of SV40 in mesothelial cells. After asbestos exposure, all these mice developed MM, with a very low incidence of other tumors, so they are suitable for testing new therapeutic or chemopreventive strategies [65].

6.3.5 *In Vivo* Imaging of Orthotopic Models

Subcutaneous tumors can be easily monitored using a caliper giving an immediate estimate of the tumor growth and consequently of drug response. This is not possible for orthotopic models where the tumor burden could only be evaluated at autopsy.

In recent years the development of imaging techniques suitable for small animals, such as computed tomography, positron emission tomography (PET), magnetic resonance imaging (MRI), and optical imaging, has made possible to measure tumor growth in orthotopic models overcoming one of the main disadvantages of these models, which is, of course, that one cannot measure tumor growth directly as in the subcutaneous models.

The first attempt to follow the tumor growth after intrathoracic injection of MM cells in rats used chest X-ray analysis to confirm the occurrence of the disease and to detect pulmonary and pleural abnormalities. A radiographic score was applied and correlated with the clinical status of the animals [46]. More recently, PET has been used to image tumor growth in preclinical MM models [66, 67]. Unfortunately, despite its translational potential from small animals to humans, this technique requires expensive equipment and a cyclotron for radionuclide production limiting its application to facilities associated with clinical centers. Optical imaging can visualize tumor growth by detecting fluorescent or luminescent signals from tumor cells genetically modified to express luciferase or fluorescent proteins. Although this approach is not translationable to the clinic, optical imaging is more suitable for small laboratories since it is more cost-effective and allows rapid and sensitive imaging. Different models of MM were established that can be visualized with bioluminescence [68, 69] or fluorescence [70]. An interesting approach was described by Meerang et al. combining bioluminescence and MRI, the latter providing reliable quantification of the tumor burden together with anatomical information [71].

6.3.6 Applications for *In Vivo* Malignant Mesothelioma Models

MM has a complex microenvironment, with a complicated network between tumor cells, stromal cells, and infiltrating immune cells. Cytokines and growth factors reciprocally influence the behavior of the different cell populations, resulting in a very aggressive and poorly chemosensitive neoplasm. Vázquez et al. observed a discrepancy between the *in vitro* and *in vivo* sensitivity of human MM models, further supporting the important role of the tumor microenvironment [72]. Therefore animal models are needed to study the mechanism of the pathogenesis of MM, the contribution of genetic mutation and inflammation to tumor progression, and new therapeutic or chemopreventive strategies. Animal models are also used to confirm biomarkers or molecular targets identified *in vitro,* before their clinical validation. The animal models described here, with their advantages, disadvantages, and main applications, are summarized in Table 6.2.

Table 6.2 Summary of the main pros and cons of MM animal models and their main application in preclinical research

		Advantages	Disadvantages	Main applications
Transplantable models	*Site of inoculum*			
	Subcutaneous	• Easy grafting procedure • Easy assessment of tumor growth	• Different microenvironment • No metastasis • Drug response may be different from orthotopic models	*Pharmacological studies*: efficacy, pharmacokinetic, and pharmacodynamic evaluation Identification of predictive biomarkers (xenograft models) Development of new immunotherapies (syngeneic models)
	Orthotopic	• Anatomical site that allows more patient-like tumor growth and dissemination • Microenvironment more similar to the clinic • Pleural effusion or ascites may occur	• Technical procedure for intrapleural grafting may be difficult and risky • Impossible to measure tumor size directly • Needs of *in vivo* imaging techniques to follow tumor growth	
	Animal background			
	Cell line-derived xenografts	• Human cell lines maintain most of the molecular features of the human tumor. • Reproducible tumor growth	• Immortalized cell lines may lose the heterogeneity typical of human tumors • Long-term culturing may lead to a genetic drift, limiting clinical predictivity • Immunocompromised host does not fully reproduce the complex tumor microenvironment	
	Patient-derived xenografts (PDX)	• Maintain the main histological features of the human disease, even the stromal component • The heterogeneity of the original tumor is at least partly preserved • Less genetic drift	• Establishment of PDX biobank is expensive and time-consuming • Progressive drift from primarily human to primarily mouse stroma component • Immunocompromised host	
	Syngeneic	• Rapid and reproducible tumor growth • Fully immunocompetent host	• *In vitro* immortalized cell lines • Response to therapy may be different from that of human mesotheliomas	

Table 6.2 (continued)

<table>
<tr><th></th><th></th><th>Advantages</th><th>Disadvantages</th><th>Main applications</th></tr>
<tr><td rowspan="2">Asbestos-induced models</td><td>Wild-type background</td><td>• Use of the same carcinogen as in humans
• The tumors reproduce the morphology, growth pattern, and clinical behavior of the human disease</td><td>• Low incidence and very long latency
• Need of in vivo imaging techniques to follow tumor growth
• Possible development of some other cancer type depending of the site of asbestos injection</td><td rowspan="2">Test the carcinogenicity of asbestos and asbestos-like fibers
Understanding the pathogenic mechanisms of mesothelioma
Identify early biomarkers of mesothelioma
Study the genetic contribution to mesothelioma development
Chemopreventive studies
Pharmacological studies (MexTAg model)</td></tr>
<tr><td>Genetically modified background</td><td>• Use of the same carcinogen as in humans
• The tumors reproduce the morphology, growth pattern, and clinical behavior of the human disease
• Higher incidence (up to 100% in MexTAg mice) and shorter lag time than wild-type mice
• Reproduce some of the most common genetic lesions observed in human mesothelioma</td><td>• Needs of in vivo imaging techniques to follow tumor growth
• Occurrence of spontaneous cancers (model-dependent)
• Response to therapy may be different from that of human mesotheliomas</td></tr>
</table>

6.4 Conclusions

Several preclinical models of MM are available *in vitro* and *in vivo,* each with its strengths and limitations. The intrinsic inability of models to adequately reproduce tumor heterogeneity and/or the tumor microenvironment, together with our inadequate knowledge of the genomic and epigenetic alterations of MM, is the main reason for the broad gap between the good results in some preclinical models and the poor outcomes in clinical studies.

While continuing our efforts to obtain optimal preclinical tools, full characterization of MM patients and *in vitro/in vivo* models is mandatory to permit correlations with drug responses. New technologies are now available that help unravel the molecular alterations behind this disease and the complex links between the neoplastic cells and the host components that appear to be vital for the clinical behavior of MM. In addition, more research is needed to clarify the mechanisms behind the chemoresistance of MM *in vivo* that could be also related to pharmacokinetic factors, such as insufficient or heterogeneous drug distribution in the tumor tissue [73].

At the moment, given the absence of "perfect" MM models, specific attention must be paid to the selection of the right test systems to be used on the basis of the research hypothesis. As a general suggestion, the experimental data should be reproduced in multiple models in order to compensate their unavoidable shortcomings, thus verifying the strength and clinical relevance of the obtained results.

Acknowledgements Our preclinical work on MM is supported by Fondazione Buzzi Unicem. We gratefully acknowledge Maurizio D'Incalci for suggestions and critically reading the manuscript.

References

1. Zalcman G, Mazieres J, Margery J, Greillier L, Audigier-Valette C, Moro-Sibilot D, et al. Bevacizumab for newly diagnosed pleural mesothelioma in the Mesothelioma Avastin Cisplatin Pemetrexed Study (MAPS): a randomised, controlled, open-label, phase 3 trial. Lancet. 2016;387:1405–14.
2. McCambridge AJ, Napolitano A, Mansfield AS, Fennell DA, Sekido Y, Nowak AK, et al. Progress in the management of malignant pleural mesothelioma in 2017. J Thorac Oncol. 2018;13:606–23.
3. Singh A, Pruett N, Hoang CD. In vitro experimental models of mesothelioma revisited. Transl Lung Cancer Res. 2017;6:248–58.
4. Robinson C, Solin JN, Lee YG, Lake RA, Lesterhuis WJ. Mouse models of mesothelioma: strengths, limitations and clinical translation. Lung Cancer Manag. 2014;3:397–410.
5. Kakiuchi T, Takahara T, Kasugai Y, Arita K, Yoshida N, Karube K, et al. Modeling mesothelioma utilizing human mesothelial cells reveals involvement of phospholipase-C beta 4 in YAP-active mesothelioma cell proliferation. Carcinogenesis. 2016;37:1098–109.
6. Rintoul RC, Rassl DM, Gittins J, Marciniak SJ. MesobanK UK: an international mesothelioma bioresource. Thorax. 2016;71:380–2.
7. Oehl K, Kresoja-Rakic J, Opitz I, Vrugt B, Weder W, Stahel R, et al. Live-cell mesothelioma biobank to explore mechanisms of tumor progression. Front Oncol. 2018;8:40.
8. Ke Y, Reddel RR, Gerwin BI, Reddel HK, Somers AN, McMenamin MG, et al. Establishment of a human in vitro mesothelial cell model system for investigating mechanisms of asbestos-induced mesothelioma. Am J Pathol. 1989;134:979–91.
9. Connell ND, Rheinwald JG. Regulation of the cytoskeleton in mesothelial cells: reversible loss of keratin and increase in vimentin during rapid growth in culture. Cell. 1983;34:245–53.
10. Sherwood AL, Mutsaers SE, Peeva VK, Robinson C, DeSilva CJ, Swanson NR, et al. Spontaneously immortalized mouse mesothelial cells display characteristics of malignant transformation. Cell Prolif. 2008;41:894–908.
11. Davis JM, Bolton RE, Miller BG, Niven K. Mesothelioma dose response following intraperitoneal injection of mineral fibres. Int J Exp Pathol. 1991;72:263–74.
12. Kellerman LC, Valeyrie L, Fernandez N, Opolon P, Sabourin J-C, Maubec E, et al. Regression of AK7 malignant mesothelioma established in immunocompetent mice following intratumoral gene transfer of interferon gamma. Cancer Gene Ther. 2003;10:481–90.
13. Mezzapelle R, Rrapaj E, Gatti E, Ceriotti C, Marchis FD, Preti A, et al. Human malignant mesothelioma is recapitulated in immunocompetent BALB/c mice injected with murine AB cells. Sci Rep. 2016;6:22850.
14. Robinson C, van Bruggen I, Segal A, Dunham M, Sherwood A, Koentgen F, et al. A novel SV40 TAg transgenic model of asbestos-induced mesothelioma: malignant transformation is dose dependent. Cancer Res. 2006;66:10786–94.
15. Blum W, Pecze L, Felley-Bosco E, Worthmüller-Rodriguez J, Wu L, Vrugt B, et al. Establishment of immortalized murine mesothelial cells and a novel mesothelioma cell line. In Vitro Cell Dev Biol Anim. 2015;51:714–21.
16. Sneddon S, Patch A-M, Dick IM, Kazakoff S, Pearson JV, Waddell N, et al. Whole exome sequencing of an asbestos-induced wild-type murine model of malignant mesothelioma. BMC Cancer. 2017;17:396.
17. Mazzocchi AR, Rajan SAP, Votanopoulos KI, Hall AR, Skardal A. In vitro patient-derived 3D mesothelioma tumor organoids facilitate patient-centric therapeutic screening. Sci Rep. 2018;8:2886.
18. Kim K-U, Wilson SM, Abayasiriwardana KS, Collins R, Fjellbirkeland L, Xu Z, et al. A novel in vitro model of human mesothelioma for studying tumor biology and apoptotic resistance. Am J Respir Cell Mol Biol. 2005;33:541–8.
19. Wilson SM, Barbone D, Yang T-M, Jablons DM, Bueno R, Sugarbaker DJ, et al. mTOR mediates survival signals in malignant mesothelioma grown as tumor fragment spheroids. Am J Respir Cell Mol Biol. 2008;39:576–83.
20. Kim H, Phung Y, Ho M. Changes in global gene expression associated with 3D structure of tumors: an ex vivo matrix-free mesothelioma spheroid model. PLoS One. 2012;7:e39556.
21. Huh D, Hamilton GA, Ingber DE. From three-dimensional cell culture to organs-on-chips. Trends Cell Biol. 2011;21:745–54.
22. Russell WMS, Burch RL. The principles of humane experimental technique. London: Methuen; 1959.
23. Wagner JC, Sleggs CA, Marchand P. Diffuse pleural mesothelioma and asbestos exposure in the North Western Cape Province. Br J Ind Med. 1960;17:260–71.
24. Gilson JC. Health hazards of asbestos. Recent studies on its biological effects. Trans Soc Occup Med. 1966;16:62–74.
25. Wagner JC, Berry G, Skidmore JW, Timbrell V. The effects of the inhalation of asbestos in rats. Br J Cancer. 1974;29:252–69.

26. Gross P, de Treville RTP, Tolker EB, Kaschak M, Babyak MA. Experimental asbestosis. The development of lung cancer in rats with pulmonary deposits of chrysotile asbestos dust. Arch Environ Health. 1967;15:343–55.
27. Gross P, de Treville RTP. Experimental asbestosis. Arch Environ Health Int J. 1967;15:638–49.
28. Wagner JC, Berry G. Mesotheliomas in rats following inoculation with asbestos. Br J Cancer. 1969;23:567–81.
29. Whitaker D, Shilkin KB, Walters MN. Cytologic and tissue culture characteristics of asbestos-induced mesothelioma in rats. Acta Cytol. 1984;28:185–9.
30. Lee Shin M, Firminger HI. Acute and chronic effects of intraperitoneal injection of two types of asbestos in rats with a study of the histopathogenesis and ultrastructure of resulting mesotheliomas. Am J Pathol. 1973;70:291–314.
31. Craighead JE, Akley NJ, Gould LB, Libbus BL. Characteristics of tumors and tumor cells cultured from experimental asbestos-induced mesotheliomas in rats. Am J Pathol. 1987;129:448–62.
32. Mohr U, Pott F, Vonnahme FJ. Morphological aspects of mesotheliomas after intratracheal instillations of fibrous dusts in Syrian golden hamsters. Exp Pathol. 1984;26:179–83.
33. Wagner JC, Griffiths DM, Hill RJ. The effect of fibre size on the in vivo activity of UICC crocidolite. Br J Cancer. 1984;49:453–8.
34. Davis JM, Addison J, Bolton RE, Donaldson K, Jones AD, Smith T. The pathogenicity of long versus short fibre samples of amosite asbestos administered to rats by inhalation and intraperitoneal injection. Br J Exp Pathol. 1986;67:415–30.
35. Miller BG, Searl A, Davis JM, Donaldson K, Cullen RT, Bolton RE, et al. Influence of fibre length, dissolution and biopersistence on the production of mesothelioma in the rat peritoneal cavity. Ann Occup Hyg. 1999;43:155–66.
36. Minardi F, Maltoni C. Results of recent experimental research on the carcinogenicity of natural and modified asbestos. Ann N Y Acad Sci. 1988;534:754–61.
37. Suzuki Y, Kohyama N. Malignant mesothelioma induced by asbestos and zeolite in the mouse peritoneal cavity. Environ Res. 1984;35:277–92.
38. Davis MR, Manning LS, Whitaker D, Garlepp MJ, Robinson BW. Establishment of a murine model of malignant mesothelioma. Int J Cancer. 1992;52:881–6.
39. Chahinian AP, Beranek JT, Suzuki Y, Bekesi JG, Wisniewski L, Selikoff IJ, et al. Transplantation of human malignant mesothelioma into nude mice. Cancer Res. 1980;40:181–5.
40. Manning LS, Whitaker D, Murch AR, Garlepp MJ, Davis MR, Musk AW, et al. Establishment and characterization of five human malignant mesothelioma cell lines derived from pleural effusions. Int J Cancer. 1991;47:285–90.
41. Griffin TW, Stocl M, Collins J, Fernandes J, Maher VE. Combined antitumor therapy with the chemotherapeutic drug doxorubicin and an anti-transferrin receptor immunotoxin: in vitro and in vivo studies. J Immunother. 1992;11:12–8.
42. Cook JW, Sterman DH, Singhal S, Smythe WR, Kaiser LR. Suramin inhibits the growth of malignant mesothelioma in vitro, and in vivo, in murine flank and intraperitoneal models. Lung Cancer. 2003;42:263–74.
43. Littlejohn JE, Cao X, Miller SD, Ozvaran MK, Jupiter D, Zhang L, et al. Bcl-xL antisense oligonucleotide and cisplatin combination therapy extends survival in SCID mice with established mesothelioma xenografts. Int J Cancer. 2008;123:202–8.
44. Colt HG, Astoul P, Wang X, Yi ES, Boutin C, Hoffman RM. Clinical course of human epithelial-type malignant pleural mesothelioma replicated in an orthotopic-transplant nude mouse model. Anticancer Res. 1996;16:633–9.
45. Astoul P, Wang X, Colt H, Boutin C, Hoffman R. A patient-like human malignant pleural mesothelioma nude-mouse model. Oncol Rep. 1996;3:483–7.
46. Pimpec-Barthes FL, Bernard I, Alsamad IA, Renier A, Kheuang L, Fleury-Feith J, et al. Pleuro-pulmonary tumours detected by clinical and chest X-ray analyses in rats transplanted with mesothelioma cells. Br J Cancer. 1999;81:1344–50.
47. Martarelli D, Catalano A, Procopio A, Orecchia S, Libener R, Santoni G. Characterization of human malignant mesothelioma cell lines orthotopically implanted in the pleural cavity of immunodeficient mice for their ability to grow and form metastasis. BMC Cancer. 2006;6:130.
48. Van TT, Hanibuchi M, Goto H, Kuramoto T, Yukishige S, Kakiuchi S, et al. SU6668, a multiple tyrosine kinase inhibitor, inhibits progression of human malignant pleural mesothelioma in an orthotopic model. Respirology. 2012;17:984–90.
49. Wu L, Allo G, John T, Li M, Tagawa T, Opitz I, et al. Patient-derived xenograft establishment from human malignant pleural mesothelioma. Clin Cancer Res. 2017;23:1060–7.
50. Hanahan D, Coussens LM. Accessories to the crime: functions of cells recruited to the tumor microenvironment. Cancer Cell. 2012;21:309–22.
51. Goodglick LA, Vaslet CA, Messier NJ, Kane AB. Growth factor responses and protooncogene expression of murine mesothelial cell lines derived from asbestos-induced mesotheliomas. Toxicol Pathol. 1997;25:565–73.
52. Jackaman C, Bundell CS, Kinnear BF, Smith AM, Filion P, van, et al. IL-2 intratumoral immunotherapy enhances CD8+ T cells that mediate destruction of tumor cells and tumor-associated vasculature: a novel mechanism for IL-2. J Immunol. 2003;171:5051–63.
53. Miselis NR, Wu ZJ, Van Rooijen N, Kane AB. Targeting tumor-associated macrophages in an orthotopic murine model of diffuse malignant mesothelioma. Mol Cancer Ther. 2008;7:788–99.
54. Miselis NR, Lau BW, Wu Z, Kane AB. Kinetics of host cell recruitment during dissemination of diffuse malignant peritoneal mesothelioma. Cancer Microenviron. 2010;4:39–50.

55. Mishalian I, Bayuh R, Levy L, Zolotarov L, Michaeli J, Fridlender ZG. Tumor-associated neutrophils (TAN) develop pro-tumorigenic properties during tumor progression. Cancer Immunol Immunother. 2013;62:1745–56.
56. Sekido Y. Molecular pathogenesis of malignant mesothelioma. Carcinogenesis. 2013;34:1413–9.
57. Marsella JM, Liu BL, Vaslet CA, Kane AB. Susceptibility of p53-deficient mice to induction of mesothelioma by crocidolite asbestos fibers. Environ Health Perspect. 1997;105:1069–72.
58. Vaslet CA, Messier NJ, Kane AB. Accelerated progression of asbestos-induced mesotheliomas in heterozygous p53+/− mice. Toxicol Sci. 2002;68:331–8.
59. Altomare DA, Vaslet CA, Skele KL, Rienzo AD, Devarajan K, Jhanwar SC, et al. A mouse model recapitulating molecular features of human mesothelioma. Cancer Res. 2005;65:8090–5.
60. Jongsma J, van Montfort E, Vooijs M, Zevenhoven J, Krimpenfort P, van der Valk M, et al. A conditional mouse model for malignant mesothelioma. Cancer Cell. 2008;13:261–71.
61. Bott M, Brevet M, Taylor BS, Shimizu S, Ito T, Wang L, et al. The nuclear deubiquitinase BAP1 is commonly inactivated by somatic mutations and 3p21.1 losses in malignant pleural mesothelioma. Nat Genet. 2011;43:668–72.
62. Testa JR, Cheung M, Pei J, Below JE, Tan Y, Sementino E, et al. Germline BAP1 mutations predispose to malignant mesothelioma. Nat Genet. 2011;43:1022–5.
63. Wiesner T, Fried I, Ulz P, Stacher E, Popper H, Murali R, et al. Toward an improved definition of the tumor spectrum associated with BAP1 germline mutations. J Clin Oncol. 2012;30:e337–40.
64. Cheung M, Testa JR. BAP1, a tumor suppressor gene driving malignant mesothelioma. Transl Lung Cancer Res. 2017;6:270–8.
65. Robinson C, Walsh A, Larma I, O'Halloran S, Nowak AK, Lake RA. MexTAg mice exposed to asbestos develop cancer that faithfully replicates key features of the pathogenesis of human mesothelioma. Eur J Cancer. 2011;47:151–61.
66. Tsuji AB, Sogawa C, Sugyo A, Sudo H, Toyohara J, Koizumi M, et al. Comparison of conventional and novel PET tracers for imaging mesothelioma in nude mice with subcutaneous and intrapleural xenografts. Nucl Med Biol. 2009;36:379–88.
67. Saito Y, Furukawa T, Arano Y, Fujibayashi Y, Saga T. Comparison of semiquantitative fluorescence imaging and PET tracer uptake in mesothelioma models as a monitoring system for growth and therapeutic effects. Nucl Med Biol. 2008;35:851–60.
68. Yanagihara K, Tsumuraya M, Takigahira M, Mihara K, Kubo T, Ohuchi K, et al. An orthotopic implantation mouse model of human malignant pleural mesothelioma for in vivo photon counting analysis and evaluation of the effect of S-1 therapy. Int J Cancer. 2010;126:2835–46.
69. Feng M, Zhang J, Anver M, Hassan R, Ho M. In vivo imaging of human malignant mesothelioma grown orthotopically in the peritoneal cavity of nude mice. J Cancer. 2011;2:123–31.
70. Yamaoka N, Kawasaki Y, Xu Y, Yamamoto H, Terada N, Okamura H, et al. Establishment of in vivo fluorescence imaging in mouse models of malignant mesothelioma. Int J Oncol. 2010;37:273–9.
71. Meerang M, Boss A, Kenkel D, Broggini-Tenzer A, Bérard K, Lauk O, et al. Evaluation of imaging techniques for the assessment of tumour progression in an orthotopic rat model of malignant pleural mesothelioma. Eur J Cardiothorac Surg. 2015;47:e34–41.
72. Vázquez R, Licandro SA, Astorgues-Xerri L, Lettera E, Panini N, Romano M, et al. Promising in vivo efficacy of the BET bromodomain inhibitor OTX015/MK-8628 in malignant pleural mesothelioma xenografts. Int J Cancer. 2017;140:197–207.
73. Giordano S, Zucchetti M, Decio A, Cesca M, Fuso Nerini I, Maiezza M, et al. Heterogeneity of paclitaxel distribution in different tumor models assessed by MALDI mass spectrometry imaging. Sci Rep. 2016;6:39284.

Pathological Diagnosis of Mesothelioma

7

Gabriella Fontanini, Greta Alì, and Rossella Bruno

7.1 Introduction

Diffuse malignant mesothelioma is an aggressive and fatal tumor that arises from the mesothelial cells lining the thoracic, pericardial, abdominal, and tunica vaginalis cavities. More than 90% of the reported cases of mesothelioma occur in the pleura, 4–7% in the peritoneum, and fewer than 1% jointly occurring in the pericardium and tunica vaginalis testis [1].

Diffuse malignant mesothelioma is a relatively rare tumor and its diagnosis is extremely uncommon for some general pathologists, who could remain unfamiliar with this diagnosis for their entire careers. This neoplasm has received a great deal of attention because of its relationship to occupational and environmental exposure to asbestos, which represents the main risk for malignant pleural mesothelioma (MPM), with a latency period of approximately 40 years between fiber exposure and onset of the disease [2, 3]. Therefore, two important aspects associated with the diagnosis of diffuse malignant mesothelioma are on the one hand the medicolegal implications and, on the other hand, the enormous prognostic weight of this diagnosis related to the dismal outcome of almost all affected patients.

The serosal tissues are home to a broad spectrum of tumors and tumor-like conditions. Primary serous tumors have been classified on the basis of the anatomic site (pleura versus peritoneum), but no ideal classification system exists. Alongside diffuse malignant mesothelioma, other even rarer mesothelial neoplasms have shown not to be caused by asbestos exposure and which have different prognoses and treatments [4, 5]. These neoplasms include localized mesothelioma, well-differentiated papillary mesothelioma, cystic mesothelioma, and adenomatoid tumor.

In the present chapter, major issues concerning the pathological diagnostic approach of mesothelioma are reviewed, with special emphasis on the use of immunohistochemical and molecular markers. In particular, the cytological features of malignancy and the histological patterns of mesothelioma (both diffuse malignant mesothelioma and other mesotheliomas) are described to assist pathologists in this challenging diagnosis. This chapter aims to address crucial diagnostic problems related to the differential diagnosis of much more common lesions that mimic diffuse malignant mesothelioma, especially fibrous pleuritis and reactive mesothelial hyperplasia, as well as metastatic malignant tumors.

G. Fontanini (✉)
Department of Surgical, Medical, Molecular Pathology, and Critical Area, University of Pisa, Pisa, Italy
e-mail: gabriella.fontanini@med.unipi.it

G. Alì · R. Bruno
Unit of Pathological Anatomy, Azienda Ospedaliero Universitaria Pisana, Pisa, Italy
e-mail: g.ali@ao-pisa.toscana.it; rossella.bruno@for.unipi.it

G. L. Ceresoli et al. (eds.), *Mesothelioma*, https://doi.org/10.1007/978-3-030-16884-1_7

7.2 Diffuse Malignant Mesothelioma

The diagnosis of diffuse malignant mesothelioma remains difficult and should use morphological assessment within an appropriate clinical and radiological context, and be supplemented by ancillary diagnostic techniques, in particular, immunohistochemistry and, more recently, molecular tests.

The most common cause of malignant mesothelioma is asbestos exposure. Other established causes include radiation, environmental exposure to mineral fiber erionite (in a localized area of Turkey), and simian virus 40 inoculation. Moreover, some mesotheliomas do not have an identifiable cause [6–8]. Therefore, in the presence of adequate pathologic tissue, a history of asbestos exposure must be irrelevant and should not be taken into consideration by the pathologist when confirming or excluding malignant mesothelioma [9].

Gross distribution of the tumor is a critical feature in the accurate diagnosis of mesothelioma and mostly depends on when a mesothelioma is observed during its natural history. Malignant pleural mesothelioma tends to grow over the surface of the pleura, predominantly on the parietal pleura. As the tumor progresses, the nodules tend to converge, and eventually encase the lung in a shell of tumor cells [4]. Although diffuse malignant pleural mesothelioma typically occurs with lung encasement and relative sparing of lung parenchyma, pathologists should be aware of unusual presentations, including mesothelioma cases with absent or scarce pleural involvement and presentation as metastatic disease or mimic of interstitial lung diseases [10].

Diffuse malignant peritoneal mesothelioma in its early stages consists of several small nodules and plaques, indiscernible from those of carcinomatosis peritonealis [11]. In advanced stages, peritoneal mesothelioma encases the abdominal viscera and the invasion of underlying structures like the outer layer of the intestine is not unusual. Occasionally, there is an involvement of both the pleural and peritoneal cavities, making it difficult or impossible to determine the primary site.

On imaging or pleuroscopy/laparoscopy, the description of the serosa (pleura, peritoneum, hydrocele) is useful in the diagnosis of mesothelial lesions in order to decide whether a proliferation is truly malignant. As regards the pleural site, circumferential pleural thickening involving the mediastinal pleura on computed tomography scan as well as nodular pleural thickening is generally malignant [12]. A pathologist should be extremely careful to diagnose a mesothelioma if the pleuroscopist or the laparoscopist assesses that the serosa does not present any lesions.

The pathological approach to diffuse malignant mesothelioma lesions should always be based on the results obtained from adequate serosal biopsies (less commonly from cytology) in terms of both tissue quality and quantity. Since the key indicator of malignancy remains the invasion of pre-existing tissue, multiple, large, and deep serosal biopsies comprising stroma are necessary (Figs. 7.1 and 7.2). Overall, the larger and more targeted is the biopsy, the more likely it is to perform a correct and definitive diagnosis. In this respect, thoracoscopy or laparoscopic biopsies are considered the preferred biopsy techniques to obtain adequate tissue samples. However, ultrasound-guided and computed-tomography-guided biopsies may have a high diagnostic yield (up to 90%) [13–15]. In cases of thoracoscopic biopsies, a minimum of five biopsies is recommended comprising soft tissues of the parietal pleura or of the lung [13].

7.2.1 Histological Features of Diffuse Malignant Mesothelioma

Diffuse malignant mesothelioma is a heterogeneous tumor, which includes three main histological subtypes divided into epithelioid (60–80%), sarcomatoid (<10%), and biphasic (mixed) (10–15%), according to the 2015 World Health Classification of Lung and Pleural Tumors [4, 9, 16]. A variety of patterns may be observed in each of these major categories and this can result in significant diagnostic problems owing to the range of tumors that can enter in differ-

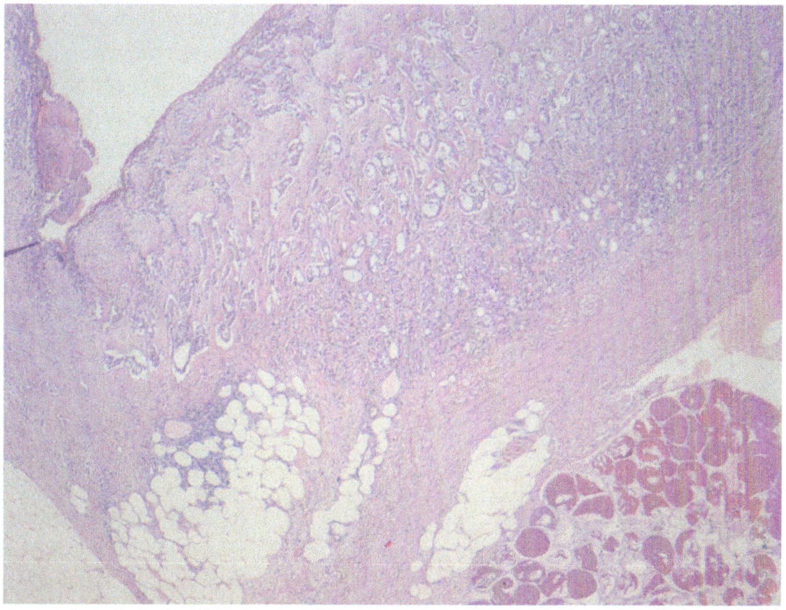

Fig. 7.1 Thoracoscopic biopsy showing frank invasion of the chest wall soft tissue by epithelioid diffuse malignant mesothelioma (hematoxylin–eosin, original magnification ×40)

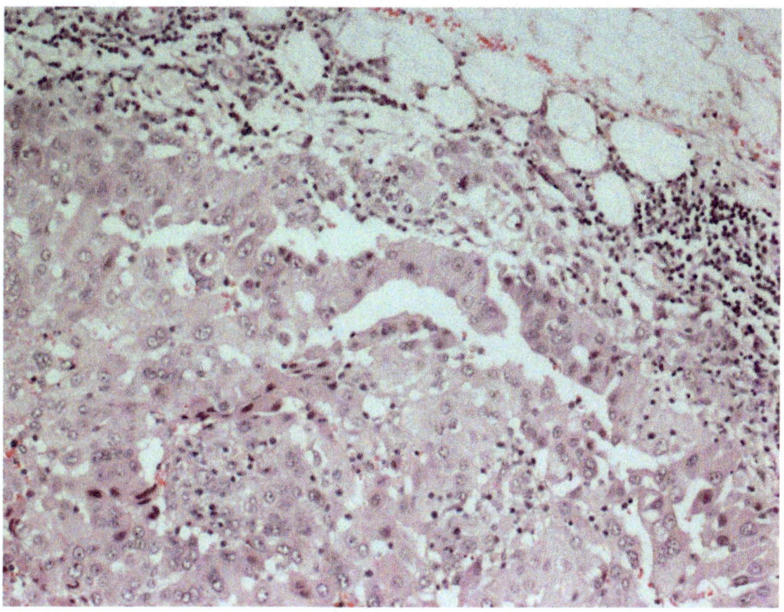

Fig. 7.2 Higher power showing epithelioid subtype of diffuse malignant pleural mesothelioma clearly invading fat (hematoxylin–eosin, original magnification ×100)

ential diagnosis. The recognition of the various patterns will guide the differential diagnosis and selection of subsequent ancillary tests. Some of these morphological variants have been shown to correlate with overall survival (see below). Therefore, a microscopic description of the patterns present in the specimen may be useful, but the major histologic subtype must be provided in the final diagnosis.

Table 7.1 reports the histological classification of diffuse malignant mesothelioma.

Epithelioid mesothelioma displays a wide range of histological patterns, and several distinct patterns have been observed in the same neoplasm, although one pattern may predominate. The most common secondary histological patterns of epithelioid diffuse malignant mesothelioma are tubulopapillary, solid, and trabecular;

psammoma bodies may be present in any of these patterns. Other less common patterns include micropapillary, adenomatoid (microcystic), clear cells, transitional, deciduoid, small cells, and lymphohistiocytoid [4, 16–18].

The morphologic features of the individual tumor cells may show mild to marked atypia and varying degrees of mitotic activity; the mitoses are infrequent except for the more poorly differentiated neoplasms, which are also uncommon [9].

Table 7.1 Histologic classification of malignant mesothelioma

Epithelioid
Tubulopapillary
Solid
Trabecular
Micropapillary
Adenomatoid (microcystic)
Clear cell
Transitional
Deciduoid
Small cell
Pleomorphic
Lymphohistiocytoid
Sarcomatoid
Fibrosarcomatoid
Heterologous elements
Lymphohistiocytoid
Desmoplastic
Biphasic (mixed)

Tubulopapillary and adenomatoid variants generally contain cuboidal or low columnar cells that are typically bland with open nuclei and eosinophilic cytoplasm, which often mimic reactive mesothelial cells occurring in response to various types of injury. In the tubulopapillary pattern, the tumor cells border the tubules or papillae and form on fibrovascular connective tissue cores or delicate epithelioid cell papillae devoid of stroma (Figs. 7.3 and 7.4). The tubules often contain thin basophilic secretions consisting of hyaluronic acid. The adenomatoid variant is characterized by tumor cells that develop microcystic areas or lace-like structures (Figs. 7.5 and 7.6). Epithelioid mesotheliomas also grow as solid sheets or nests of large polygonal tumor cells in a desmoplastic stroma (Fig. 7.7). In some cases, the tumor cells of the solid pattern may be rather pleomorphic with giant anaplastic tumor cells. When the latter are prominent (more than 10% of the tumor), the term pleomorphic variant of malignant mesotheliomas is used (Fig. 7.8). Recently, two different studies have demonstrated that this pattern has a highly aggressive behavior and poor survival, like that of sarcomatoid MPM [17, 19, 20].

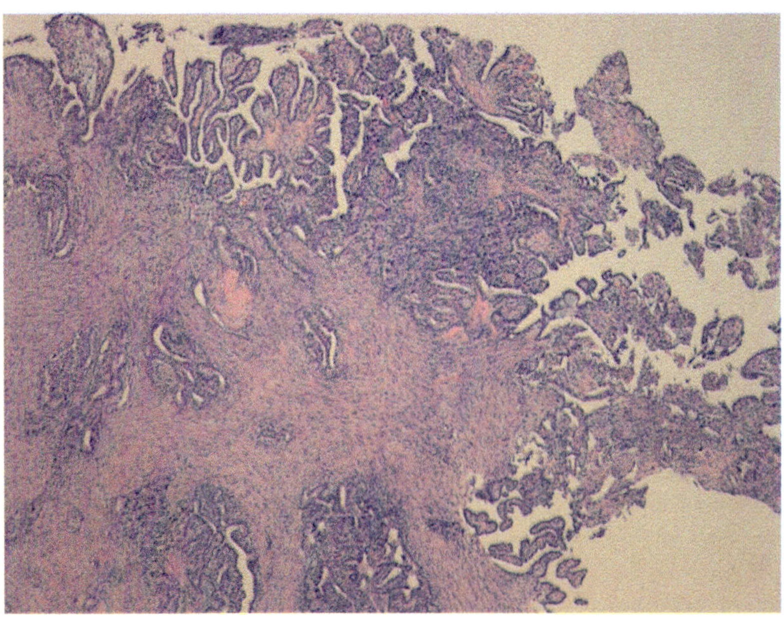

Fig. 7.3 Diffuse malignant mesothelioma, epithelioid subtype. Low power showing tubulopapillary variant (hematoxylin–eosin, original magnification ×40)

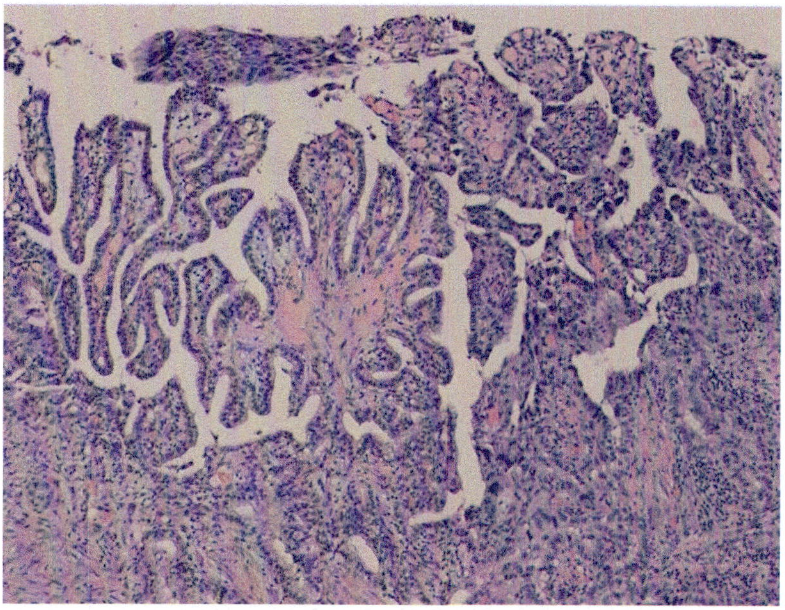

Fig. 7.4 Diffuse malignant mesothelioma, epithelioid subtype; tubulopapillary variant (hematoxylin–eosin, original magnification ×100)

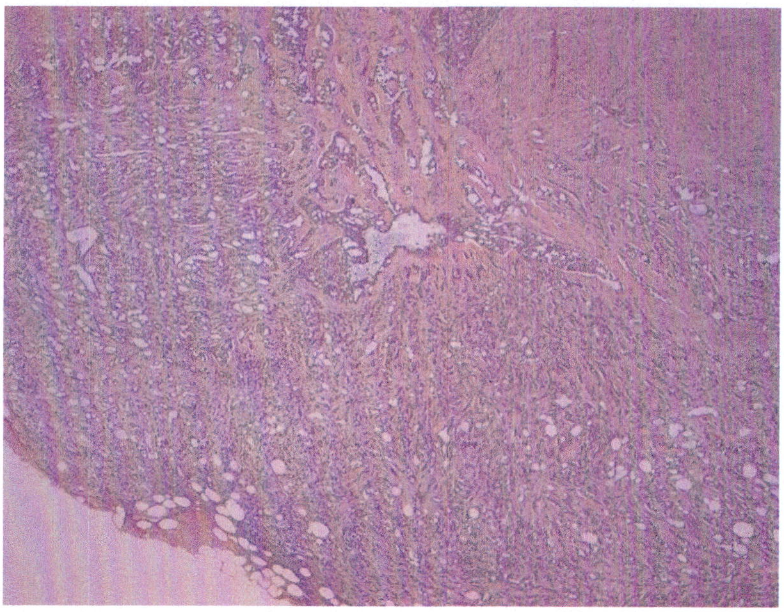

Fig. 7.5 Diffuse malignant mesothelioma, epithelioid subtype; adenomatoid variant with microcystic areas (hematoxylin–eosin, original magnification ×40)

These sheets of tumor cells may present abundant glassy eosinophilic cytoplasm with distinct cell borders. This pattern is referred to as deciduoid mesothelioma, a high-grade subgroup showing a much more aggressive clinical course [17, 21]. Although a histological grading system has not yet been validated for diffuse malignant mesothelioma, preliminary data strongly suggest that mitotic count and especially nuclear grade, including nuclear atypia, are independent poor prognostic factors [22].

Less commonly, in some epithelioid mesotheliomas, the tumor cells may be quite small, a pattern that has been described as small-cell variant [23]. These latter neoplasms look quite different from small-cell lung carcinoma with which they

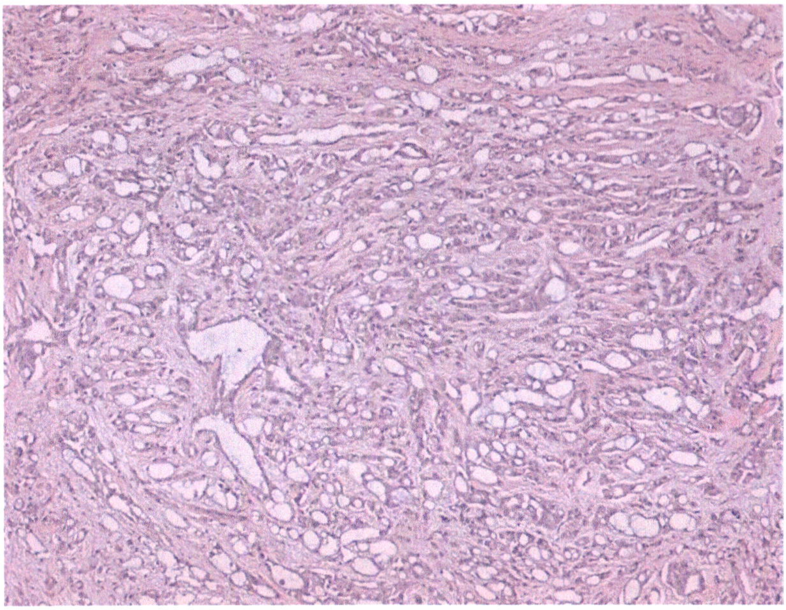

Fig. 7.6 Diffuse malignant mesothelioma, epithelioid subtype. Higher power of adenomatoid variant (hematoxylin–eosin, original magnification ×100)

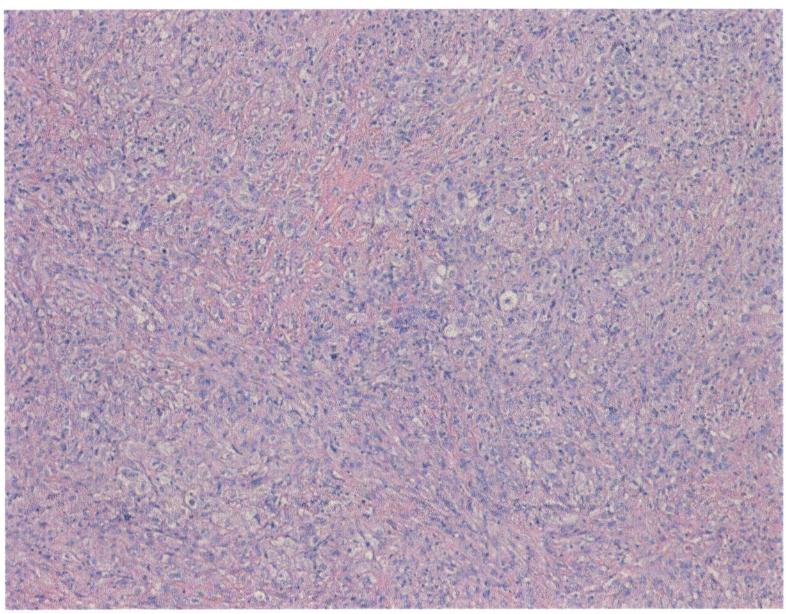

Fig. 7.7 Diffuse malignant mesothelioma, epithelioid subtype; solid variant (hematoxylin–eosin, original magnification ×40)

should not be confused. Other rare patterns show clear, signet ring, or rhabdoid cells [18].

The fibrous reactive stroma present in epithelioid mesothelioma can be scant or prominent, with various grades of cellularity that could make the distinction from true sarcomatoid component difficult. In these cases, BRCA1-associated protein 1 (BAP1) expression by immunohistochemistry can be helpful, showing a loss of expression in areas of sarcomatoid mesothelioma [24].

Sarcomatoid mesothelioma is the least common but most aggressive of the histological types of mesothelioma [25]. The sarcomatoid subtype of diffuse malignant mesothelioma is usually characterized by the proliferation of spindle cells arranged in fascicles, which can have a her-

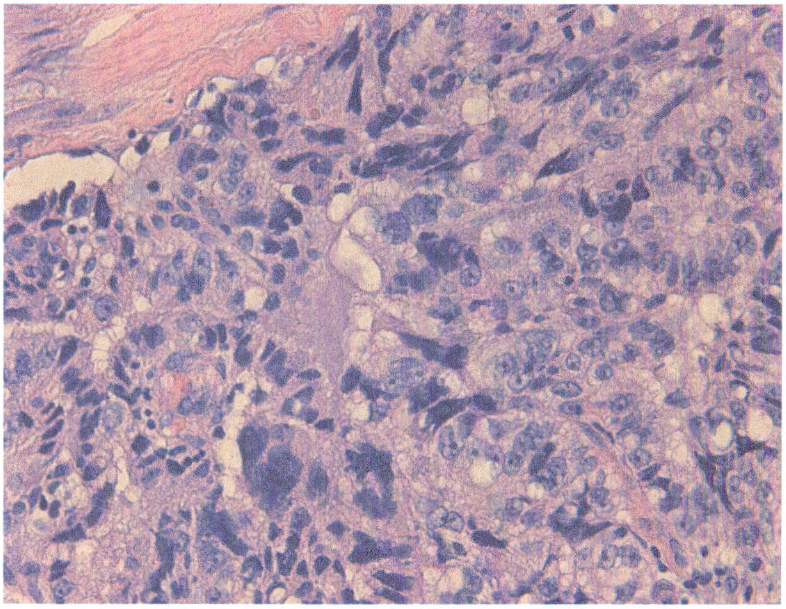

Fig. 7.8 Diffuse malignant mesothelioma, epithelioid subtype, pleomorphic variant with sheets of large, atypical epithelioid cells with giant cells (hematoxylin–eosin, original magnification ×400)

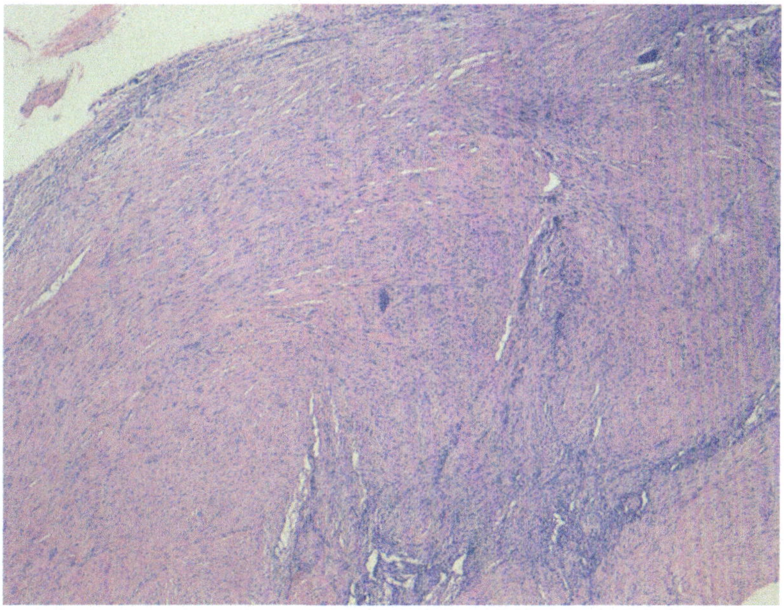

Fig. 7.9 Diffuse malignant mesothelioma, sarcomatoid subtype shows spindle cell proliferation conveying a fibrosarcomatous appearance (hematoxylin–eosin, original magnification ×40)

ringbone pattern conveying a fibrosarcomatous appearance, or can be arranged in a haphazard distribution (Figs. 7.9 and 7.10). The cells usually show fusiform or plump nuclei with various grades of atypia and mitotic activity. In a very small number of sarcomatoid diffuse malignant mesotheliomas, heterologous elements such as osteosarcomatoid, rhabdomyosarcomatous, or chondrosarcomatoid differentiation are observed [16, 26]. Some sarcomatoid mesotheliomas show atypical giant cells with large, bizarre, and hyperchromatic nuclei that can mimic undifferentiated high-grade pleomorphic sarcomas [19].

Desmoplastic diffuse malignant mesothelioma is the rarest pattern (<2%) and is characterized by proliferation of the bland spindle cells

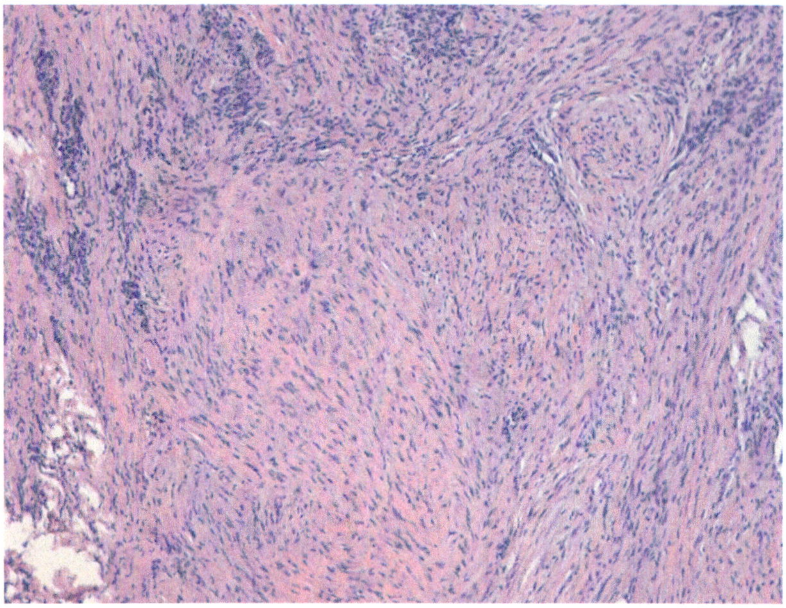

Fig. 7.10 Higher power showing diffuse malignant mesothelioma, sarcomatoid subtype (hematoxylin–eosin, original magnification ×100)

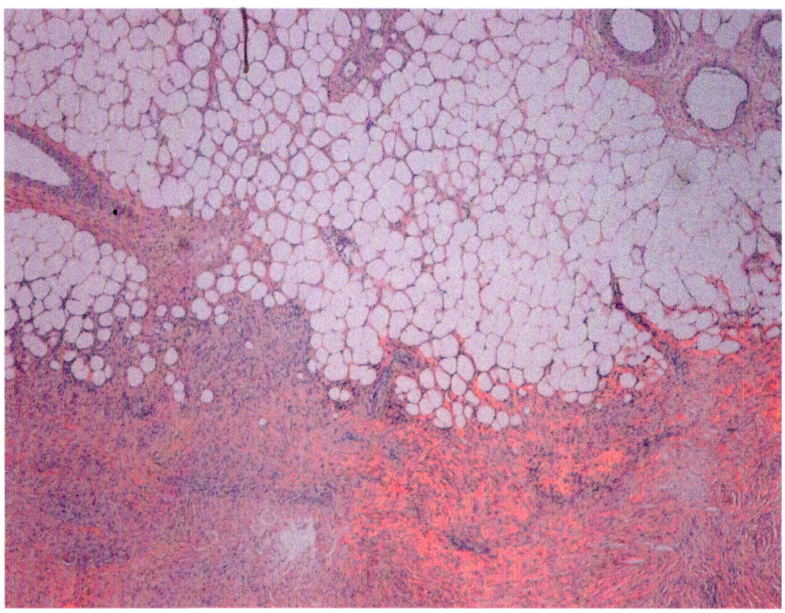

Fig. 7.11 Low-power image of diffuse malignant mesothelioma, desmoplastic, with prominent hyalinized stroma with spindle cell component clearly in invading adipose tissue (hematoxylin–eosin, original magnification ×40)

arranged in a "patternless" pattern within a band of dense collagenous stroma (Figs. 7.11 and 7.12). This proliferation should occupy at least 50% of the tumor to conform to the World Health Organization classification [4]. It is well known that the histological distinction between desmoplastic mesothelioma and benign fibrous pleuritis can be difficult, especially in small biopsy specimens. The distinction is based on the findings of cellular stromal nodules and bland necroses or clearly epithelioid or sarcomatoid foci, in addition to the invasion of chest wall soft tissue or underlying lung parenchyma [16, 27].

Biphasic malignant mesothelioma is a highly characteristic pattern of mesothelioma containing a mixture of epithelioid and sarcoma-

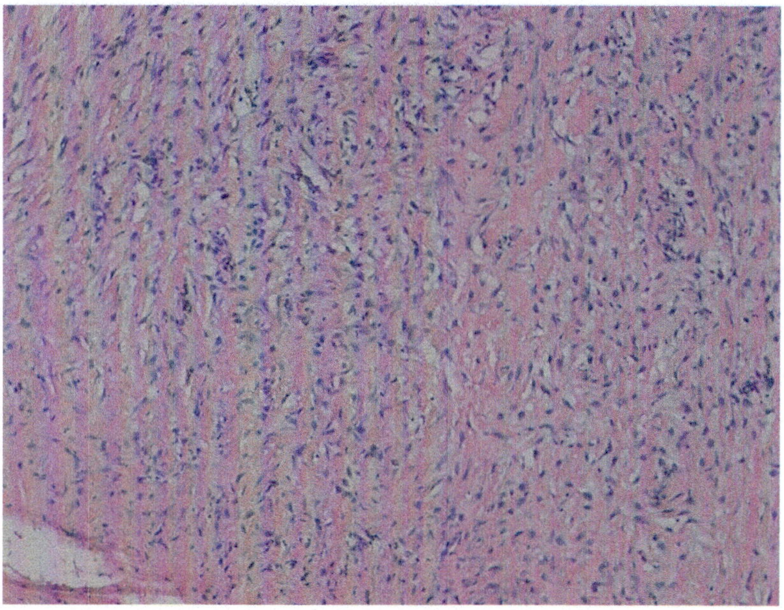

Fig. 7.12 Higher power of desmoplastic mesothelioma showing bland spindle cells (hematoxylin–eosin, original magnification ×100)

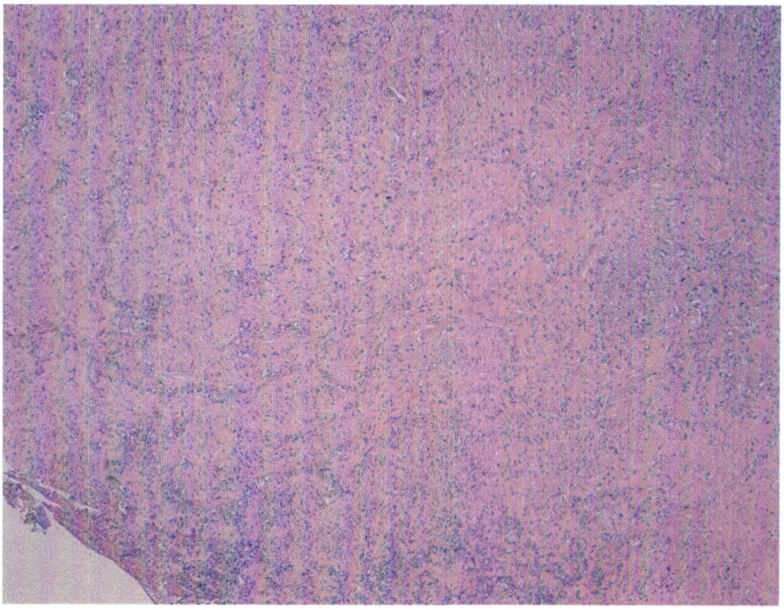

Fig. 7.13 Diffuse malignant mesothelioma, biphasic subtype, with epithelioid component and prominent sarcomatoid component (hematoxylin–eosin, original magnification ×40)

toid areas within the same tumor, often closely intermingled (Figs. 7.13 and 7.14). Although any combination of the subtypes listed in Table 7.1 is possible, these neoplasms are usually poorly differentiated so that well-differentiated elements are typically absent. Each pattern should constitute at least 10% of the neoplasm; however, when there is less of either, the malignant mesothelioma can be designated predominantly sarcomatoid or epithelioid [16]. Needless to say, the more a mesothelioma is sampled, the greater is the possibility to reveal the biphasic nature of the tumor. However, pathologists should be careful not to confuse a benign mesothelium entrapped by a sarcomatoid mesothelioma or reactive fibrous stroma in epithelioid subtypes with a

Fig. 7.14 Diffuse malignant mesothelioma, biphasic subtype, medium power (hematoxylin–eosin, original magnification ×100)

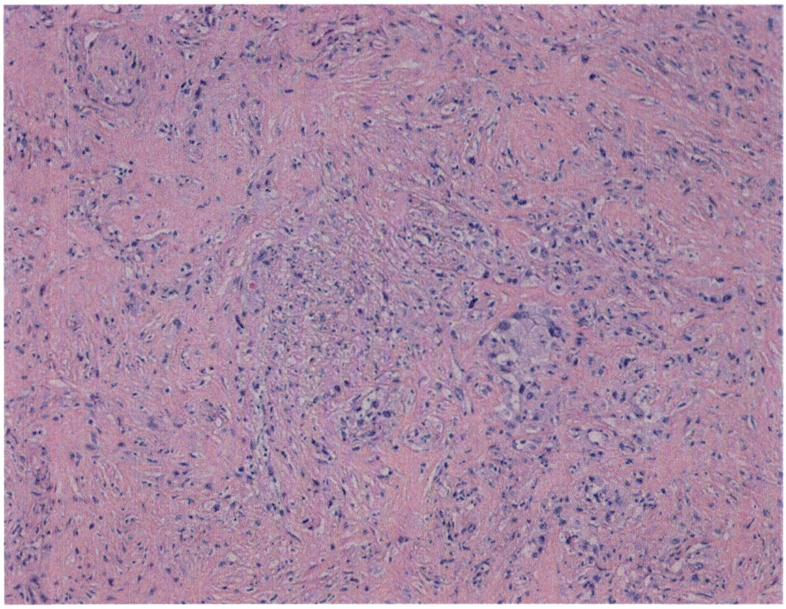

true biphasic malignant mesothelioma. Recently, the percentage of epithelioid differentiation has proved to be an independent predictor of survival in patients with biphasic malignant pleural mesothelioma and this element should probably be taken into account when recommending surgical treatment for these patients [28]. Therefore, the amount of epithelioid component should be provided by the pathologists in their microscopic description or final diagnosis.

7.2.2 Histological Features of Peritoneal Malignant Mesothelioma

The histological features of diffuse malignant peritoneal mesothelioma are similar to those of pleural mesothelioma with epithelioid and sarcomatoid aspects. The epithelioid subtypes are more frequently tubulopapillary and solid patterns [9]. However, several site-specific issues are recognized in the peritoneum. Pure sarcomatoid diffuse malignant mesothelioma is quite uncommon in the peritoneum, accounting for only 2% out of 326 sarcomatoid diffuse malignant mesotheliomas evaluated in a single study [25]. Similarly, the hypocellular, hyalinised, desmoplastic variant is exceptional in this site and the incidence of biphasic tumors is lower than in the pleural disease; however, as in pleural mesotheliomas, the sarcomatoid and biphasic subtypes have a significantly poorer prognosis and are less suitable for treatment [29, 30].

7.3 Localized Malignant Mesothelioma

Localized malignant mesothelioma is an extremely rare tumor of the serosal membranes with microscopic, immunohistochemical, and ultrastructural features of diffuse malignant mesothelioma, but lacking the diffuse growth pattern [31]. Fewer than 50 cases have been reported [31–34] and this tumor has been described more frequently in the pleura than in the peritoneum or pericardium. The mean age is approximately 60 years and there is a slight male predisposition [4]. At present, the association of localized malignant mesothelioma with asbestos exposure is not proven. Macroscopically, localized malignant mesothelioma is a solitary, circumscribed mass attached to the surface of the serosa (pleura, peritoneum, and pericardium) in a sessile or pedunculated manner. This tumor has a more favorable prognosis than diffuse malignant mesothelioma and requires a different type of treatment, usually surgical excision [31].

7.4 Well-Differentiated Papillary Mesothelioma

Well-differentiated papillary carcinoma is a rare tumor arising predominantly in the female peritoneum or less frequently in the tunica vaginalis testis in men, although similar neoplasms have recently been reported in the pericardium and pleura [4, 35–37]. No association with asbestos exposure has been identified. Macroscopically, the tumor is often characterized by multiple pelvic and omental nodules, ranging from 0.5 cm to several centimeters in size. The tumor is not characterized by the diffuse bulky spread of diffuse malignant mesothelioma. Microscopically, the tumor consists of papillary structures and of a superficial growth pattern. The papillae show a more-or-less myxoid fibrovascular core and are lined by a single layer of uniform flattened to cuboidal mesothelial cells. These epithelioid cells often show mild atypia and have inconspicuous mitotic activity. The papillary lining cells stain appropriately with mesothelial immunohistochemical markers.

Well-differentiated papillary mesothelioma can be differentiated from diffuse malignant mesothelioma by the lack of a diffuse growth pattern, prominent uniform papillary architecture, lack of cellular stratification and cytologic atypia, and relative lack of invasion. Differentiation may thus be impossible on small biopsies. In general, well-differentiated papillary mesotheliomas follow either a benign indolent or low-grade malignant course with progressive disease extending over a 5- to 10-year period [4, 38].

7.5 Cystic Mesothelioma

Cystic mesothelioma or peritoneal inclusion cysts are alternative names given to this lesion, which represents a rare tumor nearly always encountered in the peritoneum, although rare pleural multicystic mesotheliomas have been described [39–42]. The lesion occurs more predominantly in reproductive age women, and a history of past pelvic surgery, endometriosis, or inflammatory pelvic disease is present in the majority of cases. There is no documented evidence that cystic mesothelioma is related to asbestos exposure. Almost all cystic mesotheliomas are benign and do not metastasize, although the tumor may recur after surgery [43].

Briefly, this tumor is composed of single or multiple thin-walled cysts containing gelatinous fluid and varying in size from a few millimeters to several centimeters. Histologically, the cysts are lined by a single layer of cuboidal or flattened mesothelial cells, which do not show invasion. The lack of histological complexity and invasion as well as the localized nature distinguishes this lesion from diffuse malignant mesothelioma.

7.6 Cytological Diagnosis of Malignant Mesothelioma

Recurrent serosal effusions, pleural effusions or ascites, are a common symptom of mesothelioma, and these specimens are routinely submitted for cytological examination (smears and/or cell-blocks). Extreme caution should be taken when diagnosing diffuse malignant mesothelioma on cytologic grounds alone, since exfoliative cytologic preparations do not allow the evaluation of clear invasion, the only absolute criterion for malignancy. A definitive diagnosis of malignant mesothelioma by cytological examination alone remains controversial, especially in the light of the medicolegal implications correlated with the diagnosis of diffuse malignant mesothelioma [9, 44]. However, in selected cases in which more invasive procedures are contraindicated, the cytological diagnosis of diffuse malignant mesothelioma, which relies on a different set of both cellular and architectural features and is supported by ancillary techniques, can be performed, although the sensitivity of cytology is low compared to that of histology. In fact, the reported sensitivity of the mesothelioma cytology diagnosis ranges from 30% to 75% [45–48]. In the cases in which histology is not available, a close correlation with clinical and imaging findings is also essential for a definitive diagnosis.

Not all mesothelial tumor cells exfoliate in the serosal cavity and mesothelioma cells in malignant effusions are virtually always of epithelioid type. Indeed, the malignant cells in sarcomatoid mesothelioma are unlikely to be shed into the effusion fluid. Sarcomatoid mesothelioma may cause serosal effusions, but these are typically not malignant and contain only reactive epithelioid mesothelial cells, which may mislead the pathologist. Presumably, these effusions are caused by the local effects of sarcomatoid mesothelioma on serosal membranes and obstructive lymphatics. In such cases, a core biopsy or larger specimens are necessary to establish a definitive diagnosis, especially when surgery is considered, because the presence of a sarcomatoid component may influence therapeutic management [49].

Several cytological features in serosal effusions raise varying levels of suspicion for malignant mesothelioma, such as the extent of mesothelial proliferation, the presence of papillary structures, scalloped borders of cell clumps, intercellular windows, variation of cytoplasmic staining and its density, and low nuclear-to-cytoplasmic ratios (Fig. 7.15). However, some of the cytomorphological findings of MPM are shared between reactive and malignant epithelioid mesothelial cells (Fig. 7.16). As a matter of fact, the malignant mesothelioma cells lack the significant degree of pleomorphism observed with carcinoma cells (Fig. 7.17) and are in some cases bland. Therefore, the differential diagnosis of mesothelial proliferations may be very difficult or even impossible to make in cytological specimens, underscoring the importance of ancillary techniques to clarify diagnosis [9, 44].

The application of immunocytochemistry and molecular methods, such as fluorescent in situ hybridization (FISH) performed preferentially on cellblocks, increases the diagnostic accuracy of cytology [12, 50–52]. The differential diagnosis of malignant mesothelioma and the use of immunohistochemistry and molecular markers in cytological samples are the same as in histological specimens. Several immunohistochemical markers, such as desmin, tumor protein p53 (p53), epithelial membrane antigen (EMA), glucose transporter protein 1 (GLUT-1), insulin-like growth factor 2 messenger RNA-binding protein 3 (IMP-3), and CD146, have been proposed to assist in uncertain cases [53–60]. However, none of these markers, alone or in combination, has

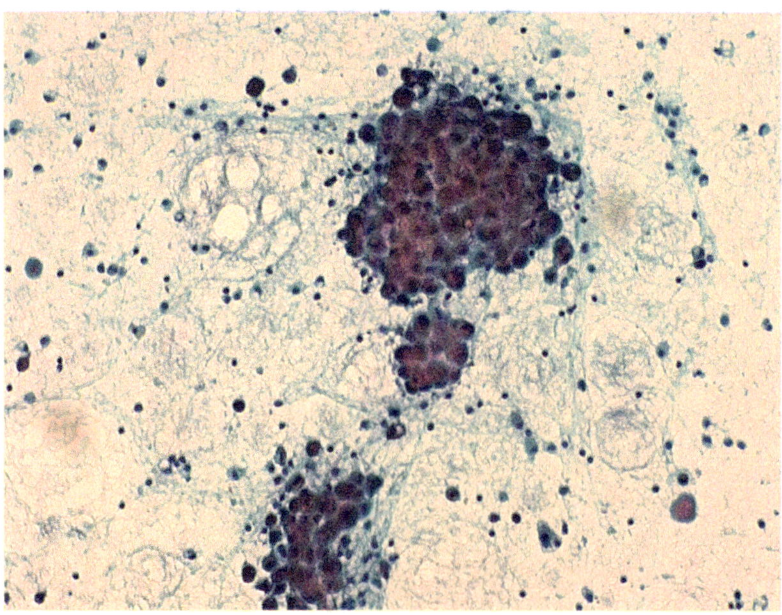

Fig. 7.15 Effusion with epithelioid mesothelioma. The specimen is highly cellular with malignant mesothelial cells forming papillary tissue fragments (Papanicolau, original magnification ×200)

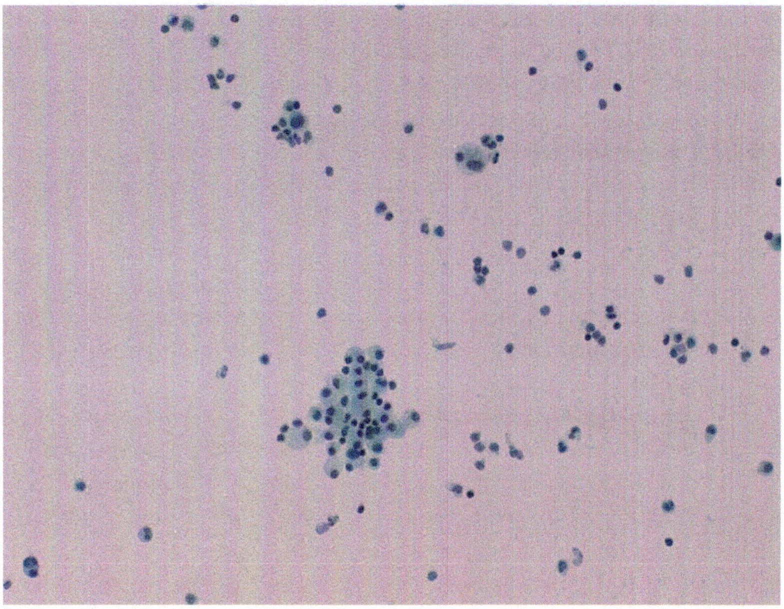

Fig. 7.16 Reactive mesothelial hyperplasia in effusion from a patient with lung infection (Papanicolau, original magnification ×200)

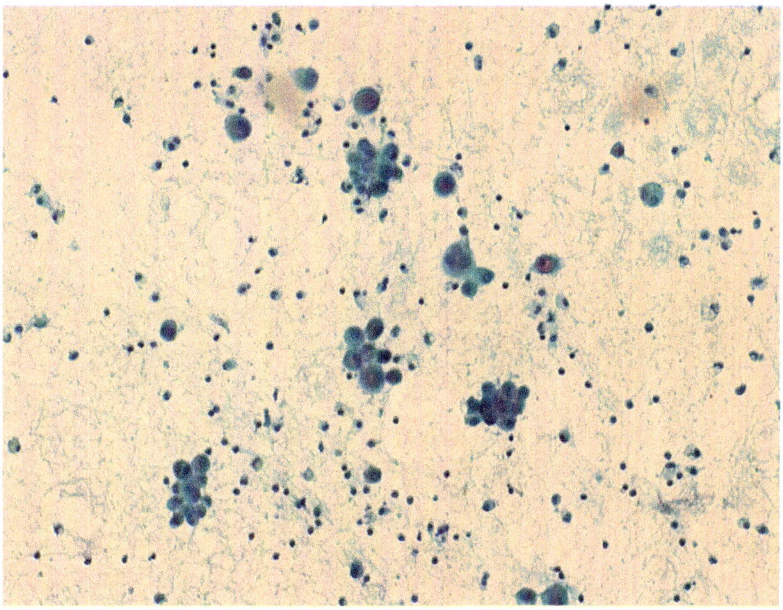

Fig. 7.17 Effusion from a patient with lung adenocarcinoma (Papanicolau, original magnification ×200)

appeared to be useful with sufficient confidence in the routine diagnosis of diffuse malignant mesothelioma [9].

Among the new ancillary tests, the homozygous deletion of *p16* (*CDKN2A*) detected by FISH and the loss of BAP1 expression by immunocytochemistry are particularly helpful to differentiate mesothelial hyperplasia from malignant mesothelioma. These two markers were shown to be highly specific for mesothelioma; however, their low sensitivity limits their clinical utility [24, 61–67].

The cytological distinction between mesothelioma and secondary carcinoma is less problematic now than in earlier decades; overall, if the sample is adequate for cellblock preparation various immunohistochemical studies can be performed [16]. Owing to the frequent litigation of cases of diffuse malignant mesothelioma and to the availability of many mesothelial and adenocarcinoma markers, the guidelines strongly recommend that all cases should be confirmed by immunocytochemistry or immunohistochemistry [44].

7.7 Histochemistry in the Diagnosis of Malignant Mesothelioma

Mucin histochemistry is an inexpensive and simple method to distinguish malignant mesothelioma from metastatic adenocarcinoma [68]. Malignant mesothelioma cells contain glycogen and may have vacuoles containing hyaluronic acid detectable by Alcian blue staining at pH 2.5 and digestible by hyaluronidase. However, hyaluronic acid is found in normal mesothelial cells as well as in other non-mesothelial tumors, so that the reaction has limited specificity. Neoplastic cells of adenocarcinoma may produce neutral mucin that can be highlighted by periodic acid–Schiff (PAS) after digestion as well as by Alcian blue but it is not digested by hyaluronidase. Mucicarmine staining highlights these vacuoles but may also stain hyaluronic acid in malignant mesotheliomas; as a consequence, this type of stain should not be used for distinguishing adenocarcinoma from mesothelioma. Another pitfall for pathologists evaluating histochemical stains is represented by the evidence that there are rare epithelioid mesotheliomas able to show positive results with periodic acid–Schiff after digestion, as observed in adenocarcinomas [69]. For the recognition of these limitations and for the expansion of immunohistochemistry in recent years, the role of mucin histochemistry in the diagnosis of malignant mesothelioma has diminished. Therefore, the employment of histochemistry for the differential diagnosis of diffuse malignant mesothelioma is only occasionally indicated in tumors showing contradictory immunohistochemical stain results [9].

7.8 Immunohistochemistry in the Diagnosis of Malignant Mesothelioma

Immunohistochemistry is integral to the diagnosis of diffuse malignant mesothelioma, representing the most useful and standard ancillary procedure. Immunohistochemistry plays an important role in three different areas in mesothelioma diagnosis: to distinguish malignant epithelioid mesothelioma from metastatic epithelioid carcinoma, to distinguish malignant sarcomatoid mesothelioma from other spindle cell tumors, and to distinguish benign and malignant mesothelial proliferations.

The exact combination and number of antigens to be evaluated depends on the histopathological patterns of malignant mesothelioma (epithelioid/sarcomatoid), on the diagnostic dilemma to be resolved, and on the antibodies available in the pathology laboratory [70, 71]. Since none of the antibodies used for the diagnosis of malignant mesothelioma is 100% sensitive or specific, the International Mesothelioma Interest Group (IMIG) recommends an initial workup with an immunohistochemical panel comprising pancytokeratin (multiple keratins, such as AE1/AE3, CAM5.2) plus two mesothelial markers and two markers for the other tumors considered on the basis of morphology. If the results are concordant, the diagnosis could be considered established. If the results of this immunohistochemical panel are discordant, the pathologist should expand the panel of antibodies, again based on the differential diagnosis to be solved [9]. The immunohistochemical markers should have sensitivity or specificity greater than 80%, and the interpretation of immunostaining should consider the localization of the stain (membrane, nuclear, cytoplasmic) and the percentage of positive cells, more than 10% of which have been suggested for cytoplasmic membranous markers [9].

Immunohistochemical staining with pancytokeratin is particularly useful in the diagnosis of diffuse malignant mesothelioma, since all mesotheliomas potentially show positive results. However, few (approximately 5–10%) sarcomatoid mesotheliomas are keratin-negative; in these cases, other mesothelial markers, such as

Table 7.2 Immunohistochemical markers more often used in the diagnosis of mesothelioma

Mesothelial markers	Carcinoma markers	Organ-specific markers
Calretinin	BerEP4	*Lung*: TTF1, Napsin A
WT1	mCEA	*Breast*: ER, PGR, GCDFP15, Mammaglobin
Podoplanin (D2-40)	MOC31	*Renal*: PAX8, PAX2
Cytokeratin 5/6	B72.3	*Gastrointestinal*: CDX2, cytokeratin 20, mCEA
	BG8 (Lewis Y)	*Prostate*: PSA, PSMA
	CD15 (LeuM1)	
	Claudin-4	

WT1 Wilms' tumor gene, *mCEA* monoclonal carcinoembryonic antigen, *TTF1* thyroid transcription factor 1, *ER* estrogen receptor, *PGR* progesterone receptor, *GCDFP15* gross cystic disease fluid protein, *PSA* prostate-specific antigen, *PSMA* prostate-specific membrane antigen

calretinin and podoplanin (D2-40), could rule out the exact diagnosis [17, 25]. Based on their sensitivity and specificity, the most useful mesothelial markers for MPM diagnosis are calretinin, Wilms' tumor gene (WT1), cytokeratin 5/6 (CK5/6), and D2-40 [9, 16]. However, negativity for the mentioned mesothelial antibodies does not exclude the diagnosis of malignant mesothelioma, since 30% of these tumors present a "null" phenotype [13]. Table 7.2 lists the most common mesothelial immunohistochemical markers used.

The choice of the other immunohistochemical markers included in the diagnostic panel depends on the tumor in differential diagnosis (see next paragraphs for more details).

7.9 Differential Diagnosis of Malignant Mesothelioma

7.9.1 Differential Diagnosis of Benign and Malignant Mesothelial Proliferations

The differential diagnosis of benign and malignant mesothelial proliferations is crucial for patient care and has medicolegal implications because of the occupational relationship between diffuse malignant mesothelioma and asbestos exposure [12, 71].

When histology and appropriate immunohistochemical stains have shown the mesothelial origin of a proliferation, it is necessary to determine whether the proliferation is malignant or benign reactive, mostly for pleural lesions. Reactive benign mesothelial proliferations comprise lesions composed by both epithelioid cells and spindle cells; benign reactive spindle cell proliferations are generally fibrous pleuritis. Differential diagnosis is in both cases challenging, especially in small biopsy specimens. As emphasized earlier in this chapter, the definitive diagnosis of malignant mesothelioma requires stromal invasion and relies mostly on histological examination, with the exception of some cytological specimens. Fat is the most frequently encountered stroma; the presence of mesothelial cells within fat makes the proliferation malignant as well as the presence of mesothelial cells in muscle tissue or invasion of lung or another organ. However, care should be taken that the mesothelial cells are really in the tissue because occasionally artifactual "carry" can mimic invasion [12].

7.9.1.1 Reactive Mesothelial Hyperplasia Versus Epithelioid/Mixed Malignant Mesothelioma

Although reactive mesothelial proliferations are noninvasive, the entrapment of benign mesothelial cells within fibrous tissue can simulate neoplastic invasion. In the pleura and in the peritoneum, reactive mesothelial cell entrapment may be observed in patients with recurrent effusions of any causation due to the successive cycles of inflammatory stimulation, mesothelial proliferation, and reparative fibrosis. In the pleura, reactive mesothelial cell entrapment may be seen in association with pneumothorax, previous surgery, collagen vascular disease, and infections (Fig. 7.18). The entrapment of mesothelial cells in the peritoneum may be found in association with liver cirrhosis, ascites, and endometriosis.

Morphologic features that help distinguish reactive mesothelial hyperplasia from epithelioid

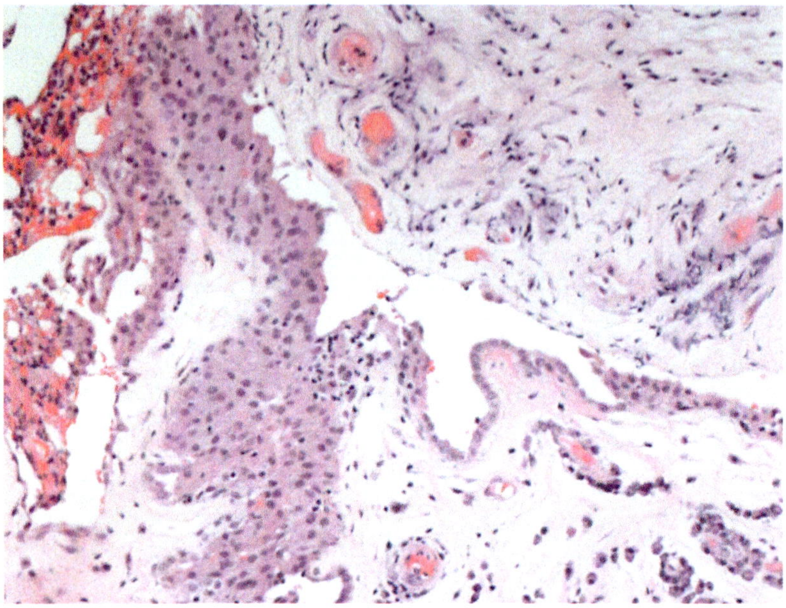

Fig. 7.18 Reactive mesothelial hyperplasia in a pleural biopsy with superficial proliferation of benign mesothelial cells (hematoxylin–eosin, original magnification ×100)

mesothelioma are zonation, extent and complexity of cellular proliferation, cytologic atypia, numerous mitoses, and necrosis. However, these features may be shared between hyperplasia and mesothelioma [4]. Therefore, this differential diagnosis is often morphologically difficult, making it necessary to resort to various ancillary tests. First, keratin immunostaining may assist in highlighting invasive diffuse malignant mesothelioma cells. However, as mentioned above, several immunohistochemical markers are more likely to be positive in benign proliferations, others in malignant ones. These markers include desmin, p53, EMA, GLUT-1, IMP-3, and CD146 [53–60]. EMA, p53, GLUT-1, IMP-3, and CD146 are preferentially expressed in neoplastic mesothelium, whereas desmin is preferentially expressed in the reactive one. Table 7.3 summarizes the most commonly expected staining results with these antibodies. However, they at best are able to provide statistical differences in large series of cases and there is insufficient evidence they can be relied upon in single case [9, 52].

At present, BAP1 immunohistochemistry and *p16* FISH represent the most effective analyses to discriminate between benign and malignant mesothelial lesions [24, 52, 61–66].

Table 7.3 Immunohistochemical markers differentiating benign from malignant mesothelial proliferations

Desmin	Claimed to mark benign proliferations
EMA	Claimed to mark mesotheliomas
P53	Claimed to mark mesotheliomas
GLUT-1	Claimed to mark mesotheliomas
BAP1	Claimed to mark benign proliferation
IMP-3	Claimed to mark mesotheliomas
CD146	Claimed to mark mesotheliomas

EMA epithelial membrane antigen, *GLUT-1* glucose transporter-1, *IMP-3* insulin-like growth factor 2 messenger RNA-binding protein-3, *BAP1* BRCA1-associated protein 1

BAP1 somatic mutations resulting in protein loss appear to be common in hereditary and sporadic malignant pleural mesotheliomas [61]. There is considerable variability in the reported frequency of BAP1 protein loss; epithelioid/mixed mesotheliomas lose BAP1 more frequently than the sarcomatoid pattern, approximately 60–70% and 15%, respectively. Interestingly, recent studies have shown BAP1 protein expression in all benign mesothelial proliferations. Although more data are needed, the specificity of BAP1 loss is 100%, making BAP1 an excellent biomarker in the distinction between benign and malignant mesothelial proliferations [24, 52, 64–66].

Several recent studies have shown that the homozygous deletion of *p16* by FISH is found only in malignant pleural mesotheliomas, whereas none of benign mesothelial proliferations has demonstrated a loss of *p16* with a specificity of 100% [52, 61–63]. However, not all mesotheliomas harbor this deletion, and the sensitivity for epithelioid/biphasic mesothelioma ranges from approximately 45% to 85%. The sensitivity of the *p16* FISH test is much higher in sarcomatoid mesothelioma; in some works, the deletion is documented in up to 100% of cases, but other studies have reported a lower proportion of *p16*-deleted sarcomatous tumors [52]. However, apart from the excellent specificity of these two markers, their low sensitivity limits their clinical utility, as the failure to identify *p16* loss by FISH, or BAP1 loss by immunohistochemistry, is insufficient to make a process benign. On the other hand, the limited sensitivity of each test may be improved by running both tests [67, 72, 73].

Besides BAP1 and p16, recently the immunohistochemical analysis of methylthioadenosine (MTAP) has also been evaluated for separating benign from malignant pleural lesions. *MTAP* encodes for a tumor suppressor and is located at the 9p21.3 locus very close to *CDKN2A;* its expression is frequently lost in MPM and as regards as the discrimination between malignant and benign pleural lesions, the reported specificity is high with a satisfying sensitivity, comparable with BAP1 and *p16* testing [74, 75]. Moreover, the availability of new techniques and the increasing knowledge about the mesothelioma genetic landscape has led to the definition of some molecular panels, including genes or microRNAs specifically deregulated or altered in MPM that proved to be valuable in this kind of differential diagnosis, both on pleural tissues and effusions [74, 76, 77].

Anyway, although new effective biomarkers and tools for the differential diagnosis between malignant and benign pleural lesions have been successfully identified and tested, further validation is warranted. Currently, the best biomarkers recommended in the clinical practice to differentiate malignant from benign pleural lesions remain BAP1 and *p16* [9, 50, 74].

7.9.1.2 Fibrous Organizing Pleuritis Versus Desmoplastic Malignant Pleural Mesothelioma

Benign reactive sarcomatoid proliferations are mainly represented by fibrous pleuritis, so that the separation of benign fibrous entities from desmoplastic malignant pleural mesothelioma could be extremely difficult [9, 16, 27, 78]. Desmoplastic mesotheliomas are paucicellular processes that resemble scars or organizing pleuritis at low power. The invasion into adjacent tissue by neoplastic cells is often more difficult to visualize than in other histological types of malignant mesothelioma. Immunohistochemistry has little value between benign spindle cell proliferation and desmoplastic mesothelioma, except for pancytokeratin immunostaining, which helps to highlight the presence of malignant cells in the stromal tissue (Fig. 7.19). However, the pathologist should be careful not to confuse the true invasion of desmoplastic malignant mesothelioma with the fatlike spaces that may be present in some organizing pleuritis, the so-called "fat fake" phenomenon (Fig. 7.20) [79]. This change is the result of the traction artifact caused by inflammation and of the organization in the fibrous connective tissue. S-100 immunohistochemistry can be useful to distinguish true fat from "fake fat," which can be both positive and negative [79]. Alongside stromal invasion, useful histological features in this differential diagnosis could include the uniformity of growth in organizing pleuritis with typical zonation formed by increased cellular infiltrate under the effusion, and less cellular infiltrates with more fibrosis toward the chest wall. Another feature is the presence of pleuritis with small capillaries oriented perpendicular to the surface opposite to the inconspicuous capillaries in the tumor. Moreover, desmoplastic malignant pleural mesothelioma could show nodular stromal expansions, foci of clear sarcomatoid or epithelioid subtypes, and bland tumor necroses [12]. The molecular analysis of *p16* by FISH could ameliorate the differential diagnosis of desmoplastic mesothelioma, owing to the high frequency of *p16* homozygous deletion reported in the literature in this variant of diffuse malignant mesothelioma. On the contrary, immunohistochemical BAP1 loss is rarely present

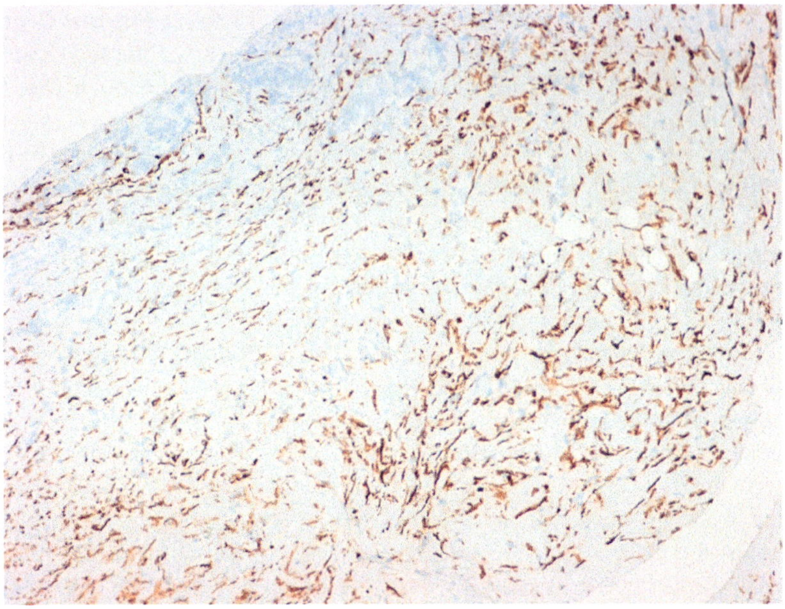

Fig. 7.19 Immunohisto chemical study for pancytokeratin highlighting the presence of malignant cells in the adipose tissue (original magnification ×40)

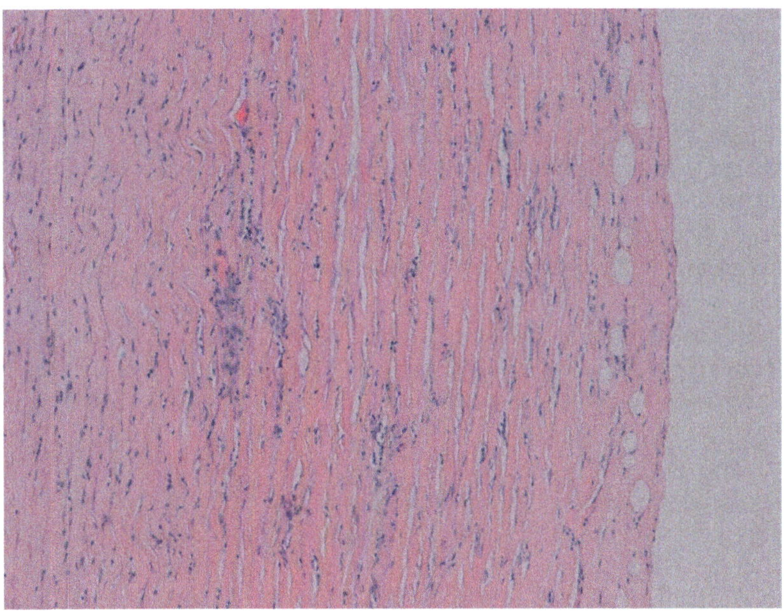

Fig. 7.20 Fake fat in a pleural biopsy from a patient with effusion and fibrosis (hematoxylin–eosin, original magnification ×100)

in sarcomatous and desmoplastic mesothelioma, demonstrating its limited value in this setting [80].

7.9.2 Differential Diagnosis of Malignant Mesothelioma and Secondary Tumors Involving the Serosa

Because of the broad spectrum of histologic patterns of diffuse malignant mesothelioma and the difficulty in the distinction from secondary neoplasms involving the serosa a variety of immunostains have been developed to assist in this kind of differential diagnosis. No single antibody is sufficiently specific and sensitive to diagnose mesothelioma; consequently, the various panels of antibodies have been proposed to aid in the differential diagnosis between mesothelioma and other diseases with which it may be confused. The most important antibody of these panels is pancytokeratin not only to highlight the invasion of malignant cells, but also to exclude some rare malignant neoplasms involving the serosa (lymphoma, melanoma, and sarcomas). Indeed, epithelioid/biphasic and most sarcomatoid mesotheliomas stain diffusely and are strongly positive with this antibody.

7.9.2.1 Epithelioid/Mixed Malignant Mesothelioma Versus Carcinoma

The differential diagnosis between epithelioid/mixed malignant mesothelioma and metastatic carcinoma to the serosa varies in relation to the morphological and clinical information, which guides the selection of the immunohistochemistry panel, since immunohistochemistry can greatly improve this diagnostic topic [9, 16, 70]. The most useful general carcinoma markers are the monoclonal carcinoembryonic antigen (CEA), BerEP4, CD15 (LeuM1), MOC31, BG8, claudin-4, and B72.3 [16, 60, 70, 71]. These markers fail to stain the majority of mesotheliomas, while other immunohistochemical markers can be used to confirm the origin of carcinoma. The main differential diagnosis is certainly between epithelioid malignant mesothelioma and adenocarcinoma. For pleural malignant mesothelioma, differential diagnosis is predominantly pulmonary adenocarcinoma, which either spreads directly to the pleura or metastasizes. In this case, the immunohistochemical panel should include the markers of lung adenocarcinoma, such as the thyroid transcription factor 1 (TTF-1) and Napsin A [81]. In this context, CEA and BerEP4 may be useful in occasional cases showing discordant immunohistochemical staining. For several malignant epithelioid proliferations in the pleura, differential diagnosis also comprises squamous cell carcinoma. p40 is the best marker to distinguish malignant pleural mesothelioma from squamous cell carcinoma, whereas CK5/6 is also expressed in mesothelioma and for this reason does not solve this diagnostic dilemma [82, 83].

Differential diagnosis for peritoneal diffuse malignant mesothelioma includes peritoneal carcinomatosis from the intestinal tract, pancreas, and primary and secondary (female) mullerian system, especially serous carcinoma. Similarly to pleural mesothelioma, immunohistochemical studies are helpful to support or exclude peritoneal mesothelioma, but the panel of antibodies must be different. Adenocarcinoma of the gastrointestinal tract can be differentiated by CDX2 nuclear positivity, a marker of intestinal differentiation, cytokeratin 20, and monoclonal CEA [71]. In the female peritoneum, the differential diagnosis between epithelioid mesothelioma and serous carcinoma may be particularly complex, since the two tumors share clinical presentation, pattern of peritoneal involvement, and morphologic features. In this case, the most appropriate panel may be the combination of calretinin, estrogen receptor (ER), BerEP4, and TAG-72 [84–86]. In males, prostate-specific antigen (PSA) and prostate-specific membrane antigen (PSMA)-positive cytoplasmic staining indicate an adenocarcinoma of the prostate [71]. ER, progesterone receptor (PGR), gross cystic disease fluid protein (GCDFP15), and mammaglobin, if positive markers, can help distinguish malignant mesothelioma from metastatic breast carcinoma [87]. Other useful immunohistochemical markers are PAX8 or PAX2, which show nuclear positivity in renal cell carcinoma as they are not expressed in mesothelial neoplasms [88]. Table 7.2 lists the immunohistochemical markers more commonly used in the differential diagnosis between epithelioid/mixed malignant mesothelioma and carcinoma.

7.9.2.2 Sarcomatoid Malignant Mesothelioma Versus Spindle Cell Malignancy

The major differential diagnoses for sarcomatoid malignant mesothelioma are primary and secondary sarcoma and metastatic sarcomatoid carcinoma [18]. The clinical history and anatomic distribution of the tumor are important considerations; some non-mesothelial tumors, such as sarcomatoid carcinoma or synovial sarcoma, tend to be localized, while sarcomatoid mesotheliomas have a diffuse distribution. Immunohistochemistry has a more restricted role for the differential diagnosis of sarcomatoid malignant mesothelioma than for the epithelioid/mixed form, since mesothelial markers often show weak and focal expression, or fail to identify mesothelial differentiation. The most useful markers for sarcomatoid mesothelioma are calretinin and D2-40, which are expressed in a variable percentage of cases and which can recognize the mesothelial origin of the neoplasm [13, 70]. Most sarcomatoid/desmoplastic malignant mesotheliomas are strongly positive for cytokeratins, whereas most sarcomas are keratin-negative; thus, consistent keratin immunostaining combined with calretinin and D2-40 could be useful to distinguish spindle cell mesothelioma from sarcoma of a different lineage [89–91]. Occasionally, the expression of muscle markers (muscle-specific actin, smooth muscle actin, desmin) and/or neural markers (S-100, neuron-specific enolase) can be observed in sarcomatoid mesothelioma. It follows that the demonstration of positive staining for keratin and mesothelial markers is essential to confirm the diagnosis of malignant mesothelioma [26]. Positive results for keratins alone do not rule out a metastatic sarcomatoid carcinoma; in this regard, the positivity for mesothelial markers (calretinin, D2-40) supports the diagnosis of sarcomatoid mesothelioma [70]. There are some keratin-positive sarcomas, such as angiosarcoma and monophasic synovial sarcoma and in these cases, the expression of specific lineage markers and the presence of characteristic genetic changes could solve some diagnostic issues [89–91]. For example, the differential diagnosis between sarcomatoid diffuse malignant mesothelioma and synovial sarcoma is extremely complex; indeed, monophasic synovial sarcoma may express keratin as well as some mesothelial markers, such as calretinin and CK5/6. However, a definitive diagnosis can only be made by cytogenetic analysis for the demonstration of the translocation between chromosomes X and 18. This translocation is present in over 90% of synovial sarcomas and is not reported in diffuse malignant mesothelioma. For this reason, the identification of the *t(X;18)* translocation is of great aid when this entity enters differential diagnosis [92].

7.10 Conclusions

The diagnostic process of malignant mesothelioma is complex and can be one of the greatest challenges faced by the practicing surgical pathologist. Although mesothelioma is a rare tumor, its diagnosis has a severe prognosis and always entails important medicolegal implications. The pathologist should carefully evaluate the clinical, radiological, and pathological features. However, a history of asbestos exposure should not be taken into consideration when confirming or excluding mesothelioma. Diffuse malignant mesotheliomas must be differentiated from localized malignant mesotheliomas, which have different clinical behaviors. The definitive pathological diagnosis of diffuse malignant mesothelioma usually requires a tissue specimen (and, less frequently, cytology) to demonstrate that the tumor has a mesothelial phenotype and that it shows neoplastic invasion as opposed to reactive mesothelial hyperplasia. Evidence of malignant mesothelioma on cytological examination should be confirmed by histological analysis, or if biopsy is not feasible, cytological diagnosis should be always supported by clinical, radiological, and surgical findings. Identification of the histological appearance (epithelioid, biphasic, sarcomatoid) of diffuse malignant mesothelioma should be a standard histopathological practice. Indeed, it could facilitate diagnosis and provide important information about the clinical outcome since the histological subtype is still the best predictor of prognosis.

Immunohistochemistry is fundamental for the diagnosis and differential diagnosis of malignant mesothelioma. The immunohistochemical approach should rely on the application of a panel including positive (mesothelial-related) and negative markers, as suggested by morphology and clinical information when available. Moreover, molecular analysis, such as a fluorescent in situ hybridization assay for the *p16* homozygous deletion, is more widely available and could be useful in selected cases, distinguishing benign from malignant pleural proliferations.

References

1. Henderson DW, Whitaker D, Shilkin KB. The differential diagnosis of malignant messothelioma: a practical approach to diagnosis during life. In: Henderson DW, Shilkin KB, Langlois SLP, et al., editors. Malignant mesothelioma. New York: Hemisphere; 1992. p. 184.

2. Scherpereel A, Astoul P, Baas P, Berghmans T, Clayson H, de Vuyst P, et al. Guidelines of the European Respiratory Society and the European Society of Thoracic Surgeons for the management of malignant pleural mesothelioma. Eur Respir J. 2010;35:479–95.
3. Sekido Y. Molecular pathogenesis of malignant mesothelioma. Carcinogenesis. 2013;34:1413–9.
4. Travis WD, Brambilla E, Burke AP, Marx A, Nicholson AG. In: Travis WD, Brambilla E, Burke AP, Marx A, Nicholson AG, editors. WHO classification of tumours of the lung, pleura, thymus and heart, vol. 7. 4th ed. Lyon: WHO, IARC; 2015.
5. Tavassoli FA, Devilee P. In: Tavassoli FA, Devilee P, editors. Pathology and genetics: tumours of the breast and female genital organs, WHO classification of tumours series, vol. IV. Lyon: IARC Press; 2003.
6. Peterson JT, Greenberg SD, Buffler PA. Non-asbestos-related malignant mesothelioma. A review. Cancer. 1984;54:951–60.
7. Carbone M, Pass HI, Rizzo P, Marinetti M, Di Muzio M, Mew DJ, et al. Simian virus 40-like DNA sequences in human pleural mesothelioma. Oncogene. 1994;9:1781–90.
8. Selçuk ZT, Cöplü L, Emri S, Kalyoncu AF, Sahin AA, Bariş YI. Malignant pleural mesothelioma due to environmental mineral fiber exposure in Turkey. Analysis of 135 cases. Chest. 1992;102:790–6.
9. Husain AN, Colby TV, Ordóñez NG, Allen TC, Attanoos RL, Beasley MB, et al. Guidelines for pathologic diagnosis of malignant mesothelioma: 2017 update of the consensus statement from the International Mesothelioma Interest Group. Arch Pathol Lab Med. 2018;142:89.
10. Larsen BT, Klein JRH, Hornychová H, Nuti R, Thirumala S, Leslie KO, et al. Diffuse intrapulmonary malignant mesothelioma masquerading as interstitial lung disease: a distinctive variant of mesothelioma. Am J Surg Pathol. 2013;37:1555–64.
11. Asensio JA, Goldblatt P, Thomford NR. Primary malignant peritoneal mesothelioma. A report of seven cases and a review of the literature. Arch Surg. 1990;125:1477–81.
12. Churg A, Galateau-Salle F. The separation of benign and malignant mesothelial proliferations. Arch Pathol Lab Med. 2012;136:1217–26.
13. Novello S, Pinto C, Torri V, Porcu L, Di Maio M, Tiseo M, et al. The third Italian consensus conference for malignant pleural mesothelioma: state of the art and recommendations. Crit Rev Oncol Hematol. 2016;104:9–20.
14. Pinto C, Novello S, Torri V, Ardizzoni A, Betta PG, Bertazzi PA, et al. Second Italian consensus conference on malignant pleural mesothelioma: state of the art and recommendations. Cancer Treat Rev. 2013;39:328–39.
15. van Zandwijk N, Clarke C, Henderson D, Musk AW, Fong K, Nowak A, et al. Guidelines for the diagnosis and treatment of malignant pleural mesothelioma. J Thorac Dis. 2013;5:E254–307.
16. Travis WD, Brambilla E, Burke AP, Marx A, Nicholson AG. Introduction to the 2015 World Health Organization classification of tumors of the lung, pleura, thymus, and heart. J Thorac Oncol. 2015;10:1240–2.
17. Arif Q, Husain AN. Malignant mesothelioma diagnosis. Arch Pathol Lab Med. 2015;139:978–80.
18. Gibbs AR. Tumours of the serosal membranes. Armed forces Institute of Pathology Atlas of Tumour Pathology. Occup Environ Med. 2006;64:288.
19. Kadota K, Suzuki K, Sima CS, Rusch VW, Adusumilli PS, Travis WD. Pleomorphic epithelioid diffuse malignant pleural mesothelioma: a clinicopathological review and conceptual proposal to reclassify as biphasic or sarcomatoid mesothelioma. J Thorac Oncol. 2011;6:896–904.
20. Ordóñez NG. Pleomorphic mesothelioma: report of 10 cases. Mod Pathol. 2012;25:1011–22.
21. Ordóñez NG. Deciduoid mesothelioma: report of 21 cases with review of the literature. Mod Pathol. 2012;25:1481–95.
22. Kadota K, Suzuki K, Colovos C, Sima CS, Rusch VW, Travis WD, et al. A nuclear grading system is a strong predictor of survival in epitheloid diffuse malignant pleural mesothelioma. Mod Pathol. 2012;25:260–71.
23. Ordóñez NG. Mesotheliomas with small cell features: report of eight cases. Mod Pathol. 2012;25:689–98.
24. Cigognetti M, Lonardi S, Fisogni S, Balzarini P, Pellegrini V, Tironi A, et al. BAP1 (BRCA1-associated protein 1) is a highly specific marker for differentiating mesothelioma from reactive mesothelial proliferations. Mod Pathol. 2015;28:1043–57.
25. Klebe S, Brownlee NA, Mahar A, Burchette JL, Sporn TA, Vollmer RT, et al. Sarcomatoid mesothelioma: a clinical-pathologic correlation of 326 cases. Mod Pathol. 2010;23:470–9.
26. Klebe S, Mahar A, Henderson DW, Roggli VL. Malignant mesothelioma with heterologous elements: clinicopathological correlation of 27 cases and literature review. Mod Pathol. 2008;21:1084–94.
27. Mangano WE, Cagle PT, Churg A, Vollmer RT, Roggli VL. The diagnosis of desmoplastic malignant mesothelioma and its distinction from fibrous pleurisy: a histologic and immunohistochemical analysis of 31 cases including p53 immunostaining. Am J Clin Pathol. 1998;110:191–9.
28. Vigneswaran WT, Kircheva DY, Ananthanarayanan V, Watson S, Arif Q, Celauro AD, et al. Amount of epithelioid differentiation is a predictor of survival in malignant pleural mesothelioma. Ann Thorac Surg. 2017;103:962–6.
29. Sebbag G, Yan H, Shmookler BM, Chang D, Sugarbaker PH. Results of treatment of 33 patients with peritoneal mesothelioma. Br J Surg. 2000;87:1587–93.
30. Sugarbaker PH, Welch LS, Mohamed F, Glehen O. A review of peritoneal mesothelioma at the Washington Cancer Institute. Surg Oncol Clin N Am. 2003;12:605–21, xi.

31. Allen TC, Cagle PT, Churg AM, Colby TV, Gibbs AR, Hammar SP, et al. Localized malignant mesothelioma. Am J Surg Pathol. 2005;29:866–73.
32. Crotty TB, Myers JL, Katzenstein AL, Tazelaar HD, Swensen SJ, Churg A. Localized malignant mesothelioma. A clinicopathologic and flow cytometric study. Am J Surg Pathol. 1994;18:357–63.
33. Nakas A, Martin-Ucar AE, Edwards JG, Waller DA. Localised malignant pleural mesothelioma: a separate clinical entity requiring aggressive local surgery. Eur J Cardiothorac Surg. 2008;33:303–6.
34. Asioli S, Dal Piaz G, Damiani S. Localised pleural malignant mesothelioma. Report of two cases simulating pulmonary carcinoma and review of the literature. Virchows Arch. 2004;445:206–9.
35. Daya D, McCaughey WT. Well-differentiated papillary mesothelioma of the peritoneum. A clinicopathologic study of 22 cases. Cancer. 1990;65:292–6.
36. Butnor KJ, Sporn TA, Hammar SP, Roggli VL. Well-differentiated papillary mesothelioma. Am J Surg Pathol. 2001;25:1304–9.
37. Galateau-Sallé F, Vignaud JM, Burke L, Gibbs A, Brambilla E, Attanoos R, et al. Well-differentiated papillary mesothelioma of the pleura: a series of 24 cases. Am J Surg Pathol. 2004;28:534–40.
38. Malpica A, Sant'Ambrogio S, Deavers MT, Silva EG. Well-differentiated papillary mesothelioma of the female peritoneum: a clinicopathologic study of 26 cases. Am J Surg Pathol. 2012;36:117–27.
39. Weiss SW, Tavassoli FA. Multicystic mesothelioma. An analysis of pathologic findings and biologic behavior in 37 cases. Am J Surg Pathol. 1988;12:737–46.
40. Ross MJ, Welch WR, Scully RE. Multilocular peritoneal inclusion cysts (so-called cystic mesotheliomas). Cancer. 1989;64:1336–46.
41. Ball NJ, Urbanski SJ, Green FH, Kieser T. Pleural multicystic mesothelial proliferation. The so-called multicystic mesothelioma. Am J Surg Pathol. 1990;14:375–8.
42. Katsube Y, Mukai K, Silverberg SG. Cystic mesothelioma of the peritoneum: a report of five cases and review of the literature. Cancer. 1982;50:1615–22.
43. Rapisarda AMC, Cianci A, Caruso S, Vitale SG, Valenti G, Piombino E, et al. Benign multicystic mesothelioma and peritoneal inclusion cysts: are they the same clinical and histopathological entities? A systematic review to find an evidence-based management. Arch Gynecol Obstet. 2018;297:1353–75.
44. Hjerpe A, Ascoli V, Bedrossian C, Boon M, Creaney J, Davidson B, et al. Guidelines for cytopathologic diagnosis of epithelioid and mixed type malignant mesothelioma. Complementary statement from the International Mesothelioma Interest Group, also endorsed by the International Academy of Cytology and the Papanicolaou Society of Cytopathology. Cytojournal. 2015;12:26.
45. Rakha EA, Patil S, Abdulla K, Abdulkader M, Chaudry Z, Soomro IN. The sensitivity of cytologic evaluation of pleural fluid in the diagnosis of malignant mesothelioma. Diagn Cytopathol. 2010;38:874–9.
46. Paintal A, Raparia K, Zakowski MF, Nayar R. The diagnosis of malignant mesothelioma in effusion cytology: a reappraisal and results of a multi-institution survey. Cancer Cytopathol. 2013;121:703–7.
47. Segal A, Sterrett GF, Frost FA, Shilkin KB, Olsen NJ, William Musk A, et al. A diagnosis of malignant pleural mesothelioma can be made by effusion cytology: results of a 20 year audit. Pathology (Phila). 2013;45:44–8.
48. Henderson DW, Reid G, Kao SC, van Zandwijk N, Klebe S. Challenges and controversies in the diagnosis of mesothelioma: part 1. Cytology-only diagnosis, biopsies, immunohistochemistry, discrimination between mesothelioma and reactive mesothelial hyperplasia, and biomarkers. J Clin Pathol. 2013;66:847–53.
49. Ismail-Khan R, Robinson LA, Williams CC, Garrett CR, Bepler G, Simon GR. Malignant pleural mesothelioma: a comprehensive review. Cancer Control. 2006;13:255–63.
50. Galateau-Salle F, Churg A, Roggli V, Travis WD. World Health Organization Committee for tumors of the pleura. The 2015 World Health Organization classification of tumors of the pleura: advances since the 2004 classification. J Thorac Oncol. 2016;11:142–54.
51. Husain AN. Mesothelial proliferations: useful marker is not the same as a diagnostic one. Am J Clin Pathol. 2014;141:152–3.
52. Churg A, Sheffield BS, Galateau-Salle F. New markers for separating benign from malignant mesothelial proliferations: are we there yet? Arch Pathol Lab Med. 2016;140:318–21.
53. Attanoos RL, Griffin A, Gibbs AR. The use of immunohistochemistry in distinguishing reactive from neoplastic mesothelium. A novel use for desmin and comparative evaluation with epithelial membrane antigen, p53, platelet-derived growth factor-receptor, P-glycoprotein and Bcl-2. Histopathology. 2003;43:231–8.
54. Minato H, Kurose N, Fukushima M, Nojima T, Usuda K, Sagawa M, et al. Comparative immunohistochemical analysis of IMP3, GLUT1, EMA, CD146, and desmin for distinguishing malignant mesothelioma from reactive mesothelial cells. Am J Clin Pathol. 2014;141:85–93.
55. Shi M, Fraire AE, Chu P, Cornejo K, Woda BA, Dresser K, et al. Oncofetal protein IMP3, a new diagnostic biomarker to distinguish malignant mesothelioma from reactive mesothelial proliferation. Am J Surg Pathol. 2011;35:878–82.
56. Lee AF, Gown AM, Churg A. IMP3 and GLUT-1 immunohistochemistry for distinguishing benign from malignant mesothelial proliferations. Am J Surg Pathol. 2013;37:421–6.
57. Husain AN, Mirza MK, Gibbs A, Hiroshima K, Chi Y, Boumendjel R, et al. How useful is GLUT-1 in differentiating mesothelial hyperplasia and fibrosing pleuritis from epithelioid and sarcomatoid mesotheliomas? An international collaborative study. Lung Cancer. 2014;83:324–8.

58. Ikeda K, Tate G, Suzuki T, Kitamura T, Mitsuya T. Diagnostic usefulness of EMA, IMP3, and GLUT-1 for the immunocytochemical distinction of malignant cells from reactive mesothelial cells in effusion cytology using cytospin preparations. Diagn Cytopathol. 2011;39:395–401.
59. Ikeda K, Tate G, Suzuki T, Kitamura T, Mitsuya T. IMP3/L523S, a novel immunocytochemical marker that distinguishes benign and malignant cells: the expression profiles of IMP3/L523S in effusion cytology. Hum Pathol. 2010;41:745–50.
60. Lonardi S, Manera C, Marucci R, Santoro A, Lorenzi L, Facchetti F. Usefulness of Claudin 4 in the cytological diagnosis of serosal effusions. Diagn Cytopathol. 2011;39:313–7.
61. Ladanyi M. Implications of P16/CDKN2A deletion in pleural mesotheliomas. Lung Cancer. 2005;49(Suppl 1):S95–8.
62. Illei PB, Ladanyi M, Rusch VW, Zakowski MF. The use of CDKN2A deletion as a diagnostic marker for malignant mesothelioma in body cavity effusions. Cancer. 2003;99:51–6.
63. Chung CT-S, Santos GDC, Hwang DM, Ludkovski O, Pintilie M, Squire JA, et al. FISH assay development for the detection of p16/CDKN2A deletion in malignant pleural mesothelioma. J Clin Pathol. 2010;63:630–4.
64. Nasu M, Emi M, Pastorino S, Tanji M, Powers A, Luk H, et al. High incidence of somatic BAP1 alterations in sporadic malignant mesothelioma. J Thorac Oncol. 2015;10:565–76.
65. Bott M, Brevet M, Taylor BS, Shimizu S, Ito T, Wang L, et al. The nuclear deubiquitinase BAP1 is commonly inactivated by somatic mutations and 3p21.1 losses in malignant pleural mesothelioma. Nat Genet. 2011;43:668–72.
66. Yoshikawa Y, Sato A, Tsujimura T, Emi M, Morinaga T, Fukuoka K, et al. Frequent inactivation of the BAP1 gene in epithelioid-type malignant mesothelioma. Cancer Sci. 2012;103:868–74.
67. Sheffield BS, Hwang HC, Lee AF, Thompson K, Rodriguez S, Tse CH, et al. BAP1 immunohistochemistry and p16 FISH to separate benign from malignant mesothelial proliferations. Am J Surg Pathol. 2015;39:977–82.
68. Cibas ES, Corson JM, Pinkus GS. The distinction of adenocarcinoma from malignant mesothelioma in cell blocks of effusions: the role of routine mucin histochemistry and immunohistochemical assessment of carcinoembryonic antigen, keratin proteins, epithelial membrane antigen, and milk fat globule-derived antigen. Hum Pathol. 1987;18:67–74.
69. Hammar SP, Bockus DE, Remington FL, Rohrbach KA. Mucin-positive epithelial mesotheliomas: a histochemical, immunohistochemical, and ultrastructural comparison with mucin-producing pulmonary adenocarcinomas. Ultrastruct Pathol. 1996;20:293–325.
70. Betta P-G, Magnani C, Bensi T, Trincheri NF, Orecchia S. Immunohistochemistry and molecular diagnostics of pleural malignant mesothelioma. Arch Pathol Lab Med. 2012;136:253–61.
71. Ordóñez NG. Application of immunohistochemistry in the diagnosis of epithelioid mesothelioma: a review and update. Hum Pathol. 2013;44:1–19.
72. Hwang HC, Pyott S, Rodriguez S, Cindric A, Carr A, Michelsen C, et al. BAP1 immunohistochemistry and p16 FISH in the diagnosis of sarcomatous and desmoplastic mesotheliomas. Am J Surg Pathol. 2016;40:714–8.
73. Hida T, Hamasaki M, Matsumoto S, Sato A, Tsujimura T, Kawahara K, et al. BAP1 immunohistochemistry and *p16* FISH results in combination provide higher confidence in malignant pleural mesothelioma diagnosis: ROC analysis of the two tests: BAP1 IHC and *p16* FISH in mesothelioma. Pathol Int. 2016;66:563–70.
74. Churg A, Nabeshima K, Ali G, Bruno R, Fernandez-Cuesta L, Galateau-Salle F. Highlights of the 14th international mesothelioma interest group meeting: pathologic separation of benign from malignant mesothelial proliferations and histologic/molecular analysis of malignant mesothelioma subtypes. Lung Cancer. 2018;124:95–101.
75. Hida T, Hamasaki M, Matsumoto S, Sato A, Tsujimura T, Kawahara K, et al. Immunohistochemical detection of MTAP and BAP1 protein loss for mesothelioma diagnosis: comparison with 9p21 FISH and BAP1 immunohistochemistry. Lung Cancer. 2017;104:98–105.
76. Bruno R, Alì G, Fontanini G. Molecular markers and new diagnostic methods to differentiate malignant from benign mesothelial pleural proliferations: a literature review. J Thorac Dis. 2018;10:S342–52.
77. Micolucci L, Akhtar MM, Olivieri F, Rippo MR, Procopio AD. Diagnostic value of microRNAs in asbestos exposure and malignant mesothelioma: systematic review and qualitative meta-analysis. Oncotarget. 2016;7(36):58606–37.
78. Churg A, Colby TV, Cagle P, Corson J, Gibbs AR, Gilks B, et al. The separation of benign and malignant mesothelial proliferations. Am J Surg Pathol. 2000;24:1183–200.
79. Churg A, Cagle P, Colby TV, Corson JM, Gibbs AR, Hammar S, et al. The fake fat phenomenon in organizing pleuritis: a source of confusion with desmoplastic malignant mesotheliomas. Am J Surg Pathol. 2011;35:1823–9.
80. Hwang HC, Sheffield BS, Rodriguez S, Thompson K, Tse CH, Gown AM, et al. Utility of BAP1 immunohistochemistry and p16 (CDKN2A) FISH in the diagnosis of malignant mesothelioma in effusion cytology specimens. Am J Surg Pathol. 2016;40:120–6.
81. Bishop JA, Sharma R, Illei PB. Napsin A and thyroid transcription factor-1 expression in carcinomas of the lung, breast, pancreas, colon, kidney, thyroid, and malignant mesothelioma. Hum Pathol. 2010;41:20–5.
82. Ordóñez NG. The diagnostic utility of immunohistochemistry in distinguishing between epithelioid mesotheliomas and squamous carcinomas of the lung: a comparative study. Mod Pathol. 2006;19:417–28.

83. Tatsumori T, Tsuta K, Masai K, Kinno T, Taniyama T, Yoshida A, et al. p40 is the best marker for diagnosing pulmonary squamous cell carcinoma: comparison with p63, cytokeratin 5/6, desmocollin-3, and sox2. Appl Immunohistochem Mol Morphol. 2014;22:377–82.
84. Bollinger DJ, Wick MR, Dehner LP, Mills SE, Swanson PE, Clarke RE. Peritoneal malignant mesothelioma versus serous papillary adenocarcinoma. A histochemical and immunohistochemical comparison. Am J Surg Pathol. 1989;13:659–70.
85. Ordóñez NG. Value of immunohistochemistry in distinguishing peritoneal mesothelioma from serous carcinoma of the ovary and peritoneum: a review and update. Adv Anat Pathol. 2006;13:16–25.
86. Attanoos RL, Webb R, Dojcinov SD, Gibbs AR. Value of mesothelial and epithelial antibodies in distinguishing diffuse peritoneal mesothelioma in females from serous papillary carcinoma of the ovary and peritoneum. Histopathology. 2002;40:237–44.
87. Ordóñez NG, Sahin AA. Diagnostic utility of immunohistochemistry in distinguishing between epithelioid pleural mesotheliomas and breast carcinomas: a comparative study. Hum Pathol. 2014;45:1529–40.
88. Ordóñez NG. Value of PAX8, PAX2, napsin A, carbonic anhydrase IX, and claudin-4 immunostaining in distinguishing pleural epithelioid mesothelioma from metastatic renal cell carcinoma. Mod Pathol. 2013;26:1132–43.
89. Lucas DR, Pass HI, Madan SK, Adsay NV, Wali A, Tabaczka P, et al. Sarcomatoid mesothelioma and its histological mimics: a comparative immunohistochemical study. Histopathology. 2003;42:270–9.
90. Rdzanek M, Fresco R, Pass HI, Carbone M. Spindle cell tumors of the pleura: differential diagnosis. Semin Diagn Pathol. 2006;23:44–55.
91. Beasley MB. Immunohistochemistry of pulmonary and pleural neoplasia. Arch Pathol Lab Med. 2008;132:1062–72.
92. Miettinen M, Limon J, Niezabitowski A, Lasota J. Calretinin and other mesothelioma markers in synovial sarcoma: analysis of antigenic similarities and differences with malignant mesothelioma. Am J Surg Pathol. 2001;25:610–7.

8 Tissue and Circulating Biomarkers in Mesothelioma

Paolo Andrea Zucali

8.1 Introduction

In the worldwide, many million people have been exposed to asbestos leading to a continuous increase of morbidity and mortality by malignant pleural mesothelioma and a high number of individuals at risk of developing this fatal pleural disease [1].

It was demonstrated that early diagnosis significantly improves overall survival [2–4]. Unfortunately, malignant pleural mesothelioma is mostly diagnosed at an advanced stage when it is untreatable with the available therapeutic strategies.

The search for the malignant pleural mesothelioma biomarkers has been ongoing for the last 30 years. In fact, tumor biomarkers can play an important role not only in the screening (for the early detection of disease), diagnosis, and prognosis, but also in the predictive and monitoring treatment response.

Currently, the available tissue and serological diagnostic biomarkers are characterized by relatively poor sensitivity and specificity preventing the use of reliable tools both for identification of individuals exposed to asbestos and other carcinogenic fibers and for early detection in patients who are developing malignant mesothelioma [5].

P. A. Zucali (✉)
Department of Oncology, Humanitas Clinical and Research Hospital, Milano, Italy
e-mail: paolo.zucali@humanitas.it

It is possible to categorize the diagnostic biomarkers as the following: historical tissue biomarkers of malignant mesothelioma, including immunohistochemical ones, such as glucose transporter 1 (GLUT-1), tumor protein p53 (p53), desmin, epithelial membrane antigen (EMA), insulin like-growth factor II messenger RNA-binding protein 3 (IMP-3) [6–14]; emerging tissue biomarkers such as the BRCA1 associated protein 1 (BAP-1) and the cyclin dependent kinase inhibitor 2A (*CDKN2A*) gene, better known as *p16* [15]; soluble biomarkers, such as mesothelin and fibulin-3 [16–22]. More recently, a list of new biomarkers, including signature based on microRNA and messenger RNA expression, DNA, molecular panels and classification algorithms, and antibody targets, are being proposed for malignant mesothelioma [5, 23–28]. Moreover, with the advent of targeted therapy and the rapid progress in immunotherapy for the treatment of malignant mesothelioma, it is required to extend biomarker discovery and validation to an individualized approach to assess a patient's suitability to these treatments.

8.2 Tissue Biomarkers

In agreement with the current studies and consensus reports, the most important markers in the diagnosis of malignant pleural mesothelioma are the tissue "mesothelioma markers" calretinin (CR), cytokeratin 5 (CK 5), podoplanin (PDP),

G. L. Ceresoli et al. (eds.), *Mesothelioma*, https://doi.org/10.1007/978-3-030-16884-1_8

Table 8.1 Tumor tissue biomarkers

Biomarker	Methods	Role	Results
Calretinin	IHC – TM	Diagnostic/prognostic	Diagnosis epithelioid histology; worse prognosis
Cytokeratin 5	IHC	Diagnostic	Diagnosis MPM
Podoplanin	IHC	Diagnostic	Differentiate MPM from ADK
WT1-Protein	IHC	Diagnostic/predictive	Differentiate MPM from ADK; potential therapeutic target
GLUT1	IHC	Diagnostic	Diagnosis of malignancy
p53 Protein	IHC	Diagnostic	Diagnosis of malignancy
Desmin	IHC	Diagnostic	Diagnosis of benignity
EMA	IHC	Diagnostic	Diagnosis of malignancy
IMP-3	ICH	Diagnostic/prognostic	Diagnosis of malignancy; worse prognosis
p16 gene	FISH	Diagnostic	Diagnosis of MPM
BAP-1	IHC - FISH	Diagnostic/prognostic	Diagnosis of MPM; good prognosis
Mesothelin	IHC	Diagnostic/predictive	Diagnosis of MPM; therapeutic target
CD8+TILs	IHC	Prognostic	Good prognosis
CD20+Ls	IHC	Prognostic	Good prognosis
CD163+TAMs	IHC	Prognostic	Worse prognosis
IL-7R+	IHC	Prognostic	Worse prognosis
PD-L1	IHC	Prognostic/predictive	Worse prognosis; therapeutic target

IHC immunohistochemistry, *TM* Tissue Microarray, *MPM* malignant pleural mesothelioma, *ADK* adenocarcinoma

and Wilms' tumor-1 protein (WT1) (Table 8.1). Other tissue mesothelioma markers with a diagnostic/prognostic role are mesothelin, GLUT-1, p53, desmin, EMA, IMP-3, BAP-1, and *p16*. Moreover, a plethora of downregulated and upregulated genes and regions of chromosomal gains and losses were discovered with the aim to identify specific tumor signatures versus normal tissue. Finally, it was shown that immunoscore is a potential prognostic biomarker also in malignant pleural mesothelioma.

8.2.1 Calretinin

Calretinin is a calcium-binding protein belonging to the EF-hand family [29]. Among the immunomarkers, CR seems to be the most valuable in differentiating malignant mesothelioma from lung and breast adenocarcinoma, provided that only widespread nuclear reaction is considered positive [30, 31]. Calretinin is useful for the diagnosis of epithelioid malignant mesothelioma because its expression is low in the areas with sarcomatous differentiation and it has limited value in discriminating malignant mesothelioma from serous or squamous carcinomas [30, 32].

8.2.2 Cytokeratin 5

Cytokeratins are intermediates filaments (more than 70 CK subtypes have been identified) located in the cytoplasm of epithelial cells and subsets of non-epithelial cells (including mesothelial cells) [32]. The positivity of CK5 is detectable in the large majority of malignant mesotheliomas but also in squamous cell carcinoma, basal-like breast carcinoma, ovarian serous and endometrioid carcinoma whereas lung and breast adenocarcinomas are mostly negative [33, 34].

8.2.3 Podoplanin

Podoplanin is a sialoglycoprotein detectable in podocytes, involved in embryogenesis and expressed in several normal tissues, including lymphatic endothelial cells and mesothelium [35]. The expression of PDP is frequent in malignant pleural mesothelioma, seminoma, and angiosarcoma while it is less frequent in breast adenocarcinomas and rare in lung carcinomas [35]. For this reason, PDP has an important role in differentiating malignant pleural mesothelioma from adenocarcinoma [36, 37]. The expression of

PDP is possible in squamous and serous carcinoma whereas it is contradictory in areas with sarcomatous differentiation, limiting its discriminatory value in these cases [35, 38–40].

8.2.4 Wilms' Tumor-1 Protein

The WT1 is a tumor suppressor gene that encodes the nuclear WT1 protein. The suppressor role of WT1 protein is dependent on the presence of wild-type p53. In fact, in the absence of p53, WT1 protein acts as an activator [41]. Its expression is normally detectable in developing human organs but overexpressed in leukemia and some solid tumors, such as breast cancer and malignant mesothelioma [42–44]. For this reason, WT1 protein is a biomarker for malignant mesothelioma useful to differentiate lung adenocarcinoma but not breast adenocarcinoma [34]. Moreover, WT1 expression is contradictory in non-epithelial mesothelioma and of limited discriminatory value to distinguish between malignant mesothelioma and serous carcinoma [31, 45, 46]. The WT1 has also been suggested as a potential therapeutic target for malignant mesothelioma considering its unique overexpression, as well as a negative prognostic factor in peritoneal malignant mesothelioma [47].

8.2.5 Glucose Transporter 1 GLUT-1

The glucose transporter 1 is a member of the mammalian facilitative GLUT family of passive carriers functioning as an energy-independent system for the glucose transport. GLUT-1 is considered a marker of malignancy and it is overexpressed in a variety of tumors [48]. This biomarker showed a high specificity for malignant pleural mesothelioma (90–100%), while its sensitivity values ranged from 21% to 85% [7–9, 49]. If positive, GLUT-1 is informative for malignancy only because the absence of immune-reactivity does not exclude malignant pleural mesothelioma diagnosis.

8.2.6 Tumor Protein p53

The protein p53 is a tumor suppressor with a crucial role in the development of cancer. Its nuclear accumulation has been suggested as supporting evidence of malignancy. Nevertheless, its efficacy in clinical practice is minimal due to the contradictory literature data [11, 12].

8.2.7 Desmin

Desmin is a muscle-specific class III intermediate filament. Its homopolymers constitute a stable intra-cytoplasmic filamentous network connecting myofibrils to each other and to the plasma membrane. Desmin is a marker of benignity. Its sensitivity ranges from 48% to 84% whereas its specificity reaches 97% in some studies [7, 11]. However, a proportion of malignant pleural mesothelioma (as high as 50%) has been reported to be positive as well [48]. Therefore, its use in clinical practice is very limited.

8.2.8 Epithelial Membrane Antigen

The EMA is a membrane-bound protein, member of the mucin family including O-glycosylated proteins essential in construction of protective mucous barriers on epithelial surfaces and in intracellular signaling. The EMA is a biomarker of malignancy. Its sensitivity ranges from 41% to 79% and its specificity from 88% to 100% [7, 49]. Unfortunately, this marker was found positive also in atypical mesothelial hyperplasia and in benign lesions and for this reason its use is minimal [12].

8.2.9 Insulin Like-Growth Factor II Messenger RNA-Binding Protein 3

The IMP-3 is an onco-fetal cytoplasmic protein expressed in fetal tissues. It acts as an oncogene and its staining is observed in many carcinomas.

The IMP3 is a biomarker of tumor aggressiveness and its expression correlates with a worse prognosis in human malignancies [13]. It is a highly specific biomarker for malignancy and it was suggested for the differentiation of malignant pleural mesothelioma from reactive mesothelial proliferations [13]. Its sensitivity ranges from 37% to 94%, regardless of subtype and location. Nevertheless, some benign alterations, such as atypical hyperplasia, stain for this marker as well [7, 12, 14, 49].

8.2.10 Gene *p16*

The International Mesothelioma Interest Group (IMIG) guidelines for histological and cytological diagnosis of MPM suggested the analysis of two relatively new markers either on FFPE tissues from biopsies or on cytological specimens: p16 by FISH and BAP1 by immunohistochemistry [15, 50, 51]. The p16 is a cyclin-dependent kinase inhibitor and it acts as a tumor suppressor [52]. It is frequently deleted (locus 9p21) in malignant lesions and it has never been reported as altered in benign lesions. Its specificity for malignant pleural mesothelioma is 100% whereas its sensitivity ranges between 43% and 93% [53, 54]. The loss of p16 occurs in all histologic subtypes, but it is particularly characteristic of cases with biphasic and sarcomatoid morphology and it is known to be associated with poor outcome in comparison with cases with retained p16 [55]. In contrast, the loss of BAP1 is more frequently associated with epithelioid morphology and it is largely retained in cases with sarcomatoid morphology [55]. The combination of p16 by FISH and BAP1 by immunohistochemistry has been reported to increase sensitivity for malignant pleural mesothelioma diagnosis up to 90% in some studies whereas the specificity is always 100% [50, 53, 56]. Nevertheless, BAP1 and p16 examinations do not allow the detection of all MPM cases, even when the combined assay approach is utilized, because the two markers are only deleted in a proportion of mesotheliomas and the failure to find their alterations does not assure the benign nature of a mesothelial process.

8.2.11 BRCA1-Associated Protein 1

The BAP1 is a nuclear de-ubiquitinase protein targeting histones and the host cell factor 1 (HCF1) transcriptional cofactor. It has several functions, including chromatin regulation, transcriptional regulation, and participating in multiprotein complexes that regulate gluconeogenesis, repair of cellular differentiation, cell cycle checkpoints, transcription, and apoptosis [57]. As a result, BAP1 acts as a tumor suppressor and it plays an important role in damage response [57, 58]. The BAP1 gene is located on chromosome 3p21: it is frequently deleted in numerous malignant tumors but it has never been reported as altered in benign lesions. Its specificity for malignant pleural mesothelioma is 100% whereas its sensitivity ranges between 61% and 67% [59]. A significantly higher incidence of malignant tumors than observed in the general population (more often developed in an earlier age than expected) is reported among families carrying the mutation of BAP1 [57]. A BAP1 cancer syndrome, including cutaneous melanoma, uveal melanoma, renal cell carcinoma, malignant mesothelioma, and other potential malignant tumors, has been proposed [60]. Germline BAP1 mutations are observed among families with an extraordinary high incidence of malignant mesothelioma and in 25% of sporadic malignant mesothelioma, reporting BAP1 as a gene to predispose for malignant pleural mesothelioma and possibly modulate mineral fiber carcinogenesis [58, 60]. Moreover, several studies showed that BAP1 mutations are significantly more common in epithelioid malignant mesothelioma than sarcomatoid and biphasic tumors [58, 61]. Several reports associated loss of BAP1 with improved prognosis [55]. However, although this is clearly the case in patients with germline BAP1 mutation, it appears that in sporadic cases this effect is at least in part due to its association with epithelioid histology, which itself portends a more favorable prognosis than non-epithelioid morphology [55]. If a significant association of p16 loss with poor outcomes was observed and it is independent of histologic subtype, BAP1 expression by immunohistochemistry is not an independent risk factor [55]. Although

BAP1 expression by immunohistochemistry is not independently predictive of survival across malignant pleural mesothelioma as a whole, when placed in the context of histologic subtype and p16 status, risk stratification was evident [55]. In particular, patients with CDKN2A disomy and loss of BAP1 expression had improved outcomes compared with those with CDKN2A disomy and retained BAP1 expression, especially among epithelioid cases.

Recently, in vitro study showed that BAP1 loss favors cell proliferation by the up-regulation of the enhancer of zeste 2 polycomb repressive complex 2 subunit (EZH2), a histonelysine *N*-methyltransferase overexpressed in various cancers [62, 63]. In a series of 32 malignant pleural mesothelioma and 44 benign mesothelial proliferations, BAP1 loss and EZH2 high expression were observed in 53% and 66% of malignant pleural mesothelioma, respectively. None of the benign lesions presented BAP1 loss or EZH2 high expression, suggesting that the markers together had a diagnostic sensitivity of 90% and a specificity of 100% [64].

8.2.12 Mesothelin

Mesothelin is a 40-kDa glycoprotein attached to the cell surface by a glycosylphosphatidylinositol anchor and expressed on mesothelioma, pancreatic, ovarian, and other tumor malignancies, with limited expression on normal tissue. Its regulation and role are not completely clear. However, it has been suggested its role for the wnt/b-catenin pathway and it has been demonstrated that promoter methylation could control its expression [65–67]. Mesothelin is preferentially elevated in the serum of patients with mesothelioma with high specificity for mesothelioma [68]. In fact, mesothelin can be shed from the cell surface by tumor necrosis factor-a-converting enzyme [69].

The limited expression of mesothelin on normal tissues has led to test mesothelin as a target by immune-based therapies in mesothelioma. The efficacy of several mesothelin-directed treatment approaches is under investigation [69].

8.2.13 Gene Expression Profiling

In an attempt to understand malignant pleural mesothelioma molecular pathogenesis, several studies have used microarray technologies. A lot of gene expression profiling trials have discovered a plethora of downregulated and upregulated genes and regions of chromosomal gains and losses, while most studies have analyzed gene expression in tumor versus normal tissue [70–73]. Among the downregulated genes there are the growth-factor genes affecting the apoptotic pathway, cell adhesion, cytoskeletal anchoring, and tumor suppressor genes [70–73]. Among the over-expressed genes and pathways there are anti-apoptotic genes, metabolic regulating genes, angiogenesis, cell adhesion, detoxification genes, several DNA repair gene pathways, chemokines, chemo-, radio-, and multidrug resistant genes, oncogenes and generally genes driving all phases of cell cycle [70–74]. Furthermore, differentially expressed genes involved in tumor invasiveness and the circadian clock, cell protection, and resistance have been identified [73, 75].

Although several gene signatures with a prognostic role have been proposed, there is not a consensus on single genes or gene signatures helpful for clinical decision due to minimal agreement among study results [76]. Differences in gene expression between epithelioid and sarcomatous malignant mesothelioma were observed in several studies, with all favorable genes being associated with epithelioid histology and unfavorable genes with sarcomatous histology [76, 77].

Reyniès et al. used unsupervised hierarchical clustering on a transcriptomic data from 38 cultures of malignant mesothelioma as well as mutation analysis of the BAP1, CDKN2A, CDKN2B, NF2, and TP53 genes [78]. Three-gene signature (PPL, UPK3B, and TFPI) were identified and these are able to distinguish two subgroups of epithelioid malignant pleural mesothelioma, C1 and C2. The subgroup C1 showed more frequent BAP1 alterations. The subgroup C2 included sarcomatoid and desmoplastic malignant pleural mesotheliomas and had most dismal prognosis. In fact, analyzing the markers of epithelial-to-mesenchymal transition (EMT), the subgroup C2 was characterized by a mesenchymal phenotype, in agreement with the knowledge that sarcomatoid malignant mesothelioma has the worse prognosis.

Gordon et al. developed a gene expression ratio-based prognostic and diagnostic test for malignant pleural mesothelioma [79–81]. Using mRNA expression profiling data from patients with malignant pleural mesothelioma with different survival outcomes, they were able to define two different groups of patients and to train an expression ratio-based outcome predictor model. In particular, they identified the genes that had statistically significant inversely correlated expression levels among the two outcome groups determining with their use the prognostic expression ratios. Finally, they developed a four-gene expression ratio test able to predict statistically significantly treatment-related patient outcome after radical surgery independent of the histologic mesothelioma subtype. They also acquired RNA from malignant pleural mesothelioma with fine-needle aspiration biopsies in order to perform diagnostic gene expression tests using the relative expression level of the 6 genes (CALB2, CLDN7, ANXA8, EPCAM, CD200, and NKX2-1) determined by RT-PCR to calculate a combined score (i.e., geometric mean) of 3 individual gene pair expression ratios (CALB2/CLDN7, ANXA8/EPCAM, CD200/NKX2-1) [81]. The diagnostic test between malignant pleural mesothelioma and lung adenocarcinoma had a sensitivity of 100% and specificity of 90%.

Bueno et al. identified four distinct molecular subtypes analyzing transcriptomes, whole exomes, and targeted exomes with RNA-seq data from 216 patients with malignant pleural mesothelioma: epithelioid (with the longest survival), biphasic-epithelioid (biphasic-E), biphasic-sarcomatoid (biphasic-S), and sarcomatoid [82]. Two-thirds of the histological epithelioid samples were reclassified into other molecular categories. Through exome analysis, BAP1, NF2, TP53, SETD2, DDX3X, ULK2, RYR2, CFAP45, SETDB1, and DDX51 were found significantly mutated in malignant mesothelioma while recurrent mutations such as SF3B1 and TRAF7 were identified. Furthermore, recurrent gene fusions and splice alterations were found to be frequent mechanisms for inactivation of NF2, BAP1, and SETD2. Through integrated analyses, alterations in Hippo, mTOR, histone methylation, RNA helicase, and p53 signaling pathways were identified. These mutational rates and signatures specific for malignant pleural mesothelioma are different from other cancers and these differences, along with mutations, expression profiles and gene fusions, could potentially improve the diagnosis of malignant mesothelioma [82].

8.2.14 Stromal Immune Microenvironment

The presence of tumor-infiltrating macrophages and lymphocytes (TILs) has been shown to correlate with the clinical outcome of multiple solid tumors (including malignant mesothelioma), and with outcomes based on type, density, and location of immune cell infiltrates [83–89].

Several studies reported correlations between the presence of CD8+ TILs and malignant pleural mesothelioma survival [90, 91]. In particular, patients with a high density of CD8+ TILs in tumors tended to exhibit improved survival and reduced frequency of mediastinal lymph node metastases [88, 92].

If the role of B lymphocytes during tumor immunity still remains controversial, the tumor-infiltrating CD20+ B lymphocytes were found to have a role in constraining epithelioid malignant pleural mesothelioma resulting in improved patient survival [88].

Emerging evidences have shown the clinical significance of tumor associated macrophages (TAMs) in several malignant tumors [93–95]. In particular, M1 TAMs have shown immune-stimulatory properties and conferred enhanced tumor resistance and cytotoxicity, while M2 TAMs (CD163+) have demonstrated an immune-suppressive role by inducing specific cytokines secretion, promoting angiogenesis, supporting tumor progression, invasion, and metastasis [94, 96]. In patients with epithelioid malignant pleural mesothelioma, the elevated M2 TAMs (CD163+) correlated with worse prognosis suggesting that the adaptive humoral immune response may play a crucial role in disease progression [88]. Moreover, it was found that the sarcomatoid malignant pleural mesothelioma had highest estimates for T cells and M2 TAMs (CD163+) while the M2 TAMs (CD163+) and their ratio to biologically relevant TILs (CD8+ T-cell and CD20+ B-cell) were independent markers of worse prognosis [82, 88].

The IL-7R expression was reported as a poor prognostic marker in early stage lung adenocarcinoma and breast cancer. In fact, IL-7R is suggested to induce tumor growth and lymphangiogenesis via upregulation of vascular endothelial growth factor D and, therefore, IL-7 may promote tumor progression via the activation of IL-7R on both tumor cells and Tregs. In a large series of epithelial malignant pleural mesothelioma, tumoral IL-7R expression levels were associated with unfavorable prognosis [88].

In general, the PD-L1 expression was shown in approximately 20–40% of malignant pleural mesothelioma [82, 97–99]. PD-L1 expression is measured most commonly by immunohistochemistry. However, no test is uniformly accepted as the standard and the thresholds for positivity have not been yet defined for all the PD-L1 antibodies. Moreover, a different and more reproducible methodology for evaluating PD-L1 has been evaluated with the measurement of mRNA showing association with better outcomes. In a series of 211 patients with malignant pleural mesothelioma, Bueno et al. determined the positivity of PD-L1 in 39% of patients by CD274, as assessed by RNA-seq (reads per kilobase of target per million mapped reads >2.3) [82]. The clinical significance of localization of PD-L1 expression is not yet known. In fact, PD-L1 can be expressed by multiple components of the tumor microenvironment, including infiltrating immune cells and tumor cells themselves. Furthermore, the biological consequences of PD-L1 expression depend on cell membrane localization while cytoplasmic staining may represent intracellular stores of PD-L1 which may be developed to the cell surface depending on appropriate stimulation. In a series of 106 patients with malignant pleural mesothelioma, 40% of patients resulted positive for PD-L1 by immunohistochemistry and PD-L1 expression was only cytoplasmic in 43% of cases, cytoplasmic and membranous in 33%, and exclusive membranous in 24% [98]. In another series, all patients presented cytoplasmic and majority of them membrane staining of PD-L1 [99]. The association of PD-L1 expression with histology has been reported. In general, the sarcomatoid histotype has shown a higher expression of PD-L1 (50–100%) compared with other histotypes (9–23%) [82, 97–99]. Finally, a strong correlation between PD-L1 expression on tumor cells and prognosis has been observed in malignant pleural mesothelioma. The effect of PD-L1 status on prognosis resulted independent of the histology. If the PD-L1 expression in malignant pleural mesothelioma is more frequent in no epithelial patients, PD-L1 negative patients had a significantly better prognosis than the PD-L1 positive patients [82, 97–99].

8.3 Circulating Biomarkers

Blood and pleural effusion are the ideal sample types for detecting biomarkers (Table 8.2). The soluble biomarkers in blood and peritoneal/pleural effusion are interesting tools for rapid diagnosis also in malignant mesothelioma. The most important ones include soluble mesothelin-related peptides (SMRP), osteopontin, fibulin-3, high-mobility group box 1 (HMGB1). Recently, the discovery of protein signatures and aberrant expression of miRNA in tissue and body fluids in tumor could significantly improve the diagnostic accuracy in malignant mesothelioma.

8.3.1 Soluble Mesothelin-Related Peptides (SMRP)

To date, SMRP is the only biomarker for diagnostic and prognostic purposes approved by the FDA and suggested by several consensuses [100, 101]. In particular, FDA approved the MESOMARK assay as a humanitarian use device for the monitoring of epithelioid and biphasic mesothelioma using serum as an analyte [102]. The SMRP are

Table 8.2 Circulating biomarkers

Biomarker	Methods	Role	Results
SMRP	ELISA/MESOMARK (blood, pleural effusion)	Diagnostic/prognostic/predictive	Diagnosis of MPM; worse prognosis; clinical monitoring of response
Osteopontin	ELISA (blood)	Diagnostic/prognostic	Diagnosis of MPM; worse prognosis; clinical monitoring of response
Fibulin-3	ELISA (blood, pleural effusion)	Diagnostic/prognostic	Diagnosis of MPM; worse prognosis
HMGB-1	ELISA (serum)	Diagnostic/prognostic	Diagnosis of MPM; worse prognosis
MicroRNA	HM—qRT-PCR (serum)	Diagnostic/prognostic	Diagnosis of MPM; different miRNA or signature of miRNA showed good or poor prognosis
Proteomic	SOMAmer—SRM (serum)	Diagnostic	Diagnosis of MPM

HM Hybridization based miRNA microarray, *qRT-PCR* quantitative reverse transcription polymerase chain reaction, *SRM* selected reaction monitoring assay technology

membrane-bound peptides processed to yield megakaryocyte-potentiating factor (MPF) and mesothelin, which remains attached to the cell membrane via glycophosphatidylinositol linkage [103]. By activation of NF-kB pathway, resulting in increase of interleukin-6 level, mesothelin promotes tumor cell survival and proliferation [104]. In 2003, Robinson et al. proposed the determination of serum SMRP as a marker for diagnosis of malignant mesothelioma and monitoring disease progression [105]. Subsequent studies confirmed SMRP dosage as a potential tool for screening asbestos exposed individuals for early diagnosis of malignant pleural mesothelioma suggesting serum SMRP as a promising marker not only for diagnosis but also for prognosis and clinical monitoring [106–112]. However, all studies detected high SMRP concentrations only in the epithelioid and mixed malignant mesothelioma. As a diagnostic marker, mesothelin has shown high specificity (96%) but low sensitivity (47%) [68]. On the other hand, as a prognostic marker, the literature data are inconclusive. In fact, if several studies have shown no correlation between serum mesothelin levels and survival outcomes, other studies have shown that SMRP levels are inversely associated with overall survival [109, 112–117]. In multivariate analysis limited to epithelial MPM, the prognostic impact of SMRP on overall survival was lost, suggesting that histology remains a critical determinant of prognosis [68]. Possible explanations for the mixed results on mesothelin as a prognostic marker include small sample sizes and heterogeneous treatment among the different studies [118]. Finally, several data suggest SMRP as a useful tumor marker for detecting the progression of malignant mesothelioma and evaluating tumor response to treatment [119]. Nevertheless, the poor sensitivity of mesothelin (35–50%) limits its value [120].

8.3.2 Osteopontin

Osteopontin is an extracellular cell adhesion glycoprotein that plays key roles in different biological processes such as immunological regulation, cell–matrix interaction, and cell-signaling via interaction with integrin and CD44 receptors, cell migration, and tumor development [121, 122]. Osteopontin resulted up-regulated in cells exposed to asbestos in-vitro, as well as in rat models of asbestos-induced carcinogenesis [123]. The serum osteopontin levels are increased in malignant pleural mesothelioma and therefore osteopontin has been considered as a potential biomarker for early detection of the disease. Comparing patients with asbestos-related non-malignant pulmonary disease with patients without asbestos exposure and patients with surgically staged pleural mesothelioma, Pass et al. found that serum osteopontin levels were significantly higher in patients with malignant pleural mesothelioma than in those with exposure to asbestos, with a sensitivity of 77.6% and a specificity of 85.5% (cutoff value: 48.3 ng/mL) [124]. Moreover, comparing patients with stage I mesothelioma and patients with asbestos exposure, the sensitivity and specificity were 84.6% and 88.4%, respectively (cutoff value 62.4 ng/mL). Some studies confirmed the role of osteopontin as a potential diagnostic biomarker for patients with malignant mesothelioma whereas several other studies were not able to confirm these results [115, 125–128].

These controversial results could be explained by several reasons, such as different ELISA essays used for osteopontin and different control populations evaluated, which may not be reflective of high-risk screening populations. Nevertheless, to definitively assess the diagnostic power of this biomarker, further studies with larger sample size and better design are needed. Despite controversy over diagnostic value, some studies have investigated the role of osteopontin as a prognostic biomarker. In general, low immunohistochemical expression and low baseline plasma levels of osteopontin were independently associated with favorable survival outcomes [112, 129]. Pass et al. combined plasma biomarkers of malignant pleural mesothelioma with EORTC prognostic index founding that higher levels of osteopontin and mesothelin were individually associated with a worse prognosis after adjusting for this specific prognostic index [130]. Moreover, they observed that the incorporation of either plasma osteopontin or mesothelin into the predictive prognostic index model led to a statistically significant improvement in Harrell's C-statistic and the log-osteopontin level, the EORTC clinical prognostic index and the hemoglobin level remained as independently significant predictors in the final prognostic model.

8.3.3 Fibulin-3

The human fibulin-3 is a member of the extracellular glycoprotein fibulin family encoded by the gene epidermal growth factor (EGF), containing fibulin-like extracellular matrix protein 1 (EFEMP1) [131]. Fibulin-3 has been implicated in the regulation of cell proliferation and migration in malignant pleural mesothelioma by its involvement with cell morphology, growth, adhesion, and motility. The diagnostic value of fibulin-3 for malignant pleural mesothelioma has been investigated. Pass et al. found that plasma fibulin-3 levels were significantly higher in patients with malignant pleural mesothelioma compared to patients with only asbestos exposure, with a sensitivity of 96.7% and specificity of 95.5% [20]. Moreover, fibulin-3 levels in the pleural effusion were found significantly higher in patients with malignant pleural mesothelioma compared to patients with pleural effusion unrelated to malignant pleural mesothelioma. In a retrospective analysis of two cohorts of patients with malignant pleural mesothelioma, plasma fibulin-3 levels showed low diagnostic accuracy because it was significantly elevated in one (Sydney cohort) but not in the other (Vienna cohort) [22]. Prospective data are needed to validate fibulin-3 as a potential biomarker for patients with malignant pleural mesothelioma.

8.3.4 High-Mobility Group Box 1 (HMGB1)

The high-mobility group box 1 (HMGB1) is a typical damage-associated molecular pattern (DAMP) and it is a mediator of several biological processes such as transcription, cell proliferation, DNA repair, and inflammation [132, 133]. It was shown that the exposure of primary human mesothelial cells to asbestos fibers induces programmed necrosis and consequent release of HMGB1, triggering the process of cell transformation [134]. Moreover, malignant mesothelioma cells on one hand has shown an active autocrine production of HMGB1 and on the other they were resulted addicted to HMGB1 for growth and invasion [134]. Several studies found that serum and plasma HMGB1 levels were higher in patients with malignant mesothelioma compared to healthy individuals or individuals with benign asbestos-related disease [134–136]. The prognostic role of HMGB1 was established in a systematic review and meta-analysis because a significant negative correlation between serum HMGB1 level and survival was observed [135, 137]. Napolitano et al. discovered that hyper-acetylated HMGB1 levels were significantly higher in patient with malignant mesothelioma compared to asbestos-exposed individuals and healthy controls with a sensitivity and specificity of 100% [1]. Moreover, the HMGB1 levels resulted not influenced by tumor stage and the combination of HMGB1 and fibulin-3 produced better sensitivity and specificity in differentiating patients with malignant mesothelioma from patients with benign or malignant pleural effusion not related to malignant mesothelioma [1]. These results suggest a role for hyper-acetylated HMGB1 as a potential diagnostic marker to differentiate patients with malignant pleural mesothelioma. However, prospective validation studies are needed.

8.3.5 MicroRNA

The MicroRNAs (miRNAs) are non-coding RNA molecules of 18–22 nucleotides that regulate gene expression at the post-transcriptional level by binding the 3′-untranslated regions of target miRNAs inhibiting translation of target messenger RNAs by pairing with messenger RNA recognition elements [138]. Thus, miRNAs are expected to regulate many cellular activities, such as proliferation, differentiation, metabolism, apoptosis, senescence, angiogenesis, and invasion. It was shown that deregulated miRNAs frequently occur in several cancers, malignant mesothelioma included. The miRNAs are considered excellent biomarkers due to their stability and the possibility to be analyzed in routinely processed tissue samples as well as in blood samples. A lot of trials evaluated the miRNA expression in tissues of malignant mesothelioma using microarrays and several series of miRNAs specifically overexpressed or downregulated in malignant mesothelioma compared to normal tissue were identified [139–144]. Among over-expressed miRNAs, miR-30b∗, miR-32∗, miR-483-3p, miR-584, and miR-885-3p were predicted to regulate the tumor suppressor genes CDKN2A and NF2, while downregulated miRNAs such as miR-9, miR-7-1∗ and miR-203 were expected to target the oncogenes HGF, PDGFA, EGF, and JUN [143]. Moreover, the expression of miR-17-5p and miR-30c was correlated with survival in patients with sarcomatoid malignant mesothelioma [142]. Another study observed that the elevated miR-29C∗ expression was linked with a significantly higher survival of patients with malignant mesothelioma whereas the loss of miR-31 (linked with frequent homozygous loss of 9p21.3 chromosome in malignant mesothelioma) was associated with tumor suppressor activity [145]. A miR-Score, a signature of 6 miRNAs (miR-21-5p, miR-23a-3p, miR-30e-5p, miR-221-3p, miR-222-3p, and miR-31-5p) predicting long survival, was identified among patients with malignant mesothelioma undergoing surgery (extra pleural pneumonectomy or palliative surgery) [146]. Also cell-free, circulating miRNAs have been suggested as biomarkers for malignant mesothelioma. Bononi et al. identified three circulating miRNAs (miRNA 197-3p, miRNA-1281, and miRNA 32-3p) upregulated in patients with malignant pleural mesothelioma compared to the control group [147]. In particular, miR-197 and miRNA 32-3p were found to downregulate the FOXO3 gene and tumor suppressor gene pTEN plus anti-proliferative factor BTG2, respectively, suggesting a role in carcinogenesis of malignant mesothelioma. All these data suggested that deregulated miRNAs could be considered as promising diagnostic biomarkers and prognostic factors for malignant mesothelioma as well. Nevertheless, their clinical utility should be further explored in large prospective trials.

8.3.6 Proteomics

The proteome is the whole full set of proteins expressed by an organism or a system in a particular time and under defined physiological or pathological conditions. The discovery of protein signatures, which have been recently exploited for the effective screening of a high number biomarkers, could significantly improve the diagnostic accuracy in several cancers, malignant mesothelioma included [148–150]. To screen serological diagnostic markers of malignant mesothelioma, the SOMAmer protein technology has been used in a multicenter case–control study including 117 patients with malignant mesothelioma and 142 control subjects with asbestos exposure [150, 151]. A 13-marker random forest classifier was developed from 64 candidate biomarkers extrapolated from more than 1000 screened proteins. This random forest model was able to differentiate malignant mesothelioma from controls (AUC 0.99, sensitivity >90%, specificity >90%) better than mesothelin (AUC 0.82, sensitivity 66%, specificity 88%) [150]. The potency of this proteomics approach, providing a multiplex biomarker signature, is likely a promising diagnostic tool for malignant pleural mesothelioma [152].

Using a selected reaction monitoring (SRM) assay technology, a seven glycopeptide signature in cells of malignant mesothelioma was identified and used to investigate surfaceoma derived serum candidate biomarker panels for malignant mesothelioma [153].

This seven glycopeptide signature was able to accurately discriminate malignant mesothelioma from healthy controls and to significantly improve the diagnostic accuracy of mesothelin (if combined) in differentiating malignant mesothelioma from non-small-cell lung cancer [153].

8.4 Future Perspectives

Developments in biomarker research for malignant mesothelioma prognosis and diagnosis have seen in recent years. Likely, a combination of the most performing and valuable markers validated by the ongoing studies will potentially allow more accurate diagnosis of malignant mesothelioma and earlier detection in the near future. Ideally, potential biomarkers should be non-invasive and easy-to-use; test-related costs should be minimal; time to analytical result should be sufficiently short. Further to some tissue and circulating biomarkers, also breathomics seems to meet these requirements. Breathomics is an increasingly investigated research field showing promising results for early stage diagnosis of malignant pleural mesothelioma [154]. However, several limitations common to many studies, such as lack of standardized treatments and assays, affect results and analysis. Moreover, low patient numbers limit the conclusiveness of results. To overcome these limitations, selection of homogenous series of patients, standardization of assays, and increased cooperation among research centers in combining cohorts and increasing study sizes are needed.

References

1. Napolitano A, Antoine DJ, Pellegrini L, et al. HMGB1 and its hyperacetylated isoform are sensitive and specific serum biomarkers to detect asbestos exposure and to identify mesothelioma patients. Clin Cancer Res. 2016;22:3087–96.
2. Carbone M, Kanodia S, Chao A, et al. Consensus report of the 2015 Weinman International Conference on mesothelioma. J Thorac Oncol. 2016;11:1246–62.
3. Rusch VW, Chansky K, Kindler HL, et al. The IASLC Mesothelioma Staging Project: Proposals for the M descriptors and for revision of the TNM stage groupings in the forthcoming (eighth) edition of the TNM classification for mesothelioma. J Thorac Oncol. 2016;11:2112–9.
4. Nowak AK, Chansky K, Rice DC, et al. The IASLC Mesothelioma Staging Project: proposals for revisions of the T descriptors in the forthcoming eighth edition of the TNM classification for pleural mesothelioma. J Thorac Oncol. 2016;11:2089–99.
5. Micolucci L, Akhtar MM, Olivieri F, et al. Diagnostic value of microRNAs in asbestos exposure and malignant mesothelioma: systematic review and qualitative meta-analysiš. Oncotarget. 2016;7:58606–37.
6. Chang S, Oh MH, Ji SY, et al. Practical utility of insulin-like growth factor II mRNA-binding protein 3, glucose transporter 1, and epithelial membrane antigen for distinguishing malignant mesotheliomas from benign mesothelial proliferations: IMP3, GLUT-1, and EMA in mesothelioma. Pathol Int. 2014;64:607–12.
7. Minato H, Kurose N, Fukushima M, et al. Comparative immunohistochemical analysis of IMP3, GLUT1, EMA, CD146, and desmin for distinguishing malignant mesothelioma from reactive mesothelial cells. Am J Clin Pathol. 2014;141:85–93.
8. Monaco SE, Shuai Y, Bansal M, et al. The diagnostic utility of p16 FISH and GLUT-1 immunohistochemical analysis in mesothelial proliferations. Am J Clin Pathol. 2011;135:619–27.
9. Lagana SM, Taub RN, Borczuk AC. Utility of glucose transporter 1 in the distinction of benign and malignant thoracic and abdominal mesothelial lesions. Arch Pathol Lab Med. 2012;136:804–9.

10. Kato Y, Tsuta K, Seki K, et al. Immunohistochemical detection of GLUT-1 can discriminate between reactive mesothelium and malignant mesothelioma. Mod Pathol. 2007;20:215–20.
11. Hasteh F, Lin GY, Weidner N, et al. The use of immunohistochemistry to distinguish reactive mesothelial cells from malignant mesothelioma in cytologic effusions. Cancer Cytopathol. 2010;118:90–6.
12. Churg A, Galateau-Salle F. The separation of benign and malignant mesothelial proliferations. Arch Pathol Lab Med. 2012;136:1217–26.
13. Shi M, Fraire AE, Chu P, et al. Oncofetal protein IMP3, a new diagnostic biomarker to distinguish malignant mesothelioma from reactive mesothelial proliferation. Am J Surg Pathol. 2011;35:878–82.
14. Ikeda K, Tate G, Suzuki T, et al. IMP3/L523S, a novel immunocytochemical marker that distinguishes benign and malignant cells: the expression profiles of IMP3/L523S in effusion cytology. Hum Pathol. 2010;41:745–50.
15. Husain AN, Colby TV, Ordóñez NG, et al. Guidelines for pathologic diagnosis of malignant mesothelioma: 2017 update of the consensus statement from the International Mesothelioma Interest Group. Arch Pathol Lab Med. 2018;142:89–108.
16. Creaney J, Robinson BW. Malignant mesothelioma biomarkers. Chest. 2017;152:143–9.
17. Cui A, Jin XG, Zhai K, et al. Diagnostic values of soluble mesothelin-related peptides for malignant pleural mesothelioma: updated meta-analysis. BMJ Open. 2014;4:e004145.
18. Blanquart C, Gueugnon F, Nguyen JM, et al. CCL2, galectin-3, and SMRP combination improves the diagnosis of mesothelioma in pleural effusions. J Thorac Oncol. 2012;7:883–9.
19. Mundt F, Nilsonne G, Arslan S, et al. Hyaluronan and N-ERC/mesothelin as key biomarkers in a specific two- step model to predict pleural malignant mesothelioma. PLoS One. 2013;8:e72030.
20. Pass HI, Levin SM, Harbut MR, et al. Fibulin-3 as a blood and effusion biomarker for pleural mesothelioma. N Engl J Med. 2012;367:1417–27.
21. Battolla E, Canessa PA, Ferro P, et al. Comparison of the diagnostic performance of fibulin-3 and mesothelin in patients with pleural effusions from malignant mesothelioma. Anticancer Res. 2017;37:1387–91.
22. Kirschner MB, Pulford E, Hoda MA, et al. Fibulin-3 levels in malignant pleural mesothelioma are associated with prognosis but not diagnosis. Br J Cancer. 2015;113:963–9.
23. Andersen M, Grauslund M, Ravn J, et al. Diagnostic potential of miR-126, miR-143, miR-145, and miR-652 in malignant pleural mesothelioma. J Mol Diagn. 2014;16:418–30.
24. Ak G, Tomaszek SC, Kosari F, et al. MicroRNA and mRNA features of malignant pleural mesothelioma and benign asbestos-related pleural effusion. Biomed Res Int. 2015;2015:635748.
25. De Rienzo A, Richards WG, Yeap BY, et al. Sequential binary gene ratio tests define a novel molecular diagnostic strategy for malignant pleural mesothelioma. Clin Cancer Res. 2013;19:2493–502.
26. Parodi S, Filiberti R, Marroni P, et al. Differential diagnosis of pleural mesothelioma using logic learning machine. BMC Bioinformatics. 2015;16(Suppl 9):S3.
27. Tosun AB, Yergiyev O, Kolouri S, et al. Detection of malignant mesothelioma using nuclear structure of mesothelial cells in effusion cytology specimens. Cytometry A. 2015;87:326–33.
28. Bruno R, Alì G, Giannini R, et al. Malignant pleural mesothelioma and mesothelial hyperplasia: a new molecular tool for the differential diagnosis. Oncotarget. 2017;8:2758–70.
29. Gotzos V, Vogt P, Celio MR. The calcium binding protein calretinin is a selective marker for malignant pleural mesotheliomas of the epithelial type. Pathol Res Pract. 1996;192:137–47.
30. King JE, Thatcher N, Pickering CAC, Hasleton PS. Sensitivity and specificity of immunohistochemical markers used in the diagnosis of epithelioid mesothelioma: a detailed systematic analysis using published data. Histopathology. 2006;48:223–32.
31. Ordóñez NG. What are the current best immunohistochemical markers for the diagnosis of epithelioid mesothelioma? A review and update. Hum Pathol. 2007;38:1–16.
32. Shield PW, Koivurinne K. The value of calretinin and cytokeratin 5/6 as markers for mesothelioma in cell block preparations of serous effusions. Cytopathology. 2008;19:218–23.
33. Mohammad T, Garratt J, Torlakovic E, Gilks B, Churg A. Utility of a CEA, CD15, calretinin, and CK5/6 panel for distinguishing between mesotheliomas and pulmonary adenocarcinomas in clinical practice. Am J Surg Pathol. 2012;36:1503–8.
34. Pu RT, Pang Y, Michael CW. Utility of WT-1, p63, MOC31, mesothelin, and cytokeratin (K903 and CK5/6) immunostains in differentiating adenocarcinoma, squamous cell carcinoma, and malignant mesothelioma in effusions. Diagn Cytopathol. 2008;36:20–5.
35. Padgett DM, Cathro HP, Wick MR, Mills SE. Podoplanin is a better immunohistochemical marker for sarcomatoid mesothelioma than calretinin. Am J Surg Pathol. 2008;32:123–7.
36. Saad RS, Lindner JL, Lin X, Liu YL, Silverman JF. The diagnostic utility of D2–40 for malignant mesothelioma versus pulmonary carcinoma with pleural involvement. Diagn Cytopathol. 2006;34:801–6.
37. Deniz H, Kibar Y, Güldür ME, Bakir K. Is D2–40 a useful marker for distinguishing malignant mesothelioma from pulmonary adenocarcinoma and benign mesothelial proliferations? Pathol Res Pract. 2009;205:749–52.
38. Ordóñez NG. Podoplanin: a novel diagnostic immunohistochemical marker. Adv Anat Pathol. 2006;13:83–8.
39. Hinterberger M, Reineke T, Storz M, Weder W, Vogt P, Moch H. D2-40 and calretinin – a tissue microar-

ray analysis of 341 malignant mesotheliomas with emphasis on sarcomatoid differentiation. Mod Pathol. 2007;20:248–55.

40. Ordóñez NG. D2-40 and podoplanin are highly specific and sensitive immunohistochemical markers of epithelioid malignant mesothelioma. Hum Pathol. 2005;36:372–80.
41. Oates J, Edwards C. HBME-1, MOC-31, WT1 and calretinin: an assessment of recently described markers for mesothelioma and adenocarcinoma. Histopathology. 2000;36:341–7.
42. Tsuta K, Kato Y, Tochigi N, Hoshino T, Takeda Y, Hosako M, et al. Comparison of different clones (WT49 versus 6F-H2) of WT-1 antibodies for immunohistochemical diagnosis of malignant pleural mesothelioma. Appl Immunohistochem Mol Morphol. 2009;17:126–30.
43. Amin KM, Litzky LA, Smythe WR, Mooney AM, Morris JM, Mews DJ, et al. Wilms' tumor 1 susceptibility (WT1) gene products are selectively expressed in malignant mesothelioma. Am J Pathol. 1995;146:344–56.
44. Langerak AW, Williamson KA, Miyagawa K, Hagemeijer A, Versnel MA, Hastie ND. Expression of the Wilms' tumor gene WT1 in human malignant mesothelioma cell lines and relationship to platelet-derived growth factor A and insulin-like growth factor 2 expression. Genes Chromosom Cancer. 1995;12:87–96.
45. Kumar-Singh S, Segers K, Rodeck U, Backhovens H, Bogers J, Weyler J, et al. WT1 mutation in malignant mesothelioma and WT1 immunoreactivity in relation to p53 and growth factor receptor expression, cell-type transition, and prognosis. J Pathol. 1997;181:67–74.
46. Kushitani K, Takeshima Y, Amatya VJ, Furonaka O, Sakatani A, Inai K. Differential diagnosis of sarcomatoid mesothelioma from true sarcoma and sarcomatoid carcinoma using immunohistochemistry. Pathol Int. 2008;58:75–83.
47. Scattone A, Serio G, Marzullo A, Nazzaro P, Corsi F, Cocca MP, et al. High Wilms' tumour gene (WT1) expression and low mitotic count are independent predictors of survival in diffuse peritoneal mesothelioma. Histopathology. 2012;60:472–81.
48. Churg A, Sheffield BS, Galateau-Salle F. New markers for separating benign from malignant mesothelial proliferations: are we there yet? Arch Pathol Lab Med. 2016;140:318–21.
49. Chang S, Oh MH, Ji SY, et al. Practical utility of insulinlike growth factor II mRNA-binding protein 3, glucose transporter 1, and epithelial membrane antigen for distinguishing malignant mesotheliomas from benign mesothelial proliferations: IMP3, GLUT-1, and EMA in mesothelioma. Pathol Int. 2014;64:607–12.
50. Sheffield BS, Hwang HC, Lee AF, et al. BAP1 immunohistochemistry and p16 FISH to separate benign from malignant mesothelial proliferations. Am J Surg Pathol. 2015;39:977–82.
51. Walts AE, Hiroshima K, McGregor SM, et al. BAP1 immunostain and CDKN2A (p16) FISH analysis: clinical applicability for the diagnosis of malignant mesothelioma in effusions. Diagn Cytopathol. 2016;44:599–606.
52. Nabeshima K, Matsumoto S, Hamasaki M, et al. Use of p16 FISH for differential diagnosis of mesothelioma in smear preparations. Diagn Cytopathol. 2016;44:774–80.
53. Hida T, Matsumoto S, Hamasaki M, et al. Deletion status of p16 in effusion smear preparation correlates with that of underlying malignant pleural mesothelioma tissue. Cancer Sci. 2015;106:1635–41.
54. Hiroshima K, Wu D, Hasegawa M, et al. Cytologic differential diagnosis of malignant mesothelioma and reactive mesothelial cells with FISH analysis of p16. Diagn Cytopathol. 2016;44:591–8.
55. McGregor SM, McElherne J, Minor A, et al. BAP1 immunohistochemistry has limited prognostic utility as a complement of CDKN2A (p16) fluorescence in situ hybridization in malignant pleural mesothelioma. Hum Pathol. 2017;60:86–94.
56. Hwang HC, Sheffield BS, Rodriguez S, et al. Utility of BAP1 immunohistochemistry and p16 (CDKN2A) FISH in the diagnosis of malignant mesothelioma in effusion cytology specimens. Am J Surg Pathol. 2016;40:120–6.
57. Carbone M, Yang H, Pass HI, Krausz T, Testa JR, Gaudino G. BAP1 and cancer. Nat Rev Cancer. 2013;13:153–9.
58. Bott M, Brevet M, Taylor BS, et al. The nuclear deubiquitinase BAP1 is commonly inactivated by somatic mutations and 3p21.1 losses in malignant pleural mesothelioma. Nat Genet. 2011;43:668–72.
59. Cigognetti M, Lonardi S, Fisogni S, et al. BAP1 (BRCA1-associated protein 1) is a highly specific marker for differentiating mesothelioma from reactive mesothelial proliferations. Mod Pathol. 2015;28:1043–57.
60. Testa JR, Cheung M, Pei J, Below JE, Tan Y, Sementino E, et al. Germline BAP1 mutations predispose to malignant mesothelioma. Nat Genet. 2012;43:1022–5.
61. Yoshikawa Y, Sato A, Tsujimura T, Emi M, Morinaga T, Fukuoka K, et al. Frequent inactivation of the BAP1 gene in epithelioid-type malignant mesothelioma. Cancer Sci. 2012;103:868–74.
62. LaFave LM, Béguelin W, Koche R, et al. Loss of BAP1 function leads to EZH2-dependent transformation. Nat Med. 2015;21:1344–9.
63. Kim KH, Roberts CW. Targeting EZH2 in cancer. Nat Med. 2016;22:128–34.
64. Shinozaki-Ushiku A, Ushiku T, Morita S, et al. Diagnostic utility of BAP1 and EZH2 expression in malignant mesothelioma. Histopathology. 2017;70:722–33.
65. Prieve MG, Moon RT. Stromelysin-1 and mesothelin are differentially regulated by Wnt-5a and Wnt-1 in C57mg mouse mammary epithelial cells. BMC Dev Biol. 2003;3:2.
66. Hollevoet K, Mason-Osann E, Muller F, Pastan I. Methylation associated partial down-regulation

of mesothelin causes resistance to anti-mesothelin immunotoxins in a pancreatic cancer cell line. PLoS One. 2015;10(3):e0122462.
67. Creaney J, Robinson BW. Malignant mesothelioma biomarkers from discovery to use in clinical practice for diagnosis, monitoring, screening, and treatment. Chest. 2017;152(1):143–9.
68. Hollevoet K, Reitsma JB, Creaney J, et al. Serum mesothelin for diagnosing malignant pleural mesothelioma: an individual patient data meta-analysis. J Clin Oncol. 2012;30(13):1541–9.
69. Pastan I, Hassan R. Discovery of mesothelin and exploiting it as a target for immunotherapy. Cancer Res. 2014;74(11):2907–12.
70. Røe OD, Anderssen E, Sandeck H, Christensen T, Larsson E, Lundgren S. Malignant pleural mesothelioma: genome-wide expression patterns reflectin general resistance mechanisms and a proposal of novel targets. Lung Cancer. 2010;67:57–68.
71. Nymark P, Lindholm PM, Korpela MV, Lahti L, Ruosaari S, Kaski S, et al. Gene expression profiles in asbestos-exposed epithelial and mesothelial lung cell lines. BMC Genomics. 2007;8:62.
72. Kettunen E, Nicholson AG, Nagy B, Wikman H, Seppänen JK, Stjernvall T, et al. L1CAM, INP10, P-cadherin, tPA and ITGB4 over-expression in malignant pleural mesotheliomas revealed by combined use of cDNA and tissue microarray. Carcinogenesis. 2005;26:17–25.
73. Røe OD, Anderssen E, Helge E, Pettersen CH, Olsen KS, Sandeck H, et al. Genome-wide profile of pleural mesothelioma versus parietal and visceral pleura: the emerging gene portrait of the mesothelioma phenotype. PLoS One. 2009;4:e6554.
74. Gordon GJ, Rockwell GN, Jensen RV, Rheinwald JG, Glickman JN, Aronson JP, et al. Identification of novel candidate oncogenes and tumor suppressors in malignant pleural mesothelioma using large-scale transcriptional profiling. Am J Pathol. 2005;166:1827–40.
75. Mohr S. Cell protection, resistance and invasiveness of two malignant mesotheliomas as assessed by 10K-microarray. Biochim Biophys Acta. 2004;1688:43–60.
76. López-Ríos F, Chuai S, Flores R, Shimizu S, Ohno T, Wakahara K, et al. Global gene expression profiling of pleural mesotheliomas: overexpression of aurora kinases and P16/CDKN2A deletion as prognostic factors and critical evaluation of microarray-based prognostic prediction. Cancer Res. 2006;66:2970–9.
77. Usami N, Fukui T, Kondo M, Taniguchi T, Yokoyama T, Mori S, et al. Establishment and characterization of four malignant pleural mesothelioma cell lines from Japanese patients. Cancer Sci. 2006;97:387–94.
78. De Reynie SA, Jaurand MC, Renier A, Couchy G, Hysi I, Elarouci N, et al. Molecular classification of malignant pleural mesothelioma: identification of a poor prognosis subgroup linked to the epithelial-to-mesenchymal transition. Clin Cancer Res. 2014;20:1323–34.
79. Gordon GJ, Dong L, Yeap BY, Richards WG, Glickman JN, Edenfield H, et al. Four-gene expression ratio test for survival in patients undergoing surgery for mesothelioma. J Natl Cancer Inst. 2009;101:678–86.
80. Gordon GJ, Jensen RV, Hsiao L, Gullans SR, Blumenstock JE, Richards WG, et al. Using gene expression ratios to predict outcome among patients with mesothelioma. J Natl Cancer Inst. 2003;95:598–605.
81. De Rienzo A, Dong L, Yeap BY, Jensen RV, Richards WG, Gordon GJ, et al. Fine needle aspiration biopsies for gene expression ratio-based diagnostic and prognostic tests in malignant pleural mesothelioma. Clin Cancer Res. 2011;17:310–6.
82. Bueno R, Stawiski EW, Goldstein LD, et al. Comprehensive genomic analysis of malignant pleural mesothelioma identifies recurrent mutations, gene fusions and splicing alterations. Nat Genet. 2016;48(4):407–16.
83. Galon J, Costes A, Sanchez-Cabo F, et al. Type, density, and location of immune cells within human colorectal tumors predict clinical outcome. Science. 2006;313:1960–4.
84. Bograd AJ, Suzuki K, Vertes E, et al. Immune responses and immunotherapeutic interventions in malignant pleural mesothelioma. Cancer Immunol Immunother. 2011;60:1509–27.
85. Pages F, Berger A, Camus M, et al. Effector memory T cells, early metastasis, and survival in colorectal cancer. N Engl J Med. 2005;353:2654–66.
86. Zhang L, Conejo-Garcia JR, Katsaros D, et al. Intratumoral T cells, recurrence, and survival in epithelial ovarian cancer. N Engl J Med. 2003;348:203–13.
87. Mahmoud SM, Paish EC, Powe DG, et al. Tumor-infiltrating CD8C lymphocytes predict clinical outcome in breast cancer. J Clin Oncol. 2011;29:1949–55.
88. Ujiie H, et al. The tumoral and stromal immune microenvironment in malignant pleural mesothelioma: a comprehensive analysis reveals prognostic immune markers. Oncoimmunology. 2015;4:e1009285.
89. Cornelissen R, et al. Ratio of intratumoral macrophage phenotypes is a prognostic factor in epithelioid malignant pleural mesothelioma. PLoS One. 2014;9:e106742.
90. Anraku M, Cunningham KS, Yun Z, et al. Impact of tumor-infiltrating T cells on survival in patients with malignant pleural mesothelioma. J Thorac Cardiovasc Surg. 2008;135:823–9.
91. Yamada N, Oizumi S, Kikuchi E, et al. CD8C tumor-infiltrating lymphocytes predict favorable prognosis in malignant pleural mesothelioma after resection. Cancer Immunol Immunother. 2010;59:1543–9.
92. Suzuki K, Kadota K, Sima CS, et al. Chronic inflammation in tumor stroma is an independent predictor of prolonged survival in epithelioid malignant pleural mesothelioma patients. Cancer Immunol Immunother. 2011;60:1721–8.
93. Lissbrant IF, Stattin P, Wikstrom P, Damber JE, Egevad L, Bergh A. Tumor associated macro-

phages in human prostate cancer: relation to clinicopathological variables and survival. Int J Oncol. 2000;17:445–51.
94. Solinas G, Germano G, Mantovani A, Allavena P. Tumor-associated macrophages (TAM) as major players of the cancer-related inflammation. J Leukoc Biol. 2009;86:1065–73.
95. Bingle L, Brown NJ, Lewis CE. The role of tumourassociated macrophages in tumour progression: implications for new anticancer therapies. J Pathol. 2002;196:254–65.
96. Sica A, Larghi P, Mancino A, et al. Macrophage polarization in tumour progression. Semin Cancer Biol. 2008;18:349–55.
97. Cedrés S, Ponce-Aix S, Zugazagoitia J, et al. Analysis of expression of programmed cell death 1 ligand 1 (pd-l1) in malignant pleural mesothelioma (MPM). PLoS One. 2015;10(3):e0121071.
98. Mansfield A, Roden A, Peikert T, et al. B7-H1 expression in malignant pleural mesothelioma is associated with sarcomatoid histology and poor prognosis. J Thorac Oncol. 2014;9:1036–40.
99. Combaz-Lair C, Galateau-Sallé F, McLeer-Florin A, et al. Immune biomarkers PD-1/PD-L1 and TLR3 in malignant pleural mesotheliomas. Hum Pathol. 2016;52:9–18.
100. Creaney J, Dick IM, Robinson BW. Discovery of new biomarkers for malignant mesothelioma. Curr Pulmonol Rep. 2015;4:15–21.
101. Cristaudo A, Bonotti A, Guglielmi G, Fallahi P, Foddis R. Serum mesothelin and other biomarkers: what have we learned in the last decade? J Thorac Dis. 2018;10(Suppl 2):S353–9.
102. Li ZQ, Verch T, Allard WJ. MESOMARK(®) in vitro diagnostic test for mesothelioma. Expert Opin Med Diagn. 2007;1(1):137–42.
103. Hassan R, Bera T, Pastan I. Mesothelin: a new target for immunotherapy. Clin Cancer Res. 2004;10:3937–42.
104. Tang Z, Qian M, Ho M. The role of mesothelin in tumor progression and targeted therapy. Anti Cancer Agents Med Chem. 2013;13:276–80.
105. Robinson BW, Creaney J, Lake R, et al. Mesothelin family proteins and diagnosis of mesothelioma. Lancet. 2003;362:1612–6.
106. Robinson BW, Creaney J, Lake R, et al. Soluble mesothelin-related protein--a blood test for mesothelioma. Lung Cancer. 2005;49:S109–11.
107. Hassan R, Remaley AT, Sampson ML, et al. Detection and quantitation of serum mesothelin, a tumor marker for patients with mesothelioma and ovarian cancer. Clin Cancer Res. 2006;12:447–53.
108. Scherpereel A, Grigoriu B, Conti M, et al. Soluble mesothelin-related peptides in the diagnosis of malignant pleural mesothelioma. Am J Respir Crit Care Med. 2006;173:1155–60.
109. Cristaudo A, Foddis R, Vivaldi A, et al. Clinical significance of serum mesothelin in patients with mesothelioma and lung cancer. Clin Cancer Res. 2007;13:5076–81.
110. Grigoriu BD, Scherpereel A. Diagnostic value of soluble mesothelin in malignant mesothelioma. Thorax. 2008;63:87–8.
111. Wheatley-Price P, Yang B, Patsios D, et al. Soluble mesothelin-related peptide and osteopontin as markers of response in malignant mesothelioma. J Clin Oncol. 2010;28:3316–22.
112. Hollevoet K, Nackaerts K, Gosselin R, et al. Soluble mesothelin, megakaryocyte potentiating factor, and osteopontin as markers of patient response and outcome in mesothelioma. J Thorac Oncol. 2011;6:1930–7.
113. Hollevoet K, Nackaerts K, Thas O, et al. The effect of clinical covariates on the diagnostic and prognostic value of soluble mesothelin and megakaryocyte potentiating factor. Chest. 2012;141:477–84.
114. Creaney J, Dick IM, Meniawy TM, et al. Comparison of fibulin-3 and mesothelin as markers in malignant mesothelioma. Thorax. 2014;69:895–902.
115. Grigoriu BD, Scherpereel A, Devos P, et al. Utility of osteopontin and serum mesothelin in malignant pleural mesothelioma diagnosis and prognosis assessment. Clin Cancer Res. 2007;13:2928–35.
116. Schneider J, Hoffmann H, Dienemann H, et al. Diagnostic and prognostic value of soluble mesothelin-related proteins in patients with malignant pleural mesothelioma in comparison with benign asbestosis and lung cancer. J Thorac Oncol. 2008;3:1317–24.
117. Linch M, Gennatas S, Kazikin S, et al. A serum mesothelin level is a prognostic indicator for patients with malignant mesothelioma in routine clinical practice. BMC Cancer. 2014;14:674.
118. Sun H, Vaynblat A, Pass H. Diagnosis and prognosis—review of biomarkers for mesothelioma. Ann Transl Med. 2017;5(11):244.
119. Franko A, Dolzan V, Kovac V, et al. Soluble mesothelin related peptides levels in patients with malignant mesothelioma. Dis Markers. 2012;32:123–31.
120. Van Zandwijk N, Clarke C, Henderson D, et al. Guidelines for the diagnosis and treatment of malignant pleural mesothelioma. J Thorac Dis. 2013;5:E254–307.
121. Chen RX, Xia YH, Xue TC, et al. Osteopontin promotes hepatocellular carcinoma invasion by up-regulating MMP-2 and uPA expression. Mol Biol Rep. 2011;38:3671–7.
122. Ohashi R, Tajima K, Takahashi F, et al. Osteopontin modulates malignant pleural mesothelioma cell functions in vitro. Anticancer Res. 2009;29:2205–14.
123. Sandhu H, Dehnen W, Roller M, et al. mRNA expression patterns in different stages of asbestos-induced carcinogenesis in rats. Carcinogenesis. 2000;21:1023–9.
124. Pass HI, Lott D, Lonardo F, et al. Asbestos exposure, pleural mesothelioma, and serum osteopontin levels. N Engl J Med. 2005;353:1564–73.
125. Cristaudo A, Bonotti A, Simonini S, et al. Combined serum mesothelin and plasma osteopontin measurements in malignant pleural mesothelioma. J Thorac Oncol. 2011;6:1587–93.

126. Cristaudo A, Foddis R, Bonotti A, et al. Comparison between plasma and serum osteopontin levels: usefulness in diagnosis of epithelial malignant pleural mesothelioma. Int J Biol Markers. 2010;25:164–70.
127. Rai AJ, Flores RM, Mathew A, et al. Soluble mesothelin related peptides (SMRP) and osteopontin as protein biomarkers for malignant mesothelioma: analytical validation of ELISA based assays and characterization at mRNA and protein levels. Clin Chem Lab Med. 2010;48:271–8.
128. Paleari L, Rotolo N, Imperatori A, et al. Osteopontin is not a specific marker in malignant pleural mesothelioma. Int J Biol Markers. 2009;24:112–7.
129. Cappia S, Righi L, Mirabelli D, et al. Prognostic role of osteopontin expression in malignant pleural mesothelioma. Am J Clin Pathol. 2008;130:58–64.
130. Pass HI, Goparaju C, Espin-Garcia O, et al. Plasma biomarker enrichment of clinical prognostic indices in malignant pleural mesothelioma. J Thorac Oncol. 2016;11:900–9.
131. Zhang Y, Marmorstein LY. Focus on molecules: fibulin-3 (EFEMP1). Exp Eye Res. 2010;90:374–5.
132. Scaffidi P, Misteli T, Bianchi ME. Release of chromatin protein HMGB1 by necrotic cells triggers inflammation. Nature. 2002;418:191–5.
133. Bianchi ME, Beltrame M, Paonessa G. Specific recognition of cruciform DNA by nuclear protein HMG1. Science. 1989;243:1056–9.
134. Jube S, Rivera ZS, Bianchi ME, et al. Cancer cell secretion of the DAMP protein HMGB1 supports progression in malignant mesothelioma. Cancer Res. 2012;72:3290–301.
135. Tabata C, Kanemura S, Tabata R, et al. Serum HMGB1 as a diagnostic marker for malignant peritoneal mesothelioma. J Clin Gastroenterol. 2013;47:684–8.
136. Ying S, Jiang Z, He X, et al. Serum HMGB1 as a potential biomarker for patients with asbestos-related diseases. Dis Markers. 2017;2017:5756102.
137. Wu T, Zhang W, Yang G, et al. HMGB1 overexpression as a prognostic factor for survival in cancer: a meta-analysis and systematic review. Oncotarget. 2016;7:50417–27.
138. Di Leva G, Garofalo M, Croce CM. MicroRNAs in cancer. Annu Rev Pathol. 2014;9:287–314.
139. Lamberti M, Capasso R, Lombardi A, et al. Two different serum MiRNA signatures correlate with the clinical outcome and histological subtype in pleural malignant mesothelioma patients. PLoS One. 2015;10:e0135331.
140. Weber DG, Johnen G, Bryk O, et al. Identification of miRNA-103 in the cellular fraction of human peripheral blood as a potential biomarker for malignant mesothelioma--a pilot study. PLoS One. 2012;7:e30221.
141. Kirschner MB, Cheng YY, Badrian B, et al. Increased circulating miR-625-3p: a potential biomarker for patients with malignant pleural mesothelioma. J Thorac Oncol. 2012;7:1184–91.
142. Busacca S, Germano S, De Cecco L, et al. MicroRNA signature of malignant mesothelioma with potential diagnostic and prognostic implications. Am J Respir Cell Mol Biol. 2010;42:312–9.
143. Guled M, Lahti L, Lindholm PM, et al. CDKN2A, NF2, and JUN are dysregulated among other genes by miRNAs in malignant mesothelioma -A miRNA microarray analysis. Genes Chromosom Cancer. 2009;48:615–23.
144. Xu Y, Zheng M, Merritt RE, et al. miR-1 induces growth arrest and apoptosis in malignant mesothelioma. Chest. 2013;144:1632–43.
145. Ivanov SV, Goparaju CM, Lopez P, et al. Pro-tumorigenic effects of miR-31 loss in mesothelioma. J Biol Chem. 2010;285:22809–17.
146. Kirschner MB, Cheng YY, Armstrong NJ, et al. MiRscore: a novel 6-microRNA signature that predicts survival outcomes in patients with malignant pleural mesothelioma. Mol Oncol. 2015;9:715–26.
147. Bononi I, Comar M, Puozzo A, et al. Circulating microRNAs found dysregulated in ex-exposed asbestos workers and pleural mesothelioma patients as potential new biomarkers. Oncotarget. 2016;7:82700–11.
148. Borrebaeck CA. Precision diagnostics: moving towards protein biomarker signatures of clinical utility in cancer. Nat Rev Cancer. 2017;17:199–204.
149. Giusti L, Da Valle Y, Bonotti A, et al. Comparative proteomic analysis of malignant pleural mesothelioma evidences an altered expression of nuclear lamin and filament-related proteins. Proteomics Clin Appl. 2014;8:258–68.
150. Ostroff RM, Mehan MR, Stewart A, et al. Early detection of malignant pleural mesothelioma in asbestos-exposed individuals with a noninvasive proteomics-based surveillance tool. PLoS One. 2012;7:e46091.
151. Gold L, Ayers D, Bertino J, et al. Aptamer-based multiplexed proteomic technology for biomarker discovery. PLoS One. 2010;5:e15004.
152. Bonotti A, Foddis R, Landi S, et al. A novel panel of serum biomarkers for MPM diagnosis. Dis Markers. 2017;2017:3510984.
153. Cerciello F, Choi M, Nicastri A, et al. Identification of a seven glycopeptide signature for malignant pleural mesothelioma in human serum by selected reaction monitoring. Clin Proteomics. 2013;10:16.
154. Lagniau S, Lamote K, van Meerbeeck JP, Vermaelen KY. Biomarkers for early diagnosis of malignant mesothelioma: Do we need another moonshot? Oncotarget. 2017;8(32):53751–62.

Diagnostic Imaging of Mesothelioma

9

Christopher M. Straus and Samuel G. Armato III

9.1 Introduction

Radiologic imaging is critical to the diagnosis, staging, clinical management, and surveillance of patients with malignant pleural mesothelioma. Chest radiography, computed tomography (CT), magnetic resonance imaging (MRI), and positron emission tomography (PET) have all been used to assess the structure, extent, or physiology of mesothelioma. Over the years, however, the relative importance of these imaging modalities has evolved with technology and the introduction of new therapeutic regimens. Invariably, the discovery and initial diagnosis of this disease centers on imaging. Furthermore, assessment of the efficacy of current treatments requires serial radiologic examinations over time: almost every mesothelioma patient receives numerous imaging exams during the course of treatment, as this is the best method to track treatment response and evaluate for known concomitant associated secondary issues. Although traditional imaging defines the morphology and extent of mesothelioma tumor, increasingly more advanced imaging options are being deployed to evaluate tumor physiology and allow for earlier detection of disease that has originated or moved beyond the pleural space. Computer software has become a more useful tool for the quantitative analysis of the acquired image data (known as "radiomics"); together with enhanced visualization approaches, the extraction of additional objective information from radiologic images can have a positive impact on patient care decisions. This chapter describes the imaging modalities that have been employed for the evaluation of mesothelioma and explores current and future directions in the imaging of this complex tumor.

9.2 Chest Radiography

Chest radiography remains the most common radiologic procedure performed in the United States, and, consequently, initial detection of mesothelioma is likely to originate from an abnormal preliminary radiographic chest examination. Evaluation and even detection of this complex pathology in the two-dimensional radiographic projection is neither a sensitive nor a specific diagnosis. Subsequent study with another imaging modality is invariably required. Overlapping anatomy and technical limitations of projection radiography also prevent identification of disease extent, specifically the involvement of critical structures. Most often the radiologist is alerted only to secondary radiographic signs of mesothelioma, including unilateral pleural effusion, ipsilateral shift of the mediastinum, underlying asymmetric lung volume loss with or without

C. M. Straus · S. G. Armato III (✉)
Department of Radiology, The University of Chicago, Chicago, IL, USA
e-mail: cstraus@uchicago.edu; s-armato@uchicago.edu

G. L. Ceresoli et al. (eds.), *Mesothelioma*, https://doi.org/10.1007/978-3-030-16884-1_9

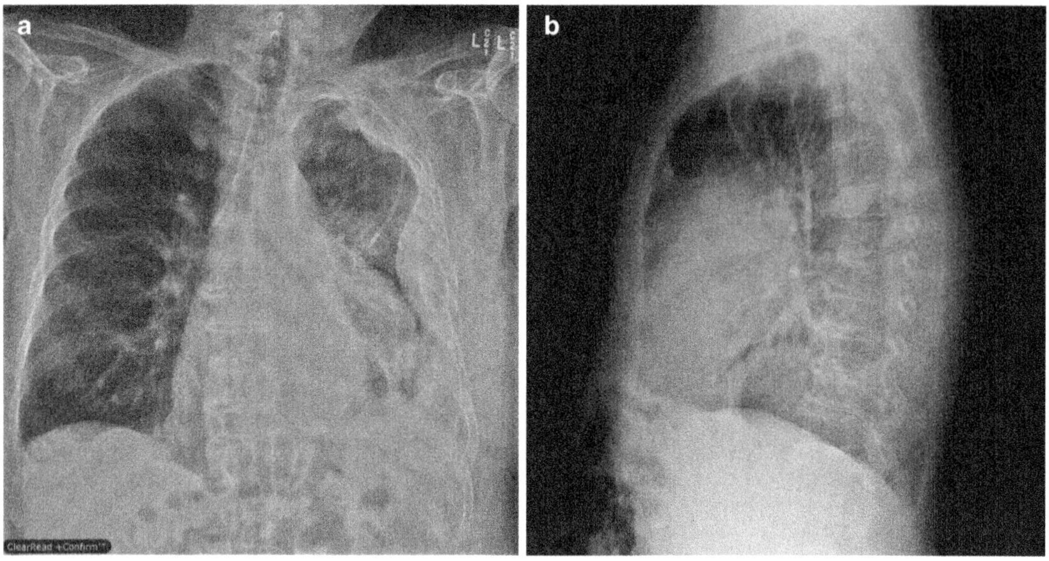

Fig. 9.1 (**a**) Posteroanterior (**b**) and lateral chest radiographs of a patient with left-sided malignant pleural mesothelioma. Note unilateral irregular pleural thickening (representing both tumor and pleural fluid), left-to-right mediastinal shift, and ipsilateral volume loss

calcified pleural plaques, and diffuse lobulated pleural thickening [1–3] (Fig. 9.1); these findings, however, are not necessarily specific to mesothelioma and could represent a wide range of etiologies, most commonly secondary findings related to other malignancies or pleural infection.

In practice, the ability to diagnose mesothelioma on chest radiography is only possible at more advanced stages (related to more pronounced secondary changes associated with the disease) when the presence of metastatic lung nodules or lymph nodes, pulmonary interstitial disease (e.g., thickening of interlobular septa), and destruction of ribs or vertebral bodies may be more easily noted [4]. Contralateral pleural abnormalities generally reflect asbestos exposure rather than metastases [5], since mesothelioma tends to spread directly by contiguous growth (Fig. 9.2) [6]. Radiography can contribute to patient surveillance in the post-therapy and post-surgery settings. While radiography may be used to monitor patients for postsurgical complications, ipsilateral tumor recurrence requires CT evaluation once the lung has reaerated [5]; CT also would be required to differentiate among recurrent disease, infection, or postsurgical complications in the presence of radiographic findings such as mediastinal shift, ipsilateral air-fluid level, or contralateral lung nodules [5]. Furthermore, given its increased sensitivity for early detection of post-procedural complications, CT is increasingly being used as the sole imaging modality for post-therapy evaluation beyond the most immediate time period.

9.3 Computed Tomography

A fundamental limitation of radiography is its projection of inherently three-dimensional structures to a single two-dimensional imaging plane. The resulting superposition of anatomy and any embedded pathologic process creates a visual scene in which subtle abnormalities might lack sufficient contrast with adjacent structures and therefore remain undetected. The series of transaxial images that comprise a CT scan provides radiologists with a vast amount of information that far exceeds that offered by radiography. The information provided by standard transaxial images is augmented by the ability of CT to generate reformatted images in the coronal and sagittal planes as a result of the near-isotropic voxels captured by state-of-the-art scanners with sub-millimeter slice thickness. This complement

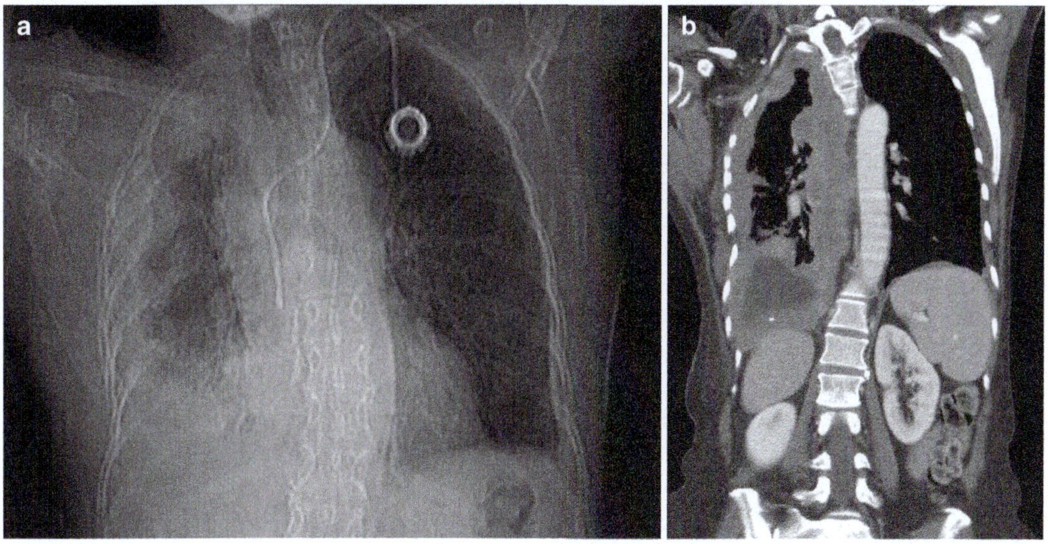

Fig. 9.2 (**a**) Posteroanterior chest radiograph of a patient with right-sided disease manifesting as irregular pleural thickening. (**b**) Coronal reformatting of a CT scan from the same patient further delineates irregular pleural thickening throughout the right hemithorax with both mediastinal invasion and loculated fluid (*). Note smooth, relatively thin plaque along the contralateral diaphragmatic pleura (arrows) representing benign disease rather than contralateral malignancy

of images is especially relevant to the visualization of mesothelioma with its irregular shape, complex growth pattern, and potentially extensive disease burden that might involve neighboring structures (Fig. 9.3). Consequently, CT has become the imaging modality with the greatest impact on mesothelioma detection, staging, and treatment response assessment.

The spatial extent and tissue characteristics of mesothelioma tumor are accentuated with CT relative to radiography, although the range of pixel values spanned by mesothelioma tumor can be very similar to that of adjacent tissues even on CT [7]. The radiologic manifestation of pleural abnormalities falls into three broad categories: pleural effusion, pleural thickening, and pleural calcification [8] (and is often a combination thereof). CT, and especially contrast-enhanced CT, demonstrates all three categories of abnormal pleural findings with high sensitivity and has the potential to distinguish the relative contributions of these three components if present in combination. These abnormal pleural findings on CT, however, are not specific to mesothelioma and must be differentiated from a variety of other diseases, both benign and malignant, including

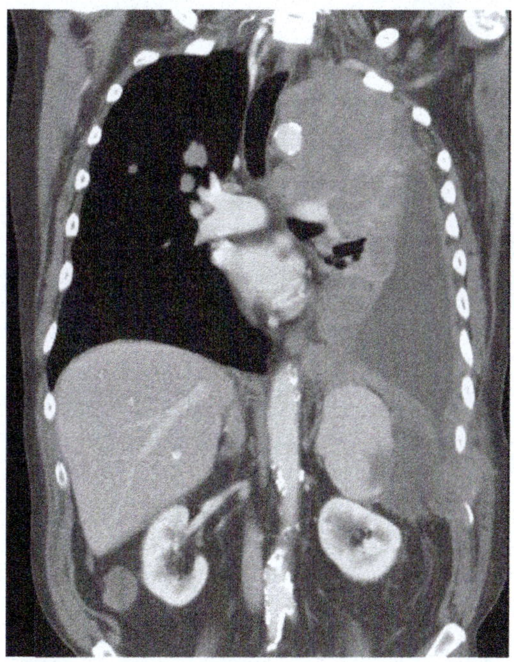

Fig. 9.3 Coronal CT section from a patient with left-sided disease highlighting extensive effusion (*), invasion of the aortic arch and great vessels (black arrows), chest wall invasion (arrowhead), and transdiaphragmatic extension involving splenic displacement and invasion (white arrows)

(non-mesothelioma) asbestos-related pleural disease, tuberculous pleurisy, empyema, and metastatic disease [9, 10].

On CT, mesothelioma is often characterized by a circumferential, nodular soft-tissue pleural thickening that can involve interlobar fissures [2] (Fig. 9.4). Pleural effusions (Fig. 9.5) and associated changes preferentially in the lower hemithorax are typical CT findings [5, 11]. The use of intravenous contrast optimizes the identification of lymphadenopathy and highlights invasion of critical adjacent vascular structures [11]. An acknowledged shortcoming of CT is its relatively limited sensitivity for hilar lymph node involvement [11], which impacts the utility of CT in the assessment of N stage. Pleural plaques and thickening are also common CT findings in mesothelioma patients but, when present in combination with mesothelioma, are thought to reflect asbestos exposure and not active mesothelioma; the pathogenesis of either lesion and the possible preneoplastic nature of mesothelioma-associated pleural plaques remains unproven [12, 13].

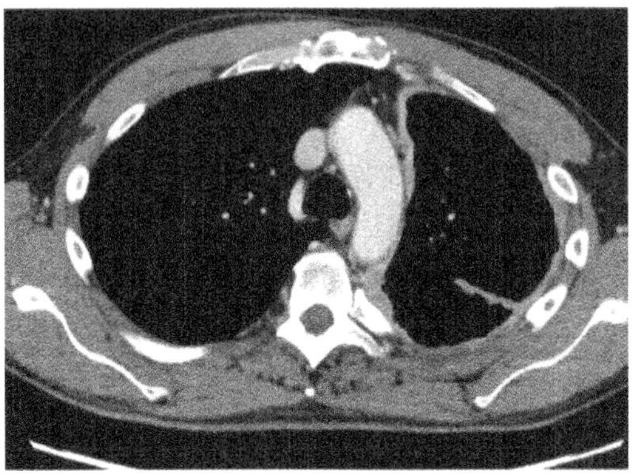

Fig. 9.4 Axial CT section demonstrating left-sided nodular pleural thickening with direct extension into the left major interlobar fissure (arrow)

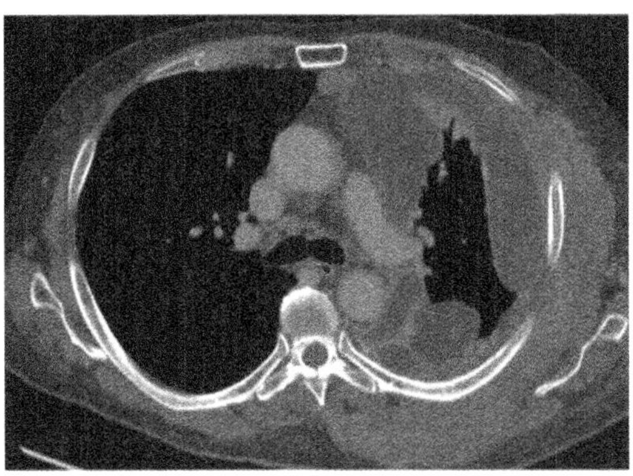

Fig. 9.5 Axial CT section demonstrating mild-to-moderate left-sided pleural nodular disease with more extensive associated hypodense regions (*) representing non-contiguous loculated effusions

To provide a clinical context for these CT findings, pleural effusions were identified in 76% of the initial CT scans obtained from a cohort of 50 mesothelioma patients [14], with the majority of these effusions occupying less than one-third of the affected hemithorax. In this same cohort, 94% of the patients demonstrated pleural thickening, with 72% of these cases classified as nodular thickening, 50% classified as predominantly lower zone, and 47% with a thickness that exceeded 1 cm (Fig. 9.6). Thickening in the superior mediastinum was identified in 70% of cases, diaphragmatic crural thickening was observed in 84% of cases, and interlobar fissural thickening was noted in 84% of cases. In a report from another cohort of 50 mesothelioma patients [15], pleural effusions were identified in 74% of patients, 92% of the patients demonstrated pleural thickening, and interlobar fissural thickening was noted in 86% of cases. Focal pleural intrapulmonary masses were demonstrated in 8% of

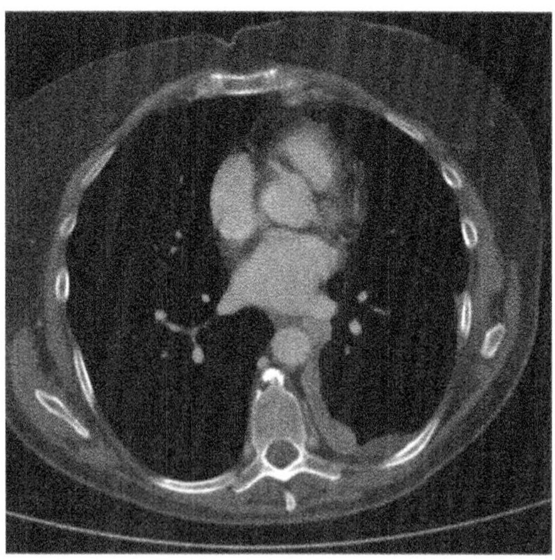

Fig. 9.6 Axial CT section capturing left-sided paraspinal disease with discrete regions of pleural soft-tissue thickening measuring more than 1 cm (arrows)

the cases, half of which involved or abutted the chest wall [15] (Fig. 9.7).

"Cone beam CT" directly captures three-dimensional information from the patient; cone beam CT, however, is not the current standard for diagnostic radiology purposes. Instead, the clinical standard, spiral (or helical) CT, is considered a 2.5-dimensional imaging modality in that the individually captured image planes may be viewed separately, viewed in succession to span the anatomic region, or stacked together to create a single volumetric representation of the imaged anatomy. Accordingly, assessment of anatomic volumes or the volumetric extent of disease burden is an important contribution of CT to patient management. One such CT-based assessment of volume is the impact of mesothelioma on the volume of the affected hemithorax. In particular, with volume loss of the ipsilateral lung secondary to extensive pleural disease, ipsilateral mediastinal shift may or may not be demonstrated; ipsilateral lung volume loss without mediastinal shift is referred to as the "fixed mediastinum." Ipsilateral volume loss may also be observed on CT due to narrowed intercostal spaces ("rib crowding") [11] with elevation of the ipsilateral hemidiaphragm [15] (Fig. 9.8). This appearance can be complicated by substantial pleural effusion or pleural thickening causing contralateral mediastinal shift without an ipsilateral increase in aerated lung volume.

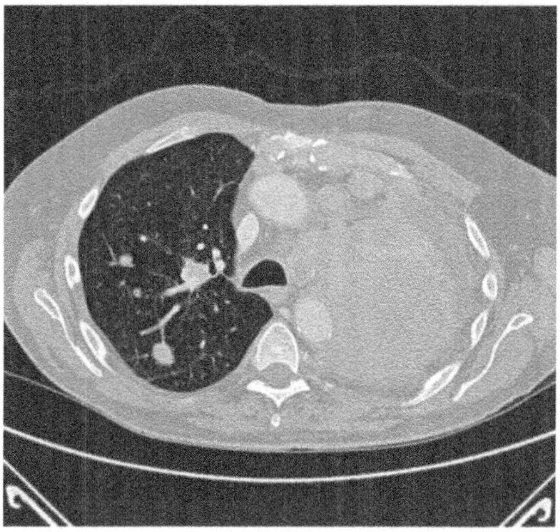

Fig. 9.7 Axial CT section from the same patient as in Fig. 9.3 demonstrates contralateral lung nodules (arrows), which are best visualized with the image displayed using a "lung window"

CT is generally used to assist in the identification of findings that distinguish diffuse pleural pathology from benign pleural changes. A pleural rind in excess of 1 cm thick, mediastinal pleural involvement, and pleural nodularity

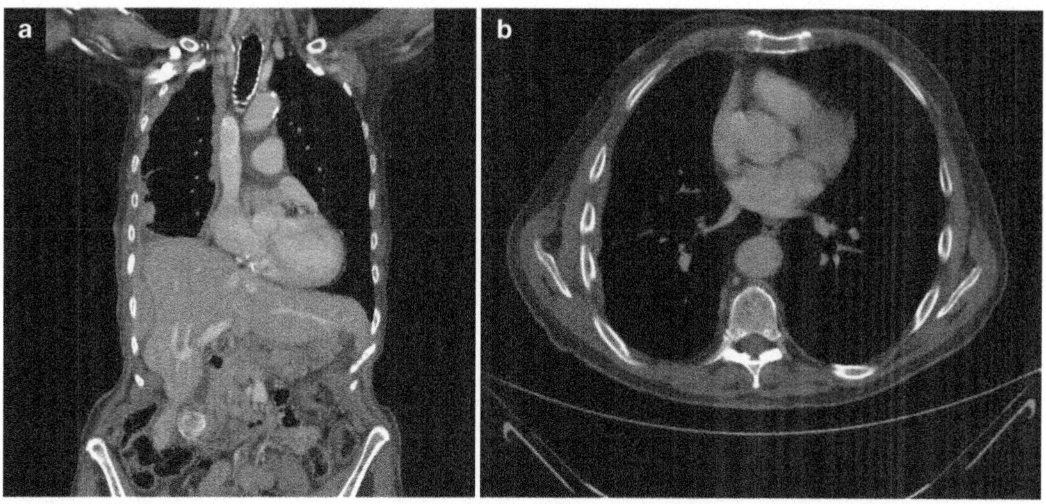

Fig. 9.8 Right-sided disease resulting in (**a**) ipsilateral volume loss and elevated hemidiaphragm in the coronal CT section and (**b**) rib crowding captured in the axial CT section. Note extension of tumor deep into the costophrenic angle laterally with the distinct preservation of subdiaphragmatic fat indicating integrity of the peritoneal cavity in (**a**) (arrow)

have been associated specifically with malignant pleural diseases [1]. These key findings of malignancy are all generally well depicted on CT, as is progression beyond the pleural cavity (invasion of the chest wall, invasion of the mediastinum, or transdiaphragmatic extension) (Fig. 9.9), lymph node metastasis (Fig. 9.10), and displacement or destruction of ribs or vertebral bodies (Fig. 9.11) [1]. Among a cohort of 71 patients with diffuse pleural disease presenting as pleural thickening [8], findings observed to be significantly more common in patients with malignant pleural disease than in patients with benign pleural disease were nodular pleural thickening, parietal pleural thickening (in excess of 1 cm), mediastinal pleural involvement, and the presence of a pleural rind. Three additional diffuse pleural disease patients without pleural thickening, however, demonstrated unilateral pleural effusion as the sole indicator of pleural malignancy in this minority subpopulation of patients. In this cohort, only pleural calcifications were specific to a benign process (Fig. 9.12). Although benign pleural disease may present unilaterally, a unilateral presenta-

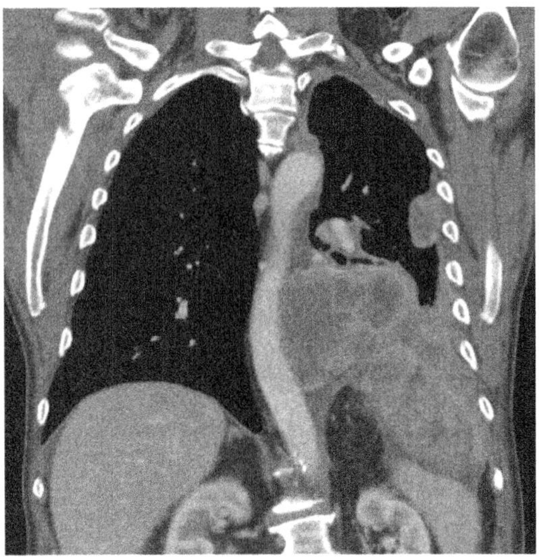

Fig. 9.9 Extensive left-sided disease with clear destruction of, and extension through, the left hemidiaphragm displacing the spleen inferiorly (arrow) on this coronal CT section

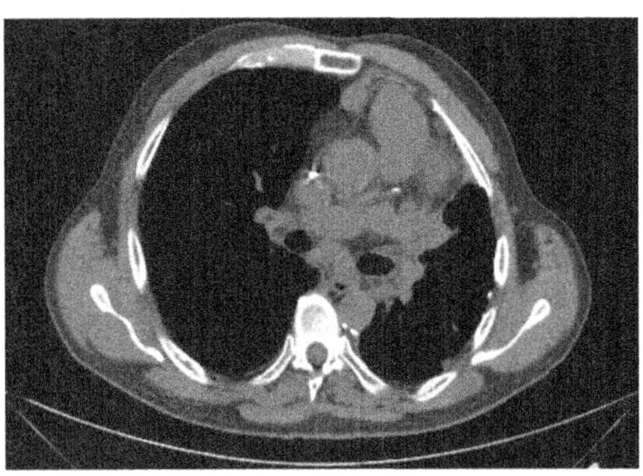

Fig. 9.10 Midthoracic axial CT section demonstrating subcarinal conglomerate nodal mass (arrows) and perivascular lymphadenopathy (arrowhead)

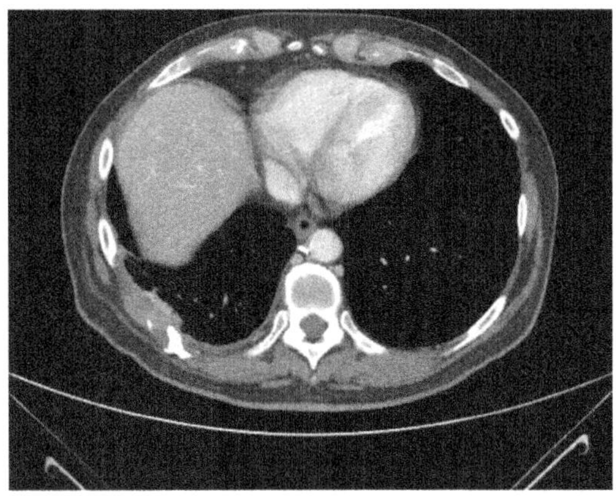

Fig. 9.11 Axial CT section capturing osseous involvement and tumor extension as demonstrated by destruction of the right eighth rib (arrow) with an expansible mass

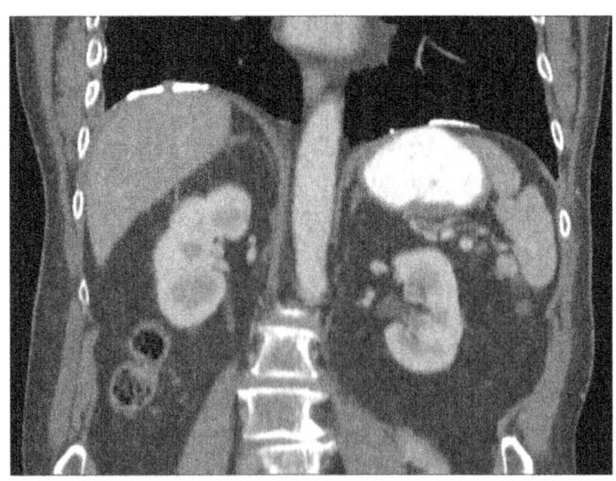

Fig. 9.12 Coronal CT section demonstrating thick pleural calcifications (arrows) and the relative absence of additional soft-tissue pleural thickening

tion of pleural disease within asbestos-exposed patients was highly specific for malignant disease in general (and, in particular, suggestive of mesothelioma) [8].

CT has the potential to differentiate mesothelioma from other malignant pleural diseases, yet this task is generally inconsistent and challenging. In a cohort of 215 patients with mesothelioma, metastatic pleural disease, and benign pleural disease [9], the following were identified as independent findings to differentiate (1) mesothelioma from metastatic pleural disease and (2) all malignant pleural diseases from benign pleural disease: the presence of a pleural rind, mediastinal pleural involvement, and pleural thickness exceeding 1 cm. These findings differentiating malignant pleural disease from benign pleural disease are consistent with those of the study discussed in the previous paragraph [8], which, interestingly, reported that the CT findings in mesothelioma patients were the same as in patients with metastatic pleural disease from other causes. Pleural nodularity is a characteristic CT finding in mesothelioma patients and in patients with other malignant pleural diseases that can be used to differentiate these patients from patients with benign pleural disease; however, pleural nodularity does not differentiate mesothelioma from metastatic pleural disease [9].

CT effectively captures intrapulmonary findings that are known to be associated generally with asbestos exposure or known to accompany mesothelioma specifically: lung nodules, rounded atelectasis, and ipsilateral atelectasis [14]. Associated compressive atelectasis secondary to large tumor or effusion is also a common presentation feature in mesothelioma patients (Fig. 9.13). Invasion of the pericardium by mesothelioma can be captured on CT as pericardial thickening (with or without pericardial effusion) [5] (Fig. 9.14); nevertheless, the ability to distinguish pericardial involvement from mediastinal pleural disease remains difficult given their immediate adjacent relationship [15]. Pericardial involvement is most evident when there is extension into the pericardium outlined by mediastinal fat. Effort has been made to assimilate findings from the literature into an evidence-based guideline on reading CT scans of mesothelioma patients to improve the proficiency of radiologists and physicians in the diagnosis of this disease [16], but widespread adoption of such guidelines has not been achieved.

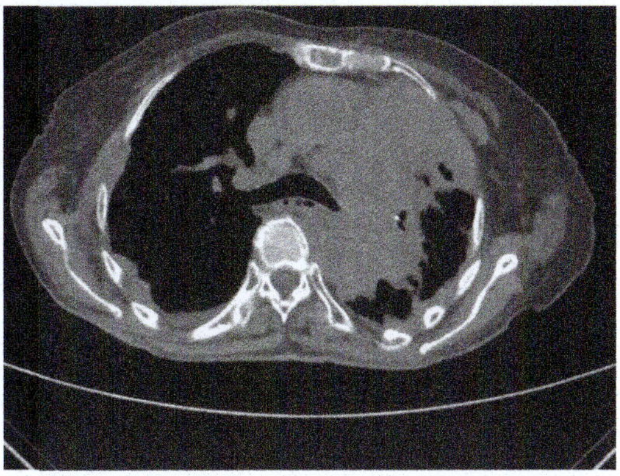

Fig. 9.13 Axial CT section demonstrating extensive left-sided disease with tumor and compressive atelectasis; similar density between tumor and collapsed lung prevents clear demarcation of lung boundary and tumor margin

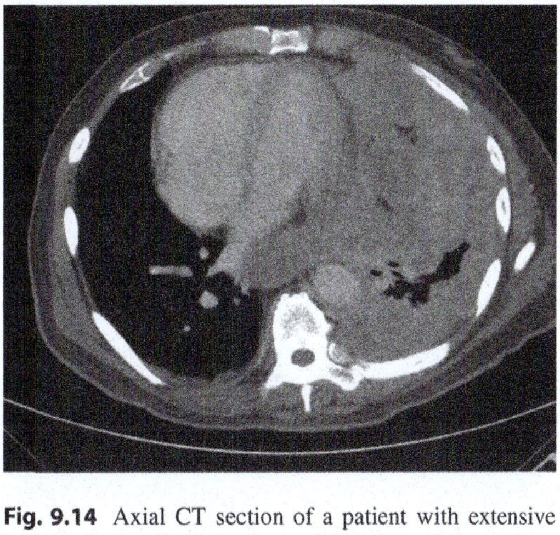

Fig. 9.14 Axial CT section of a patient with extensive left-sided pleural thickening and invasion of the pericardium (and likely the left ventricle); note the small crescent of fluid representing an associated pericardial effusion (arrow)

The accepted use of low-dose CT for the screening of asymptomatic individuals for lung cancer provides an opportunity for the early detection of other thoracic abnormalities that might be captured. The identification of other pathologies besides lung cancer on these low-dose CT screening studies is so relevant that the term "lung cancer screening" is being replaced simply by the term "lung screening." Screening for any disease requires a well-defined subpopulation of individuals who are, to some degree, "at risk" for that disease. Naturally, by extension, any effort to screen specifically for mesothelioma should target asbestos workers or those related to the industry. To date, reports on low-dose CT as a screening tool for the detection of mesothelioma in asbestos-exposed workers have been mixed in terms of diagnostic yield [17, 18].

The standard acquisition of a CT scan captures a static representation of patient anatomy at a fixed time. The intravenous injection of an iodinated contrast agent serves to accentuate the vasculature (and heavily vascularized tissues) from adjacent structures that would otherwise be indistinguishable. Enhanced images are best obtained after a specified time delay to allow for the contrast to disburse systemically; the images acquired after that delay period also are static but are "enhanced" by the presence of the contrast agent. Dynamic, contrast-enhanced CT (DCE-CT) scans incorporate a temporal component by acquiring images of the patient while the contrast agent is initially coursing through the patient's blood vessels and into (and subsequently out of) vascularized structures but before significant dilution throughout the blood pool and removal by the kidneys; this dynamic image acquisition approach allows CT to capture physiologic information about blood flow, although this information is constrained to a more limited axial range of anatomy as the patient table does not move during the dynamic acquisition. A number of hemodynamic parameters (such as tissue blood flow, tissue blood volume, tissue peak enhancement, time to peak enhancement, and mean transit time) may be computed from image data acquired in this manner. A recent study used hemodynamic parameters computed from DCE-CT scans of mesothelioma patients to investigate the correlation of these parameters with patient response and to explore whether changes in tumor hemodynamics might precede changes in physical tumor bulk [19].

9.4 Magnetic Resonance Imaging

Magnetic resonance imaging (MRI) is substantially different from CT, from the physics that governs image acquisition to the biological mechanisms that can be analyzed through the captured images. While CT captures information about how patient tissues and disease processes attenuate X-rays (with manipulation of the X-ray beam's energy spectrum the only practical way for the technologist to alter the signal detected by the scanner), MRI allows for a large array of pulse sequences, each designed to capture information about different physiologic processes, often on the cellular level. Consequently, MRI can depict not only patient anatomy with soft-tissue contrast that exceeds that of CT but also water diffusion (through the apparent diffusion coefficient (ADC) calculated from diffusion-weighted imaging (DWI)), blood flow (through dynamic contrast-enhanced (DCE) MRI), and vascular permeability (through the volume transfer constant, Ktrans, computed from DCE-MRI). Proper attention to image acquisition parameters is essential to generating MRI images that allow for optimal assessment of the pleura [20].

Although of relatively limited use in the chest given associated artifacts from aerated lung, MRI benefits the clinical evaluation of mesothelioma patients [21] by optimizing distinction between mesothelioma tumor and adjacent and commonly involved tissues such as chest wall, ribs, and diaphragm. Specifically, a substantial percentage of patients presents with indistinguishable findings in, for example, the pericardial and diaphragmatic regions, where both malignant and benign diseases can demonstrate subtle CT changes. In such cases, MRI can be used to identify secondary findings associated with early tumor invasion (e.g., edema in the overlying ribs) that specifically exclude benign abnormalities. As noted previously, MRI has a much greater sensitivity for capturing soft-tissue differences relative to CT. MRI is specifically well suited for identifying distinct unaltered fat planes between critical structures, as expected, for example, along the caudal diaphragmatic surface and adjacent

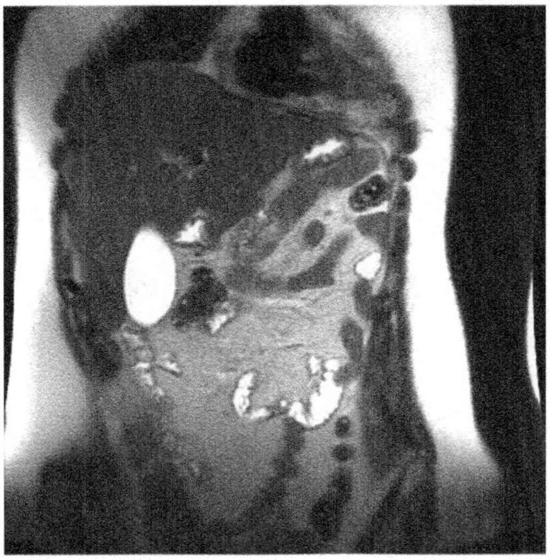

Fig. 9.15 T1-weighted sagittal MR image demonstrates clear undersurface of the diaphragm (arrows) indicating that disease has not penetrated the peritoneal cavity

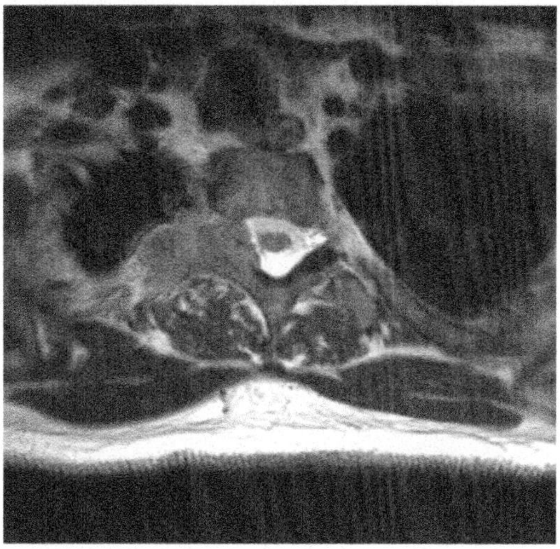

Fig. 9.16 Right-apical mesothelioma along the posterior medial aspect with direct invasion into the spinal canal demonstrated on an axial T2-weighted MR image (arrow); note invasion and displacement of the thecal sac (arrowhead)

abdominal organs; a smooth inferior diaphragmatic surface on MRI remains one of the most reliable indicators of potential resectability and likewise of tumor invasion into the mediastinal fat (Fig. 9.15). While minimal pleural thickening may be a challenge to diagnose on CT, MRI offers creative ways to manipulate the signal detected from different tissues in the scanner, such as through "early contrast enhancement," which may offer potential as a perfusion-based biomarker of pleural malignancy [22].

Although MRI does not match CT in its ability to depict pleural calcifications and to detect enlarged lymph nodes with pathologic suspicion, it is important to note that neither CT nor MRI can achieve accurate lymph node staging due to both low sensitivity and low specificity. Contrast-enhanced T1-weighted MRI is more sensitive to detection of vertebral body or rib invasion, subdiaphragmatic extension, and fissural spread of tumor. T2-weighted MRI without fat suppression allows for the differentiation of mesothelioma tumor from pleural fluid, a distinction that confounds the assessment of tumor burden on CT. Both modalities remain grossly similar in depicting invasion of the chest wall, mediastinum, and lung parenchyma, while mesothelioma generates increased signal strength relative to the normal chest wall on T2-weighted MRI [5, 23, 24], with particular advantages if tumor invasion of the spinal canal must be excluded [1] (Fig. 9.16). Focal thickening and enhancement of interlobar fissures additionally occur more frequently in malignant pleural disease (mesothelioma or other malignancies) than in benign pleural disease, and this potential subtle finding is more likely to be appreciated on MRI. Thus, use of MRI remains largely relegated to specific circumstances unique to a particular patient, despite some studies comparing CT and MRI scans that showed that pleural fluid, pleural enhancement, focal pleural thickening, and enhancement of focal pleural thickening were significantly more frequent in mesothelioma patients than in patients with other pleural malignancies or benign pleural disease [25, 26].

The value of DWI in the assessment of mesothelioma has increased in recent years. DWI, in which specific pulse sequences allow MRI to capture the diffusion of water across cell membranes (membrane integrity), has been reported to demonstrate a "pleural pointillism" sign with diagnostic ability in the differentiation between malignant pleural disease and benign conditions that is superior to mediastinal pleural thickness and shrinking of the lung [27]. DWI has shown an

ADC value (computed from DWI images) that is significantly higher for the epithelioid histological subtype of mesothelioma than for the sarcomatoid subtype, presumably due to the increased water diffusion that occurs in epithelioid disease as a result of cells that are less densely packed than the cells of the sarcomatoid subtype [28]. The ability of MRI to extract information from mesothelioma tumors that could previously only be obtained from an invasive biopsy offers great promise for the future role of imaging in this disease.

9.5 Positron Emission Tomography

Positron emission tomography (PET) with the radiotracer fluorine-18-labeled 2-deoxyglucose (FDG) provides functional images of metabolic activity that are used throughout oncology to differentiate malignant from benign lesions, provide tumor staging, and evaluate tumor response. It is important to note that almost all PET studies performed clinically today are actually PET-CT studies in which, during a single examination, both the functional information of PET and the anatomic detail of CT are acquired in a manner that simplifies co-registration, thus allowing for a more complete assessment. In the mesothelioma setting, the predominant role of PET is in the identification of the anatomic extent of disease. In addition to the qualitative, visual assessment of PET images, semiquantitative metrics such as the standardized uptake value (SUV) (the ratio of radiotracer uptake in a defined region, corrected for decay, to the injected dose normalized for body weight) and total glycolytic volume (TGV) (a parameter that considers total metabolic activity in the context of the volume of a defined region) enhance the benefit of this imaging modality. FDG-PET measures tissue metabolic activity of any nature, since FDG is not a specific tumor marker [29]; as a result, FDG-PET is unable to discriminate mesothelioma from other malignant pleural diseases or other tissues that are highly metabolically active such as inflammatory diseases. Thus, PET interpretation is particularly dependent on clinical context: mesothelioma patients with a prior talc pleurodesis, for example, are especially susceptible to potentially misleading PET scans.

PET may be effective in guiding biopsy site selection and obtaining the most relevant tissue samples for analysis (Fig. 9.17). One study based on SUV values reported 91% sensitivity with 100% specificity in the differentiation of benign and malignant pleural disease [29], a finding that could improve the yield of (and confidence in) acquired biopsy samples obtained with the ben-

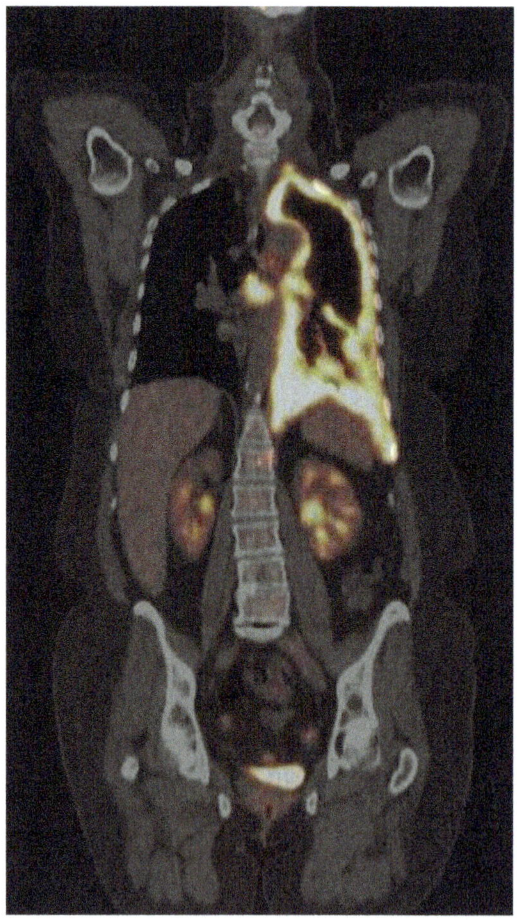

Fig. 9.17 Fused coronal PET-CT scan image (CT displayed as grayscale; PET displayed as red temperature scale) demonstrating extensive left-sided pleural disease representing primary tumor; distinct additional focal mediastinal uptake reveals a subcarinal nodal mass (arrow), which represents a potential biopsy site associated with relatively diminished risk in sampling transbronchially

efit of PET images. Although the potential contribution of PET in tumor staging has been reported [29], the ability of PET to depict local extent of mesothelioma is not considered reliable and remains inferior to its ability to identify extrathoracic metastases [30].

The unique functional nature of the information captured by PET has made this modality the subject of studies investigating novel uses of imaging. One such study explored the prognostic value of PET and identified volumetric FDG-PET parameters (specifically tumor volume and glycolytic activity) as being more predictive of survival than TNM staging [31]. Another study used FDG-PET to predict the early response of patients to chemotherapy [32], a task with important implications for patient management and the conduct of clinical trials, and a task that establishes PET imaging as a potentially powerful biomarker. Moving beyond FDG (the most common radiopharmaceutical), other radiotracers have been investigated for mesothelioma. Fluorine-18-labeled fluoromisonidazole (FMISO) PET captures information about tumor hypoxia, a parameter that is key to understanding tumor resistance to therapy. Mesothelioma tumor has been found to contain substantial areas of hypoxia based on FMISO-PET imaging [33]. Other groups have developed preclinical models to evaluate the efficacy of fluorine-18-labeled fluorothymidine (FLT) PET as a marker for tumor cell proliferation in mesothelioma [34].

9.6 Tumor Measurement

Assessment of disease progression or response to therapy is critical for patient management decisions and the evaluation of drug efficacy during clinical trials. Tumor measurements obtained from medical images provide the basis for this assessment. Although CT has become the standard modality for the image-based assessment of tumor response, there might be a future role for other modalities such as FDG-PET and DWI in this domain [35]. To be useful, these quantitative measurements of tumor burden must be reproducible with low variability across and within readers and they must be acquired in a standardized manner for consistency across multiple sites. The issue of standardization has evolved over the years. For historical reference, in 1981 the World Health Organization (WHO) recommended the bidimensional measurement (the product of (1) the longest axial diameter of the lesion and (2) the longest diameter constructed perpendicular to this longest axial diameter) of tumors on imaging studies [36]; tumor response was determined from the relative change of bidimensional measurements across temporally sequential images [36]. In 2000, the Response Evaluation Criteria in Solid Tumors (RECIST) guidelines replaced the bidimensional measurement of a tumor with a single tumor measurement, the longest axial diameter [37, 38], and classified patients as demonstrating (1) "partial response", (2) "progressive disease", (3) "stable disease", or (4) "complete response" [38].

Both the WHO and the RECIST guidelines were meant to accommodate typical tumors that tend to be spherical in shape and tend to growth (or shrink) in a roughly isotropic manner; mesothelioma, however, with its circumferential extent around the lung and a growth pattern directed inward toward the center of the affected hemithorax, renders such guidelines inadequate [39, 40]. In 2004, "modified RECIST" introduced a measurement paradigm specifically tailored to the morphology and growth pattern of pleural mesothelioma tumor [41]. Although this article was published as a research study, the modified RECIST approach was quickly adopted by the mesothelioma clinical trials community as a de facto guideline in which two unidimensional measurements of pleural thickness are obtained on each of three distinct CT sections, with the sum of these tumor thickness measurements representing tumor burden; the RECIST tumor response classification then is applied to the change in the summed measurements across temporally sequential CT scans. The modified RECIST measurement process can be detailed as (1) the selection of three CT sections in which tumor is most prominent, (2) the identification of two specific locations (sites) within these sections, and (3) the measurement of tumor thickness at these sites, a step that may be subdivided as follows: (1) selection of a specific point along the outer tumor margin at which to initiate the measurement, (2) determination of the direction that captures the most appropriate dimension of the tumor, and (3) location of the inner tumor margin encountered in that direction; the distance between the outer and inner tumor margin points at each measurement site then represents tumor thickness at that site [42]. Recently, modified RECIST 1.1 guidelines were published to "collate and apply research published since the development of modified RECIST, align modified RECIST with RECIST 1.1, address those aspects of tumor measurement that were neglected or not well characterized in the modified RECIST paper, and clarify ambiguous or difficult measurement issues that have been highlighted through the subsequent decade of clinical trials research" [43]. So important is the topic of tumor measurement in mesothelioma that it is the subject of the next chapter in this book, which presents a more thorough treatment of the issues involved with image-based tumor measurements; applications to staging, prognosis, and tumor response assessment; the potential for measurements of tumor volume; and the role of different imaging modalities.

9.7 Conclusions

Radiologic imaging is an essential tool for tumor assessment and patient management in malignant pleural mesothelioma. With an array of available imaging modalities, each designed to capture specific structural and/or functional characteristics of anatomy and disease, the strengths (and limitations) of these various modalities must be understood by the healthcare provider to maximize patient benefit from the imaging examination and reduce the potential for erroneous interpretation of the imaging findings. CT, MRI, and PET (or, more correctly, PET-CT) play distinct and often complementary roles in mesothelioma diagnosis, staging, response assessment, surgical planning, and surveillance. Advancements in imaging technology over the years have enhanced the contributions of radiology to the multidisciplinary assessment of mesothelioma; future developments remain to be explored and incorporated into patient care.

References

1. Eibel R, Tuengerthal S, Schoenberg SO. The role of new imaging techniques in diagnosis and staging of malignant pleural mesothelioma. Curr Opin Oncol. 2003;15:131–8.
2. Aberle DR, Balmes JR. Computed tomography of asbestos-related pulmonary parenchymal and pleural diseases. Clin Chest Med. 1991;12:115–31.
3. Gefter WB, Epstein DM, Miller WT. Radiographic evaluation of asbestos related chest disorders. Crit Rev Diagn Imaging. 1984;21:133–81.
4. Wechsler RJ, Rao VM, Steiner RM. The radiology of thoracic malignant mesothelioma. Crit Rev Diagn Imaging. 1984;20:283–310.
5. Marom EM, Erasmus JJ, Pass HI, Patz EF Jr. The role of imaging in malignant pleural mesothelioma. Semin Oncol. 2002;29:26–35.
6. Wanebo HJ, Martini N, Melamed MR, Hilaris B, Beattie EJ Jr. Pleural mesothelioma. Cancer. 1976;38:2481–8.
7. Corson N, Sensakovic WF, Straus C, Starkey A, Armato SG III. Characterization of mesothelioma and tissues present in contrast-enhanced thoracic CT scans. Med Phys. 2011;38:942–7.
8. Leung AN, Müller NL, Miller RR. CT in differential diagnosis of diffuse pleural disease. AJR. 1990;154:487–92.
9. Metintas M, Ucgun I, Elbek O, et al. Computed tomography features in malignant pleural mesothelioma and other commonly seen pleural diseases. Eur J Radiol. 2002;41:1–9.
10. Müller NL. Imaging of the pleura. Radiology. 1993;186:298–309.
11. Yilmaz UM, Utkaner G, Yalniz E, Kumcuoglu Z. Computed tomographic findings of environmental asbestos-related malignant pleural mesothelioma. Respirology. 1998;3:33–8.
12. Müller KM, Fischer M. Malignant pleural mesotheliomas: an environmental health risk in southeast Turkey. Respiration. 2000;67:608–9.
13. Rabinowitz JG, Efremidis SC, Cohen B, et al. A comparative study of mesothelioma and asbestos using computed tomography and conventional chest radiography. Radiology. 1982;144:453–60.
14. Ng CS, Munden RF, Libshitz HI. Malignant pleural mesothelioma: the spectrum of manifestations on CT in 70 cases. Clin Radiol. 1999;54:415–21.
15. Kawashima A, Libshitz HI. Malignant pleural mesothelioma: CT manifestations in 50 cases. AJR Am J Roentgenol. 1990;155:965–9.

16. Zhou H, Tamura T, Kusaka Y, Suganuma N, Subhannachart P, Vijitsanguan C, Noisiri W, Hering KG, Akira M, Itoh H, Arakawa H, Ishikawa Y, Kumagai S, Kurumatani N. Development of a guideline on reading CT images of malignant pleural mesothelioma and selection of the reference CT films. Eur J Radiol. 2012;81:4203–10.
17. Roberts HC, Patsios DA, Paul NS, DePerrot M, Teel W, Bayanati H, Shepherd F, Johnston MR. Screening for malignant pleural mesothelioma and lung cancer in individuals with a history of asbestos exposure. J Thorac Oncol. 2009;4:620–8.
18. Fasola G, Belvedere O, Aita M, Zanin T, Follador A, Cassetti P, Meduri S, De Pangher V, Pignata G, Rosolen V, Barbone F, Grossi F. Low-dose computed tomography screening for lung cancer and pleural mesothelioma in an asbestos-exposed population: baseline results of a prospective, nonrandomized feasibility trial—an Alpe-adria Thoracic Oncology Multidisciplinary Group Study (ATOM 002). Oncologist. 2007;12:1215–24.
19. Gudmundsson E, Labby Z, Straus CM, Sensakovic WF, Li F, Rose B, Cunliffe A, Kindler HL, Armato SG III. Dynamic contrast-enhanced CT for the assessment of tumor response in malignant pleural mesothelioma: a pilot study. Eur Radiol. 2018;29(2):682–8.
20. Patel AM, Berger I, Wileyto EP, Khalid U, Torigian DA, Nachiappan AC, Barbosa EM Jr, Gefter WB, Galperin-Aizenberg M, Gupta NK, Simone CB 2nd, Haas AR, Alley EW, Singhal S, Cengel KA, Katz SI. The value of delayed phase enhanced imaging in malignant pleural mesothelioma. J Thorac Dis. 2017;9:2344–9.
21. Knuuttila A, Halme M, Kivisaari L, Kivisaari A, Salo J, Mattson K. The clinical importance of magnetic resonance imaging versus computed tomography in malignant pleural mesothelioma. Lung Cancer. 1998;22:215–25.
22. Tsim S, Humphreys CA, Cowell GW, Stobo DB, Noble C, Woodward R, Kelly CA, Alexander L, Foster JE, Dick C, Blyth KG. Early contrast enhancement: a novel magnetic resonance imaging biomarker of pleural malignancy. Lung Cancer. 2018;118:48–56.
23. Bonomo L, Feragalli B, Sacco R, Merlino B, Storto ML. Malignant pleural disease. Eur J Radiol. 2000;34:98–118.
24. Lorigan JG, Libshitz HI. MR imaging of malignant pleural mesothelioma. J Comput Assist Tomogr. 1989;13:617–20.
25. Kinoshita T, Ishii K, Miyasato S. Localized pleural mesothelioma: CT and MR findings. Magn Reson Imaging. 1997;15:377–9.
26. Knuuttila A, Kivisaari L, Kivisaari A, Palomäki M, Tervahartiala P, Mattson K. Evaluation of pleural disease using MR and CT. Acta Radiol. 2001;42:502–7.
27. Coolen J, De Keyzer F, Nafteux P, De Wever W, Dooms C, Vansteenkiste J, Derweduwen A, Roebben I, Verbeken E, De Leyn P, Van Raemdonck D, Nackaerts K, Dymarkowski S, Verschakelen J. Malignant pleural mesothelioma: visual assessment by using pleural pointillism at diffusion-weighted MR imaging. Radiology. 2015;274:576–84.
28. Gill RR, Umeoka S, Mamata H, Tilleman TR, Stanwell P, Woodhams R, Padera RF, Sugarbaker DJ, Hatabu H. Diffusion-weighted MRI of malignant pleural mesothelioma: preliminary assessment of apparent diffusion coefficient in histologic subtypes. AJR Am J Roentgenol. 2010;195:W125–30.
29. Bénard F, Sterman D, Smith RJ, Kaiser LR, Albelda SM, Alavi A. Metabolic imaging of malignant pleural mesothelioma with fluorodeoxyglucose positron emission tomography. Chest. 1998;114:713–22.
30. Flores RM, Akhurst T, Gonen M, Larson SM, Rusch VW. Positron emission tomography defines metastatic disease but not locoregional disease in patients with malignant pleural mesothelioma. J Thorac Cardiovasc Surg. 2003;126:11–6.
31. Nowak AK, Francis RJ, Phillips MJ, Millward MJ, van der Schaaf AA, Boucek J, Musk AW, McCoy MJ, Segal A, Robins P, Byrne MJ. A novel prognostic model for malignant mesothelioma incorporating quantitative FDG-PET imaging with clinical parameters. Clin Cancer Res. 2010;16:2409–17.
32. Francis RJ, Byrne MJ, van der Schaaf AA, et al. Early prediction of response to chemotherapy and survival in malignant pleural mesothelioma using a novel semiautomated 3-dimensional volume-based analysis of serial 18F-FDG PET scans. J Nucl Med. 2007;48:1449–58.
33. Francis RJ, Segard T, Morandeau L, Lee YC, Millward MJ, Segal A, Nowak AK. Characterization of hypoxia in malignant pleural mesothelioma with FMISO PET-CT. Lung Cancer. 2015;90:55–60.
34. Tsuji AB, Sogawa C, Sugyo A, Sudo H, Toyohara J, Koizumi M, Abe M, Hino O, Harada YN, Furukawa T, Suzuki K, Saga T. Comparison of conventional and novel PET tracers for imaging mesothelioma in nude mice with subcutaneous and intrapleural xenografts. Nucl Med Biol. 2009;36:379–88.
35. Cheng L, Tunariu N, Collins DJ, Blackledge MD, Riddell AM, Leach MO, Popat S, Koh DM. Response evaluation in mesothelioma: beyond RECIST. Lung Cancer. 2015;90:433–41.
36. Miller AB, Hogestraeten B, Staquet M, Winkler A. Reporting results of cancer treatment. Cancer. 1981;47:207–14.
37. James K, Eisenhauer E, Christian M, et al. Measuring response in solid tumors: unidimensional versus bidimensional measurement. J Natl Cancer Inst. 1999;91:523–8.
38. Therasse P, Arbuck SG, Eisenhauer EA, et al. New guidelines to evaluate the response to treatment in solid tumors. J Natl Cancer Inst. 2000;92:205–16.
39. Monetti F, Casanova S, Grasso A, Cafferata MA, Ardizzoni A, Neumaier CE. Inadequacy of the new Response Evaluation Criteria in Solid Tumors (RECIST) in patients with malignant pleural mesothelioma: report of four cases. Lung Cancer. 2004;43:71–4.

40. van Klaveren RJ, Aerts JGJV, de Bruin H, Giaccone G, Manegold C, van Meerbeeck JP. Inadequacy of the RECIST criteria for response evaluation in patients with malignant pleural mesothelioma. Lung Cancer. 2004;43:63–9.
41. Byrne MJ, Nowak AK. Modified RECIST criteria for assessment of response in malignant pleural mesothelioma. Ann Oncol. 2004;15:257–60.
42. Armato SG III, Oxnard GR, MacMahon H, et al. Measurement of mesothelioma on thoracic CT scans: a comparison of manual and computer-assisted techniques. Med Phys. 2004;35:1105–15.
43. Armato SG III, Nowak AK. Revised modified RECIST criteria for assessment of response in malignant pleural mesothelioma (version 1.1). J Thorac Oncol. 2018;13:1012–21.

Measuring Malignant Pleural Mesothelioma

10

Anna K. Nowak and Samuel G. Armato III

10.1 Introduction

Measurement of the volume or bulk of tumor has three key purposes. First, when tumor bulk is measured at one timepoint, such as at the time of presentation, it may provide prognostic information. Second, when tumor bulk is measured longitudinally, the rate of change may also refine prognostication. Third, tumor bulk measured longitudinally in the context of treatment provides a measure of treatment efficacy, and indirectly, additional prognostic information incorporating information from response or progression on treatment. Hence, measurement of disease underpins important activities which inform clinical trials and epidemiological research—robust staging and measurement of response in groups of patients and determine individual patient care (assessing prognosis and evaluating treatment effectiveness). This chapter will cover the history and current status of measurement of mesothelioma for these purposes and will highlight the most important challenges and areas for further research.

A. K. Nowak (✉)
National Centre for Asbestos Related Diseases and Medical School, University of Western Australia, Nedlands, WA, Australia
e-mail: anna.nowak@uwa.edu.au

S. G. Armato III
Department of Radiology, The University of Chicago, Chicago, IL, USA
e-mail: s-armato@uchicago.edu

Measuring malignant pleural mesothelioma has posed many difficulties for radiologists, researchers, and clinicians. The goal of most tumor measurement, as stated above, is to elicit a metric that can represent a patient's tumor bulk. While most non-mesothelioma tumors grow in a somewhat spherical morphology from an initial nidus of tumor (Fig. 10.1), malignant pleural mesothelioma grows as a rind around the interior of the chest wall and the exterior of the lung, forming a circumferential plaque that is rarely uniform and may involve adjacent structures (Fig. 10.2). Although the volume of a spherical lesion can be

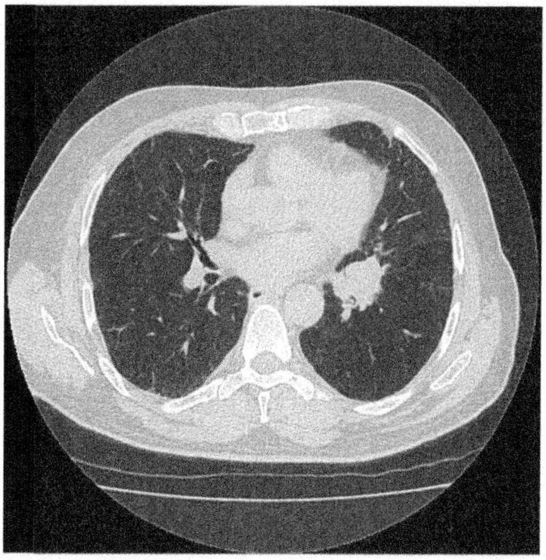

Fig. 10.1 Many cancers grow in a relatively spherical morphology from a central nidus. This example demonstrates a left-sided peri-hilar non-small cell lung cancer

G. L. Ceresoli et al. (eds.), *Mesothelioma*, https://doi.org/10.1007/978-3-030-16884-1_10

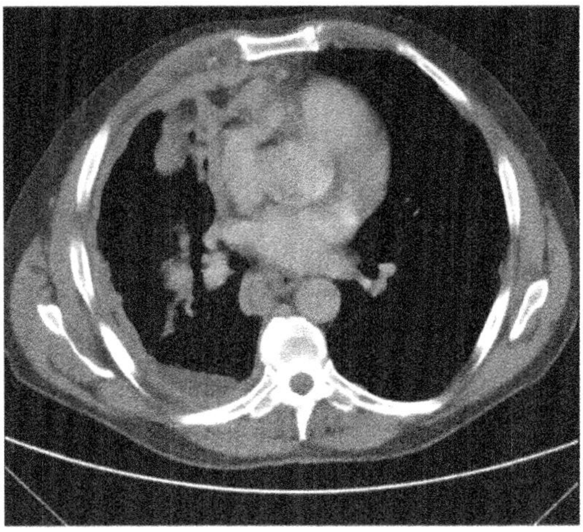

Fig. 10.2 Complex morphology of malignant pleural mesothelioma, with circumferential disease around the pleural cavity and infiltration into mediastinal fat, with involvement of the pulmonary fissure

approximately quantified through simple mathematics, clearly this is a more difficult proposition for pleural mesothelioma. Furthermore, there are a number of potential confounders when attempting to measure pleural mesothelioma. For example, it may be difficult to distinguish atelectasis, pleural scarring, pleural plaques, or effusion from tumor rind, particularly when pleural effusion is loculated or dense and may appear very similar in density to pleural tumor. These challenges caused by the growth pattern of mesothelioma and the similar density of adjacent structures will impact any form of tumor measurement in this disease.

10.2 Measuring Tumor for Cancer Staging

Cancer staging aims to stratify patient survival using anatomical tumor characteristics to describe the bulk of the disease and the involvement of organs or other structures. By definition, stage is determined from imaging performed at or around the time of diagnosis, prior to treatment initiation. The relationship among overall cancer burden, metastatic potential, and patient survival is well established in many cancers. Most cancer staging and prognostic systems include some estimate or surrogate of tumor burden within the T stage, often as categories based on unidimensional tumor diameter [1]. In many cancers, particularly those that are readily surgically resectable, cancer stage determines subsequent treatment. Cancer stage may also be an important inclusion or stratification factor in clinical trials, and it allows for comparisons among datasets such as treatment or population registries. The AJCC/UICC cancer staging manuals, which undergo revisions every 5–7 years, form an internationally consistent platform for staging, with T, N, and M descriptors defined for each cancer and each stage. Clinical T categorization, or CT stage, incorporates imaging and physical examination performed prior to the start of any treatment. Historically, mesothelioma T staging has not included any surrogate of tumor volume but has instead detailed the anatomical structures infiltrated by disease, including the chest wall, lung parenchyma, mediastinum, and other adjacent structures [2–4]. Certainly, potential surgical management of mesothelioma may be more appropriately determined by anatomical extent of invasion rather than tumor size, but there may be a role for tumor measurements in mesothelioma staging, particularly to aid prognostication where surgical intervention is not proposed (Fig. 10.3a and b).

The relationship between tumor burden and survival in mesothelioma has been known for two decades, with a 1997 paper describing the prognostic value of tumor volume in patients undergoing surgical resection. Tumors were measured using three-dimensional reconstructions of chest CT scans, with a measured tumor volume <100 cc predicting better survival [5]. These findings have been reproduced in a number of studies of CT imaging-derived volume, most commonly in the context of extrapleural pneumonectomy [6, 7]. Semi-automated quantification of tumor volume using FDG-PET scanning also provides prognostic information, although only when histological subtype is excluded from the model. In patients with epithelioid mesothelioma, total glycolytic volume (TGV), a composite of standardized uptake value intensity and tumor volume, was prognostic on both univariate and multivariate analysis [8]. These findings have been confirmed using a similar methodology that

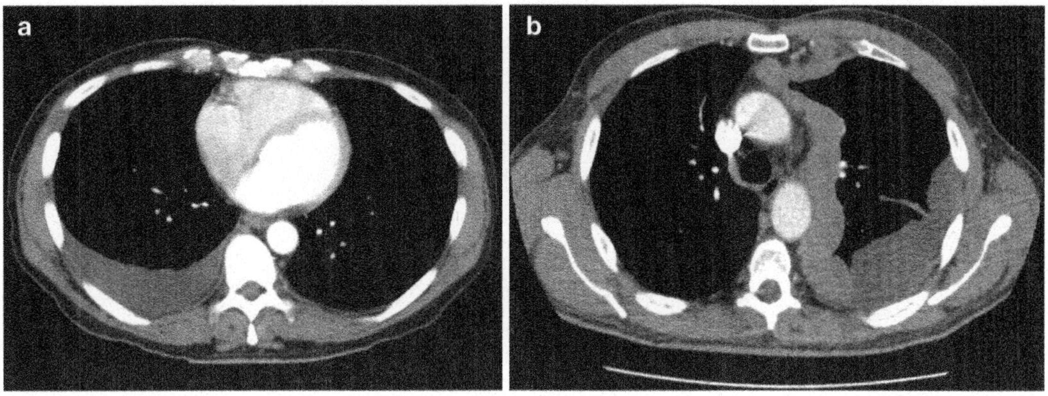

Fig. 10.3 (**a**) No visible pleural tumor at presentation. Patient presents with pleural effusion only and has a more favorable prognosis. (**b**) Bulky mediastinal mesothelioma at presentation. Patient would be expected to have a less favorable prognosis

incorporated volumetric aspects with intensity of FDG uptake [9]. Hence, there is substantial evidence for the importance of tumor volume as a prognostic factor in the context of surgery, chemotherapy, and supportive care.

In an effort to provide a stronger evidence basis for the staging of mesothelioma, the International Association for the Study of Lung Cancer (IASLC) developed a prospective staging database that collected, in addition to the usual T staging descriptors of anatomical invasion, three unidimensional measurements of pleural tumor thickness. These measurements were prospectively collected for the purpose of this database from 472 of the total 3519 patients. Unidimensional measurements of tumor thickness were acquired to provide a semi-quantitative surrogate of tumor bulk. An important strength of this approach was its simplicity as a technique that could be readily applied in any setting, including when the software, expertise, or time for CT-based volumetry was not available. Measurements of pleural tumor were obtained perpendicular to the chest wall or mediastinum at the point of maximum tumor thickness, with one measurement acquired each in the upper, middle, and lower third of the thorax (Fig. 10.4a and b) [10]. Individual pleural tumor thickness measurements ranged from 0 to 153 mm, and the median thickness increased from the upper to the middle zone and from the middle to the lower zone. These pleural thickness measurements correlated with T stage categories—as the mean sum of the pleural thickness increased, so did the T stage. These exploratory data were statistically examined in three ways: using the maximum of the three thickness measurements, summing the three measurements, and ranking the measurement sum by quartile to identify prognostic cut points. Survival decreased as quartile of summed pleural thickness measurement increased, with the median survival of the lowest quartile (<16 mm) being 23.4 months, and the median survival of the highest quartile (>50 mm) being 13.2 months (p = 0.005). Data-driven cut points of summed measurement below 13 mm, 13–60 mm, and above 60 mm sum also stratified for survival (p = 0.0001), and increasing thickness category was associated with increased clinical T category, nodal stage, and overall stage. Even a single data-driven cut point for maximal tumor thickness had prognostic significance, with patients in whom no measured tumor thickness exceeded 5.1 mm having a median survival of 24.2 months, and those in whom any pleural thickness exceeded 5.1 mm having a median survival of 17.7 months (p = 0.014). Moreover, the coarse categorization of tumor morphology into "minimal," "nodular," and "rind-like" yielded a significant difference in survival between those categorized as having minimal disease and those considered to have nodular or rind-like tumor (Fig. 10.5) (18.2 vs. 14.5 months, respectively).

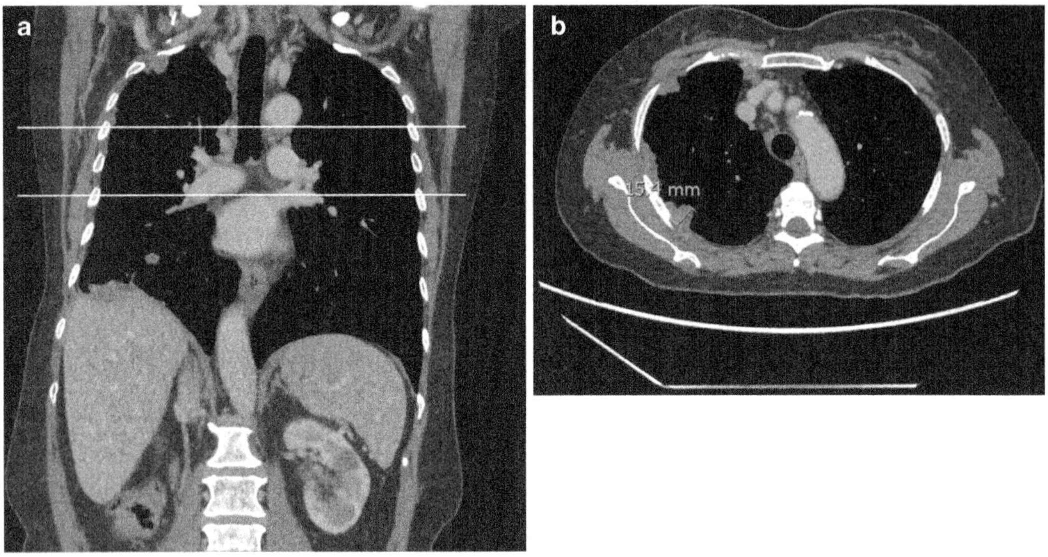

Fig. 10.4 (**a**) The thickest area of tumor is measured above the bottom of the aortic arch, between the aortic arch and top of the right atrium, and below the right atrium. (**b**) The maximal thickness at any slice within these "thirds" of the hemithorax is taken as the measurement for the purpose of staging

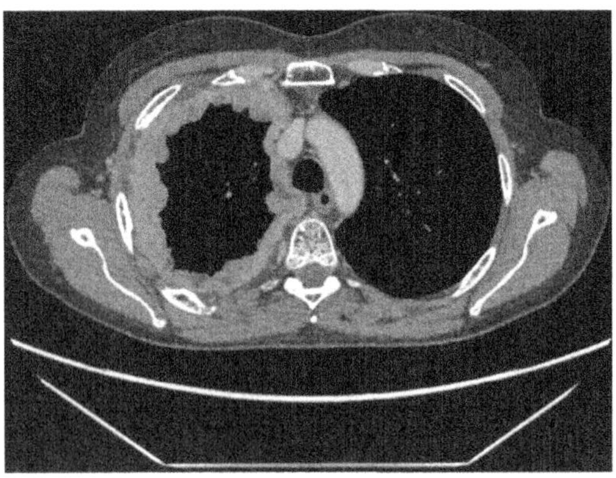

Fig. 10.5 An example of "rind-like" morphology, with circumferential tumor of similar thickness encasing the pleural cavity

Although these IASLC mesothelioma staging project data provide initial evidence to support the importance of tumor bulk in mesothelioma staging, there is currently insufficient evidence to support a move toward measurement-based staging, and T staging for now remains based on anatomical invasion [10]. Nevertheless, the next iteration of the IASLC mesothelioma prospective staging database will again include unidimensional measurements as a surrogate for tumor bulk and will incorporate a pilot study on volumetric measurements. These data are expected to be collected over the next 3 years.

Further support for the relationship among unidimensional measurement of thickness, tumor volume, and survival was provided in a recent publication that examined these questions in patients undergoing radiotherapy on the SMART protocol prior to definitive surgery for mesothelioma [11]. The investigators obtained three structured measurements from each of the mediastinal, chest wall, and diaphragmatic tumors, yielding a total of nine unidimensional tumor measurements. Tumor volume was estimated from the gross tumor volume derived from a radiation boost volume calculation. The total of these nine measurements correlated significantly ($p < 0.0001$) with tumor volume. The thickness of diaphragmatic tumor was most strongly associated with time to recurrence ($p < 0.0001$) and survival ($p = 0.001$), while the association with both was weaker for mediastinal tumor thickness and absent when only chest wall thickness was considered.

Hence, evidence clearly points to the prognostic value of tumor volume, or surrogates of tumor volume such as unidimensional measurements, in mesothelioma. It remains unclear as to whether tumor volume or other measurements will be more strongly prognostic than the current T stage and whether these measurements should be incorporated into T staging in addition to, or instead of, descriptors of anatomical invasion. For routine clinical practice, however, the simplicity of unidimensional measurements is clearly attractive.

10.3 Measuring Tumor to Assess Response to Treatment

Tumor response assessment underpins a number of key outcome measures in clinical trials. Not only is objective radiological response a surrogate outcome measure for the biological activity of treatments, but progression-free survival, time to progression, and duration of response are time-to-event measures that also require a robust and validated method of defining response and progression. The first widely used tumor response criteria were the WHO response criteria, which were very poorly suited to the unique growth pattern of pleural mesothelioma. The WHO response criteria were most suited to measuring lesions with well-defined bidimensional axes, with each lesion measurement comprising the product of the longest diameter of the lesion and its longest perpendicular diameter [12]. Lesion measurements then were summed to produce a total baseline tumor measurement, and these measurements were repeated at each imaging timepoint. A partial response was defined as a 50% decrease in the sum of these measurements with respect to baseline. Although unidimensional measurements were allowed, a partial response also required a 50% decrease in any unidimensional measurement, equating mathematically to a 75% decrease in the sum of the products of perpendicular diameters. Hence, this measurement system, if used for unidimensional measurements in mesothelioma, required a correspondingly greater reduction in tumor to be considered a "partial response" and may have contributed to the historical lack of measured chemotherapy efficacy in this disease.

In 2000, the RECIST 1.0 criteria for assessment of tumor response were developed, an important modification of which was the use of unidimensional tumor measurements only [13]. Unidimensional measurements have been theorized to be more closely related to cell kill by chemotherapy than the bidimensional product, at least with respect to spherical tumor masses [14]. There is also agreement between the sum of the product of diameters and the sum of unidimensional measurements for spherical tumors [14], although others identified discordance between response categories allocated using WHO vs. RECIST 1.0 criteria [15]. Nevertheless, it is important to remember that the unidimensional measurements of RECIST 1.0 evolved from the measurement of essentially spherical lesions and assumed relatively symmetrical changes in all tumor diameters.

RECIST 1.0 is limited in its application to mesothelioma. The unit of measurement is the "lesion," and given that mesothelioma often comprises one contiguous tumor mass, there is no guidance as to which part of this mass would be considered a "lesion" and whether the mass could be measured in more than one area. Furthermore, the requirement to record '"all" other lesions or sites of disease as nontarget lesions imposes a difficult documentation burden on those measuring mesothelioma. RECIST 1.0 requires the measurement of each lesion's "longest diameter," which is clearly problematic in mesothelioma as the growth of mesothelioma usually follows the curvature of the chest wall, with no clear endpoint to the longest diameter (Fig. 10.6a). Furthermore, when mesothelioma responds to therapy, that response usually demonstrates as a reduction in tumor thickness, rarely as a reduction in the extent of tumor along the chest wall or mediastinum (Fig. 10.6b). The "longest diameter" could also be applied to measurements of structures of fixed length, for example, tumor infiltrating the pulmonary fissures or tumor between two fixed structures such as the carina and thoracic vertebrae; however, clearly this presentation would again be inappropriate for assessment by longest diameter, as any reduction in tumor burden would reduce the

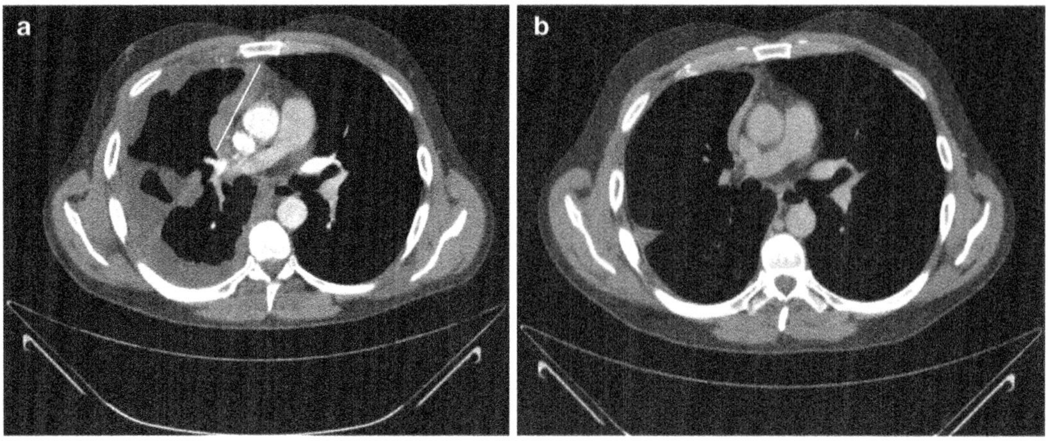

Fig. 10.6 (**a**) The "longest diameter" of this tumor site could ostensibly be measured as shown (white line) in this image. (**b**) the area measured in Fig. 10.6a. has reduced in thickness with a very significant tumor response; however, the "longest diameter" measurement from Fig. 10.6a. would be unchanged

thickness of pulmonary fissure involvement, for example, rather than the longest diameter of the tumor.

Following the publication and adoption of RECIST 1.0, shortcomings of these criteria as applied to mesothelioma were rapidly highlighted in the literature [16–18]. However, prior to the development of RECIST 1.0, an adaptation of response criteria that utilized unidimensional measurements of the tumor rind thickness had been described and used in two phase II clinical trials [19, 20]. A similar set of criteria also was adopted for the pivotal randomized phase III clinical trial of cisplatin and pemetrexed, which first demonstrated benefits of chemotherapy in advanced mesothelioma and promoted the utility of incorporating unidimensional measurements of tumor rind thickness as a surrogate for overall survival benefit [21]. Widespread acceptance of the results of this important clinical trial laid the foundation for acceptance of modified RECIST for mesothelioma, published in 2004 [22].

10.4 RECIST Modified for Mesothelioma

Modified RECIST for mesothelioma (mRECIST) was published as a research paper and subsequently became the de-facto standard methodology for response assessment in mesothelioma, a fact often overlooked when noting gaps in the measurement and response assessment approaches outlined in this paper [22]. In the context of specific guidance on implementation of tumor measurement protocols, mRECIST did not include, or did not specify in detail, some key points. Essentially, mRECIST for mesothelioma did not propose a new set of response criteria and was implicitly intended to align with RECIST 1.0 when considering issues such as minimum measurable disease, categories of response, and handling of non-pleural lesions; however, it described a set of guidelines around *how* to obtain tumor measurements in this disease. Most notably, mRECIST proposed two measurements perpendicular to the chest wall or mediastinum at each of three levels (CT sections) to capture tumor *thickness* in the affected hemithorax (Fig. 10.7a–c). The sum of these measurements then became the unidimensional pleural measurement for any given CT scan, with the sum of the unidimensional measurements of any additional non-pleural lesions being treated as per RECIST 1.0 and added to the pleural measurement. Criteria for response (a reduction of at least 30% in the summed tumor thickness measurements) and progression (a summed measurement increase of at least 20%) were unchanged by mRECIST. Despite some ambiguities, mRECIST has

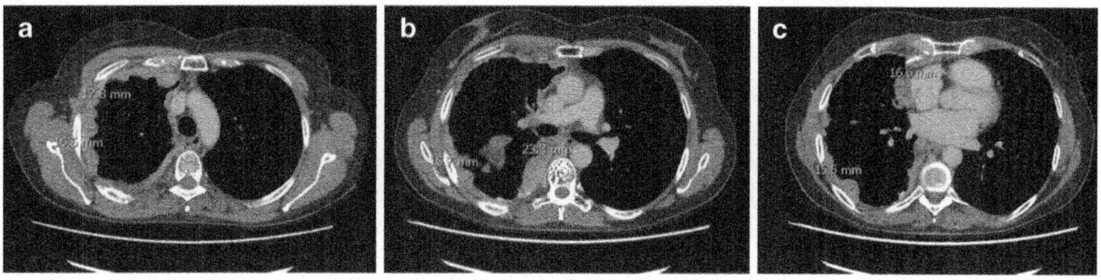

Fig. 10.7 (a–c) Two unidimensional measurements have been taken perpendicular to the chest wall or mediastinum on each of three axial CT slices, to give six measurements in total which form the sum of unidimensional pleural measurements

generally been applied as intended and has now been widely used in mesothelioma clinical trials for over a decade [23–29]. Although the extent of reduction in unidimensional measurements that should be considered "partial response" in mesothelioma has been debated, the original mRECIST paper did demonstrate improved patients outcomes with a 30% reduction in unidimensional measurements. More recently, Labby et al. used tumor thickness as a continuous variable in an independent cohort and validated that change in mRECIST-acquired tumor thickness measurements was independently associated with patient prognosis [30].

10.5 Updating RECIST Modified for Mesothelioma

In 2009, RECIST was updated to version 1.1, with a suite of publications detailing not only the updated guidelines but also reporting in detail the research supporting the proposed changes [31–38]. Notable changes included reducing the number of lesions to be measured per organ, providing specific guidelines for the measurement of pathological lymph nodes, changes to requirements for confirmation of response, and incorporation of a minimum increase in tumor measurement when determining response in order to mitigate the risk of overcalling progression based on small changes in tumor measurement. These changes had not yet been applied to mesothelioma, as mRECIST remained the standard response guidelines in this disease. Some elements of RECIST 1.1 were intuitively appropriate to incorporate in the mesothelioma setting, for example, measurement of pathologically involved lymph nodes had excellent validity for use in mesothelioma. The requirements for confirmation of response only when response was a primary endpoint were also relevant; however, to consider a reduction in the number of lesions measured from an involved hemithorax from six (per mRECIST) to two (per RECIST 1.1) would substantially reduce the representativeness of any measured area of tumor.

To clarify ambiguities in mRECIST and incorporate important and relevant updates from RECIST 1.1, modified RECIST 1.1 for mesothelioma (mRECIST 1.1) was developed [39]. This paper provides more detailed guidance on the application of measurements in mesothelioma, adds updated recommendations in the context of RECIST 1.1, and incorporates intervening research, as well as clarifications from a decade of experience. Aspects that required specific clarification included definition of minimal measureable disease and measurable lesions, more guidance around location of measurements and descriptions of nonmeasurable pleural disease, and incorporation of specific considerations around pathological lymph nodes, non-pleural disease, bilateral pleural disease, and progressive disease.

RECIST 1.0 and 1.1 conceptualize the "lesion" as the unit to be measured, but this concept is difficult to apply to mesothelioma. While many other tumors are discrete foci that can be measured in a longest dimension, the growth pattern of mesothelioma as a circumferential sheet or rind around the lung means that a patient's tumor could actually comprise one continuous tumor mass, potentially a single "lesion," extending through multiple levels of the hemithorax and across multiple CT sections. However, to consider that the complexities of tumor growth or response in mesothelioma could be captured by one measurement from this single lesion is overly simplistic. Modified RECIST 1.1, hence, formalizes the concept of a "measurement site" on the pleura, allowing the observer to select a number of appropriate measurement sites irrespective of the number of separate physical lesions. The observer first selects CT sections with the greatest pleural thickness and identifies sites on these sections that are most suitable to reproducible longitudinal measurements. When measuring tumor thickness, the observer must select a point on the outer margin of the tumor to initiate the measurement and then measure in a direction that best captures the thickness of the tumor at the site, extending the measurement to the inner margin of the tumor [40]. Ideally, these measurements would be made using a computer interface and will be, as per mRECIST, perpendicular to a tangent to the curve of the pleura on the chest wall or mediastinum. Even when the same point on the outer tumor margin is selected, different observers may construct measurement lines either in different directions or with differing interpretations of the inner margin of the tumor, thus leading to interobserver variability [40, 41]. Hence, in order to reduce variability, mRECIST 1.1 recommends that once a baseline measurement has been obtained at a specific measurement site, all subsequent measurements at that site should be oriented in the same direction. Furthermore, the same image display parameters should be used at each timepoint, which may provide more consistency in selecting the inner margin of the tumor. mRECIST 1.1 also suggests that the same observer acquire measurements across timepoints. To maximize temporal consistency, even when the same observer is obtaining measurements sequentially, it is highly recommended that observers capture annotated images for use as a visual reference when future measurements are acquired.

The original mRECIST did not explicitly state the minimum tumor thickness measurement but was intended to accord with the RECIST 1.0 definition of 10 mm as the minimum measurable disease thickness. The concept underpinning this minimum lesion size recommendation was that the minimum size for a measurable lesion should be twice the CT scan section thickness, which was 5 mm at the time RECIST was published; despite section thicknesses of 1–3 mm now standard on contemporary CT scanners, this 10-mm recommendation was not updated by RECIST 1.1. CT scanner resolution combined with the typical presentation of mesothelioma tumor as a sheet that extends across multiple contiguous axial CT sections seemed to suggest that this size recommendation could be reduced; however, as the size of an object to be measured decreases, the variability of measurement increases, thus increasing the chance of incorrect classification of response [42]. As an intervening study in mesothelioma measurement demonstrated that observer variability was acceptable down to tumor thickness measurements of 5 or 7.5 mm [43], mRECIST 1.1 now proposes a decrease in the requirement for minimally measurable tumor thickness from 10 to 7 mm. This change has the potential to increase the proportion of patients with earlier disease who may become eligible for clinical trials based on measurable tumor and will redress, in part, the disadvantage that patients with mesothelioma face through the 10-mm-thickness requirement, which equates to a very substantial tumor burden in this disease due to its unique morphology [44]. This change may also increase the number of sites available for measurement in clinical trial participants, potentially decreasing measurement variability through incorporation of more discrete measurement sites.

mRECIST 1.1 also clarifies the number of sites that should be measured for assessment of response. While RECIST 1.0 proposed measurement of up to 10 lesions in total with up to 5 in any one organ, RECIST 1.1 reduced the number of lesions to be measured to two per organ. mRECIST for mesothelioma originally specified the selection of six measurement sites but was ambiguous as to whether all six sites were required or whether the six sites represented a maximum number. mRECIST 1.1 for mesothelioma now specifies that *up to* six pleural measurement sites may be selected and that the measurement at each site must meet the criterion for minimally measurable disease. Each CT section for measurement is ideally selected on the basis of measurement reproducibility, with anatomic landmarks being readily identifiable for matching axial measurement levels in scans at subsequent timepoints. Nevertheless, mRECIST 1.1 also recognizes that the presence of measurable tumor is of primary importance. Because sites superior to the level of the left atrium are less vulnerable to the impact of inspiratory effort, and those below the level of the aortic arch reduce the impact of volume averaging and pleural curvature, these considerations should be incorporated into selection of measurement sites.

mRECIST 1.1 specifically addresses circumstances such as measurement of bilateral disease, non-pleural lesions, and measurement of nodal disease. Bilateral disease should be measured as if the pleura is a single organ, with a maximum of six pleural measurement sites distributed across both pleurae. Similarly, non-pleural lesions are handled as per RECIST 1.1; however, the up to six pleural measurement sites will be counted as the contribution from one organ (i.e., nominally as two measurements) toward the sum of measurements specified by RECIST 1.1. Furthermore, non-pleural lesions can be considered "measurable disease," even if no measurable pleural disease is apparent. Nodal disease should be measured unidimensionally as per RECIST 1.1, with any nodes identified as target lesions having a short axis of ≥15 mm and with the nodal short-axis measurement added to the overall measurement of tumor burden. mRECIST 1.1 acknowledges that some nodal sites, for example, internal mammary nodes and intercostal nodes, are unlikely to be seen at all unless pathological; however, at the moment there is insufficient data to make any recommendations that differ from RECIST 1.1.

Because mesothelioma is often circumferential, there may be many areas of tumor that cannot be incorporated into specific measurement sites or may not meet criteria for measurable disease. The morphology of mesothelioma does not allow for these areas to be individually noted; hence, mRECIST 1.1 allows for other foci of disease to be described as a whole with descriptive terms such as "extensive pleural thickening," "extensive pleural nodularity," or "circumferential pleural thickening." There is no expectation that numerous individual pleural lesions be specifically identified as nontarget lesions.

Under mRECIST 1.1, tumor response criteria for partial and complete response and stable disease mirror those of RECIST 1.1, as does a requirement for partial or complete response to be confirmed by a follow-up scan at least 4 weeks later; however, while progressive disease still requires an increase in the summed measurement of at least 20% over the nadir measurement, an absolute increase of the summed measurement of at least 5 mm over the nadir summed measurement is also required, consistent with RECIST 1.1. Assessment of "unequivocal" new lesions also requires careful review of adjacent CT sections to ensure that the "new" lesion has not been displaced, for example, from an adjacent section with change in inspiratory effort or thoracic contraction. Regarding a measurement site that demonstrates reduced thickness, RECIST 1.1 specifies that a default value of 5 mm is to be assigned if an actual measurement cannot be acquired; however, given that the sheet-like structure of mesothelioma has one margin that generally abuts normal structures and that the partial volume effect in the axial dimension does not need to be considered, mRECIST 1.1 recommends a default value of 2 mm if tumor is present at a measurement site but is too thin to accurately measure.

Because mesothelioma is nonspherical, the RECIST response classification criteria may not reflect the same changes in volume for the unidimensional changes that categorize response. This notion has been demonstrated in geometric modeling [44] and also using patient imaging data. In fact, the response criteria that were most highly correlated with survival were a reduction of 64% in unidimensional measurement for partial response and an increase of 50% for progressive disease [30]. Nevertheless, until alternative criteria are fully validated in a prospective clinical trial, no changes have been recommended for mRECIST 1.1.

10.6 Measurement of Mesothelioma in Immunotherapy Clinical Trials

The advent of immunotherapy has required some reframing of response criteria developed to assess response to chemotherapy. As with other cancers, mesothelioma is the subject of numerous immunotherapy clinical trials, with the key challenge in response assessment being immune-related pseudoprogression. Pseudoprogression is believed to develop when the immunological response to tumor leads to an influx of immune cells, which may result in an apparent increase in the bulk of the tumor as seen on imaging. This process has been considered in a number of modifications to the RECIST criteria, most recently with a consensus-based modification of RECIST 1.1 for immune-based therapeutics published by the RECIST working group [45]. These iRECIST guidelines, which are based on RECIST 1.1 measurements, allow patients to continue on clinical trials despite development of apparent new lesions or suspected initial progression of baseline target lesions, which initially would be considered "unconfirmed progressive disease" (iUPD). With continued imaging, iUPD can subsequently become "confirmed progressive disease" (iCPD). This approach allows patients to continue treatment when there is suspicion of pseudoprogression. iRECIST did not specify any considerations around pleural mesothelioma; however, mRECIST 1.1 recommends that the general principles of iRECIST be adopted for immunotherapy clinical trials in which pseudoprogression or delayed response may occur. Each clinical trial protocol should include adequate specific guidance on the application of iRECIST, informed by the general principles of mRECIST 1.1.

10.7 Incorporating FDG-PET-CT into Response Assessment for Mesothelioma

^{18}F-FDG-PET/CT is an important cancer imaging modality that has proven useful in response assessment in other cancers. FDG-PET and FDG-PET-CT have been studied in response assessment in pleural mesothelioma; however, PET-based imaging has not been well validated as a surrogate measure of outcome in large patient cohorts or in a prospective randomized clinical trial [46–49]. There are also important limitations to the measurement of response using FDG-PET, most notably the difficulty in interpreting changes in FDG uptake and SUV in the context of postoperative changes, inflammation or infection, or prior pleurodesis [8, 50, 51]. mRECIST 1.1 does not currently recommend incorporating FDG-PET-CT into measurement of response, and it is likely that the difficulties in applying FDG-PET criteria to a large subgroup of patients who have had pleural surgery or pleurodesis mean that this will not become a validated standard in the future (Fig. 10.8). Other PET tracers such as FLT-PET have been tested but also suffer from limitations [52].

10.8 Using CT Volumetry in Measurement of Pleural Mesothelioma

The potential of volumetry in the assessment of tumor response has also been studied and, if consistent and validated, would render the need for tumor measurement guidelines obsolete. Tumor volume also has potential use in staging. Clearly, the clinical use of change in volume would require a different response and progression metric. Mathematically, the RECIST response criteria, 30% reduction in tumor diameter for partial response and 20% increase in tumor diameter for progressive disease, equate to a 66% reduction in tumor volume and a 73% increase in tumor volume, respectively, using the spherical model for which these criteria were derived [44]. When these proposed volumetric "response criteria" were applied to pre- and

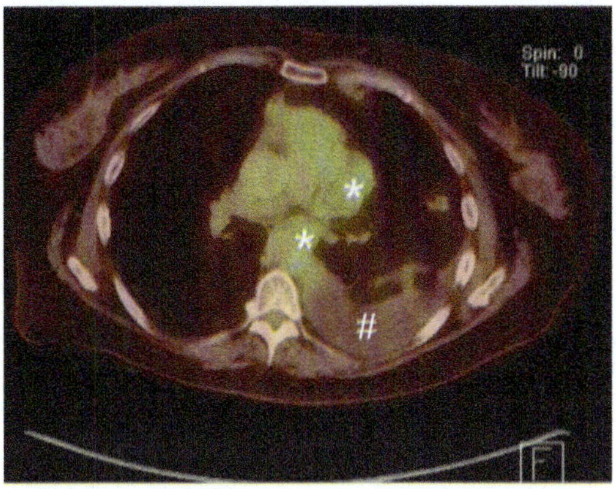

Fig. 10.8 FDG-PET-CT can help distinguish tumor (*) from pleural effusion (#); however, the use of FDG-PET-CT in assessment of response to treatment has not yet been validated

post-chemotherapy CT scans in one study, there was no significant difference among three readers in derived tumor volume ($p > 0.42$) and a high intraclass correlation coefficient (0.99) for agreement among readers in response category [53]. This was not the case for response categories derived from mRECIST measurements, for which there was poor agreement among three readers. Other investigators have found significant variability in tumor volume measurements for mesothelioma [54]. Although there is an acknowledged association between mesothelioma tumor volume and survival [55, 56], the use of response categories translated directly from unidimensional measurements has not been validated, nor have any new volumetric response metrics been developed with sufficient clinical validation to be used in clinical trials or clinical decision making [57]. Consistent application of tumor volume measurements would require use of the same image analysis software, patient setup, and image acquisition parameters; however, it remains difficult to standardize radiologist perception. Even in the simpler context of lung nodule volumetry, these issues have been challenging to standardize [58].

Measurement of tumor volume in mesothelioma is very challenging. The difficulties in distinguishing mesothelioma from adjacent structures, pleural effusion, and atelectasis are not confined to the human eye; computerized systems also struggle to differentiate between tumor and other structures that may mimic the texture and imaging characteristic of tumor [59]. Correlation between physical tumor bulk of postoperative specimens and CT-obtained tumor volumes was also lower than expected [60]. Indeed, an advantage of selecting individual representative sites of tumor for measurement, as per mRECIST, is that ambiguous areas and regions that are difficult to measure with confidence can be avoided. Furthermore, there are no tumor volume measurement software systems that do not require radiologist expertise and input; this need would pose a challenge in clinical trials, in which site clinical investigators commonly acquire measurements. MRI volumetry has also been studied, but MRI is more time consuming than CT and remains a more scarce resource in most settings; there has been limited research in this space [61].

It is worth noting that while the accuracy of tumor volume measurements as a representation of tumor bulk and change in tumor bulk may, in the future, be superior to unidimensional measurements, the goal of tumor measurement for response is not necessarily accuracy per se, but rather the use of a reproducible, simple, and adequate surrogate of patient outcomes. Taking these considerations into account, mRECIST 1.1 does not recommend the use of tumor volume for the current response criteria and proposes that mesothelioma tumor volumetry remains a research tool at the moment.

10.9 Conclusion

In conclusion, measurement of pleural tumor in malignant mesothelioma is a key part of clinical management and clinical trial interpretation. Clinicians, radiologists, and investigators, however, are challenged by the unique rind-like growth pattern of this disease, which leads to difficulty in applying staging and response criteria that perform well in tumors of a more spherical morphology. Nevertheless, more appropriate measurement guidelines for response have been developed for this disease and are in widespread use in clinical trials. These guidelines recently have been comprehensively updated to harmonize with RECIST 1.1 and to clarify aspects that were ambiguous in the original mRECIST publication. The use of tumor measurement in staging is under investigation, and although preliminary data support the prognostic potential of tumor measurements, they have not yet been formally incorporated into staging in this disease. CT scans remain the mainstay of imaging for tumor measurement in mesothelioma. Techniques such as CT volumetrics are promising research tools but have not yet been incorporated into routine clinical or clinical trial use since optimal, reproducible platforms and techniques remain unclear. MRI and FDG-PET scans have specific limitations in this context and are not routinely used in the measurement of tumor for response assessment. mRECIST 1.1 now should be considered the standard criteria for the assessment of tumor response to treatment in pleural mesothelioma.

References

1. Ball D, et al. Effect of tumor size on prognosis in patients treated with radical radiotherapy or chemoradiotherapy for non-small cell lung cancer. An analysis of the staging project database of the International Association for the Study of Lung Cancer. J Thorac Oncol. 2013;8(3):315–21.
2. Edge SB, Byrd DR, editors. AJCC cancer staging handbook. 7th ed. New York: Springer; 2010.
3. Rusch VW. A proposed new international TNM staging system for malignant pleural mesothelioma from the International Mesothelioma Interest Group. Lung Cancer. 1996;14(1):1–12.
4. Rusch VW, Giroux D. Do we need a revised staging system for malignant pleural mesothelioma? Analysis of the IASLC database. Ann Cardiothorac Surg. 2012;1(4):438–48.
5. Pass HI, et al. Preoperative tumor volume is associated with outcome in malignant pleural mesothelioma. J Thorac Cardiovasc Surg. 1998;115(2):310–7; discussion 317-8.
6. Olt G, Berchuck A, Bast RC Jr. The role of tumor markers in gynecologic oncology. Obstet Gynecol Surv. 1990;45(9):570–7.
7. Gill RR, et al. Epithelial malignant pleural mesothelioma after extrapleural pneumonectomy: stratification of survival with CT-derived tumor volume. AJR Am J Roentgenol. 2012;198(2):359–63.
8. Nowak AK, et al. A novel prognostic model for malignant mesothelioma incorporating quantitative FDG-PET imaging with clinical parameters. Clin Cancer Res. 2010;16(8):2409–17.
9. Klabatsa A, et al. The association of 18F-FDG PET/CT parameters with survival in malignant pleural mesothelioma. Eur J Nucl Med Mol Imaging. 2014;41(2):276–82.
10. Nowak AK, et al. The IASLC mesothelioma staging project: proposals for revisions of the T descriptors in the forthcoming eighth edition of the TNM classification for pleural mesothelioma. J Thorac Oncol. 2016;11(12):2089–99.
11. de Perrot M, et al. Impact of tumour thickness on survival after radical radiation and surgery in malignant pleural mesothelioma. Eur Respir J. 2017;49(3):1601428.
12. Miller A, et al. Reporting results of cancer treatment. Cancer. 1981;47:207–14.
13. Therasse P, et al. New guidelines to evaluate the response to treatment in solid tumors. J Natl Cancer Inst. 2000;92(3):205–16.
14. James K, et al. Measuring response in solid tumors: unidimensional versus bidimensional measurement. J Natl Cancer Inst. 1999;91(6):523–8.
15. Mazumdar M, Smith A, Schwartz LH. A statistical simulation study finds discordance between WHO criteria and RECIST guideline. J Clin Epidemiol. 2004;57(4):358–65.
16. van Klaveren RJ, et al. Inadequacy of the RECIST criteria for response evaluation in patients with malignant pleural mesothelioma. Lung Cancer. 2004;43(1):63–9.
17. Hillerdal G. Staging and evaluating responses in malignant pleural mesothelioma. Lung Cancer. 2004;43(1):75–6.
18. Monetti F, et al. Inadequacy of the new Response Evaluation Criteria in Solid Tumors (RECIST) in patients with malignant pleural mesothelioma: report of four cases. Lung Cancer. 2004;43(1):71–4.
19. Nowak AK, et al. A multicentre phase II study of cisplatin and gemcitabine for malignant mesothelioma. Br J Cancer. 2002;87(5):491–6.
20. Byrne MJ, et al. Cisplatin and gemcitabine treatment for malignant mesothelioma: a phase II study. J Clin Oncol. 1999;17(1):25–30.
21. Vogelzang NJ, et al. Phase III study of pemetrexed in combination with cisplatin versus cisplatin alone in patients with malignant pleural mesothelioma. J Clin Oncol. 2003;21(14):2636–44.
22. Byrne MJ, Nowak AK. Modified RECIST criteria for assessment of response in malignant pleural mesothelioma. Ann Oncol. 2004;15(2):257–60.
23. Maio M, et al. Tremelimumab as second-line or third-line treatment in relapsed malignant mesothelioma (DETERMINE): a multicentre, international, randomised, double-blind, placebo-controlled phase 2b trial. Lancet Oncol. 2017;18(9):1261–73.
24. Zalcman G, et al. Bevacizumab for newly diagnosed pleural mesothelioma in the Mesothelioma

Avastin Cisplatin Pemetrexed Study (MAPS): a randomised, controlled, open-label, phase 3 trial. Lancet. 2016;387:1405–14.
25. Kindler HL, et al. Multicenter, double-blind, placebo-controlled, randomized phase II trial of gemcitabine/cisplatin plus bevacizumab or placebo in patients with malignant mesothelioma. J Clin Oncol. 2012;30(20):2509–15.
26. Krug LM, et al. VANTAGE 014: vorinostat (V) in patients with advanced malignant pleural mesothelioma (MPM) who have failed prior pemetrexed and either cisplatin or carboplatin therapy: a phase III, randomized, doubleblind, placebo-controlled trial. Eur J Cancer. 2011;47:2–3.
27. Nowak AK, et al. A phase 1b clinical trial of the CD40-activating antibody CP-870,893 in combination with cisplatin and pemetrexed in malignant pleural mesothelioma. Ann Oncol. 2015;26(12):2483–90.
28. Nowak AK, et al. A phase II clinical trial of the vascular disrupting agent BNC105P as second line chemotherapy for advanced malignant pleural mesothelioma. Lung Cancer. 2013;81(3):422–7.
29. Nowak AK, et al. A phase II study of intermittent sunitinib malate as second-line therapy in progressive malignant pleural mesothelioma. J Thorac Oncol. 2012;7(9):1449–56.
30. Labby ZE, et al. Optimization of response classification criteria for patients with malignant pleural mesothelioma. J Thorac Oncol. 2012;7(11):1728–34.
31. Eisenhauer EA, et al. New response evaluation criteria in solid tumours: revised RECIST guideline (version 1.1). Eur J Cancer. 2009;45(2):228–47.
32. Bogaerts J, et al. Individual patient data analysis to assess modifications to the RECIST criteria. Eur J Cancer. 2009;45(2):248–60.
33. Schwartz LH, et al. Evaluation of lymph nodes with RECIST 1.1. Eur J Cancer. 2009;45(2):261–7.
34. Ford R, et al. Lessons learned from independent central review. Eur J Cancer. 2009;45(2):268–74.
35. Dancey JE, et al. Recommendations for the assessment of progression in randomised cancer treatment trials. Eur J Cancer. 2009;45(2):281–9.
36. Moskowitz CS, et al. A simulation study to evaluate the impact of the number of lesions measured on response assessment. Eur J Cancer. 2009;45(2):300–10.
37. Verweij J, et al. Cancer clinical trial outcomes: any progress in tumour-size assessment? Eur J Cancer. 2009;45(2):225–7.
38. Sargent DJ, et al. Validation of novel imaging methodologies for use as cancer clinical trial end-points. Eur J Cancer. 2009;45(2):290–9.
39. Armato SG 3rd, Nowak AK. Revised modified response evaluation criteria in solid tumors for assessment of response in malignant pleural mesothelioma (version 1.1). J Thorac Oncol. 2018;13(7):1012–21.
40. Armato SG 3rd, et al. Measurement of mesothelioma on thoracic CT scans: a comparison of manual and computer-assisted techniques. Med Phys. 2004;31(5):1105–15.
41. Armato SG 3rd, et al. Evaluation of semiautomated measurements of mesothelioma tumor thickness on CT scans. Acad Radiol. 2005;12(10):1301–9.
42. Oxnard GR, et al. Variability of lung tumor measurements on repeat computed tomography scans taken within 15 minutes. J Clin Oncol. 2011;29(23):3114–9.
43. Armato SG 3rd, et al. Observer variability in mesothelioma tumor thickness measurements: defining minimally measurable lesions. J Thorac Oncol. 2014;9(8):1187–94.
44. Oxnard GR, Armato SG 3rd, Kindler HL. Modeling of mesothelioma growth demonstrates weaknesses of current response criteria. Lung Cancer. 2006;52(2):141–8.
45. Seymour L, et al. iRECIST: guidelines for response criteria for use in trials testing immunotherapeutics. Lancet Oncol. 2017;18(3):e143–52.
46. Veit-Haibach P, et al. Combined FDG-PET/CT in response evaluation of malignant pleural mesothelioma. Lung Cancer. 2010;67:311. Epub ahead of print May 30.
47. Schaefer NG, et al. Response evaluation by CT and FDG-PET/CT in malignant pleural mesothelioma. J Clin Oncol. 2008;26(18S):11098.
48. Ceresoli GL, et al. Early response evaluation in malignant pleural mesothelioma (MPM) by total glycolytic volume (TGV) analysis of serial FDG-PET scans. 2008.
49. Francis RJ, et al. Early prediction of response to chemotherapy and survival in malignant pleural mesothelioma using a novel semiautomated 3-dimensional volume-based analysis of serial 18F-FDG PET scans. J Nucl Med. 2007;48(9):1449–58.
50. Kwek BH, Aquino SL, Fischman AJ. Fluorodeoxyglucose positron emission tomography and CT after talc pleurodesis. Chest. 2004;125(6):2356–60.
51. Genestreti G, et al. FDG PET/CT response evaluation in malignant pleural mesothelioma patients treated with talc pleurodesis and chemotherapy. J Cancer. 2012;3:241–5.
52. Segard T, et al. FLT PET for response assessment in malignant pleural mesothelioma (MPM) using a semi-automated volume-based region growing algorithm. Eur J Nucl Med Mol Imaging. 2012;39:S457.
53. Frauenfelder T, et al. Volumetry: an alternative to assess therapy response for malignant pleural mesothelioma? Eur Respir J. 2011;38(1):162–8.
54. Gill RR, et al. North American multicenter volumetric CT study for clinical staging of malignant pleural mesothelioma: feasibility and logistics of setting up a quantitative imaging study. J Thorac Oncol. 2016;11(8):1335–44.
55. Gill RR, Richards WG, Yeap BY, Matsuoka S, Wolf AS, Gerbaudo VH, Bueno R, Sugarbaker DJ, Hatabu H. Epithelial malignant pleural mesothelioma after extrapleural pneumonectomy: stratification of survival with CT-derived tumor volume. Am J Roentgenol. 2012;198(2):359–63.

56. Pass HI, Kranda K, Temeck BK, Feuerstein I, Steinberg SM. Surgically debulked malignant pleural mesothelioma: results and prognostic factors. Ann Surg Oncol. 1997;4(3):215–22.
57. Armato SG 3rd, et al. Imaging in pleural mesothelioma: a review of the 12th International Conference of the International Mesothelioma Interest Group. Lung Cancer. 2015;90(2):148–54.
58. Sullivan DC, et al. Metrology standards for quantitative imaging biomarkers. Radiology. 2015;277(3):813–25.
59. Corson N, et al. Characterization of mesothelioma and tissues present in contrast-enhanced thoracic CT scans. Med Phys. 2011;38(2):942–7.
60. Armato SG 3rd, et al. Radiologic-pathologic correlation of mesothelioma tumor volume. Lung Cancer. 2015;87(3):278–82.
61. Plathow C, et al. Therapy response in malignant pleural mesothelioma-role of MRI using RECIST, modified RECIST and volumetric approaches in comparison with CT. Eur Radiol. 2008;18(8):1635–43.

11 Role of Metabolic Imaging in Mesothelioma

Fabrizia Gelardi, Andrea Marciano, Paola Anna Erba, and Arturo Chiti

11.1 Introduction

Early diagnosis and clinical staging in patients affected by malignant pleural mesothelioma (MPM) is necessary to manage individual therapy strategies.

Imaging plays an important role in the diagnostic assessment of patients with MPM disease: in particular, computed tomography (CT) and magnetic resonance imaging (MRI) are routinely used for non-invasive clinical staging.

The most common CT features of malignant pleural mesothelioma consist of pleural effusion, pleural thickening, ipsilateral lung volume loss, loco regional invasion, lymphadenopathy and metastatic disease [1].

Because of the complex growth pattern of MPM, it is difficult to make a clinical judgement only based on morphological imaging, so ^{18}F-FDG PET-CT represent an important additional imaging tool in these patients.

Comparative assessment of imaging results is necessary to evaluate all the areas of possible invasion and to select those patients who may benefit from multimodality treatment.

CT is readily accessible and provides a large number of anatomic information: this imaging practice can be used to recognize patients with clearly unresectable MPM (diffuse extension of tumour into the chest wall, mediastinum, or peritoneum or metastatic disease). Though, MRI or PET can be used as preoperative non-invasive imaging techniques to integrate CT results in controversial cases [2].

11.2 PET-CT

Positron emission tomography-computed tomography (PET-CT) is a non-invasive imaging technique used to generate quantitative parameters regarding the metabolic activity of target pathologic tissues.

PET-CT combines, in a single gantry, a positron emission tomography (PET) scanner and a computed tomography (CT) scanner. This hybrid device allows to acquire sequential images and generates metabolic and morphological features in the same session, combining these into a single image.

F. Gelardi
Department of Biomedical Sciences, Humanitas University, Milan, Italy
e-mail: fabrizia.gelardi@humanitas.it

A. Marciano · P. A. Erba
Nuclear Medicine, Department of Translational Research and New Technology in Medicine, University of Pisa, Pisa, Italy
e-mail: paola.erba@unipi.it

A. Chiti (✉)
Department of Biomedical Sciences, Humanitas University, Milan, Italy

Nuclear Medicine, Humanitas Research Hospital, Milan, Italy
e-mail: arturo.chiti@hunimed.eu

G. L. Ceresoli et al. (eds.), *Mesothelioma*, https://doi.org/10.1007/978-3-030-16884-1_11

Anatomic imaging is complementary to functional imaging: when combined, the two modalities can both identify and localize functional abnormalities, a feature that was lacking in pure PET imaging. In general, CT adds specificity to the method, whereas PET adds mostly sensitivity.

Therefore, combined PET-CT allows the distinction between normal physiologic uptake and pathologic uptake, providing an accurate localization and characterization of tissues. The result is a significant reduction of the incidence of false positive and false negative imaging studies.

PET-CT improved medical diagnosis in many fields: in particular, hybrid imaging is playing an important role in the diagnosis and staging of malignant diseases, in therapy planning and assessment of metabolic response to treatment [3, 4].

In clinical practice, ^{18}F-fluoro-deoxy-glucose (FDG) is the most used radiopharmaceutical: FDG is an analogue of glucose, consequently it is absorbed, phosphorylated and retained by tissues with high uptake of glucose, working as a marker of tissue metabolic activity.

Although FDG uptake is not specific to cancer, it is well known that there is an over-expression of the GLUT glucose transporters into malignant cells and an upregulation of enzymatic activity resulting in increased tracer uptake.

Before the examination, the patient has to follow some preparation rules. The main objective is to decrease the tracer uptake in normal structures, like skeletal muscle, while maintaining and optimizing the tracer uptake in the target tissues. Therefore, non-diabetic patients should fast for at least 6 h before the FDG PET-CT study [5].

FDG uptake value has been revealed to be useful as imaging biomarker, but it is related not so directly to the proliferative activity. SUVmax is the most commonly used parameter to analyse PET/CT images: it is a semi quantitative measure, corresponding to the maximum standardized FDG uptake value of the tumour. This parameter takes into account the influence of the injected FDG activity and the patient size on FDG uptake measurement [6].

11.3 Differential Diagnosis Between Malignant and Benign Pleural Lesions

Exposure to asbestos causes asbestos-related malignant diseases, like malignant pleural mesothelioma, and a large number of benign lesions, as well as pleural plaques, benign asbestos-related pleural effusion (BAPE) and diffuse pleural thickening (DPT) [7].

The most common manifestations of malignant pleural mesothelioma are pleural effusion and pleural thickening. These are very common patterns, which can be related to a large number of malignant and benign diseases.

Pathologic confirmation by pleural biopsies is always required to make a definitive diagnosis. However, these are invasive techniques; non-invasive methods, such as imaging techniques, are important to identify the lesion to submit to biopsy and especially to avoid unnecessary invasive procedures in patients with a poor performance status.

Computed tomography (CT) identifies properly the location and dissemination of pleural lesions but is not always able to differentiate between malignant and benign disease.

^{18}F-FDG PET-CT could be useful in detecting malignant pleural lesions in patients exposed to asbestos with pleural injuries [8].

Indeed ^{18}F-FDG PET-CT provides functional and morphologic imaging at the same time, allowing a better interpretation combining the morphologic feature of the lesions on CT with the ^{18}F-FDG uptake on PET.

Terada et al. demonstrated that patients with MPM had significantly higher SUVmax (maximum Standardized Uptake Value) levels than non-MPM population, including patients with a history of asbestos exposure and a group that was not exposed to asbestos. Therefore, the authors hypothesized that levels of SUVmax could be also useful in the diagnosis of mesothelioma [8].

Another observational study by Yildirim et al. demonstrated that SUVmax levels of the pleural lesions upper than 2.2 are strongly related to malignant disease, with a sensitivity of 94.1% and a specificity of 100%. Therefore, these patients need to be investigated by invasive procedures. At the same time SUVmax shows a negative predictive value of 93.3%, and values <2.2 probably suggest non-malignant pleural disease and these patients are spared invasive procedures [6].

Another study by Sun et al. investigated the role of the ^{18}F-FDG PET-CT in the differential diagnosis between benign and malignant pleural effusion. Malignant pleural mesothelioma has to be always supposed in patients affected by pleural effusion with a history of asbestos exposure. On CT imaging pleural effusion is suspected when associated to nodular, focal and irregular pleural thickening. They suggested that is possible to increase CT evidences with ^{18}F-FDG uptake values. Indeed ^{18}F-FDG uptake increases in malignant lesions, and it should be diagnostic when SUVmax values are higher than mediastinal activity.

This study demonstrated that the sensitivity in detecting malignant effusion of CT imaging is 75%, of ^{18}F-FDG PET-CT is 91% and with integrated PET-CT increases to 93.5%. Specificities of CT imaging, ^{18}F-FDG PET imaging and ^{18}F-FDG PET/CT integrated imaging were 94.1%, 63.2% and 92.6% in detecting benign effusion. In conclusion, Sun et al. confirmed that ^{18}F-FDG PET/CT is more reliable than ^{18}F-FDG PET and CT imaging in differential diagnosis of malignant and benign pleural effusion [9].

A large number of non-malignant diseases could simulate MPM pattern and may lead to an incorrect diagnosis. Indeed, infections and inflammatory processes involving lungs, pleura and mediastinal lymph nodes cause an accumulation of inflammatory cells: these elements present an augmented metabolism state and show an increased FDG uptake. When also CT images are suspicious, a biopsy is recommended. Common manifestations that have to be differentiated from MPM are the following:

- Caseating granulomas: these structures are typical of *Mycobacterium Tuberculosis* and affect lungs and bronchopulmonary lymph nodes. Histologically, granulomas are formed by epithelioid macrophages and lymphocytes surrounding a cellular necrotic centre.
- Non-caseating granulomas: sarcoidosis is a systemic inflammatory disease that involves multiple organs, but mostly pulmonary parenchyma and lymph nodes. Granulomas present an increased FDG uptake, but it usually normalizes after steroid treatment.
- Amyloidosis: amyloid is a proteinaceous material and may settle in multiple organs, such as lungs and pleura. Amyloid deposits appear on CT like multiple nodules with sharp borders and containing calcifications.
- Talc pleurodesis: this procedure is generally performed to prevent the recurrence of malignant pleural effusions, establishing a local chronic inflammation. Pleurodesis is indicated also in patients affected by advanced MPM, therefore, is essential to distinguish this pattern from MPM recurrence. It appears as a pleural thickening and talc nodules on CT.
- Pleural fibrosis: asbestos or beryllium exposure could induce benign bilateral fibrosis and multifocal pleural plaques. These are typically lower than 1 cm and calcific on CT [10].

11.4 Non-invasive Preoperative Staging

In patients affected by MPM a correct staging of the disease anatomic extension is essential for selecting patients with resectable lesions: these patients would benefit from multimodality treatment, including chemotherapy, surgery with extra pleural pneumonectomy (EPP) and adjuvant radiation therapy.

According to the International Mesothelioma Interest Group (IMIG) staging system for MPM, only patients with stages I, II and III disease are suitable for surgery and have a better survival after EPP. Instead, patients with stage IV (any T4, any T3 and any M1) are not fit for surgical procedures and are directly addressed to chemotherapy [11].

Computed tomography (CT) and magnetic resonance imaging (MRI) are the imaging techniques of choice for studying the local extension and nodal invasion of the MPM disease [12].

Nonetheless, CT is often unsuccessful to recognize locally advanced and metastatic disease. Indeed, this technique usually underappreciates the extension of the tumour and is not always reliable to discriminate microscopic tumour invasion in the chest wall, mediastinal structures (especially in pericardium area) or through the diaphragm (Figs. 11.1 and 11.2). Consequently, approximately 20–30% of patients undergo invasive VATS (Video Assisted Thoracoscopy) and are identified as not suitable for extra pleural pneumonectomy [13, 14].

Flores et al. supposed that functional imaging might be considered in staging for improving performance in detecting unresectable disease and avoid inappropriate invasive investigation. However, PET imaging alone shows a lack of spatial resolution and cannot discriminate patients with T3 or T4 disease [12].

The introduction of combined PET/CT, with co-registration of anatomic and metabolic imaging, increases the detection of areas with augmented FDG uptake and the accuracy of preoperative IMIG staging [15].

In a report by Sørensen et al., the sensitivity of PET/CT in detecting T4 disease was 78%, compared to 67% in a study by Erasmus et al. and 19% using PET alone by Flores et al. [14, 16].

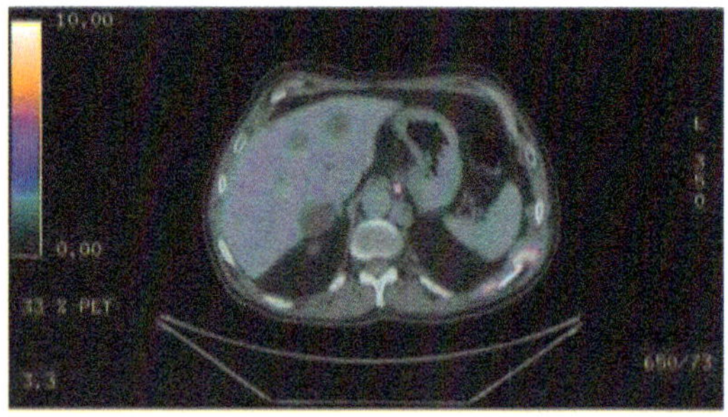

Fig. 11.1 PET/CT discriminate locally advanced disease. This practice permits the description of chest wall invasion, which could be underestimated by CT

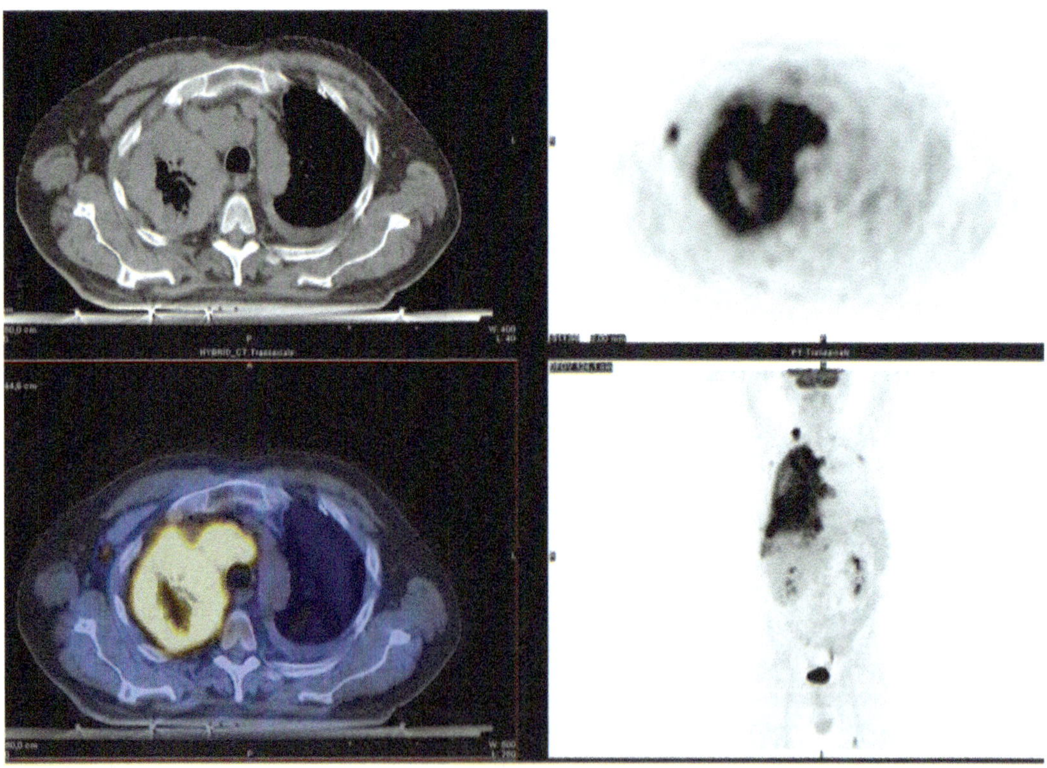

Fig. 11.2 PET/CT discriminate locally advanced disease. This practice permits the description of mediastinum structures invasion, which could be underestimated by CT

The high morbidity and mortality of the EPP practice necessarily requires invasive staging with VATS, which is decisive and essential when incongruities among CT, PET/CT and MRI occur in patient candidate to surgery [14].

Unfortunately, low spatial resolution of PET/CT combined with strong FDG uptake by the pleural lesion can make it hard to differentiate the primary lesion from bronchopulmonary and hilar lymph nodes involvement (stage N1). Although this may change the prognosis, it does not affect surgical management [16].

On the contrary, PET/CT is helpful in distinguish between N2 and N3 disease: indeed, metabolic imaging is useful for detecting mediastinum lymph node involvement (such as para-aortic region and aorticopulmonary window lymph nodes), which are not reachable by VATS and could be underestimated by non-invasive staging with CT (Fig. 11.3) [17].

In a study by Erasmus et al., PET/CT guarantees a sensitivity of 38% and a specificity of 78% in lymph node staging of sub carinal, ipsilateral internal mammary and mediastinal region (N2 disease). Every time contralateral internal mammary or hilar lymph nodes and ipsilateral supraclavicular or scalene lymph nodes (N3 disease) are swelled according to CT criteria, but do not uptake FDG, they need to be sampled in patients considered to surgery [14]. Although these evidences require a pathological confirmation in most patients, PET/CT could be useful to identify even a small number of patients in whom radical treatment may be inappropriate [12].

Furthermore, in their study Flores et al. found a correlation between high SUVmax values and mediastinal lymph nodes involvement. This relationship is not so clear, and it could be simply related to the predisposition of more metabolically active tumour to spread to mediastinal nodes [12].

At the end, PET/CT imaging is excellent in detecting distant occult metastases (SNC, lungs and bones), even when it is not possible with other morphological imaging modalities, such as CT or MRI (Figs. 11.4 and 11.5) [16].

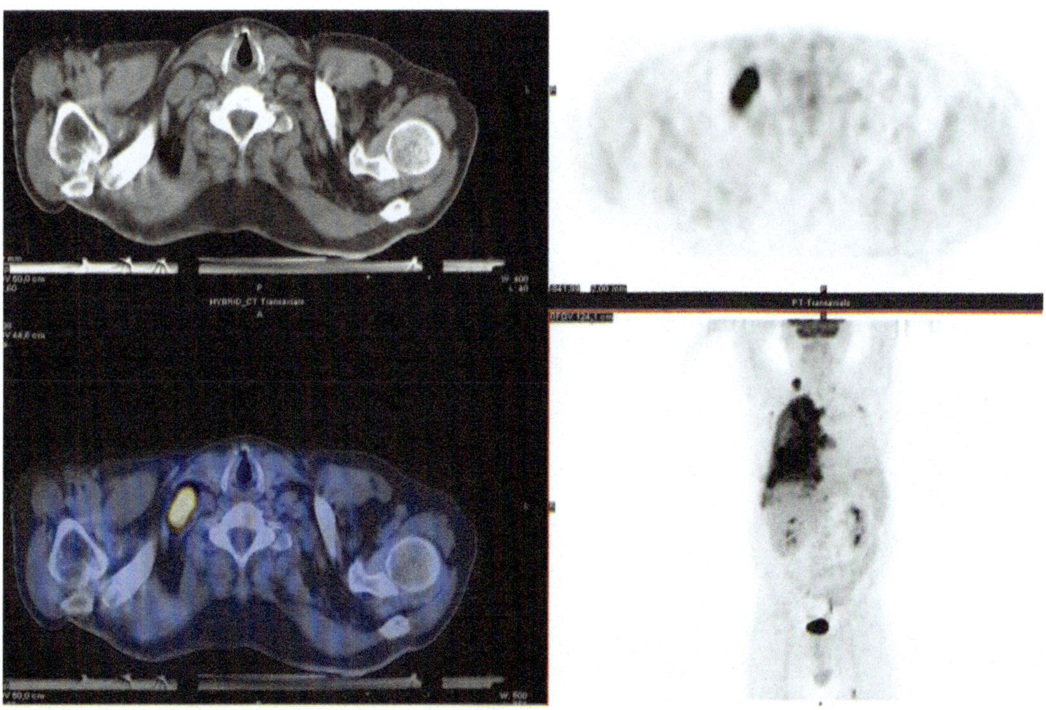

Fig. 11.3 PET/CT is helpful in distinguish between N2 and N3 disease, detecting lymph node involvement in contralateral internal mammary, contralateral hilar region, ipsilateral supraclavicular or scalene region

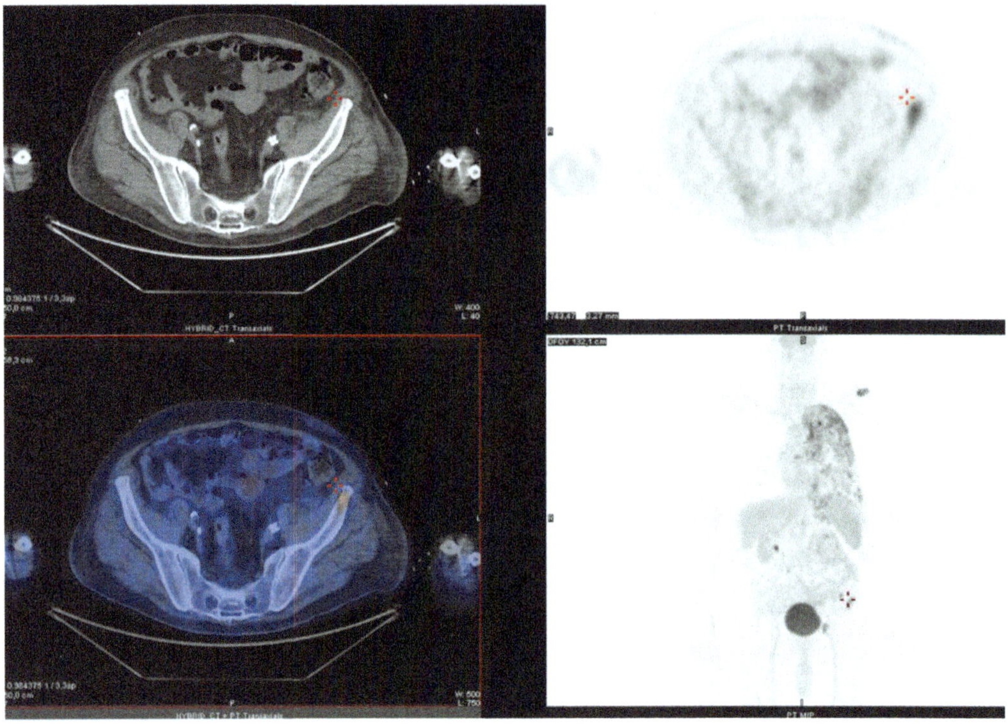

Fig. 11.4 PET/CT is useful in detecting distant occult metastases. In this patient we observe an occult metastasis located on the left iliac wing

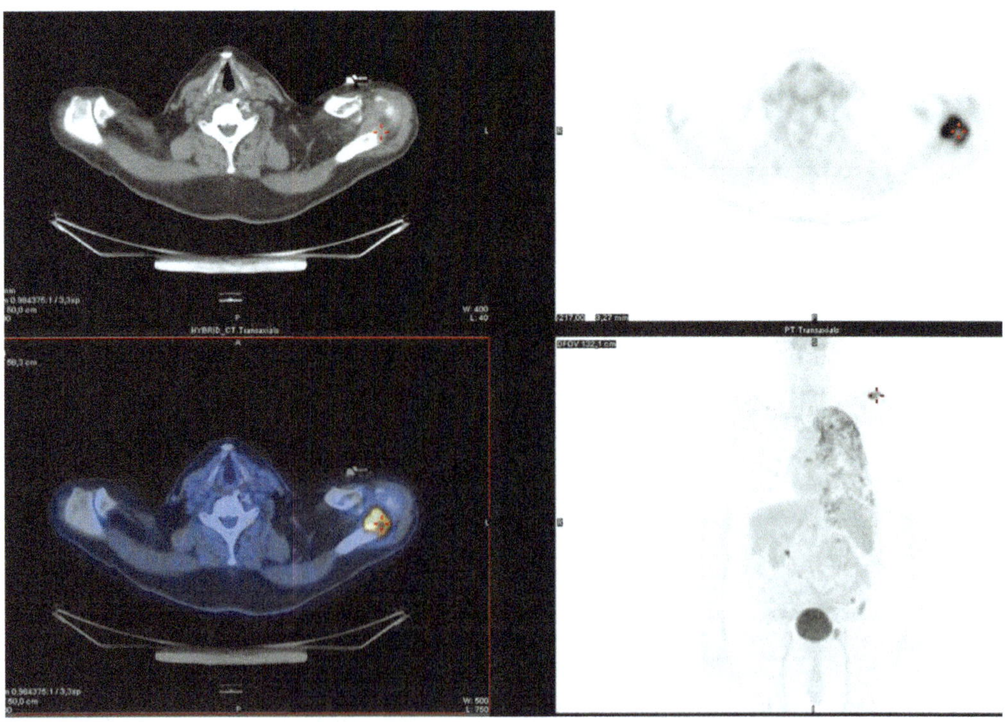

Fig. 11.5 PET/CT is useful in detecting distant occult metastases. In this patient we observe an occult metastasis located on the acromion of the left scapula

11.5 Prognosis

Patients risk stratification is essential for treatment management: ^{18}F-FDG PET-CT may be able to differentiate patients with different prognosis, avoiding aggressive treatments in cases with a bad prognosis.

A study by Lee et al. founds that the SUVmax value of the primary lesions was higher in patients with metastatic disease compared to patients without metastases. Therefore, SUVmax values could explain the aggressiveness of the disease. Instead, between the different histologic subtypes of the tumour, they didn't find any correlation with SUVmax. As a result, SUVmax values have a reliable correlation with surgical staging but not with histological grade [18].

Furthermore, several studies demonstrated that MTV (metabolic tumour volume) and TLG (total lesion glycolysis on pre-treatment imaging, could be useful prognostic biomarkers and good predictors for tumour progression.

In particular, TLG could predict overall survival better than SUVmax and MTV. Indeed, SUVmax value is a single pixel value and could be incomplete in the characterization of MPM, which is a complex and heterogeneous tumour.

Instead, MTV and TLG are three-dimensional parameters that integrate total tumour volume and metabolic activity, allowing the description of the complexity of the entire lesion.

The method used for the calculation of volume-based parameters has yet to be recognized. Unfortunately, a univocal limit value or method can't be defined in order to be universally applicable. Consequently, clear guidelines for the determination of these parameters should be established [19, 20].

11.6 Metabolic Response to Chemotherapy

The diagnosis of MPM is frequently delayed and the majority of patients are not suitable for radical surgery and systemic chemotherapy is the standard management. In these cases, an adequate assessment of tumour response to therapy is required for early identification of non-responders patients.

For this purpose, modified RECIST criteria, based on CT measurements, are recently introduced and are considered the reference for MPM [21]. The mRECIST criteria have several pitfalls and are not effective in more than 25% of the cases [22]. They have a high grade of inter-observer variability. They were not designed on malignant pleural mesothelioma growth pattern and they don't consider the metabolic activity of the remaining malignant tissue [23].

FDG PET/CT is gradually becoming essential in assessment of tumour response in patients undergoing chemotherapy, and has been included in the European Organisation for Research and Treatment of Cancer (EORTC) recommendations. Metabolic imaging analysis permits the early identification of non-responders to chemotherapy, avoiding unsuccessful treatment, which are characterized by a large number of toxicities and a high mortality risk. Several studies suggest that an early reduction of FDG uptake after chemotherapy should predict metabolic response, which can be associated with patient outcome, in particular in patients not treated with talc pleurodesis (Fig. 11.6). Moreover, ^{18}F-FDG PET is an exhaustive imaging method for differentiating residual malignant tissue from therapy-induced fibrosis [22, 24].

A study by Zucali et al. recognizes SUV and TLG after two cycles of chemotherapy as markers for correlation with progression-free survival (PFS), suggesting their predictive role in response assessment in patients treated with first-line chemotherapy.

Reductions of $\geq$25% in SUV and $\geq$30% in TLG (ΔSUV $\geq$ 25% and ΔTLG $\geq$ 30%) might have a role in defining metabolic response [22]. The additional value of the assessment of metabolic response is essential, due to its ability to predict outcome in patients who appear with stable disease (SD) or partial response (PR) on CT scan [25].

When talc pleurodesis is performed, inflammatory tissue takes-up FDG and could mask the malignant residual tissue uptake, particularly in lesions with low baseline FDG-avidity. In these patients, neither ΔSUV nor ΔTLG

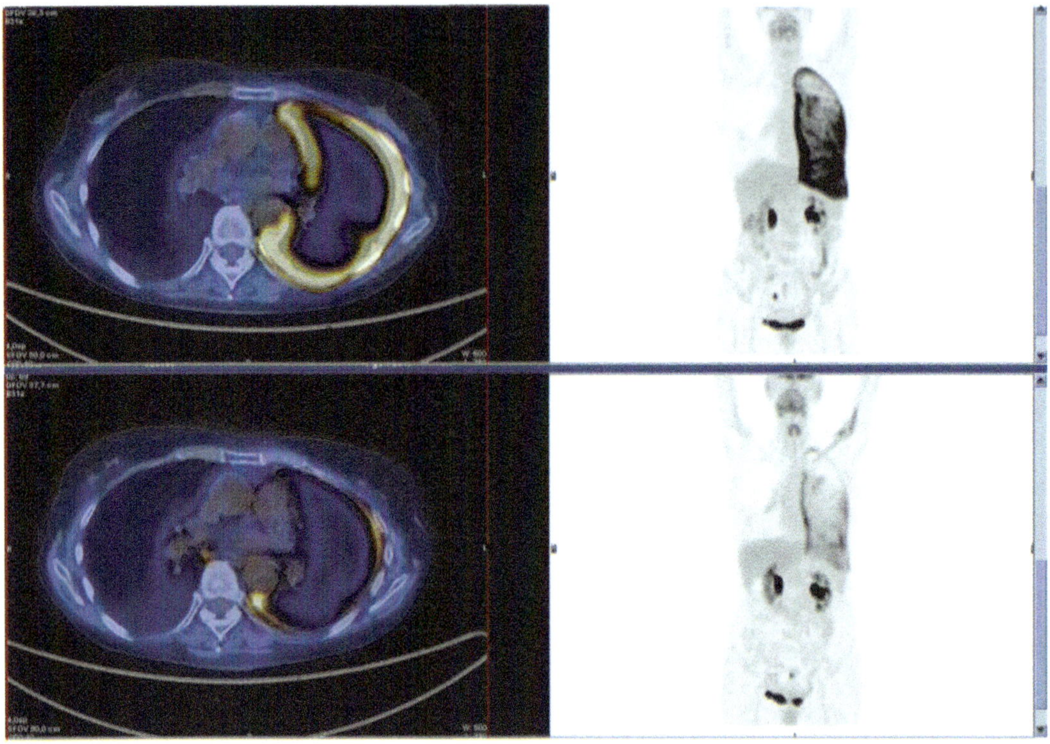

Fig. 11.6 [18]FDG PET/CT is valid in assessment of tumour response in patients undergoing chemotherapy. Upper panel shows imaging before chemotherapy. Lower panel shows significant reduction of activity after two cycles of therapy

showed a significant correlation with PFS or overall survival (OS).

In conclusion, in this study they confirm the importance of ΔSUV in clinical practice, whereas in clinical trials a combination of ΔSUV and ΔTLG could increase the association with PFS and could be more accurate in the assessment of both the parameters [26].

Kanemura et al. proposed a sequential algorithm for chemotherapy response assessment in patients affected by MPM. They suggest using mRECIST criteria in the first line for recognizing responders and stable disease patients and discriminating which patients need an additional metabolic response evaluation using PET/CT. This approach could optimize clinical efficacy and cost saving [22].

11.7 Conclusions

The complex growth pattern and the poor prognosis of MPM require an early diagnosis and accurate clinical staging. A comparative assessment of all the imaging modalities, such as CT, MR and PET/CT, is essential for patients risk stratification and for selecting patients who may benefit from multimodality treatment. ^{18}F-FDG PET-CT is gradually becoming essential in the diagnosis, non-invasive staging, therapy planning and follow-up of metabolic response to treatment.

References

1. Benamore RE, et al. Use of imaging in the management of malignant pleural mesothelioma. Clin Radiol. 2005;60:1237–47.
2. Wang ZJ, et al. Malignant pleural mesothelioma: evaluation with CT, MR imaging, and PET. Radiographics. 2004;24:105–19.
3. Blodgett TM, et al. PET/CT: form and function. Radiology. 2007;242(2):360–85.
4. Pinilla I, et al. Integrated [18]FDG PET/CT: utility and applications in clinical oncology. Clin Med Oncol. 2008;2:181–98.
5. Boellaard R, et al. FDG PET/CT: EANM procedure guidelines for tumor imaging: version 2.0. Eur J Nucl Med Mol Imaging. 2015;42:328–54.

6. Kinahan PE, et al. PET/CT standardized uptake values (SUVs) in clinical practice and assessing response to therapy. Semin Ultrasound CT MR. 2010;31:496–505.
7. Yildirim H, et al. Clinical value of fluorodeoxyglucose-positron emission tomography/computed tomography in differentiation of malignant mesothelioma from asbestos-related benign pleural disease: an observational pilot study. J Thorac Oncol. 2009;4(12):1480–4.
8. Terada T, et al. Clinical utility of 18-fluorodeoxyglucose positron emission tomography/computed tomography in malignant pleural mesothelioma. Exp Ther Med. 2012;4:197–200.
9. Sun Y, et al. The role of 18F-FDG PET/CT integrated imaging in distinguishing malignant from benign pleural effusion. PLoS One. 2016;11(8):e0161764.
10. Asad S, et al. False-positive FDG positron emission tomography uptake in nonmalignant chest abnormalities. Am J Roentgenol. 2004;182:983–9.
11. Rusch VW. A proposed new international TNM staging system for malignant pleural mesothelioma. From the international mesothelioma interest group. Chest. 1995;108(4):1122–8.
12. Patz EF Jr, et al. Malignant pleural mesothelioma: value of CT and MR imaging in predicting resectability. Am J Roentgenol. 1992;159:961–6.
13. Flores RM, et al. Positron emission tomography defines metastatic disease but not locoregional disease in patients with malignant pleural mesothelioma. J Thorac Cardiovasc Surg. 2003;126(1):11–6.
14. Frauenfelder T, et al. Use of computed tomography and positron emission tomography/computed tomography for staging of local extent in patients with malignant pleural mesothelioma. J Comput Assist Tomogr. 2014;39(2):160–5.
15. Erasmus JJ, et al. Integrated computed tomography-positron emission tomography in patients with potentially resectable malignant pleural mesothelioma: staging implications. J Thorac Cardiovasc Surg. 2005;129(6):1364–70.
16. Sørensen JB, et al. Preoperative staging of mesothelioma by 18F-fluoro-2-deoxy-D-glucose positron emission tomography/computed tomography fused imaging and mediastinoscopy compared to pathological findings after extrapleural pneumonectomy. Eur J Cardiothorac Surg. 2008;34:1090–6.
17. Schneider DB, et al. Positron emission tomography with F18-fluorodeoxyglucose in the staging and preoperative evaluation of malignant pleural mesothelioma. J Thorac Cardiovasc Surg. 2000;120(1):128–33.
18. Lee ST, et al. Prognostic value of 18F-FDG PET/CT in patients with malignant pleural mesothelioma. Mol Imaging Biol. 2009;11:473–9.
19. Kitajima K, et al. Prognostic value of pretreatment volume-based quantitative 18F-FDG PET/CT parameters in patients with malignant pleural mesothelioma. Eur J Radiol. 2017;86:176–83.
20. Lee HY, et al. Volume-based parameter of 18F-FDG PET/CT in malignant pleural mesothelioma: prediction of therapeutic response and prognostic implications. Ann Surg Oncol. 2017;17:2787–94.
21. Byrne MJ, et al. Modified RECIST criteria for assessment of response in malignant pleural mesothelioma. Ann Oncol. 2004;15:257–60.
22. Weber WA. Use of PET for monitoring cancer therapy and for predicting outcome. J Nucl Med. 2005;46:983–95.
23. Ceresoli GL, et al. Assessment of tumour response in malignant pleural mesothelioma. Cancer Treat Rev. 2007;33(6):533–41.
24. Kanemura S, et al. Metabolic response assessment with 18F-FDG-PET/CT is superior to modified RECIST for the evaluation of response to platinum-based doublet chemotherapy in malignant pleural mesothelioma. Eur J Radiol. 2017;86:92–8.
25. Lopci E, et al. Quantitative analyses at baseline and interim PET evaluation for response assessment and outcome definition in patients with malignant pleural mesothelioma. Eur J Nucl Med Mol Imaging. 2015;42:667–75.
26. Zucali PA, et al. Prognostic and predictive role of [18F]fluorodeoxyglucose positron emission tomography (FDG-PET) in patients with unresectable malignant pleural mesothelioma (MPM) treated with up-front pemetrexed-based chemotherapy. Cancer Med. 2017;6(10):2287–96.

12 Staging of Malignant Pleural Mesothelioma

Lawrence Okiror and Andrea Bille

12.1 Introduction

Malignant pleural mesothelioma (MPM) is a rare primary malignancy of the pleura. There is no known cure and prognosis is poor. Median overall survival is less than 12 months and the majority of patients are offered palliative chemotherapy and pleurodesis to manage the commonly associated pleural effusions. The disease is associated with exposure to asbestos with a latency period of two to four decades.

There have been considerable advances in understanding the aetiological mechanisms underpinning MPM, developing novel biomarkers for detecting the disease and conducting innovative clinical trials in recent years. However, these have so far not translated into significant improvement in survival reflecting the heterogeneous nature of the disease with varying clinical courses.

Unlike many solid cancers, in which tumour stage is the most important prognostic factor, the assessment of the extent of tumour in MPM presents unique difficulties in accurate staging due to the anatomical nature of the tumour. Tumour growth of MPM in the pleural cavity proceeds as a rind of uneven thickness making measurement difficult. Tools to assess and quantify this tumour bulk are not readily available. It is important to assess tumour bulk as this has been shown to have prognostic importance [1–3].

The pattern of lymphatic drainage of the pleura is complex and is significantly different from drainage pathways of the lung [4, 5]. Accurate lymph node staging in MPM is crucial as the presence of lymph node metastases adversely affects outcome [6, 7].

The initial evaluation of suspected MPM often involves clinical findings of a pleural effusion. Thoracentesis and cytological analysis may sometimes yield the diagnosis of MPM but a pleural biopsy is required in the majority of cases for accurate diagnosis and histologic subtyping. Pleural biopsy by thoracoscopy is the guideline-recommended method of diagnosis [8]. Thoracoscopy allows an excellent inspection of the pleural space and aids in staging, particularly in patients being considered for surgical resection as part of multimodality treatment as well as enabling multiple biopsies for histologic examination.

Historically, early MPM staging systems were developed from, single-institutional datasets with limited external validation and mainly derived from retrospective surgical series [9–11].

L. Okiror
Department of Thoracic Surgery, Guy's and St Thomas' Hospitals, London, UK
e-mail: l.okiror@doctors.org.uk

A. Bille (✉)
Division of Cancer Studies, King's College London, London, UK
e-mail: andrea.bille@gstt.nhs.uk

G. L. Ceresoli et al. (eds.), *Mesothelioma*, https://doi.org/10.1007/978-3-030-16884-1_12

Butchart published the first classification for mesothelioma. The system was simple but failed to provide any prognostic information as any tumour higher than stage I was considered unresectable. The Butchart mesothelioma staging system had four stages:

- Stage I: tumour confined to the parietal pleura
- Stage II: invasion of the chest wall, oesophagus, heart and contralateral pleura with or without thoracic lymph node involvement
- Stage III invasion of the diaphragm or extra-thoracic lymph nodes
- Stage IV: distant metastases

This system is no longer used, but helped to develop the staging systems currently used.

More recently, the widely adopted TNM staging system proposed by the International Mesothelioma Interest Group (IMIG) after a meeting in 1994 at which data were presented from large retrospective series and clinical trials was incorporated into the sixth edition of the Union for International Cancer Control (UICC) and the American Joint Committee on Cancer (AJCC) staging manuals [12]. The current TNM staging system was established by the International Association for the Study of Lung Cancer (IASLC) and IMIG derived from an international database that was geographically representative and included patients with MPM irrespective of treatment, pathological subtype and stage (Table 12.1). This staging system has been adopted by the UICC and AJCC for their eighth edition staging manuals.

The eighth edition TNM staging system for MPM is based on cross-sectional imaging, surgical and pathological variables. Contrast-enhanced computed tomography (CT) is the primary imaging modality for evaluation of MPM with approximation of tumour size and bulk taken from three single linear measurements

Table 12.1 Eighth edition of the TNM classification for malignant pleural mesothelioma as proposed by IASLC/IMIG and adopted by UICC/AJCC

T1	Tumour which involves the ipsilateral parietal or visceral pleura only
T2	Tumour which involves the ipsilateral pleura (parietal or visceral pleura) with invasion of at least one of the following: – Diaphragmatic muscle – Lung parenchyma
T3	Tumour which involves the ipsilateral pleura (parietal or visceral pleura) with invasion of at least one of the following: – Endothoracic fascia – Mediastinal fat – Chest wall, with or without associated rib destruction (solitary, resectable) – Pericardium (non-transmural invasion)
T4	Tumour which involves the ipsilateral pleura (parietal or visceral pleura) with invasion of at least one of the following: – Chest wall, with or without associated rib destruction (diffuse or multifocal, unresectable) – Peritoneum (direct transdiaphragmatic extension) – Contralateral pleura – Mediastinal organs (oesophagus, trachea, heart, great vessels) – Vertebrae, neuroforamen, spinal cord or brachial plexus – Pericardium (transmural invasion with or without pericardial effusion)
NX	Regional lymph nodes cannot be assessed
N0	No regional lymph-node metastases
N1	Metastases to ipsilateral intrathoracic lymph nodes (including ipsilateral bronchopulmonary, hilar, subcarinal, paratracheal, aortopulmonary, paraesophageal, peridiaphragmatic, pericardial, intercostals and internal mammary nodes)
N2	Metastases to contralateral intrathoracic lymph nodes, metastases to ipsilateral or contralateral supraclavicular lymph nodes
M0	No distant metastasis
M1	Distant metastases present

using axial CT images [3]. Magnetic resonance imaging (MRI), though not routinely used for evaluation of MPM can be used to provide additional staging information in specific clinical settings such as assessing the extent of invasion of the chest wall, mediastinum and diaphragm [13]. Integrated fluorodeoxy-D-glucose (FDG) positron emission tomography with CT (FDG-PET-CT) provides additional functional imaging which is useful for staging and is now extensively used for mesothelioma staging [14]. The addition of quantitative FDG-PET-CT parameters to clinical variables may provide additional prognostic information particularly in patients with non-sarcomatoid histology [2, 15, 16].

Additional invasive staging techniques such as mediastinoscopy, thoracoscopy and laparoscopy may be applied in selected cases of mesothelioma, particularly in patients for whom radical treatment including surgery as part of multimodality treatment is planned.

12.2 TNM Classification

There have been several systems proposed and used for staging MPM over the years. These were mainly based on data from small retrospective, single-institution surgical series. In 1994 the IASLC and IMIG proposed a TNM-based staging system developed from multiple surgical databases and this was adopted by the UICC and AJCC for their sixth edition manuals [12]. This was subsequently updated in 2009 (seventh edition). Criticism of this staging system has centred on its limited derivation cohort as well as concerns regarding the validity of lymph node descriptors [17]. The current eighth edition staging system was published in 2016 by the IASLC and IMIG and derived from an international database of over 3500 cases [3, 4, 18]. The complete dataset merged cases of clinical and postsurgical pathological stages to obtain the best TNM classification. Analysis of known prognostic variables was performed and included parameters such as tumour stage, histological subtype, sex, age and type of surgery (curative vs. palliative) which all had a statistically significant impact on overall survival. There was no statistically significant discrimination of overall survival between patients with ipsilateral parietal pleural involvement (T1a) versus those with ipsilateral visceral pleural involvement (T1b) on either clinical or pathological staging. Based on this the new eighth edition staging system merged this into a single T1 category (Table 12.1).

In the eighth edition, T1 was assigned when involvement of the parietal pleura with or without involvement of the visceral pleura is detected. T2 category was mainly assigned when lung parenchyma or fissure were involved. T3 is assigned for pericardial invasion followed by chest wall invasion. Description of T3 due to mediastinal fat invasion without pericardial invasion was less common. T4 is assigned for diffuse chest wall involvement, on diaphragmatic involvement or transmural pericardial involvement (Table 12.1).

The upstaging from clinical T1, T2 and T3 to higher pathological T stage was 56%, 54% and 39%, respectively, and the downstaging was reported in only 4% of cases.

The lymph nodal categories in the previous mesothelioma staging system were adopted from the lung cancer lymph nodal map with very little mesothelioma-specific evidence. This is problematic because of the varied lymphatic drainage pathways of the pleura and lung parenchyma. Subsequent to this some retrospective series have failed to demonstrate a prognostic difference between patients with pathologic N1 and those with pN2 disease [5]. For the eighth edition staging, clinically and pathologically staged patients were grouped together. There was a significant survival difference between patients with N0 vs. those with combined N1 and N2 metastases but not between N1 and N2. As there was no significant survival difference for patients with N1 vs. those with N2 metastases, these were grouped together into one single new N1 category. Patients with contralateral lymph node metastases (N3) are now classified as N2. Exploratory analysis of further parameters, such as pleural thickness, presence of N2 skip metastases, number of involved nodes, node ratio and distribution (upper vs. lower mediastinal vs. non-mediastinal), and site and number of distant

Table 12.2 Stage groupings of the eighth edition TNM classification for malignant pleural mesothelioma as proposed by IASLC/IMIG and adopted by UICC/AJCC

Stage	T	N	M
IA	T1	N0	M0
IB	T2, T3	N0	M0
II	T1, T2	N1	M0
IIIA	T3	N1	M0
IIIB	T1–T3	N2	M0
	T4	N0–N2	M0
IV	Any T4	Any N	M1

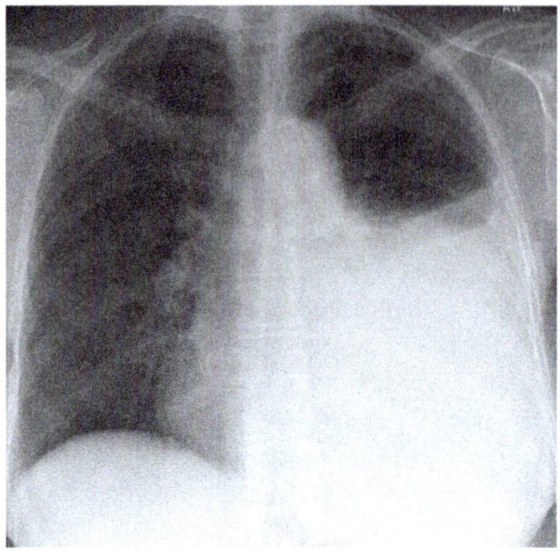

Fig. 12.1 Chest X ray shows left sided malignant pleural effusion

metastases was performed, but the number of patients included in each group was too small to derive any definitive conclusions.

Changes to the stage groupings reflect differences in overall survival hence stage IV only contains patients with metastatic disease (M1) with T4 and N3, M0 which were previously considered as stage IV now reverting to stage IIIB (Table 12.2) [18].

12.3 Radiological Imaging

The radiographic features of MPM are variable and related to the stage of the malignancy at diagnosis. Pleural effusions, pleural thickening, ipsilateral contracted chest with volume loss, lymphadenopathy, local invasion or metastases are the commonest radiological findings of MPM. Ipsilateral or contralateral pleural plaques may be seen as evidence of previous exposure to asbestos.

Chest radiography is usually the first imaging modality performed and the commonest feature of MPM on chest radiography is a unilateral pleural effusion in up to 80% of cases (Fig. 12.1) [19, 20]. Pleural thickening with ipsilateral volume loss can be seen on chest radiography. Lobulated masses with progression to a confluent rind and subsequent encasement of the lung may have the appearance of a large pleural effusion on the radiograph.

Contrast-enhanced chest CT with the upper abdomen is the imaging modality of choice for evaluation of the primary tumour and initial staging as recommended by current guidelines (Fig. 12.2) [21]. It defines the primary tumour, local invasion, intrathoracic lymphadenopathy and extrathoracic spread. A unilateral pleural effusion will be seen in three quarters of cases (Fig. 12.2a) [17]. Calcified pleural plaques which relate to previous exposure to asbestos are observed in approximately 20% of cases and should not be mistaken for osteocartilagenous differentiation (Fig. 12.2b) [17]. Diffuse pleural thickening particularly of the mediastinal pleura or diffuse pleural thickening of more than 1 cm particularly in the setting of prior exposure to asbestos is nearly diagnostic of MPM (Fig. 12.2c) [20]. Extension into the mediastinal fat will manifest in loss of tissue planes in the mediastinal structures. Encasement of >50% of the circumference trachea or oesophagus usually indicates invasion of these structures [22]. Pericardial involvement will manifest in thickening, nodules, pericardial masses, pericardial effusion or invasion. Invasion of the chest wall may be partial or transmural. There will be a loss of extrapleural fat planes, invasion of the intercostal muscles and cortical reaction or destruction of the ribs (Fig. 12.2d). Transmural invasion of the chest wall manifests as extension into the chest wall muscles with distortion of these planes. Transdiaphragmatic extension of MPM may not be well characterised by CT and MRI provides

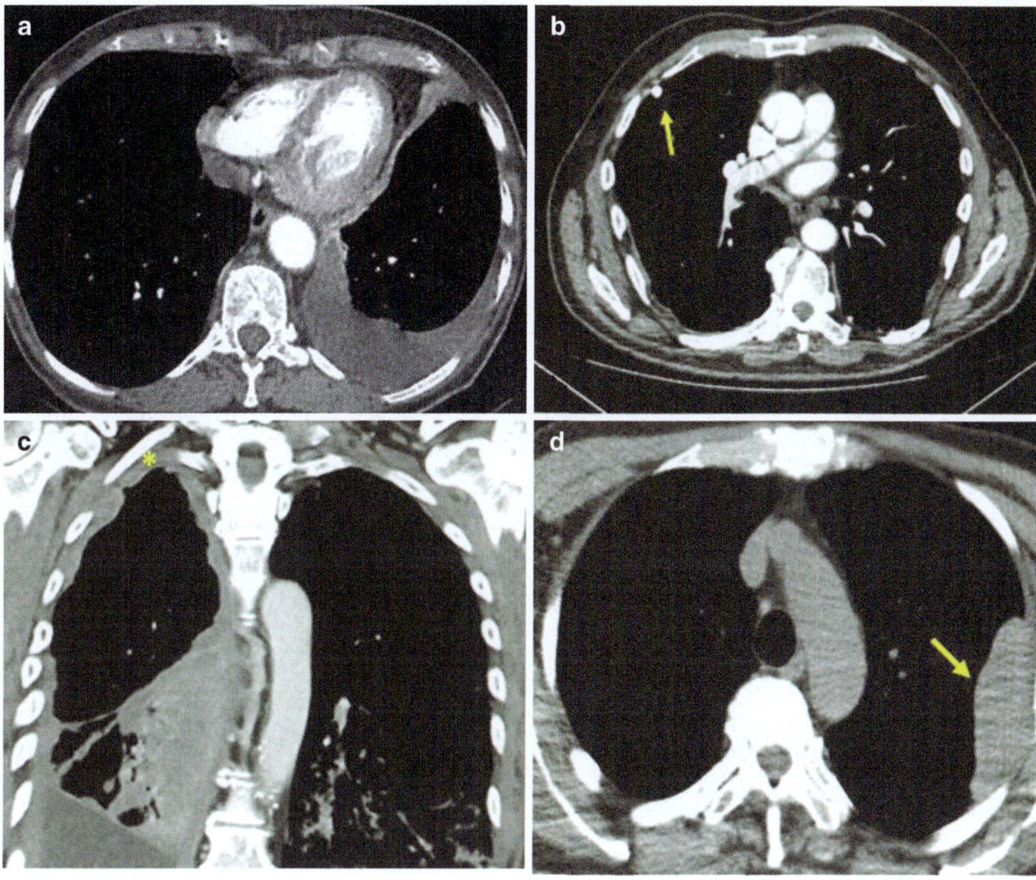

Fig. 12.2 (**a**) CT shows left sided pleural effusion. (**b**) CT shows minimal pleural thickening and pleural plaques (arrow). (**c**) CT shows extensive involvement of parietal and visceral pleura. (**d**) CT shows direct invasion in the chest wall, T4 tumour

additional information in this regard. Loss of the tissue planes on the inferior surface of the diaphragm with indentation of the liver or spleen is suggestive of invasion of the diaphragm.

Contrast-enhanced CT is the primary modality for detecting intrathoracic lymph nodal involvement with MPM. In addition to mediastinal lymph nodes, internal mammary, retrocrural and extrathoracic lymph nodes that are greater than 10 mm in diameter on short axis are considered abnormal.

Thoracic MRI is sensitive in defining chest wall, mediastinal and diaphragmatic invasion. This additional information is particularly important for patient being considered for surgical resection. A more detailed discussion on the role of MRI can be found in Chap. 9.

Functional imaging with FDG-PET-CT has been included in the preoperative staging, and some semiquantitative PET parameters have been incorporated, like the Standardized Uptake Value (SUV), as prognostic factors (Fig. 12.3a, b) [2, 14]. The superiority of PET in diagnosing malignant pleural disease is significant compared to the CT scan alone [13]. Gerbaudo et al. reported an overall accuracy of 94% (sensitivity 97%, specificity 80%) [23]. FDG-PET-CT is less accurate in detecting mediastinal lymph node involvement [24, 25] and diaphragmatic involvement (Fig. 12.3c, d).

FDG-PET-CT should be always performed before considering radical treatment options in patients with mesothelioma. Ideally it should be performed before the talc pleurodesis to reduce the risk of false positive finding.

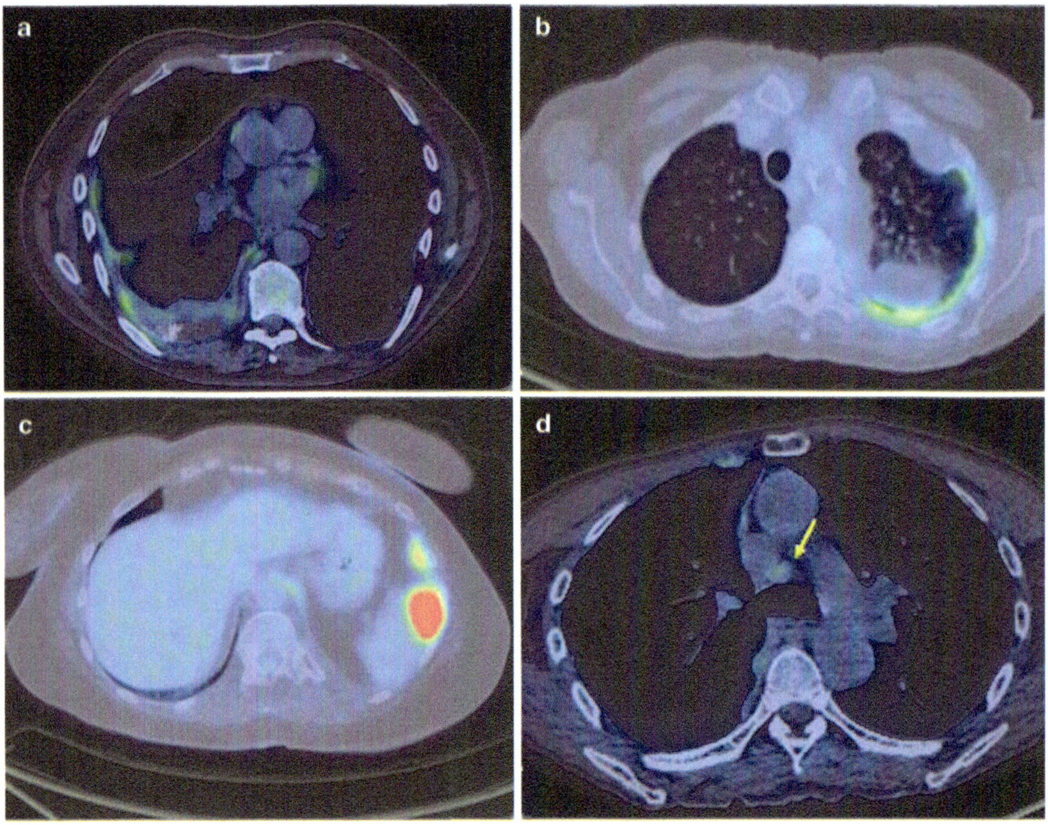

Fig. 12.3 (**a**) PET shows a cT1 tumour extension. (**b**) PET shows a tumour involving the parietal pleura and the endo thoracic fascia. (**c**) Tumour invading the diaphragm into the peritoneum, cT4. (**d**) PET shows positive para tracheal lymph node, cN1 according to eighth TNM staging

12.4 Video-Assisted Thoracoscopy

The video-assisted thoracoscopy provides a diagnosis differentiating the different subtypes of mesothelioma, but also it allows a detailed and direct assessment of the involvement of the pleural surfaces and the volume of disease. As originally reported by Boutin et al. [26] thoracoscopic features may also have a prognostic impact: extensions of disease (localized vs. diffuse) and involvement of the visceral pleura. Video-assisted thoracoscopy is recommended to assess the extension of disease and should be performed before considering a multimodality radical approach.

12.5 Endobronchial Biopsy and Video-Mediastinoscopy

Patients with pathological N1 or N2 disease have a worse prognosis compared to pN0 [4]. EBUS (endo bronchial ultrasound biopsy) and video mediastinoscopy are the most accurate staging procedures to detect mediastinal lymph node involvement. In 30% of cases mediastinal involvement can be not assessed correctly by CT or PET alone [27]. In patients with lymph node with a diameter more than 10 mm or positive on PET EBUS or video mediastinoscopy are recommended as preoperative staging in a multimodality treatment setting.

12.6 Laparoscopy

The role of laparoscopy in staging MPM is limited to selective cases in whom transdiaphragmatic involvement or peritoneal spread needs to be ruled out. This is usually in cases being considered for radical resection as part of multimodality treatment. Despite combining CT, PET and MRI, transdiaphragmatic or peritoneal involvement can be not diagnosed in up to 10% of cases (Fig. 12.3c) [28, 29].

Laparoscopy is recommended in only selected cases when therapeutic management may change depending on laparoscopic findings.

12.7 Conclusion

Clinical staging and accurate prognosis of MPM remain difficult. The latest staging scheme derives patients from a larger database drawn from a wider international pool of patients which enables a more uniform approach to benchmarking and comparison of outcomes. Histological subtype remains an important prognostic factor. There are limitations to the accuracy of imaging and with limited effective therapeutic options, outcomes from MPM are likely to remain poor. Identification of novel biomarkers and incorporation of these into staging algorithms remain a distant prospect.

References

1. Pass HI, Temeck BK, Kranda K, et al. Preoperative tumor volume is associated with outcome in malignant pleural mesothelioma. J Thorac Cardiovasc Surg. 1998;115:310–7.
2. Nowak AK, Francis RJ, Phillips MJ, et al. A novel prognostic model for malignant mesothelioma incorporating quantitative FDG-PET imaging with clinical parameters. Clin Cancer Res. 2010;16:2409–17.
3. Nowak AK, Chansky K, Rice DC, et al. The IASLC mesothelioma staging project: proposals for revisions of the T descriptors in the forthcoming eighth edition of the TNM classification for pleural mesothelioma. J Thorac Oncol. 2016;11:2089–99.
4. Rice D, Chansky K, Nowak A, Pass H, Kindler H, Shemanski L, Opitz I, Call S, Hasegawa S, Kernstine K, Atinkaya C, Rea F, Nafteux P, Rusch VW. Mesothelioma domain of the IASLC staging and prognostic factors committee, advisory boards and participating institutions. The IASLC mesothelioma staging project: proposals for revisions of the N descriptors in the forthcoming eighth edition of the TNM classification for pleural mesothelioma. J Thorac Oncol. 2016;11:2100–11.
5. Hallifax RJ, Rahman NM. Pleural embryology and gross structure, circulation, lymphatics, and nerves. In: Light RW, Gary Lee YC, editors. Textbook of pleural diseases. 3rd ed. Boca Raton: CRC Press; 2016.
6. Rusch VW, Venkatraman ES. Important prognostic factors in patients with malignant pleural mesothelioma, managed surgically. Ann Thorac Surg. 1999;68:1799–804.
7. Sugarbaker DJ, Flores RM, Jaklitsch MT, et al. Resection margins, extrapleural nodal status, and cell type determine postoperative long-term survival in trimodality therapy of malignant pleural mesothelioma: results in 183 patients. J Thorac Cardiovasc Surg. 1999;117:54–63.
8. Baas P, Fennell D, Kerr KM, Van Schil PE, Haas RL, Peters S. Malignant pleural mesothelioma: ESMO clinical practice guidelines for diagnosis, treatment and follow-up. Ann Oncol. 2015;26(Suppl 5):v31–9.
9. Butchart EG, Ashcroft T, Barnsley WC, et al. Pleuropneumonectomy in the management of diffuse malignant mesothelioma of the pleura. Experience with 29 patients. Thorax. 1976;31:15–24.
10. Sugarbaker DJ, Strauss GM, Lynch TJ, et al. Node status has prognostic significance in the multimodality therapy of diffuse, malignant mesothelioma. J Clin Oncol. 1993;11:1172–8.
11. Chahinian AP. Therapeutic modalities in malignant pleural mesothelioma. In: Chretien J, Hirsch A, editors. Diseases of the pleura. New York: Masson; 1983. p. 224–36.
12. Rusch VW. A proposed new international TNM staging system for malignant pleural mesothelioma from the international mesothelioma interest group. Lung Cancer. 1996;14:1–12.
13. Truong MT, Viswanathan C, Godoy MB, Carter BW, Marom EM. Malignant pleural mesothelioma: role of CT, MRI, and PET/CT in staging evaluation and treatment considerations. Semin Roentgenol. 2013;48:323–34.
14. Kitajima K, Doi H, Kuribayashi K. Present and future roles of FDG-PET/CT imaging in the management of malignant pleural mesothelioma. Jpn J Radiol. 2016;34:537–47.
15. Sharif S, Zahid I, Routledge T, Scarci M. Does positron emission tomography offer prognostic information in malignant pleural mesothelioma? Interact Cardiovasc Thorac Surg. 2011;12(5):806–11.

16. Bille A, Chicklore S, Okiror L, Cook GJ, Spicer J, Landau D, Lang-Lazdunski L. Patterns of disease progression on 18F-fluorodeoxyglucose positron emission tomography-computed tomography in patients with malignant pleural mesothelioma undergoing multimodality therapy with pleurectomy/decortication. Nucl Med Commun. 2013;34(11):1075–83.
17. Bonomi M, De Filippis C, Lopci E, Gianoncelli L, Rizzardi G, Cerchiaro E, Bortolotti L, Zanello A, Ceresoli GL. Clinical staging of malignant pleural mesothelioma: current perspectives. Lung Cancer (Auckl). 2017;8:127–39.
18. Rusch VW, Chansky K, Kindler HL, Nowak AK, Pass HI, Rice DC, Shemanski L, Galateau-Sallé F, BC MC, Nakano T, Ruffini E, van Meerbeeck JP, Yoshimura M. The IASLC mesothelioma staging project: proposals for the M descriptors and for revision of the TNM stage groupings in the forthcoming (eighth) edition of the TNM classification for mesothelioma. J Thorac Oncol. 2016;11(12):2112–9.
19. Wechsler RJ, Rao VM, Steiner RM. The radiology of thoracic malignant mesothelioma. Crit Rev Diagn Imaging. 1984;20(4):283–310.
20. Nickell LT Jr, Lichtenberger JP 3rd, Khorashadi L, Abbott GF, Carter BW. Multimodality imaging for characterization, classification, and staging of malignant pleural mesothelioma. Radiographics. 2014;34(6):1692–706.
21. Kindler HL, Ismaila N, Armato SG 3rd, Bueno R, Hesdorffer M, Jahan T, Jones CM, Miettinen M, Pass H, Rimner A, Rusch V, Sterman D, Thomas A, Hassan R. Treatment of malignant pleural mesothelioma: American society of clinical oncology clinical practice guideline. J Clin Oncol. 2018;36(13):1343–73.
22. Patz EF Jr, Shaffer K, Piwnica-Worms DR, et al. Malignant pleural mesothelioma: value of CT and MR imaging in predicting resectability. AJR Am J Roentgenol. 1992;159:961–6.
23. Gerbaudo VH, Sugarbaker DJ, Britz-Cunningham S, Di Carli MF, Mauceri C, Treves ST. Assessment of malignant pleural mesothelioma with 18F-FDG dual-head gamma-camera coincidence imaging: comparison with histopathology. J Nucl Med. 2002;9:1144–9.
24. Flores R. The role of PET in the surgical management of malignant pleural mesothelioma. Lung Cancer. 2005;7:S27–32.
25. Erasmus JJ, Truong MT, Smythe WR, et al. Integrated computed-tomography in patients with potentially resectable malignant pleural mesothelioma: staging implications. J Thorac Cardiovasc Surg. 2005;6:1364–70.
26. Boutin C, Rey F, Gouvernet J, Viallat JR, Astoul P, Ledoray V. Thoracoscopy in pleural malignant mesothelioma: a prospective study of 188 consecutive patients. Part 2: prognosis and staging. Cancer. 1993;72(2):394–404.
27. Sørensen JB, Ravn J, Loft A, et al. Preoperative staging of mesothelioma by 18F-fluoro-2-deoxy-D-glucose positron emission tomography/computed tomography fused imaging and mediastinoscopy compared to pathological findings after extrapleural pneumonectomy. Eur J Cardiothorac Surg. 2008;34:1090–6.
28. Rice DC, Erasmus JJ, Stevens CW, et al. Extended surgical staging for potentially resectable malignant pleural mesothelioma. Ann Thorac Surg. 2005;80:1988–92; discussion 1992–3.
29. Wald O, Groth SS, Burt BM, Sugarbaker DJ. Role of thoracoscopy, mediastinoscopy and laparoscopy in the diagnosis and staging of malignant pleural mesothelioma. J Vis Surg. 2016;2:129.

Surgery and Multimodality Treatment in Malignant Pleural Mesothelioma

13

Federico Rea, Eleonora Faccioli, and Giuseppe Marulli

13.1 Introduction

Malignant pleural mesothelioma (MPM) is an aggressive asbestos-related tumor arising from the pleural mesothelium. The incidence of this cancer in Europe is about 20 per million but a peak incidence around 2020 is expected because it is known that there is a 20–30 years' latency between asbestos exposure and disease development [1]. The reported median overall survival (OS) from diagnosis is 9–12 months, ranging from 8 months in stage IV to 40 months in stage I disease [2]. At early stages (I and II stage according to International Mesothelioma Interest Group—IMIG), when the disease is confined to the ipsilateral hemithorax, a multidisciplinary therapeutic approach with curative intent seems indicated with the aim to improve survival and quality of life. In advanced stages, where metastases in contralateral hemithorax or in distant sites are common, palliative or supportive care treatments are the first choice. Therapeutic approaches for MPM are still under debate, without a homogeneous consensus on this topic and the modern approach seems oriented to evaluate every single case in a multidisciplinary team to set the best therapy according to patients' performance status and stage of the disease.

F. Rea (✉) · E. Faccioli · G. Marulli
Thoracic Surgery Unit, Department of Cardiologic, Thoracic and Vascular Sciences, University of Padova, Padova, Italy
e-mail: federico.rea@unipd.it

The role of surgery is important in diagnosis, treatment, and staging of MPM. Because of the diffuse growth pattern and the lack of surgical margins, microscopic complete resection is theoretically impossible. Thus, a macroscopic complete resection (MCR) should be the overall aim of the resection, even though the optimal cytoreductive procedure is still controversial [3, 4].

The standard strategies for multimodality therapies are not well established, yet and the role of surgery in treatment of MPM is still unclear; many surgeons think that the goal of every surgical procedure is to leave the patient in state of no evidence of disease to improve long term outcomes [5].

There are two main surgical options to obtain MCR: pleurectomy/decortication (P/D) and extrapleural pneumonectomy (EPP); the superiority of one technique over the other is still debated and the decision to perform one or the other in multimodality approaches is based on surgeons' preference more than on robust scientific data [6].

Both surgical procedures are burdened by high morbidity, so they should be performed only in centers with a large experience in thoracic surgery [7].

Surgery often allows to obtain only cytoreduction so it must be inserted into a multimodal treatment associated with induction chemotherapy (iCT) or adjuvant chemotherapy (aCT) with or without adjuvant radiotherapy (aRT) in order

G. L. Ceresoli et al. (eds.), *Mesothelioma*, https://doi.org/10.1007/978-3-030-16884-1_13

to achieve better outcomes in term of survival and control of disease.

The best combination of these different therapeutic approaches is still matter of debate.

13.2 Surgery for MPM

13.2.1 Surgical Indications

Stage I–II MPM in patients with epithelial histotype and good performance status represents the best indication for surgery.

Sarcomatoid subtype being associated with a poor prognosis and with advanced stages of disease is a contraindication for surgery [8]. N2 disease is not an absolute contraindication in MPM as it should be considered more as "local" nodes not significantly influencing the prognosis as recently demonstrated by the results of the International Mesothelioma Interest Group (IMIG) and the International Association for the Study of Lung Cancer (IASLC) [8].

Before surgery, it is recommended to have a diagnosis not only based on cytology, because of high risk of diagnostic error, but also on tissue confirmation by pleural biopsy to allow immunohistochemical characterization to establish a certain diagnosis [9].

13.2.2 Surgical Procedures with Curative Intent

To obtain MCR the two main surgical options with curative intent are extrapleural pneumonectomy (EPP) and pleurectomy/decortication (P/D), both of them can be incorporated in multimodality regimens which include neoadjuvant or adjuvant chemotherapy and adjuvant radiotherapy.

The technique of EPP is well standardized, providing the en bloc resection of the parietal and visceral pleura, ipsilateral lung, pericardium, and hemidiaphragm [10]; it has been considered for many years the best procedure to obtain MCR and survival advantage [3].

P/D is a more limited procedure, first reported in 1975 [11] and not yet standardized in all centers; its definition has varied according to the surgical technique, therapeutic intent, and clinical indications [12]. Initially it was proposed as a cytoreductive alternative in patients who cannot tolerate EPP because it requires less cardiorespiratory reserve than EPP. In 2011, the consensus report by the International Mesothelioma Interest Group (IMIG) and the International Association for the Study of Lung Cancer (IASLC) recommended that surgical procedures for MPM should be classified into three categories: (1) extended PD (E/PD), (2) P/D, and (3) partial pleurectomy [13].

13.2.3 EPP

EPP involves en bloc resection of the visceral and parietal pleura, lung and, if necessary, ipsilateral hemidiaphragm, and pericardium (Figs. 13.1a, b and 13.2a, b). Removing the lung, it leads to a better local control of disease progression allowing the administration of a higher dose of radiotherapy without the risk of radiation pneumonitis.

This surgical technique was first reported in 1976 [14] and, since then, it has been performed as a treatment option for potentially resectable MPM.

Sugarbaker et al., in 1999, reported a 5-year survival rate of 46% and low mortality rate in patients who underwent EPP incorporated in multimodality regimens affected by epithelioid subtype and N0 disease [7].

After this report, there have been different subsequent series that have demonstrated a similar trend in median survival of 20–24 months [15, 16]. In a survey of opinions among 802 thoracic surgeons, EPP was believed to be more effective than P/D and the addition of adjuvant chemotherapy or other combinations of multimodality therapy were believed to increase the chance of cure. These beliefs were not markedly different between those who performed or did not perform each type of surgery [17].

In front of these survival advantages, EPP is burdened by several disadvantages: this surgical approach is highly debilitating for the patient with morbidity of almost 50% and mortality of 5% in centers with a large experience in the surgical management of MPM [16].

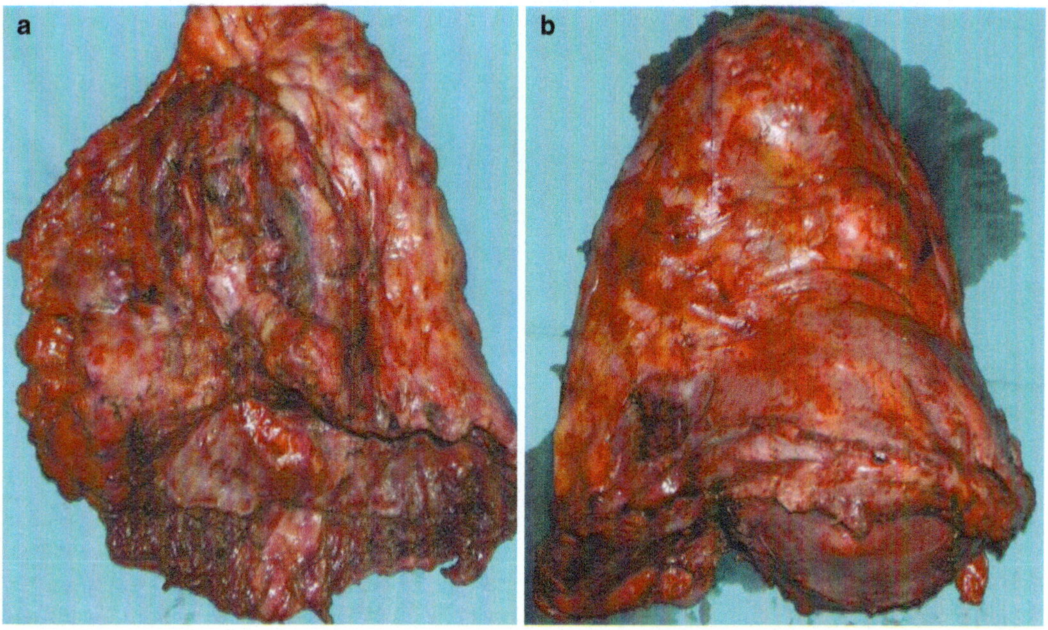

Fig. 13.1 (**a**, **b**) En bloc resection of lung, parietal, and visceral pleural after a right extrapleural pneumonectomy (EPP)

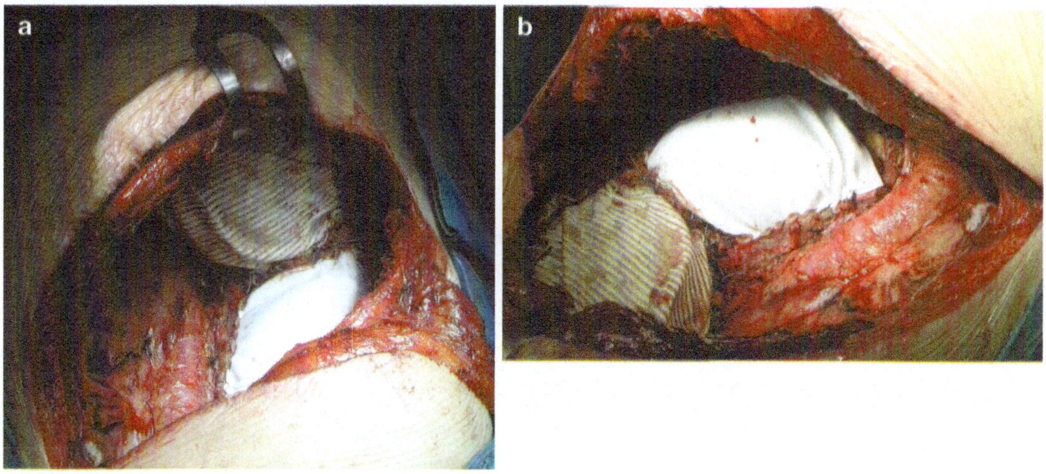

Fig. 13.2 (**a**, **b**) Resection and reconstruction with prosthesis of hemilateral pericardium and diaphragm after a right EPP

In particular, it is associated with a reduction in quality of life, a worsening of postoperative cardiorespiratory function, and difficulties in administration, tolerance, and compliance of adjuvant therapy.

The role of EPP in the treatment of MPM has been recently the subject of debate after the publication of the mesothelioma and radical surgery (MARS I). This is the largest randomized trial that compares EPP with no surgery in terms of survival and quality of life and concluded that "EPP within trimodal therapy offers no benefit and possibly harms patients" although the trial included only 16 patients in the EPP arm [18].

This trial, however, faced several problems in the enrolment of patients with few cases treated by few centers with a not acceptable high mortality rate in the EPP arm that finally conditioned the survival results.

13.2.4 P/D

P/D involves the total resection of both the parietal and visceral pleura, while the lung is spared (Fig. 13.3a, b). According to IMIG classification this surgical procedure includes:

- *Extended P/D*: parietal and visceral pleurectomy with the removal of the pericardium and/or diaphragm even though currently there is no evidence that their resection can provide a survival benefit.
- *P/D*: parietal and visceral pleurectomy without the resection of diaphragm or pericardium.
- *Partial pleurectomy*: the partial removal of the parietal and/or visceral pleura for diagnostic or palliative intent.

The first report of pleurectomy in the treatment of MPM was in 1975 by Martin et al., who described the outcome of parietal pleurectomy followed by external radiation and systemic chemotherapy in 14 patients with a median survival of 16 months [11]. This series was then extended the year later including 33 patients with MPM with a median survival of 21 months [19]. Since then, several nonrandomized studies have demonstrated the feasibility and safety of P/D with various multimodality schemes involving induction and adjuvant treatments [12, 20, 21].

P/D has some advantages compared to EPP: it preserves the ipsilateral lung parenchyma so it can be indicated in patient with a marginal cardiopulmonary reserve, making more feasible additional chemotherapy.

On the other hand, a potential disadvantage of P/D is the less cytoreductive capacity compared with EPP; in particular, the effectiveness and radicality of P/D in patients with advanced MPM is one of the main controversial points. Friedberg et al. [22] reported a MCR rate of 97% and a median survival of 21 months in their series of radical pleurectomy with intraoperative photodynamic therapy for advanced MPM. On the basis of that results, they theorized that MCR could be achieved with radical pleurectomy in all patients with MPM in whom MCR could be achieved with EPP.

In an editorial, Raja Flores [23] has pointed out the attention to a recent general shift in surgery for MPM from EPP to P/D after a comparative multicenter study by experienced mesothelioma surgeons failed to demonstrate significant survival differences between the two procedures [24]. He commented that the primary goal of surgery should not just be to obtain a MCR (R1) at the expense of pneumonectomy, but it should include the removal of as much tumor as possible while avoiding pneumonectomy, favoring lung

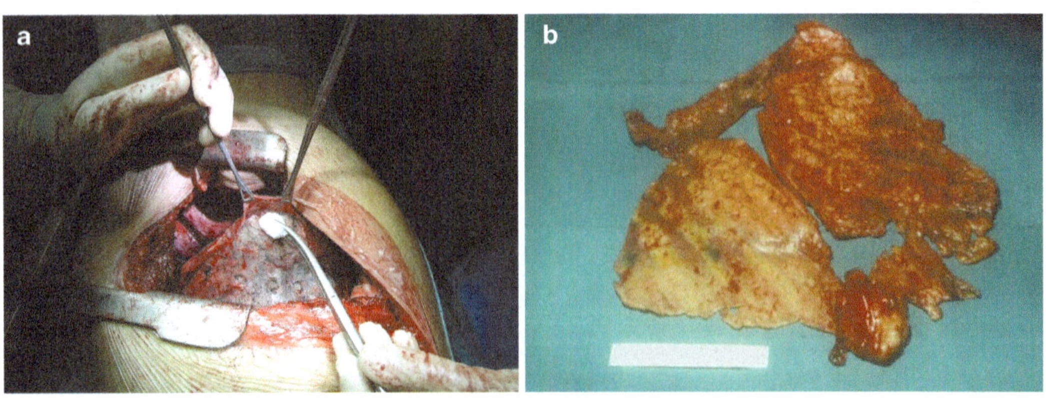

Fig. 13.3 (**a**) Pleurectomy-decortication (P/D, surgical technique). (**b**) Pathological specimen (visceral and parietal pleura) after P/D

reexpansion, prevention of fluid accumulation, and minimizing morbidity and mortality. On the basis of the currently available data the equation tips in favor of P/D rather than EPP.

13.2.5 EPP or P/D: Which One to Choose?

Many authors over the years have tried to give an answer to this question but the debate is still open.

It is a fact that the type of surgery depends on clinical factors and on individual surgical judgment and expertise [17]. The challenge is the selection of the right patient for the procedure included in a multidisciplinary setting, in order to guarantee the best benefits. Patients with histologically proven mesothelioma who would tolerate different treatment modalities including surgery should be considered for multimodal approach.

Regarding the outcomes in patients who underwent surgical procedures for MPM, the IASLC found that in patients with stage I disease, median survival time (MST) was significantly better in the EPP group than in the P/D group (40 vs. 23 months). No significant differences in survival were identified in the higher-stages patients [8].

On the other hand, some studies found that MST ranged from 13 to 29 months for P/D and from 12 to 22 months for EPP, with a trend that favored the P/D group with a lower mortality and morbidity rate [12].

Furthermore, there are increasing data in favor of P/D in terms of postoperative survival and quality of life and for all these reasons many centers are shifting their surgical approach for resectable MPM from EPP to P/D [25–27].

Some surgeons favor P/D as curative procedure in patients with minimal disease [28], others as palliative procedure in case of mediastinal structures (e.g., aorta and vertebral bodies) involvement found at thoracotomy [29].

The right surgical strategy must have the intention to achieve MCR selecting the less invasive surgical procedure so it should be initiated with the intention of performing P/D with the exception of some cases with extensive invasion of the pulmonary parenchyma.

Nevertheless, to date there are no randomized controlled trials comparing EPP with P/D, so it is still unclear which technique is better in terms of outcome or long-term survival; the type of surgery depends on clinical factors and on the expertise of individual surgeons.

13.3 Surgery and Multimodality Treatment in MPM

The past decade has seen several notable advances: effective chemotherapy regimens have been developed, various surgical approaches have been explored and refined, and various studies with multimodality therapy have been reported. Survival is clearly more promising with multimodality treatment, but the combination and timing of surgery, radiation, and chemotherapy have to be still established.

Some studies have shown that single-modality therapy [surgery or chemotherapy (CT) or radiotherapy (RT) or immunotherapy alone] did not result in advantages in term of disease free survival (DFS) or overall survival (OS) [30].

The most reasonable therapeutic approach for MPM, in the small percentage of eligible patients, is a combined treatment modality (surgery, CT, and RT) [6, 8].

The therapeutic possibilities and the specific approaches have changed enormously over time, leading the clinicians to explore new strategies and combinations of treatments.

Until the early 1920s, the cisplatin was identified as the best anticancer drug and it was routinely used in all CT regimens mainly in association with gemcitabine or doxorubicine.

This was based on the results of a meta-analysis published in 2002 [31] in which were reviewed some studies published between 1965 and 2001. This scenario has completely changed when, in 2003, a phase III study demonstrated that the combination of folate antagonists with cisplatin versus cisplatin alone in MPM led to a significantly prolonged median OS [32]. Since then, the combination of cisplatin plus pemetrexed has become the standard chemotherapeutic option also when a multidisciplinary approach is provided, both as induction or adjuvant treatment setting after surgery. Recently, new ongoing trials with biological agents are giving interesting results, with the hope to have an application in multimodality regimens in the next future [33].

As already said, surgery often allows to obtain only cytoreduction; for this reason, it must be inserted in a multimodality protocol composed by induction chemotherapy (iCT) or adjuvant chemotherapy (aCT) with/without adjuvant RT.

13.3.1 Induction Chemotherapy in a Trimodality Protocol

Chemotherapeutic regimens for MPM had some changes over the years. Berghmans et al. [31] has confirmed the efficacy of the cisplatin; the addition of the anthracyclines increases the response in the face of greater toxicity. The role of CT for this disease has completely changed with the introduction of new antimetabolites (raltitrexed and pemetrexed) that interact with the folate metabolism and lead to a real increase in survival, in particular in association with cisplatin. All these findings have led to establish that the new therapeutic standard in medical treatment of MPM is the association of pemetrexed and cisplatin [34].

iCT has some important advantages in MPM therapy: (a) it can be administered with full dosage because patients are not still "debilitated" by surgery, with a high compliance and completion of cycles rate; (b) it can lead to a downstaging of the disease, allowing to obtain a satisfactory MCR; (c) it allows for a better surgical selection based on the response to CT: a poor response to iCT may avoid an unnecessary surgical treatment; (d) a high dose of adjuvant RT, particularly after EPP may be delivered, avoiding the cumulative toxicity; (e) even though some chemotherapeutic agents may have cardiac or pulmonary toxicity, it has been reported an improvement in pulmonary function and exercise capacity after iCT [35].

On the other hand, iCT may be burdened with an increase in surgical morbidity and mortality, even if the majority of large studies have demonstrated similar mortality rates not influenced by preoperative treatments [16, 36–41].

Another potential disadvantage is the delay of surgical treatment that could negatively influence the resectability of the tumor (time from the end of CT and surgery should be 3–4 weeks).

MPM poor response rate to iCT in comparison to other tumors is documented by several studies, although occasionally a complete pathologic response has been reported [42].

The trimodality approach (iCT, plus surgery, plus aRT) has shown good results both in term of overall survival and disease free survival (DFS), superior to the results obtained in those studies in which bimodality approach was adopted.

The results of 20 studies, published between 2004 and 2015 considering the use of trimodality therapy are resumed and reported in Table 13.1.

In the most important studies OS, after trimodality treatment ranged from 8.8 months (for patients with nonepithelial histology who underwent EPP) [38] to 33.5 months [49]. Four prospective studies, in which the majority of patients were able to complete trimodality therapy on an intention to treat analysis, reported a median survival of 16.8–25.5 months [37, 45, 47, 51]. DFS ranged from 7.6 [18] to 44 months [44].

To conclude, the use of trimodality approach seems effective in prolonging survival; however, the completion of the full protocol is not easy and in those studies where intention to treat data have been reported, <50% of patients were able to complete the program [51].

13.3.2 Adjuvant Radiotherapy in a Bimodality Protocol

Adjuvant radiotherapy is administered mainly after EPP and less frequently after P/D. The most common technique reported was photons and electrons external beam radiation therapy (EBRT) with different doses or regimens.

The role of adjuvant RT with curative intent still remains unclear, even though good outcomes and reduction of local recurrence have been reported [55].

EBRT plays an important role both as adjuvant therapy or as first-line treatment in unresectable cases; in this case its aim is palliative in

Table 13.1 Studies reporting the use of induction chemotherapy in a setting of a multimodality treatment

Author	Year	Patients (*n*)	iCT regimen (*n*)	Surgery (*n*)	Adjuvant RT regimen (*n*)	IMIG stage (*n*)	Histology (*n*)	Overall survival				Disease free survival (months)	Recurrence rate (%)			
								Median (months)	1Y (%)	2Y (%)	5Y (%)		Local	L + D	Distant	Overall
Hasegawa et al. [43]	2015	42	Cis + Pem (42)	EPP (30)	54 Gy (19)	I/II (27) III (15)	Epithelial (28) Nonepithelial (14)	22.7 (EPP) 17.1 (no EPP) 27.3 (epithelial) 13.6 (nonepithelial)	NR NR NR NR	50 25 NR NR	NR NR NR NR	11	29.4	NR	35.2	64.7
De Perrot et al. [44]	2009	60	Cis + Vin (26) Cis + Pem (24) Cis + Ral (6) Cis + Gem (4)	EPP (45)	50 Gy + boost 10 Gy or 54 Gy (30)	NR	Epithelial (44) Nonepithelial (16)	14 (all) 18 (epithelial) 12 (nonepithelial)	65	18	10	NR	16.7	NR	36	53
Krug et al. [45]	2009	77	Cis + Pem (77)	EPP (57)	54 Gy (44)	I/II (39) III/IV (36) NR (2)	Epithelial (62) Nonepithelial (15)	16.8 (all) 29.1 (iCT + EPP + RT) 21.9 (iCT + EPP)	65.2 90 NR	37.2 61.2 NR	NR NR NR	10.1	14	5	21	40
Pasello et al. [46]	2012	51	Car + Pem (27) Cis + Pem (24)	EPP (36) P/D (5)	50.4 Gy (33) 21 Gy on surgical scars (3)	I/II (22) III (29)	Epithelial (38) Nonepithelial (13)	27.7 (epithelial) 11.7 (nonepithelial)	NR	NR	NR	15	NR	NR	NR	NR
Buduhan et al. [36]	2009	55	Cis/Car + Pem (24) Cis + Meth + Vin (23) Cis + Gem (5) Other (3)	EPP (46)	EBRT: 30 Gy + boost 9–18 Gy (24) IMRT: 50 Gy + boost 24 Gy (14)	I/II (13) III/IV (33) NR (9)	NR	24 (EPP) 25 (iCT + EPP + RT)	70	43	12	NR	18	24	21	63
Van Schil et al. [47]	2010	58	Cis + Pem (58)	EPP (42)	54 Gy (38)	NR	Epithelial (31) Nonepithelial (18) NR (9)	18.4 (all) 33 (iCT + EPP + RT)	70.2	NR	NR	13.9	16.2	NR	27	NR
Rea et al. [48]	2013	54	Cis + Pem (54)	EPP (41)	54–50.4 Gy (32)	I/II (21) III (33)	Epithelial (48) Nonepithelial (6)	15.5	59.2	NR	NR	8.6	20.4	NR	37	57.4

(continued)

Table 13.1 (continued)

Author	Year	Patients (*n*)	iCT regimen (*n*)	Surgery (*n*)	Adjuvant RT regimen (*n*)	IMIG stage (*n*)	Histology (*n*)	Overall survival				Disease free survival (months)	Recurrence rate (%)			
								Median (months)	1Y (%)	2Y (%)	5Y (%)		Local	L + D	Distant	Overall
Flores et al. [49]	2006	19	Cis + Gem (19)	EPP (8)	54 Gy (8)	III (13) IV (6)	Epithelial (14) Nonepithelial (5)	33.5 (EPP) 9.7 (unresectable)	NR	NR	NR	NR	0	NR	50	NR
Weder et al. [37]	2004	19	Cis + Gem (19)	EPP (16)	30 Gy + boost 20 Gy (6) 45–60 Gy (7)	NR	Epithelial (14) Nonepithelial (5)	23	79	37	NR	16.5	NR	NR	NR	92
Lang-Lazdunski et al. [38]	2012	76	Cis + Gem (11) Cis + Pem (14)	P/D (54) EPP (22)	54–45 Gy (17) 21 Gy on surgical scars (54)	I/II (23) III/IV (53)	Epithelial (50) Nonepithelial (26)	23 (EPP) 12.8 (P/D)	81.9 54.5	49 18.2	30 1	NR	52 (EPP)	NR	16	81
Okada et al. [39]	2008	65	Cis + Gem (5)	P/D (34) EPP (31)	54 Gy (9)	I/II (21) III/IV (44)	Epithelial (48) Nonepithelial (17)	13 (EPP) 17 (P/D)	57.5 59	42 30	NR 5	NR	NR	NR	NR	NR
Treasure et al. [18]	2011	50	Cis + Gem (10) Cis + Pem (8) Myt + Cis + Vin (6)	EPP (19)	54 Gy (8)	I/II (31) III (19)	Epithelial (40) Nonepithelial (10)	14.4 (EPP) 19.5 (no EPP)	52.2 73.1	NR NR	NR NR	7.6	NR	NR	NR	79
Weder et al. [16]	2007	61	Cis + Gem (61)	EPP (45)	50–60 Gy + 8 Gy on port incisions (36)	I/II (38) III (22) NR (1)	Epithelial (42) Nonepithelial (17) NR (2)	19.8 (all) 23 (EPP)	80 78	50 50	NR NR	13.5	NR	NR	NR	84
Rena and Casadio [40]	2012	77	NR (64)	EPP (40) P/D (37)	45–60 Gy (40) 21 Gy on surgical scars (37)	I (16) II (61)	Epithelial (65) Nonepithelial (12)	28 (EPP stage I) 18 (EPP stage II) 32 (P/D stage I) 23 (P/D stage II)	NR NR NR NR	57 31 67 49	NR NR NR NR	NR	21 (EPP) 56 (P/D)	26 44	53 0	NR NRNR
Trousse et al. [41]	2009	83	Cis + Pem (10)	EPP (83)	54 Gy (10) Surgical scars (25)	II (30) III/IV (44) NR (9)	Epithelial (68) Nonepithelial (15)	14.5	62.4	32.2	14.3	NR	NR	NR	NR	NR
Billé et al. [50]	2012	22	Cis + Gem/Pem (22)	EPP (22)	54 Gy + prophylactic RT 21 Gy (17)	I/II (3) III/IV (19)	Epithelial (15) Nonepithelial (7)	12.8 (EPP)	54.5	18.2	NR	NR	NR	NR	NR	77.3

Rea et al. [51]	2007	21	Car + Gem (21)	EPP (17) P/D (4)	45 Gy (15)	I/II (5) III (16)	Epithelial (20) Nonepithelial (1)	25.5	71	52	19	16.3	35.2	64.8	NR	100
Bece et al. [52]	2015	53	Cis + Pem (27)	EPP (53)	45–50.4 Gy + boost 5.4–10 Gy (31) IMRT 50.4–54 Gy + boost 5.4–12 Gy (18)	NR	Epithelial (41) Nonepithelial (8) NR (4)	30.5	83.7	57.3	NR	21.6	18.4	NR	46.9	NR
Chance et al. [53]	2014	48	Cis/Car + Pem (34)	EPP (24) P/D (24)	IMRT 45 Gy + boost to 60 Gy if necessary (48)	NR	Epithelial (37) Nonepithelial (11)	28.4 (P/D) 14.2 (EPP)	76 67	56 34	NR NR	16.4 8.2	29	13	8	NR
Thieke et al. [54]	2015	62	Cis + Pem (30) Car + Pem (23) Cis + Gem (9)	EPP (62) P/D (17)	48–54 Gy (62)	NR	Epithelial (44) Nonepithelial (18)	20.4	63	42	28	NR	NR	NR	NR	NR

EPP extrapleural pneumonectomy, *P/D*, pleurectomy/decortication, *NR* not reported, *iCT* induction chemotherapy, *RT* radiotherapy, *IMRT* intensity modulated radiation therapy, *EBRT* external beam radiation therapy, *Gy* gray, *RCT* randomized controlled trial, *Cis* cisplatin, *Pem* pemetrexed, *Car* carboplatin, *Gem* gemcitabine, *Vin* vinorelbine, *Myt* mythomicin, *Ral* raltitrexed

order to reduce pain. A total dose of 50–60 Gy (in 1.8–2 Gy daily fractions) is the most common scheme, with the possibility to increase the total dose up to 70 Gy in particular areas using boost treatments.

The three-dimensional conformational technique (EBRT) is the most used with good results when applied after EPP and less encouraging outcome when it is preceded by P/D [56], even though Lee et al. reported that P/D followed by radiation therapy is an adequate option for those who cannot tolerate EPP [57].

A relatively recent technique is intensity modulated radiation therapy (IMRT) which involves modifying the intensity of radiation in small volumes using three-dimensional treatment planning protocols; unfortunately, it is associated with severe pulmonary toxicity after EPP, with 46% reported incidence of fatal pneumonitis associated with the dose of radiation delivered to the contralateral lung [58]. On the other hand, in a recent paper, patients received EBRT or IMRT after EPP based on the preference of the treating radiotherapist. Those who underwent IMRT had significantly less local recurrence without increased complication compared to those who received EBRT (14% vs. 42%) [36]. A very recent phase II study reports good outcomes in terms of pulmonary complications in patients who received IMRT after P/D [59].

The main criticism on the use of RT in MPM are focused mainly on concerns about complications of this treatment: the challenge in adjuvant RT is the big volumes irradiated and the preservation of vital structures such as contralateral lung, heart, liver, stomach, and spinal cord.

Seven studies were published between 2001 and 2012, reporting the results of bimodality treatments with adjuvant RT (Table 13.2).

The analysis of the current literature on surgery plus adjuvant RT alone reports an OS ranging between 13.5 [56] and 18.1 [57] months and a DFS of 12.2 months [57].

The reported outcome in these studies is relatively worse, but conclusions cannot be drawn because almost all of the studies are retrospective and nonrandomized.

An ongoing single center trial (SMART, Surgery for Mesothelioma after Radiation Therapy) is employing novel protocol, which consists in a short hemithoracic high dose IMRT followed by EPP, with encouraging initial results: morbidity and mortality are acceptable with a 3-year survival rate of 84% in epithelial subtype [64], but further investigation is necessary.

13.3.3 Adjuvant Chemotherapy Plus Adjuvant Radiotherapy in a Trimodality Protocol

In the current literature there are no randomized studies capable to guide the optimal timing of CT in a multimodality setting. Eighteen studies, published between 2007 and 2015, were collected and analyzed, including a total of 1427 patients (Table 13.3).

The adoption of induction chemotherapy makes more difficult a proper dissection plane to resect visceral pleura during P/D and residual disease can be left on site. Moreover, cytoreductive surgery can increase residual tumor regrowth, in this way more vulnerable to adjuvant treatments [81].

On the other hands, potential disadvantages of the adoption of adjuvant treatments are: (a) some operable patients can escape from surgery for progression on waiting list; (b) it is impossible to verify disease response to CT, avoiding patients' selection based on disease aggressiveness; and (c) complications of surgery may cause delay or refusal of adjuvant therapies.

The review of the current literature concerning surgery plus adjuvant treatments reports an OS ranging from 11 months [78] to 56.4 months [26] (in a subgroup of patients with stage I epithelioid MPM who underwent trimodality treatment). The DFS ranged from 8 months [78] to 27 months [68].

Pemetrexed-based CT is the most common regimen used, on the other hand there is a large variability in RT adjuvant regimens over the years and according to the institution's policy. For these reasons it is not possible to compare the different multimodal regimens. In a recent study, Friedberg

Table 13.2 Studies reporting the results of bimodal protocols including surgery followed by adjuvant radiotherapy

Author	Year	Patients (*n*)	Surgery (*n*)	Adjuvant RT regimen (*n*)	IMIG Stage (*n*)	Hystology (*n*)	Overall survival				Disease free survival (months)	Recurrence (%)				Toxicity (%)
							Median (months)	1Y (%)	2Y (%)	5Y (%)		Local	L + D	Distant	Overall	
Lee et al. [57]	2002	26	P/D (26)	IORT 15 Gy + EBRT 40–50 Gy (24)	I (18) III (8)	Epithelial (19) Nonepithelial (6) NR (1)	18.1	64	32	12	12.2	NR	NR	19	NR	Pneumonitis (17) Pericarditis (4) Esophageal stricture (4)
Gomez et al. [60]	2013	136	EPP (136)	EBRT 45–50 Gy ± boost to 55–60 Gy (86)	NR	Epithelial (98) Nonepithelial (41)	14.7 (EPP + RT) 4.5 (EPP)	55	32	NR	NR	16	14	59	NR	Skin (17.4) Esophagitis/ nausea (16) Lung (11.6) Heart (2.3)
Rice et al. [61]	2007	100	EPP (100)	EBRT 45–50 Gy ± boost to 60 Gy (63)	I/II (13) III/IV (87)	Epithelial (67) Nonepithelial (33)	14 (EPP + RT) 10.2 (EPP)	NR NR	32 26	NR NR	NR NR	13 NR	NR NR	54 44	67 NR	Nausea (87.3) Dyspnea (23.8) Severe respiratory distress (1.5)
Yajnik et al. [62]	2003	35	EPP (35)	EBRT 54 Gy (35)	I/II (15) III/IV (20)	Epithelial (26) Nonepithelial (9)	NR	NR	NR	NR	NR	NR	NR	NR	NR	Lung (68.5) Nausea (62.8) Esophagus/skin (20) Vomiting (45.7)
Gupta et al. [56]	2005	123	P/D (123)	EBRT 45 Gy (123) Brachytherapy 160 Gy (54/123)	I/II (72) III/IV (51)	NR	13.5	NR	23	5	NR	32.5	23.6	11.3	67.4	Dermatitis (60) Esophagitis/ nausea (49) Dyspnea (39.8) Pneumonitis (37.3) Fatigue (34.9) Vomiting (18.6) Pericarditis (8.9) Arrhythmia (1.6)

(continued)

Table 13.2 (continued)

Author	Year	Patients (*n*)	Surgery (*n*)	Adjuvant RT regimen (*n*)	IMIG Stage (*n*)	Hystology (*n*)	Overall survival				Disease free survival (months)	Recurrence (%)				Toxicity (%)
							Median (months)	1Y (%)	2Y (%)	5Y (%)		Local	L + D	Distant	Overall	
Rusch et al. [55]	2001	88	EPP (62) P/D (5) Exploration (21)	EBRT 54 Gy (54) IORT 15–10 GY + EBRT 45–54 GY (3)	I/II (19) III/IV (69)	Epithelial (40) Nonepithelial (21) NR (27)	17	NR	NR	NR	NR	3.6	9	54.5	NR	Skin (87.7) Fatigue (85.9) Esophagus (77) Nausea (70) Vomiting (52.6) Blood (47.3) Lung (40.3) Heart (3.5)
Gupta et al. [63]	2009	86	EPP (86)	EBRT 45–54 GY (photons/ electrons) (78)	I/II (33) III/IV (45)	Epithelial (57) Nonepithelial (21)	NR	NR	NR	NR	NR	15.3	21.7	33.3	74.3	NR

IORT intraoperative radiation therapy, *RT* radiotherapy, *EBRT* external beam radiation therapy, *IMRT* intensity modulated radiation therapy, *NR* not reported, *EPP* extrapleural pneumonectomy, *P/D* pleurectomy/decortication, *GY* gray

Table 13.3 Studies reporting the use of adjuvant chemotherapy with/without RT in a setting of a multimodality treatment

Author	Pts (*n*)	Surgery (*n*)	Adjuvant CT regimen (*n*)	Adjuvant RT regimen (*n*)	IMIG stage (*n*)	Histology	Overall survival				DFS (months)	Recurrence rate (%)			
							Median (months)	1Y (%)	2Y (%)	5Y (%)		Local	L + D	Distant	Overall
Minatel et al. [65]	69	P/D (69)	Cis/Car + Pem (61)	IMRT 50 Gy + boost 10 Gy (69)	I/II (22) III/IV (47)	Epithelial (60) Nonepithelial (9)	NR NR	NR NR	65 58	NR NR	NR	19	9	19	46
Baldini et al. [66]	169	EPP (169)	HIOC: Cis ± Gem (132) Cis + Pem (77)	EPT 54 Gy IHT + 39.6 Gy mediastinum (31) IMRT 50 Gy (21) 30 Gy + boost up to 50 Gy (8)	AJCC I/II (29) III/IV (140)	Epithelial (104) Nonepithelial (65)	15	NR	NR	NR	13.1	54	NR	NR	75
Lang-Lazdunski et al. [67]	102	P/D (102)	Cis + Gem/Pem (83) Hypertermic pleural lavage povidone–iodine: Concentration 1% for 15 min (102)	21 Gy on surgical scars (102)	I/II (31) III/IV (71)	Epithelial (73) Nonepithelial (29)	32 (all) 35 (epithelial) 15 (nonepithelial)	87.2 94.5 69	62.9 76.5 31.7	23.1 30.7 7	12	69	NR	6	75
Sugarbaker et al. [68]	103	EPP (74) P/D (29)	HIOC: Cis (72) Cis concurrent with RT (3) Cis + Gem (2) Cis + Pem (39) Car + Pem (6) NR (6)	54 Gy (1) EPT 54 Gy (18) IMRT 48.6 Gy (9) NR (26)	I/II (14) III/IV (60) NR (29)	Epithelial (87) Nonepithelial (16)	35 (HIOC) 23 (control)	NR NR	NR NR	NR NR	27.1 (HIOC) 12.8 (control)	NR NR	NR NR	NR NR	38 (HIOC) 74 (control)
Bedirhan et al. [69]	76	EPP (31) P/D (45)	Car + PTX (76)	/	NR	Epithelial (60) Nonepithelial (16)	20 (all) 21 (epithelial) 12 (nonepithelial)	NR NR NR	NR NR NR	14.3 16 0	NR	NR	NR	12	64
Friedberg et al. [70]	38	P/D (38)	Pem-based CT (31)	/	AJCC I/II (1) III/IV (37)	Epithelial (31) Nonepithelial (7)	32 (all) 41 (epithelial) 7 (nonepithelial)	NR	52	NR	9.6 (all) 15.1 (epithelial) 4.8 (nonepithelial)	26	39	8	74
Nakas et al. [71]	165	EPP (98) P/D (67)	NR (58)	Radical hemithorax RT (33)	III/IV (165)	Epithelial (128) Nonepithelial (37)	15 (EPP) 13 (P/D)	58 52	30 28	6 4	10.7 (EPP) 16 (P/D)	41 44	19 12	21 6	81 62

(continued)

Table 13.3 (continued)

Author	Pts (*n*)	Surgery (*n*)	Adjuvant CT regimen (*n*)	Adjuvant RT regimen (*n*)	IMIG stage (*n*)	Histology	Overall survival				DFS (months)	Recurrence rate (%)			
							Median (months)	1Y (%)	2Y (%)	5Y (%)		Local	L + D	Distant	Overall
Patel et al. [72]	30	EPP (30)	Cis + Pem (15) Car instead of Cis (2) Gem instead of Pem (2) Addition of Bevacizumab after RT (1)	IMRT 45 Gy IHC + boost 11.8 Gy (30)	I/II (5) III (23)	Epithelial (22) Nonepithelial (8)	23.2	76	50	NR	NR	13	20	40	73
Tonoli et al. [73]	56	EPP (56)	Cis + Pem (25) HIOC: Cis (17)	External RT of surgical scars (11) IMRT 50 Gy (50) + boost up to 60 Gy (20) 3DCRT 45 Gy (4)	I/II (12) III/IV (44)	Epithelial (54) Nonepithelial (2)	46.9	79	64	50	10.7	9	NR	23	32
Bolukbas et al. [26]	35	P/D (35)	Cis + Pem (34)	21 Gy on surgical scars (29) 45 Gy + boost to 50.4 Gy (5)	I/II (16) III/IV (19)	Epithelial (27) Nonepithelial (8)	30 (all) 31.1 (epithelial) 24.8 (nonepithelial)	69	50	NR	15.8	36	6	24	67
Luckraz et al. [74]	139	EPP (49) P/D (90)	regimen changed over the years, lately Cis, Pem and Vin (66)	50–55 Gy (66)	Butchart I (38) II/III/IV (101)	Epithelial (69) Nonepithelial (70)	3.3 (EPP) 10.3 (EPP + CT) 6 (EPP RT) 19.5 (EPP + CT + RT) 8.3 (P/D) 11.9 (P/D CT) 10.4 (P/D RT) 26 (P/D + CT + RT)	NR	14 12 NR 24 9 29 24 55	NR	NR	NR	NR	NR	NR
Tilleman et al. [75]	121	EPP (96) P/D (14) Unresectable (11)	HIOC: Cis (92)	/	AJCC I/II 14 III/IV 78	Epithelial (53) Nonepithelial (39)	12.8 (all) 13.1(EPP + HIOC) 17.1 (epithelial)	NR	NR	NR	15.3	2	15	NR	51
Trousse et al. [41]	83	EPP (83)	Cis + Pem (25)	External RT (25) 54 Gy (10)	I/II (30) III/IV (44) NR (9)	Epithelial (68) Nonepithelial (15)	14.5	62.4	32.2	14.3	NR	NR	NR	NR	NR

Yan et al. [76]	70	EPP (70)	Cis/Car + Pem (16)	45 Gy + boost 9 Gy (28)	NR	Epithelial (58) Nonepithelial (12)	20 (all) 23 (epithelial) 14 (nonepithelial)	62 63 58	41	15	NR	NR	NR	NR	NR
Miles et al. [77]	13	EPP (13)	Cis + Pem (10)	IMRT 45 Gy) + boost to 60 Gy (13)	I/II (4) III/IV (9)	Epithelial (10) Nonepithelial (3)	NR	NR	NR	NR	NR	17	33	0	50
Van Sandick et al. [78]	35	P/D (12) EPP (23)	HIOC: Cis + Adr (20)	24 Gy (19) IMRT 54 Gy (12)	I/II (35) III/IV (0)	Epithelial (30) Nonepithelial (2) NR (3)	11 (HIOC) 29 (EPP/RT)	NR	NR	NR	8 (HIOC) 21 (EPP/RT)	35 7	45 27	10 40	90 73
Allen et al. [79]	39	EPP (39)	HIOC (6) Cis (14) Car + PTX (6) Cis + Gem (10) Cis + Pem (3) Others (2)	MDRT, 30 Gy + 4,0 Gy mediastinum + boost to 54 Gy (24) HDRT, 39.6 Gy (15)	Sugarbaker I (12) II (15) III (12)	Epithelial (25) Nonepithelial (14)	19	NR	NR	NR	NR	50 MDRT 27 HDRT	NR	50 MDRT 47 HDRT	NR
Lucchi et al. [80]	49	P/D (49)	Immuno-chemotherapy IL2 before and after surgery and after adjuvant CT+ HIOC with epidoxorubicin + adjuvant CT: Cis + Gem (49)	30 Gy on surgical scars (49)	II (9) III (40)	Epithelial (39) Nonepithelial (10)	26[a]	NR	60.2	23.3	NR	76	14	0	90

Pts patients, *DFS* disease free survival, *CT* chemotherapy, *RT* radiotherapy, *HIOC* heated intraoperative chemotherapy, *EPT* electron-photon technique, *IMRT* intensity modulated radiation therapy, *MDRT* moderate-dose hemithoracic radiotherapy, *IHT* ipsilateral hemithorax, *CHT* contralateral hemithorax, *Cis* cisplatin, *Pem* pemetrexed, *Car* carboplatin, *Gem* gemcitabine, *Vin* vinorelbine

[a]Since diagnosis

et al. reported a unique experience using intraoperative photodinamic therapy (PDT) associated with P/D and adjuvant CT with good outcomes in epithelial subtype [70], but more clinical trials are necessary to support these findings.

13.3.4 Heated Intraoperative Chemotherapy (HIOC)

HIOC consists in the application of chemotherapeutic agents directly to the resected surface immediately after surgery. The advantage is delivering high local dose of cytotoxic drug against microscopic disease, with decrease toxicity compared to systemic CT. The morbidity is linked to the expertise of the surgical and anesthetic team; the operations are long with high need of fluid administration, to prevent renal toxicity. In case of EPP, intraoperative caution is needed with respect to fluids infusion to prevent postpneumonectomy pulmonary edema.

There are conflicting results on this technique: some authors reported disappointing outcomes in patients who underwent surgery, HIOC, and RT compared to patients treated with EPP and RT [78], but others reported that a subgroup of patients (epithelial histology, low tumor volume, and female sex) can benefit from HIOC [68].

To date, HIOC cannot be introduced as standard treatment, because of lack of good results; nevertheless further studies are necessary to better understand its role in MPM treatment.

13.4 Conclusions

The optimal treatment of MPM is still matter of debate. It is now established that trimodality approach including CT, surgery, and RT in different combinations seems to lead to better outcome.

Each therapeutic approach has advantages and drawbacks that should be taken into consideration to optimize the best treatment for each patient, individualizing the most effective therapeutic strategy, limited side effects, and maximizing patients' quality of life. Concerning the timing of each treatment modality, both adjuvant and neoadjuvant have pros and cons and no particular treatment has shown superiority over the others. In recent years there seems to be a trend among surgeons to perform P/D more frequently than EPP.

Thus, it is important that patients be treated in a tertiary care center, where a multidisciplinary team (surgeon, oncologist, radiotherapist) can provide the highest level of quality of care to improve survival rate.

References

1. Moolgavkar SH, Meza R, Turim J. Pleural and peritoneal mesothelioma in SEER: age effects and temporal trends, 1973–2005. Cancer Causes Control. 2009;20:935–44.
2. Zucali PA, De Vincenzo F, Simonelli M, et al. Future developments in the management of malignant pleural mesothelioma. Expert Rev Anticancer Ther. 2009;9:453–67.
3. Sugarbaker DJ. Macroscopic complete resection: the goal of primary surgery in multimodality therapy for pleural mesothelioma. J Thorac Oncol. 2006;1:175–6.
4. Treasure T. What is the best approach for surgery of malignant pleural mesothelioma? It is to put our efforts into obtaining trustworthy evidence for practice. J Thorac Cardiovasc Surg. 2016;151:307–9.
5. Spaggiari L, Marulli G, Bovolato P, et al. Extrapleural pneumonectomy for malignant mesothelioma: an Italian multicenter retrospective study. Ann Thorac Surg. 2014;97:1859–65.
6. Rusch V, Baldini EH, Bueono R, et al. The role of cytoreduction in the treatment of malignant pleural mesothelioma: meeting summary of the international mesothelioma interest group congress, September 11–14, 2012, Boston, Mass. J Thorac Cardiovasc Surg. 2013;145:909–10.
7. Sugarbaker DJ, Flores RM, Jaklitsch MT, et al. Resection margins, extrapleural nodal status and cell type determine post-operative long term survival in trimodality therapy of malignant pleural mesothelioma: results in 183 patients. J Thorac Cardiovasc Surg. 1999;117:54–63.
8. Rusch VW, Giroux D, Kennedy C, et al. Initial analysis of the International Association for the Study of Lung Cancer mesothelioma database. J Thorac Oncol. 2012;7:1631–9.
9. Scherpereel A, Astoul P, Baas P, et al. Guidelines of the European Respiratory Society and the European Society of Thoracic Surgery for the management of malignant pleural mesothelioma. Eur Respir J. 2010;35:479–95.
10. Sugarbaker DJ, Jaklitsch MT, Bueno R, et al. Prevention, early detection, and management of complications after 328 consecutive extrapleu-

ral pneumonectomies. J Thorac Cardiovasc Surg. 2004;128:138–46.
11. Martini N, Bains MS, Beattie EJ Jr. Indications for pleurectomy in malignant effusion. Cancer. 1975;35:734–8.
12. Cao C, Tian DH, Pataky KA, et al. Systematic review of pleurectomy in the treatment of malignant pleural mesothelioma. Lung Cancer. 2013;81:39–27.
13. Rice D, Rusch V, Pass H, et al. Recommendation for uniform definitions of surgical techniques for malignant pleural mesothelioma. A consensus report of the International Association for the Study of Lung Cancer International Staging Committee and the International Mesothelioma Interest Group. J Thorac Oncol. 2011;6:1304–12.
14. Butchart EG, Ashcroft T, Barnsley WC, et al. Pleuropneumonectomy in the management of diffuse pleural mesothelioma of the pleura. Experience with 29 patients. Thorax. 1976;31:15–24.
15. Sugarbaker DJ, Jaklitsch MT, Bueno R, et al. Prevention, early detection, and management of complication after 328 consecutive extrapleural pneumonectomies. J Thorac Cardiovasc Surg. 2004;128:138–46.
16. Weder W, Stahel RA, Bernhard J, et al. Multicenter trial of neoadjuvant chemotherapy followed by extrapleural pneumonectomy in malignant pleural mesothelioma. Ann Oncol. 2007;18:1196–202.
17. Treasure T, Internullo E, Fiorentino F, et al. A survey of opinions and beliefs concerning surgery for malignant pleural mesothelioma amongst 802 members of the European Association for Cardio Thoracic Surgery (EACTS), the European Society of Thoracic Surgeons (ESTS) and the society of Thoracic Surgeons (STS). Interact Cardiovasc Thorac Surg. 2011;12:341–6.
18. Treasure T, Lang-lazdunski L, Waller D, et al. Extrapleural pneumonectomy versus no extrapleural pneumonectomy for patients with malignant pleural mesothelioma: clinical outcomes of the Mesothelioma and Radical Surgery (MARS) randomized feasibility study. Lancet Oncol. 2011;12:763–72.
19. Wanebo HJ, Martini N, Melamed MR, et al. Pleural mesothelioma. Cancer. 1976;38:2481–8.
20. Lim EM. MARS 2: a feasibility study comparing (extended) pleurectomy decortication versus no pleurectomy decortication in patients with malignant pleural mesothelioma (MARS2). http://www.clinicaltrials.gov/show/NCT02040272.
21. Teh E, Fiorentino F, Tan C, et al. A systematic review of lung sparing extirpative surgery for pleural mesothelioma. J R Soc Med. 2011;104:69–80.
22. Friedberg JS, Culligan MJ, Mick R, et al. Radical pleurectomy and intraoperative photodynamic therapy for malignant pleural mesothelioma. Ann Thorac Surg. 2012;93:1658–67.
23. Flores RM. The mesothelioma surgery shift. J Thorac Cardiovasc Surg. 2016;151:485–6.
24. Flores RM, Pass HI, Seshan VE, et al. Extrapleural pneumonectomy versus pleurectomy/decortication in the surgical management of malignant pleural mesothelioma: results in 663 patients. J Thorac Cardiovasc Surg. 2008;135:620–6.
25. Lang-Lazdunski L, Bille A, Belcher E, et al. Pleurectomy/decortication, hypertermic pleural lavage with povidone-iodine followed by adjuvant chemotherapy in patients with malignant pleural mesothelioma. J Thorac Oncol. 2011;6:1746–52.
26. Bolukbas S, Manegold C, Eberlein M, et al. Survival after trimodality therapy for malignant pleural mesothelioma: radical pleurectomy, chemotherapy with cisplatin/pemetrexed and radiotherapy. Lung Cancer. 2011;71:75–8.
27. Nakas A, Trousse DS, Martin-Ucar AE, et al. Open lung sparing surgery for malignant pleural mesothelioma: the benefits of a radical approach within multimodality therapy. Eur J Cardiothorac Surg. 2008;34:886–91.
28. Flores RM. Surgical options in malignant pleural mesothelioma: extrapleural pneumonectomy or pleurectomy/decortication. Semin Thorac Cardiovasc Surg. 2009;21:149–53.
29. Sugarbaker DJ, Wolf AS, Chirieac LR, et al. Surgery for malignant pleural mesothelioma. Expert Rev Respir Med. 2010;4:363–72.
30. Singhal S, Kaiser LR. Malignant pleural mesothelioma: options for management. Surg Clin N Am. 2002;82:797–831.
31. Berghmans T, Paesmans M, Lalami Y, et al. Activity of chemotherapy and immunotherapy on malignant mesothelioma: a systematic review of literature with meta-analysis. Lung Cancer. 2002;38:111–21.
32. Vogelzang NJ, Rusthoven JJ, Symanowski J, et al. Phase III study of pemetrexed in combination with cisplatin versus cisplatin alone in patients with malignant pleural mesothelioma. J Clin Oncol. 2003;21:2636–44.
33. Zalcman M, Mazieres J, Greiller L, et al. Bevacizumab for newly diagnosed pleural mesothelioma in the Mesothelioma Avastin Cisplatin Pemetrexed Study (MAPS): a randomized controlled open-label, phase 3 trial. Lancet. 2016;387:1405–14.
34. Rusch VW. Pemetrexed and cisplatin for malignant pleural mesothelioma: a new standard of care? J Clin Oncol. 2002;21:2696–30.
35. Marulli G, Rea F, Nicotra S, et al. Effect of induction chemotherapy on lung function and exercise capacity in patients affected by malignant pleural mesothelioma. Eur J Cardiothorac Surg. 2010;37:1464–9.
36. Buduhan G, Menon S, Aye R, et al. Trimodality therapy for malignant pleural mesothelioma. Ann Thorac Surg. 2009;88:870–5.
37. Weder W, Ketenholz P, Taverna C, et al. Neoadjuvant chemotherapy followed by extrapleural pneumonectomy in malignant pleural mesothelioma. J Clin Oncol. 2004;22:3451–7.
38. Lang-Lazdunski L, Bille A, Lal R, et al. Pleurectomy/decortication is superior to extrapleural pneumonectomy in the multimodality management of patients with malignant pleural mesothelioma. J Thorac Oncol. 2012;7:737–47.

39. Okada M, Mimura T, Ohbayashi C, et al. Radical surgery for malignant pleural mesothelioma: results and prognosis. Interact Cardiovasc Thorac Surg. 2008;7:102–6.
40. Rena O, Casadio C. Extrapleural pneumonectomy for early stage malignant pleural mesothelioma: a harmful procedure. Lung Cancer. 2012;77:151–5.
41. Trousse DS, Avaro JP, D'Journo XB, et al. Is malignant pleural mesothelioma a surgical disease? A review of 83 consecutive extra-pleural pneumonectomies. Eur J Cardiothorac Surg. 2009;36:759–63.
42. Bech C, Sorensen JB. Chemotherapy induced pathologic complete response in malignant pleural mesothelioma: a review and case report. J Thorac Oncol. 2010;5:735–40.
43. Hasegawa S, Okada M, Tanaka F, et al. Trimodality strategy for treating malignant pleural mesothelioma: results of a feasibility study of induction pemetrexed plus cisplatin followed by extrapleural pneumonectomy and postoperative hemithoracic radiation (Japan Mesothelioma Interest Group 0601 Trial). Int J Clin Oncol. 2016;21:523–30.
44. De Perrot M, Feld R, Cho BC, et al. Trimodality therapy with induction chemotherapy followed by extrapleural pneumonectomy and adjuvant high-dose hemithoracic radiation for malignant pleural mesothelioma. J Clin Oncol. 2009;27:1413–8.
45. Krug LM, Pass HI, Rusch VW, et al. Multicenter phase II trial of neoadjuvant pemetrexed plus cisplatin followed by extrapleural pneumonectomy and radiation for malignant pleural mesothelioma. J Clin Oncol. 2009;27:3007–13.
46. Pasello G, Marulli G, Polo V, et al. Pemetrexed plus carboplatin or cisplatin as neoadjuvant treatment of operable malignant pleural mesothelioma (MPM). Anticancer Res. 2012;32:5393–400.
47. Van Schil PE, Baas P, Gaafar R, et al. Trimodality therapy for malignant pleural mesothelioma: results from an EORTC phase II multicentre trial. Eur Respir J. 2010;36:1362–9.
48. Rea F, Favaretto A, Marulli G, et al. Phase II trial of neaodjuvant pemetrexed plus cisplatin followed by surgery and radiation in the treatment of pleural mesothelioma. BMC Cancer. 2013;13:22.
49. Flores RM, Krug LM, Rosenzweig KE, et al. Induction chemotherapy, extrapleural pneumonectomy and postoperative high-dose radiotherapy for locally advanced malignant pleural mesothelioma: a phase II trial. J Thorac Oncol. 2006;1:289–95.
50. Bille A, Belcher E, Raubenheimer H, et al. Induction chemotherapy, extrapleural pneumonectomy, and adjuvant radiotherapy for malignant pleural mesothelioma: experience of Guy's and St Thomas' hospital. Gen Thorac Cardiovasc Surg. 2012;60:289–96.
51. Rea F, Marulli G, Bortolotti L, et al. Induction chemotherapy, extrapleural pneumonectomy (EPP) and adjuvant hemi-thoracic radiation in malignant pleural mesothelioma (MPM): feasibility and results. Lung Cancer. 2007;57:89–95.
52. Bece A, Tin MM, Martin D, et al. Hemithoracic radiation therapy after extrapleural pneumonectomy for malignant pleural mesothelioma: toxicity and outcomes at an Australian institution. J Med Imaging Radiat Oncol. 2015;59:355–62.
53. Chance WW, Rice DC, Allen PK, et al. Hemithoracic intensity modulated radiation therapy after pleurectomy/decortication for malignant pleural mesothelioma: toxicity, patterns of failure, and a matched survival analysis. Int J Radiat Oncol Biol Phys. 2015;91:149–56.
54. Thieke C, Nicolay NH, Sterzing F, et al. Long-term results in malignant pleural mesothelioma treated with neoadjuvant chemotherapy, extrapleural pneumonectomy and intensity modulated radiotherapy. Radiat Oncol. 2015;10:267.
55. Rusch VW, Rosenzweig K, Venkatraman E, et al. A phase II trial of surgical resection and adjuvant high dose hemithoracic radiation for malignant pleural mesothelioma. J Thorac Cardiovasc Surg. 2001;122:788–95.
56. Gupta V, Mychalczak B, Krug LM, et al. Hemithoracic radiation therapy after pleurectomy/decortication for malignant pleural mesothelioma. Int J Radiat Oncol Biol Phys. 2005;63:1045–52.
57. Lee TT, Everett DL, Shu HG, et al. Radical pleurectomy/decortication and intraoperative radiotherapy followed by conformal radiation with or without chemotherapy for malignant pleural mesothelioma. J Thorac Cardiovasc Surg. 2002;124:1183–9.
58. Allen AM, Czerminska M, Janne PA, et al. Fatal pneumonitis associated with intensity-modulated radiation therapy for mesothelioma. Int J Radiat Oncol Biol Phys. 2006;65(3):640–5.
59. Rimner A, Zauderer MJ, Gomez DR, et al. Phase II study of hemithoracic intensity-modulated pleural radiation therapy (IMPRINT) as part of lung sparing multimodality therapy in patients with malignant pleural mesothelioma. J Clin Oncol. 2010;5:735–40.
60. Gomez DR, Hong DS, Allen PK, et al. Patterns of failure, toxicity and survival after extrapleural pneumonectomy and hemithoracic intensity-modulated radiation therapy for malignant pleural mesothelioma. J Thorac Oncol. 2013;8:238–45.
61. Rice DC, Stevens CW, Correa AM, et al. Outcomes after extrapleural pneumonectomy and intensity-modulated radiation therapy for malignant pleural mesothelioma. Ann Thorac Surg. 2007;84:1685–93.
62. Yajnik S, Rosenzweig KE, Mychalczak B, et al. Hemithoracic radiation after extrapleural pneumonectomy for malignant pleural mesothelioma. Int J Radiat Oncol Biol Phys. 2003;56:1319–26.
63. Gupta V, Krug LM, Laser B, et al. Patterns of local and nodal failure in malignant pleural mesothelioma after extrapleural pneumonectomy and photon-electron radiotherapy. J Thorac Oncol. 2009;4:746–50.
64. Cho BC, Feld R, Leighl N, et al. A feasibility study evaluating surgery for mesothelioma after radiation therapy: the "SMART" approach for resectable malignant pleural mesothelioma. J Thorac Oncol. 2014;9:397–402.

65. Minatel E, Trovo M, Bearz A, et al. Radical radiation therapy after lung-sparing surgery for malignant pleural mesothelioma: survival, pattern of failure and prognostic factor. Int J Radiat Oncol Biol Phys. 2015;93:606–13.
66. Baldini EH, Richards WG, Gill RR, et al. Updated patterns of failure after multimodality therapy for malignant pleural mesothelioma. J Thorac Cardiovasc Surg. 2015;149:1374–81.
67. Lang-Lazdunski L, Bille A, Papa S, et al. Pleurectomy/decortication, hypertermic pleural lavage with povidone-iodine, prophylactic radiotherapy and systemic chemotherapy in patient with malignant pleural mesothelioma: a 10-year experience. J Thorac Cardiovasc Surg. 2015;149:558–65.
68. Sugarbaker PH, Stuart OA, Eger C. Pharmacokinetics of hypertermic intrathoracic chemotherapy following pleurectomy and decortication. Gastroenterol Res Pract. 2012;2012:471205.
69. Bedirhan MA, Cansever L, Demir A, et al. Which type of surgery should become the preferred procedure for malignant pleural mesothelioma: extrapleural pneumonectomy or extendend pleurectomy? J Thorac Dis. 2013;5:446–54.
70. Friedberg JS, Simone CB, Culligan MJ 2nd, et al. Extended pleurectomy-decortication-based treatment for advanced stage epithelial mesothelioma yielding a median survival of nearly three years. Ann Thorac Surg. 2017;103:912–9.
71. Nakas A, von Meyenfeldt E, Lau K, et al. Long-term results after lung-sparing total pleurectomy for locally advanced (International Mesothelioma Interest Group stage T3-T4) non-sarcomatoid malignant pleural mesothelioma. Eur J Cardiothorac Surg. 2012;41:1031–6.
72. Patel PR, Yoo S, Broadwater G, et al. Effect of increasing experience on dosimetric and clinical outcomes in the management of malignant pleural mesothelioma with intensity-modulated radiation therapy. Int J Radiat Oncol Biol Phys. 2012;83:362–8.
73. Tonoli S, Vitali P, Scotti V, et al. Adjuvant radiotherapy after extra-pleural pneumonectomy for mesothelioma. Prospective analysis of a multi-institutional series. Radiother Oncol. 2011;101:311–5.
74. Luckraz H, Rahman M, Patel N, et al. Three decades of experience in the surgical multi-modality management of pleural mesothelioma. Eur J Cardiothorac Surg. 2010;37:552–6.
75. Tilleman TR, Richards WG, Zellos L, et al. Extrapleural pneumonectomy followed by intracavitary intraoperative hypertermic cisplatin with pharmacologic cytoprotection for treatment of malignant pleural mesothelioma: a phase II prospective study. J Thorac Cardiovasc Surg. 2009;138:405–11.
76. Yan TD, Boyer M, Tin MM, et al. Extrapleural pneumonectomy for malignant pleural mesothelioma: outcomes of treatment and prognostic factors. J Thorac Cardiovasc Surg. 2009;138:619–24.
77. Miles EF, Larrier NA, Kelsey CR, et al. Intensity modulated radiotherapy for resected mesothelioma: the Duke experience. Int J Radiat Oncol Biol Phys. 2008;71:1143–50.
78. Van Sandick JW, Kappers I, Baas P, et al. Surgical treatment in the management of malignant pleural mesothelioma: a single institution's experience. Ann Surg Oncol. 2008;15:1757–64.
79. Allen AM, Den R, Wong JS, et al. Influence of radiotherapy technique and dose on patterns of failure for mesothelioma patients after extrapleural pneumonectomy. Int J Radiat Oncol Biol Phys. 2007;68:1366–74.
80. Lucchi M, Chella A, Melfi F, et al. A phase II study of intrapleural immune-chemotherapy, pleurectomy/decortication, radiotherapy, systemic chemotherapy and long-term sub-cutaneous IL-2 in stage II-III malignant pleural mesothelioma. Eur J Cardiothorac Surg. 2007;31:529–35.
81. Averbach AM, Sugarbaker PH. Peritoneal mesothelioma: treatment approach based on natural history. Cancer Treat Res. 1996;81:193–211.

14 Role of Radiotherapy in Malignant Pleural Mesothelioma

Marta Scorsetti, Davide Franceschini, Fiorenza De Rose, and Vittorio Vavassori

14.1 Introduction

The role of radiotherapy (RT) in the management of malignant pleural mesothelioma (MPM) is controversial. There is a lack of evidences in favor or against RT, because only few randomized trials have been conducted until now and just few of them have completed the expected accrual. Moreover, RT in MPM is challenging from a technical point of view. Apart from the palliative setting, in all other scenarios, the target volume is significantly complex, large, and of irregular shape. The dose prescription is another major issue in MPM. On one side, mesothelioma cells are quite radioresistant, although preclinical data suggest remarkable differences in radiosensitivity [1], therefore relevant RT doses are thought to be needed for disease eradication. On the other side, due to the position and the extension of the pleura, many different healthy tissues surround or extend into the target volume, necessarily limiting RT doses delivered to avoid unacceptable toxicities.

In this chapter, we will review the possible roles of RT in MPM, highlighting pros and cons in different clinical scenarios (palliation, prevention of procedure tract metastases, adjuvant RT after surgery, radical RT, and trimodal approach). A particular attention will be paid to the technological development, highlighting how new RT techniques could improve the tolerance and efficacy of RT in MPM.

14.2 RT for Prophylaxis of Procedure Tract Metastases

Due to its nature and presentation, MPM commonly requires pleural interventions, for liquid management or for tissue diagnosis. However, these invasive procedures are related with a relevant risk of seeding of malignant cells along the procedural tract that can bring to the development of the so called "procedure tract metastases" (PTMs). These are subcutaneous nodules that also can develop many months after the procedure and can be responsible of important

M. Scorsetti (✉)
Department of Biomedical Sciences, Humanitas University, Milan, Italy

Radiotherapy and Radiosurgery Department, Humanitas Clinical and Research Hospital, Milan, Italy
e-mail: marta.scorsetti@hunimed.eu

D. Franceschini · F. De Rose
Radiotherapy and Radiosurgery Department, Humanitas Clinical and Research Hospital, Milan, Italy
e-mail: davide.franceschini@humanitas.it; fiorenza.de_rose@humanitas.it

V. Vavassori
Radiotherapy Department, Cliniche Humanitas Gavazzeni, Bergamo, Italy
e-mail: vittorio.vavassori@gavazzeni.it

G. L. Ceresoli et al. (eds.), *Mesothelioma*, https://doi.org/10.1007/978-3-030-16884-1_14

pain, affecting patients' quality of life. The incidence of PTM is not clearly established, ranging from 3.6% to 24% of patients in different series, according to the different procedures carried out [2]. RT has been advocated for the prevention of the PTMs, with controversial and contradictory results. To answer the question about the real benefit of preventive RT for PTMs, five randomized trials have been conducted and published till now. The older was published in 1995 by Boutin et al. In this trial, 40 patients were randomized to either receive 21 Gy in three fractions for 3 days to their thoracoscopy site, very soon (10–15 days) after thoracoscopy, or no radiotherapy. The PTMs incidence was 0% in the RT group versus 40% in the no RT group ($p < 0.01$). This result led the authors to strongly support the use of RT for the prevention of PTMs [3]. However, due to the very high rate of PTMs in the control group, which was significant distant from the data observed in the real clinical practice, these data were criticized.

Subsequently, an Australian trial was published showing no significant difference in PTM incidence between the treatment and control arms (PTMs incidence in the RT group 7% vs. 10% in the control group, $p = 0.53$) [4]. This study randomized 43 patients, the RT dose and fractionation was 10 Gy in single fraction. Due to the low RT dose prescribed, also the results of this trial were criticized and considered inconclusive.

Trying to solve this issue, another trial was conducted in the UK by O'Rourke et al. [5]. After a pleural intervention, 61 patients were randomized to receive 21 Gy in three fractions within 21 days or no prophylactic radiotherapy. Very few PTMs occurred (7/61, 11.5%) and there was no difference in incidence between the two arms (13 vs. 10%), leading the authors to conclude that local radiotherapy should only be used after the development of a symptomatic PTM and not as prophylaxis.

With the data coming from these trials and from other smaller not randomized studies, systematic reviews and meta-analysis were conducted [6–8]. No definitive answer in favor or against the use of prophylactic RT could be derived also from the pooled data.

More recently, the results of the Surgical and large bore procedures in Malignant pleural mesothelioma And Radiotherapy Trial (SMART) were published by Clive et al. [9]. This trial was conducted in the UK and randomized 203 patients who had undergone large-bore pleural interventions in the 35 days prior to recruitment to receive immediate radiotherapy (21 Gy in three fractions within 42 days of the pleural intervention) or deferred radiotherapy (same dose given within 35 days of PTMs diagnosis). No significant difference was seen in PTMs incidence in the immediate and deferred radiotherapy groups (9% vs. 16%; $p = 0{\cdot}14$). Median overall survival from randomization was 357 days in the immediate radiotherapy group and 365 days in the deferred radiotherapy group. The authors concluded against routine use of prophylactic irradiation of tracts in mesothelioma, provided that the patient receives regular clinical follow-up to ensure symptoms are identified and treated early.

Finally, the results of the Prophylactic Irradiation of Tracts (PIT) trial were presented at the end of 2017 [10]. Three hundred and seventy five MPM patients following a chest wall procedure were randomized 1:1 to receive PIT (within 42-days of procedure) or no PIT. PIT was delivered at a dose of 21 Gy in three fractions over three consecutive weekdays. PTMs incidence at 6 months was 6/186 (3.2%) versus 10/189 (5.3%) for the PIT versus no PIT arm respectively ($p = 0.44$) and at 12 months 15/186 (8.1%) versus 19/189 (10.1%), respectively ($p = 0.59$). Again, the authors conclude that there is no role of RT as prophylactic treatment for PTMs.

Table 14.1 summarizes randomized studies of RT for the prevention of PTMs.

According to the results of these latter trials the more recent guidelines definitely took position against the routinary use of prophylactic RT in MPM patients. Indeed, in the recent update of ASCO guidelines for MPM, it is stated that adjuvant radiation (and not prophylactic) should be offered only to patients who have resection of intervention tracts found to be histologically positive [11]. Authors also recommended further studies in epithelioid-only histologic subtypes and patients not treated with chemotherapy,

Table 14.1 Randomized studies of RT for the prevention of PTMs

Author	No. of patients	RT dose	Toxicity ≥ G3	Procedure tract metastases	Overall survival
Boutin et al. [3]	40 (20 RT vs. 20 no RT)	21 Gy in three fractions	None reported	RT: 0 No RT: 40%	Not reported
Bydder et al. [4]	58 (28 RT vs. 30 no RT)	10 Gy in one fraction	None reported	RT: 7% No RT: 10%	35% at 1 year
O'Rourke et al. [5]	61 (31 RT vs. 30 no RT)	21 Gy in three fractions	None reported	RT: 13% No RT: 10%	41 weeks (median)
Clive et al. [9]	203 (102 immediate RT vs. 101 deferred RT)	21 Gy in 3 fractions	None reported	Immediate RT: 9% Deferred RT: 16%	357 days (RT) vs. 365 days (deferred RT) (median)
Bayman et al. [10]	357 (186 RT vs. 189 no RT)	21 Gy in 3 fractions	0.5% G3 skin toxicity	RT: 8.1% No RT: 10.1%	Not reported

which in the SMART trial had a small benefit with immediate RT.

From a technical point of view, simple techniques can be used. A single direct electron beam is the preferred procedure to treat the chest wall to at least 90% (using bolus, if necessary). Alternatively, photons can be used if the depth dose to the chest wall is adequate. Twenty one Gray (Gy) in three fractions on consecutive days is the commonest dose prescribed.

14.3 Palliative Radiotherapy

During their clinical history, most patients with MPM present a combination of bone and neuropathic pain or various obstructive symptoms. Palliative radiotherapy is an effective treatment in this scenario and is often used with this intent, although we have no data that strongly support it.

MacLeod et al. reviewed literature data to assess the role of palliative RT in MPM [12]. Eight papers were included in this systematic review, but most of them were retrospective studies. Total dose and fractionation ranged from single fraction of 8–60 Gy in 30 fractions and also the recorded response rate was very heterogeneous (0–69%). Both poor study design and the small number of involved patients associated with a retrospective assessment of pain relief and the absence of reported toxicity contributed to the undefined role of palliative radiotherapy in this setting. Only data from Bisset et al.'s prospective study [13] provided the strongest evidence compared to other studies included in this review, using a clear method to evaluate the pain response and reporting a 68% response rate.

In 2015, MacLeod and colleagues published the SYSTEMS-1 study, a multicenter phase II trial designed to assess and evaluate the level of pain 5 weeks after a short course of radiotherapy (20 Gy in five fractions) [14]. Forty patients were included after an optimization of analgesia. The evaluation of pain using the Brief Pain Inventory was performed from baseline. Quality of life (QoL), fatigue, and radiotherapy toxicity were also assessed by EORTC QLQ-30, Fatigue Severity Scale (FSS) and common toxicity criteria for adverse events version 4.0, respectively. This study confirmed radiotherapy as an effective treatment for MPM-related pain (47% of patients with a clinically significant improvement of their pain at week 5), without any improvement in QoL.

Based on these results, the investigators started the SYSTEMS-2 randomized study to examine whether a dose-escalated treatment (36 Gy/6 fractions) results in clinically significant improvement of pain control compared to standard palliative radiotherapy (20 Gy/5 fractions) using advanced radiotherapy technique [15]. This trial is still ongoing and the mature data will be very useful to define the optimal schedule of radiation treatment for MPM-related pain.

Table 14.2 Selective studies of palliative RT

Author	No. of patients	RT technique	RT dose	Pain relief
Bisset et al. [13]	22	Cobalt-60	30 Gy in ten fractions	68%
MacLeod et al. [14]	40	Not reported	20 Gy in five fractions	47% at week 5
Ashton et al. [15]	112	IMRT (3DCRT if IMRT is unavailable)	20 Gy in five fractions vs. 36 Gy in six fractions	Ongoing trial

These selected studies of palliative RT are listed in Table 14.2.

Unfortunately, patients with MPM present a lot of peculiar features: poor survival, progressive decline of performance status and/or quality of life independently from pain relief, the radiotherapy planning complexity due to need for treat the entire volume of disease minimizing toxicity. All these aspects can limit the real estimate of the palliative RT efficacy.

Nevertheless, the recent update of ASCO guidelines for MPM strongly recommended that palliative radiotherapy using standard palliative schedules (8 Gy/one fraction, 20 Gy/five fractions, or 30 Gy/ten fractions) should be considered in all patients with MPM with localized disease causing pain or obstructive symptoms [11].

Any radiation technique (electrons, 2D, 3D conformal radiation therapy) can be used depending on the site of treatment volume and organs at risk.

14.4 Adjuvant RT After Extrapleural Pneumonectomy (EPP)

Extrapleural pneumonectomy (EPP) has been for years the standard surgical intervention for MPM. Briefly, EPP is a very demolitive surgical intervention, removing en bloc lung, visceral and parietal pleura, pericardium, and diaphragm [16]. The aim of this intervention is the macroscopic complete resection, however, due to the infiltrative growth pattern of MPM, local recurrence remains a significant issue also after macroscopically radical EPP [17, 18]. For this reason, postoperative hemithoracic RT has been a standard treatment for decades, until recent years. However, due to the invasiveness of this surgical procedure it has been estimated that only 52–65% of patients initially considered for trimodality therapy ultimately complete adjuvant radiation [19, 20].

From the radiation oncologist point of view, EPP facilitates the delivery of adjuvant RT, since the surgical removal of ipsilateral lung eliminates its dose constraints. Apart from this advantage, RT remains technically challenging from a dosimetric point of view. The adjacent organs at risk (OAR), particularly the contralateral lung, but also other structures such as heart, ipsilateral kidney, liver, esophagus, and spinal cord combined with the irregular size and shape of the volume to be treated represent the main obstacle in delivering effective RT doses. This is particularly relevant considering that RT doses required to sterilize the pleural cavity after EPP are probably higher than 50–54 Gy [21].

Initial experiences of adjuvant RT after EPP have been limited for decades by the available technologies that hampered a successful dose escalation without excessive toxicity. Various conventional 2D or 3D techniques are described in the literature. A combined photon–electron technique was used by Rusch et al. with promising results [21]. The authors enrolled 57 patients, 94.7% of whom had undergone EPP. Using parallel opposed photon fields up to 41.4 Gy to the hemithorax and mediastinum and a subsequent electron boost up to 54 Gy, the authors reported interesting results, with a median survival of 33.8 months in early stage disease and of 10 months in stage III or IV disease ($p = 0.04$). More interestingly, local control was achieved in 90% of cases, with a change in the common pattern of recurrence, with distant metastases noted in 64.8% of the 54 patients who underwent EPP and radiotherapy. However, in another analysis from the same group with the same technique [22] local recurrence rates resulted significantly higher up to 37%, particularly in the inferior regions of the radiotherapy volume, raising concerns about dose inhomogeneity.

A different technique known as moderate-dose-photon technique (MDRT) was described by investigators at Brigham and Women's Hospital and the Dana-Farber Cancer Institute. They used parallel opposing photon fields to deliver 30 Gy in 1.5 Gy fractions to the hemithorax and 40 Gy to the mediastinum, subsequently boosting to 54 Gy areas of particular concern (positive surgical margins or positive nodes). Used after EPP and adjuvant chemotherapy, this technique obtained acceptable toxicities rates, but local failure rates high at 35%. The reason for this high local failure rates has to be related with the delivered doses, probably insufficient to control the disease [23].

The availability of more advanced and precise technologies, like intensity modulated radiotherapy (IMRT) gave new push to the use of RT after EPP. IMRT in the setting of MPM have two possible advantages: escalation of dose to the target and reduction of toxicity. Indeed, this technique allows the increase of dose homogeneity in the target volume, while in the same time allowing a better sparing of organs at risk. A boost to areas at high risk of disease persistence or relapse can be integrated in the treatment plan and delivered simultaneously or subsequently.

Initially, dosimetric comparisons between 2D/3D technique and IMRT were conducted and published, confirming superiority of IMRT in terms of dose homogeneity [22, 24]. On the other side, IMRT increases the volumes receiving low doses, indeed one dosimetric study showed that the volume of contralateral lung receiving 20 Gy (V20) was increased by 7.2% ($p < 0.01$) with IMRT [25].

In one of the first clinical experiences of IMRT after EPP, results were very encouraging, with a 100% local control at 9 months in 28 patients treated with 45–50 Gy with boosts to 60 Gy to areas of clinical concern or positive margins [26]. On the other side, the subsequent clinical series raised a significant alarm due to the high reported rates of severe pneumonitis, even fatal in some cases [27–29]. From these experiences, stricter dose constraints for contralateral lung were derived and then applied in the clinical practice, paying special attention to mean lung dose, V5 and V20. Today the more commonly used dose constraints for lung after EPP include: mean lung dose <8 Gy, V5 < 60%, V10 < 50%, and V20 < 7% [30].

With similar constraints, pneumonitis rates decreased significantly [28, 31]. In the series by Thieke et al. [32] just two cases of pneumonitis were reported (one G3), with no G4 or G5 toxicity. Sixty two patients were treated with neoadjuvant chemotherapy, EPP and adjuvant IMRT, for a median dose of 48–54 Gy. Authors reported median OS, LRC, and DC times of 20.4, 31.4, and 21.4 months, respectively. The 1-, 2-, 3-year OS rates were 63, 42, 28%, the LRC rates were 81, 60, 40%, and the DC rates were 62, 48, 41%.

Also in the M.D. Anderson experience on 86 consecutive patients treated with EPP and adjuvant IMRT [33], pneumonitis rates were acceptable, with five patients experiencing grade 5 pulmonary toxicity (one pneumonitis and two bronchopleural fistulae). Median prescribed dose to PTV was 45–50 Gy in 25 daily fractions. Rates of locoregional recurrence-free survival, distant metastasis-free survival, and overall survival were 88%, 55%, and 55% at 1 year and 71%, 40%, and 32% at 2 years.

A phase II two-institution study evaluated adjuvant hemithoracic intensity-modulated pleural radiation therapy in 27 patients [34]. Radiation pneumonitis developed in 29.6% (six grade 2; two grade 3). Median progression-free and overall survival were 12.4 and 23.7 months, respectively. In resectable patients with MPM who received chemotherapy and intensity-modulated pleural radiation therapy, 2-year overall survival was 59%.

More advanced evolutions of IMRT, like volumetric modulated arc therapy (VMAT) and helical tomotherapy (HT) have been studied more recently in this setting. These techniques can be regarded as improvement of step and shoot IMRT, therefore they should facilitate more precise dose delivery to the tumor with increased sparing of normal tissues, potentially allowing further dose escalation and/or reduced toxicities. Various dosimetric comparisons between VMAT, HT, and IMRT have been published. Both studies from Scorsetti et al. and Kawashima et al. showed that VMAT can guarantee the same PTV coverage and dose homogeneity with less monitor units and a faster delivery, particularly important considering the target volume of a post-EPP MPM [35, 36], as shown in Fig. 14.1. A better sparing of organs at risk, particularly contralateral lung, can be obtained both with VMAT and HT, when compared with IMRT [37, 38].

Clinically, VMAT was tested on 15 patients at Hiroshima University Hospital [39] with results substantially comparable with those obtained with IMRT, in terms of toxicity and local control. Also for HT, clinical experiences have been published. A French cohort of 24 patients was treated with a dose of 50 Gy to the surgical cavity and 57 Gy to areas of clinical concern as identified by FDG-PET. With an excellent dosimetry and acceptable toxicities, 1 and 2 year overall survival were 65% and 36%, respectively [40, 41].

Table 14.3 summarizes the cited studies of RT after EPP.

Despite these technological advances, there has been a decreasing interest toward the use of RT after EPP in the last years. There are two main reasons for this. The first is the decreased use of EPP, in favor of lung conservative approaches, like pleurectomy/decortication (PD). Indeed, due to the results of the MARS trial [42] and to recent meta-analysis showing that EPP was associated with significantly higher short-term mortality rates than PD (4.5% vs. 1.7%; $p < 0.05$), patients treated with such invasive surgery are becoming more and more rare [43]. The second reason is related to the results of the SAKK 17/04 trial [44]. This was a multicenter phase II study, divided in two parts. In the first part, patients were treated with neoadjuvant chemotherapy and EPP. In the second part, patients who completed the previous treatment and underwent a macroscopic complete resection were randomized to receive RT (IMRT or 3D) or not.

The RT dose was 45–46 Gy in either 1.75, 1.8, or 2 Gy fractions, while areas at high risk for

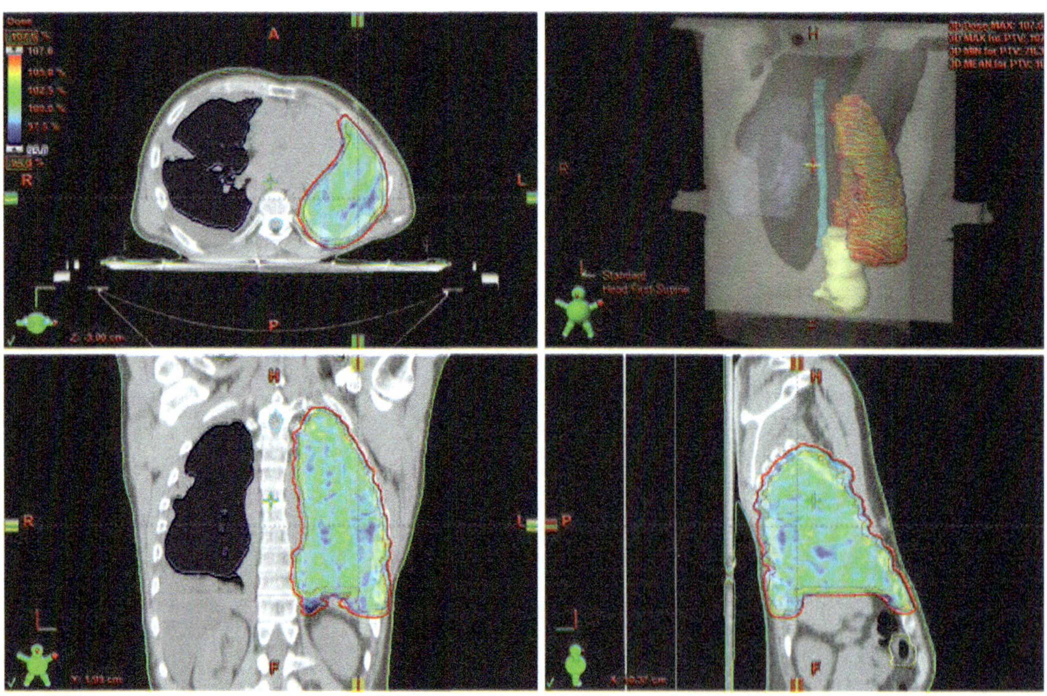

Fig. 14.1 Dose distribution (95% of prescribed dose) after EPP using *VMAT technique*

Table 14.3 Selected studies of RT after EPP

Author	No. of patients	RT technique	RT dose	Toxicity ≥ G3	Local recurrence	Distant recurrence	Overall survival
Rusch et al. [21]	54	Combined photon–electron	41.4/54 Gy	Not reported	10%	64.8%	33.8 months (stage I–II) 10 months (stage III–IV)
Baldini et al. [23]	35	Moderate dose photon technique	30/40/54 Gy	Not reported	35%	Not reported	22 months (median)
Ahamad et al. [26]	28	IMRT	45–50/60 Gy	Not reported	0	Not reported	65% at 1 year
Miles et al. [28]	13	IMRT	40–55 Gy	23%	46%	31%	77%
De Perrot et al. [31]	30	IMRT	50/60 Gy	20%	17%	37%	59 months if pN0 12 months is pN2
Thieke et al. [32]	62	IMRT	48–54 Gy	1.6%	Median locoregional control: 31.4 months	Median distant control: 21.4 months	63% at 1 year
Gomez et al. [33]	86	IMRT	45–50/55–60 Gy	Skin 17.4% Gastrointestinal 16.3% Heart 2.3% Lung 11.6%	16%	59%	55% at 1 year
Kimura et al. [39]	15	VMAT	54 Gy	20%	33.3%	46.7%	43% at 1 year
Helou et al. [41]	29	Helical Tomotherapy	50 Gy	20.7%	Not reported	Not reported	65% at 1 year

local relapse were boosted to 55.9–57.6 Gy. Fifty four patients were randomized, 25 out of 27 in the RT arm completed the treatment. Relapse free survival was 9.4 months in the RT arm (95% CI 6.5–11.9) and 7.6 months in the control arm (95% CI 4.5–10.7), although the difference was not statistically significant. The authors concluded that these data did not support the routine use of hemithoracic radiotherapy for MPM after neoadjuvant chemotherapy and EPP, further reducing data and studies in this field. However, data of the SAKK trial have been thoroughly discussed. Indeed, the trial was underpowered due to slow patient accrual and to patient dropout. For this reason it was closed earlier and did not enroll the right number of patients. Considering the technical difficulties of RT after EPP, the lack of central review and the absence of any dosimetry data biased the evaluation of the benefit that can be derived from RT in this setting. Lastly, not all patients were treated with IMRT, none with more advanced technologies [45].

For all this reason, the role of RT after EPP is still controversial. Indeed, the more recent ASCO guidelines still confirm that hemithoracic adjuvant radiation therapy may be offered to patients who undergo non–lung-sparing cytoreductive surgery (EPP), preferably in centers of excellence with experience in this modality for mesothelioma [11].

Dose of radiation for adjuvant treatment following EPP should be 50–54 Gy in 1.8–2 Gy daily fractions, with 60 Gy delivered to macroscopic residual tumors, if any. The clinical target volume (CTV) for post-EPP RT should encompass the entire pleural surface (entire surgical bed of the whole hemithorax), and any potential sites with microscopic residual disease. The gross tumor volume (GTV) should include any grossly visible tumor, with surgical clips indicative of gross residual tumor; elective nodal irradiation (regional nodes) is not recommended. The planning target volume (PTV) should consider target motion and daily set-up errors, with margins of expansion dependent on single patient and single institution assessment [46].

14.5 Adjuvant RT After Pleurectomy/Decortication (P/D)

Due to the severe perioperative complications and the significantly high short-term mortality rates, EPP was progressively less used in the clinical practice in favor of lung-sparing surgery [47]. Radical pleurectomy/decortication (P/D) is a lung-sparing surgery for MPM that represents a cytoreductive treatment option with the aim of removing all gross disease [48]. This operation includes macroscopic removal of the parietal and visceral pleural layer, sparing the underlying lung. When the diaphragm or pericardium is also resected, it should be called an extended P/D. The high possibility of having a residual microscopic disease after this kind of surgery makes the radiation treatment targeting the ipsilateral pleura a suggested adjuvant therapy.

As for radiotherapy after EPP, also in this scenario the continuous improvement of the technologies improved the opportunity to deliver effective radiotherapy for disease control.

Conventional radiotherapy techniques (2D/3D) were historically associated with high incidence of radiation pneumonitis in absence of a real survival advantage [49, 50].

With the introduction of IMRT, clinical outcome and toxicities had significant changes. The first published retrospective analysis of 36 patients who received pleural IMRT at a median dose of 46.8 Gy (range 41.4–50.4 Gy) following PD (56%) or no surgery (44%), reported a 20% grade 3 or greater pneumonitis risk, including one death. The median survival in resectable patients was 26 months [51]. In 2014, the same group analyzed retrospective data from 67 patients treated with definitive or adjuvant hemithoracic IMRT. Local failure remained the dominant form of failure pattern, with a 1- and 2-year actuarial failure rate of 56% and 74%, respectively. Patients treated with adjuvant hemithoracic pleural IMRT after P/D experienced a significantly longer time to local (1- and 2-year actuarial in-field local failure rates of 43% and 60% vs. 66% and 83%, respectively) and distant (1- and 2-year actuarial distant failure rates of 28% and 40% vs. 51% and 65%, respectively) failure than patients treated with definitive pleural IMRT [52]. The subsequent IMPRINT phase II study assessed prospectively the safety of IMRT after chemotherapy and PD delivering a total dose of 50.4 Gy in 28 fractions [34]. At a median follow up of 21.6 months, 27 patients were evaluable. Two patients experienced grade 3 radiation pneumonitis, all recovered after corticosteroid initiation, and no grade 4 or 5 radiation-related toxicities were recorded.

More recently, again the Memorial Sloan-Kettering Cancer Center, published the results of hemithoracic IMRT compared with conventional RT in patients treated with P/D. They analyzed 209 patients who underwent P/D and adjuvant RT (131 who received conventional RT and 78 who received IMPRINT) and demonstrated a statistically improved OS in the IMRT arm (median 20.2 vs. 12.3 months [$p = 0.001$]). Higher Karnofsky performance score, epithelioid histological type, macroscopically complete resection, and use of chemotherapy/IMPRINT were found to be significant factors for longer OS in multivariate analysis. Grade 2 or higher esophagitis were observed in fewer patients after IMPRINT than after conventional RT (23% vs. 47%) [53].

These selected studies of RT after PD are reported in Table 14.4.

These encouraging results favored the use of new forms of highly conformal radiotherapy, such as volumetric modulated arc therapy (VMAT) and helical tomotherapy (HT). These techniques were able to spare organs at risk (OaRs) better than IMRT with an adequate PTV coverage (Fig. 14.2).

A dosimetric comparison of VMAT and IMRT confirmed an appropriate PTV cover-

Table 14.4 Selected studies of RT after PD

Author	No. of patients	RT technique	RT dose	Toxicity ≥ G3	Local recurrence	Distant recurrence	Overall survival
Gupta et al. [50]	123	Combined photon–electron	42,5 Gy (median)	28% (grade 3–4) 1.6% (grade 5)	56%	11%	23% at 2 year
Minatel et al. [54]	28 (20 after PD or extended PD)	Tomotherapy	50–60 Gy	7% (pneumonitis) 3.5% (thrombocytopenia) 3.5% (chest wall pain)	Not reported	Not reported	Not reported
Rimner et al. [52]	28 (PD or extended PD)	IMRT	45–50.4 Gy	Not reported	43% at 1 year 66% at 2 year	28% at 1 year 51% at 2 year	89% at 1 year 82% at 2 year
Shaikh et al. [53]	209 (131 vs. 78)	Conventional photon/ electron vs. IMRT	45 Gy	four cases vs. two cases (toxicity-related deaths)	47% vs. 60% at 2 year (no significant difference)	Not reported	20% vs. 42% at 2 year

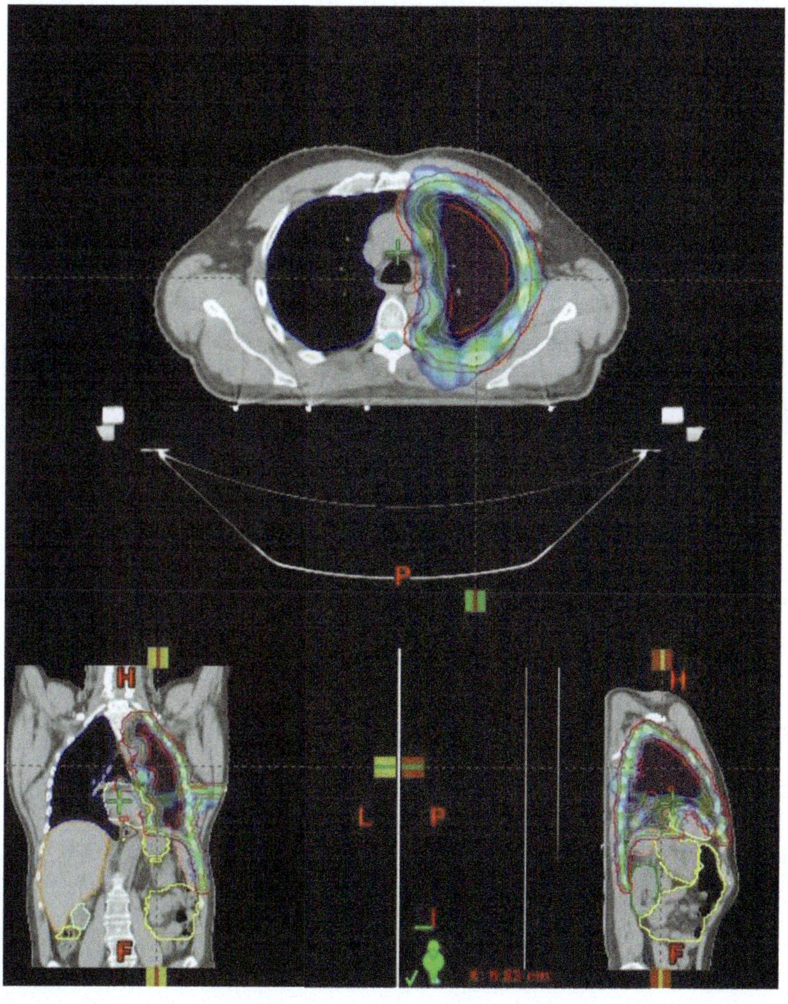

Fig. 14.2 Dose distribution (95% of prescribed dose) after PD using *VMAT technique*

age for both techniques but a better sparing of OaRs, less MU and a shorter delivery time for VMAT. This planning study involved 20 patients; the prescription dose per fraction was 1.8 Gy with a total dose ranged from 50.4 Gy to 46.8 Gy. Main planning objectives for lung and PTV were: contralateral lung, mean dose <8 Gy; PTV D95 = 94%, V95 = 94%, D05 = 115% [55]. A single dosimetric case report was published about the comparison of VMAT and HT [56] and evidenced a better sparing of contralateral lung in the HT planning study (V20, V10, V5: 0%, 2.3%, 17.1% for HT compared to 0%, 14.8%, 65.8% for VMAT).

The first clinical experience to assess the safety of high doses of radiation delivered with tomotherapy in MPM patients with intact lung was reported in 2012. Prospective data of 28 patients who had undergone PD (71%) or biopsy only (29%) were analyzed. Five of the 28 patients (17.8%) experienced severe respiratory symptoms within 5 months after the end of radiotherapy, (grade 2 pneumonitis in three cases, and grade 3 pneumonitis in two cases). No grade >3 respiratory toxicity was reported. Contralateral lung V5 was strongly correlated with the risk of pneumonitis. Patients who developed grade 2 and 3 pneumonitis had a higher contralateral lung V5 (mean V5 = 32%) than those without pneumonitis (mean V5 = 17%) ($p = 0.02$) [54].

In 2014, long term follow up data on the use of high-dose radiotherapy delivered with HT for patients who underwent radical pleurectomy/decortication (P/D) were published. Minatel et al. analyzed 20 consecutive MPM patients enrolled in a prospective study. The clinical target volume was defined as the entire hemithorax excluding the intact lung. The dose prescribed was 50 Gy in 25 fractions, while areas of FDG avidity were simultaneously boosted to 60 Gy. Cisplatin/pemetrexed chemotherapy was administered in 95% of patients. The results were among the best observed in recent studies. At a median follow up of 27 months, the median OS and PFS were 33 and 29 months, respectively, and the Kaplan–Meier estimates of OS at 2 and 3 years were 70% and 49%, respectively. No fatal toxicity was reported. Five cases of grade 3 toxicity were observed (two patients with pneumonitis, one patient with pericardial effusion, one patient with thrombocytopenia and another with pain to the chest wall). Only one patient experienced a grade 4 pericardial effusion [57].

Although the introduction of highly conformal radiotherapy techniques have improved the results in terms of toxicity and clinical outcome, adjuvant radiation treatment after lung-sparing surgery remain particularly challenging due to the risk for radiation pneumonitis, a potentially severe toxicity. Moreover, there are no randomized data about these new technologies. Therefore, the recent ASCO guidelines recommend that hemithoracic adjuvant intensity-modulated radiation therapy may be offered to patients who undergo lung-sparing surgery but only in highly experienced centers, preferably in the context of a clinical trial [11].

14.6 Definitive RT for MPM

The use of RT as definitive treatment for unresectable disease is not suggested anymore. The main limitation to this kind of approach is that the required tumoricidal dose (>60 Gy) is virtually impossible to deliver, without unacceptable risks for the healthy surrounding organs. Data in literature about this issue are generally quite old with single institution experience.

In 1988, Alberts et al. compared outcome for 262 patients treated with various combinations of RT, pleurectomy, and chemotherapy. RT was delivered to the entire hemithorax to doses of 45–80 Gy. All treatment groups had similar outcome, with a median survival time of 9.6 months; no toxicity data were described [58]. Few years later, Ball and Cruickshank reported on 12 patients treated with "radical RT." Treatment comprised 40 Gy to the entire hemithorax, after which the spinal cord was blocked and the treatment continued to a total dose of 50 Gy. Two patients experienced G5 toxicity (one hepatitis and one myelopathy), median survival time was 9 months [59]. Three different RT schedules were prescribed by Maasilta in 34 patients with unresected mesothelioma: 55 Gy in 2.2-Gy fractions (split course) to the hemithorax

Table 14.5 Selected studies of definitive RT for unresectable MPM

Author	No. of patients	RT dose	Toxicity ≥ G3	Overall survival
Ball and Cruickshank [59]	12	40/50 Gy	16.7%	9 months (median)
Maasilta [49]	34	55/70 Gy	100%	Not reported
Munter et al. [60]	11	40/50 Gy	None reported	18% at 1 year

followed by a boost to gross disease to 70 Gy; 70 Gy to the hemithorax in 1.25 twice daily fractions (split course); and 35 Gy in 1.25 twice daily fractions to the hemithorax with a boost to gross disease using 4-Gy fractions to a total dose of 71 Gy [49]. Pulmonary toxicity up to a total loss of function of ipsilateral lung was described at 12 months, while no data on local control were reported. With more advanced technologies, like IMRT, a report from Heidelberg described 11 patients treated with 40–50 Gy to the gross tumor volume. No severe acute or late effect was recorded, however no indications of efficacy was possible because of the small number of patients and the heterogeneity of the series [60].

A selected series of these cited studies are included in Table 14.5.

Based on these data, definitive RT is not recommended. Select patients with unresectable pleural disease may be considered for hemithoracic pleural IMRT at centers of excellence with expertise in this approach [11].

A different evaluation can be done in case of macroscopic asymptomatic recurrence in previously treated patients. Although no clear data can be derived from the literature, ASCO guidelines suggest that RT may be offered to these patients. Considering the high variability of clinical presentation, dose and fractionation depend on the clinical scenario, prior treatments, currently available treatment options, as well as the patient's wishes. In case of small recurrences, also high-dose hypofractionated stereotactic body radiation therapy could be taken into consideration [11].

14.7 Trimodality Treatment

While the role of each single treatment modality was investigated and the studies have confirmed significant improvements in the administration of systemic therapy, surgery, and radiotherapy, the optimal combination and therapeutic strategy for each individual patients with MPM still remains unclear and debated. The trimodality approach incudes the use of all the three strategies, with timeline and methods that vary significantly from one study to another.

In this scenario, much of the outcome data derive from EPP series.

Five multicenter studies (including three phase II trials) assessed efficacy and feasibility of the trimodality approach [19, 20, 61–63]. The small cohort of patients (range 42–77), the variety of radiotherapy techniques (not reported or 3D/IMRT) and planned radiotherapy dose (from 54 Gy to 60 Gy in 30 fractions), and the absence of control groups and randomization make the overall analysis difficult and not conclusive. Nevertheless, median overall survival rates between 15.5 and 19.9 months are reported, with a favorable prognosis for patients completing EPP (median OS range: 21.9–23 months) and a further survival benefit in patients completing radiotherapy (median OS range: 29.1–39.4 months).

The attempt to analyze a randomized sample of patients in the setting of EPP was represented by the previously cited trial SAKK 17/04. This two part multicenter randomized phase 2 trial had the purpose to assess the effect of high-dose hemithoracic radiotherapy after neoadjuvant chemotherapy and extrapleural pneumonectomy in patients with stage I–III MPM. Fifty-four patients resulted in macroscopically complete resection were randomized to receive RT or not.

The results did not support the use of adjuvant radiotherapy in the subset of patients selected for the randomization because there was no benefit in terms of locoregional relapse-free survival [44]. However, the SAKK trial conclusions cannot be considered conclusive due to the previously cited limitations of the study.

Table 14.6 Trimodality treatment (TMT) in the setting of both EPP and PD

Author	Krug et al. [20]	Van Schil et al. [19]	Minatel et al. [57]	Hasegawa et al. [62]	Rimner et al. [34]
Date of publication	2009	2010	2014	2016	2016
Type of study	Phase II	Phase II	Prospective study	Prospective feasibility	Phase II
Number of patients	77	59	20	42	45
Induction chemotherapy	Cisplatin-pemetrexed	Cisplatin-pemetrexed	Cisplatin-pemetrexed	Cisplatin-pemetrexed	Cisplatin-pemetrexed (26) or carboplatin-pemetrexed (18)
Type of surgery	EPP	EPP	PD	EPP	PD
Planned RT dose	54 Gy (30 × 1.8 Gy)	54 Gy (30 × 1.8 Gy)	50/60 Gy (25 × 2/2.4 Gy)	54 Gy (30 × 1.8 Gy)	50,4 Gy (28 × 1.8 Gy)
RT technique	Matched photon/electrons IMRT	3D conformal IMRT	Tomotherapy	3D conformal with matched photon/electrons	IMRT
Median survival for patients completing TMT	29.1 months	33 months	33 months	39.4 months	23.7 months

Other clinical data on the role of trimodality approach derive from the PD series, although less numerous.

The aforementioned experiences of the Memorial Sloan-Kettering Cancer Center and Minatel and colleagues reported encouraging data in terms of overall survival and toxicity, using IMRT and tomotherapy, respectively, after platinum/pemetrexed chemotherapy (in neoadjuvant or adjuvant setting) and lung-sparing surgery [53, 57].

Table 14.6 summarizes the main data from studies that investigated trimodality treatment in the setting of both EPP and PD, particularly regarding reported median OS.

More data are needed.

14.8 Future Directions

Intensity-modulated proton therapy (IMPT) is a new technique that, exploiting the physical characteristics of protons, could be used to escalate doses to complex target volumes, such as MPM, while improving the organs at risk sparing. Clinical data on IMPT for MPM are still lacking. Pan et al. reported on four patients with epithelioid MPM, treated with IMPT. Treatment tolerance was good, IMPT produced lower mean doses to the contralateral lung, heart, esophagus, liver, and ipsilateral kidney, with increased contralateral lung sparing when mediastinal boost was required for nodal disease [64]. More recently, Lee et al. described three cases of MPM treated with IMPT to 54 Gy after EPP, with two patients receiving boosts to 66 and 60 Gy. Treatment was well tolerated and patients received doses to OARs markedly lower than those seen in comparison VMAT or IMRT photon plans [65]. These results were comparable with dosimetric comparison studies previously published, suggesting that IMPD could reduce the doses received by liver, ipsilateral kidney, heart, and contralateral lung [66, 67].

Confirmatory clinical data are required, however protons could represent an interesting option to improve results of RT for MPM.

A completely different approach was tested in a prospective trial conducted at the Princess Margaret Hospital. In their Surgery for Mesothelioma After Radiation Therapy (SMART) trial, the researchers tested the possible role of RT as neoadjuvant treatment before surgery. In this phase I/II trial 25 patients received neoadjuvant accelerated hemithoracic

IMRT (25 Gy in five fractions with a concomitant boost of 5 Gy) followed by EPP within 1 week. IMRT was well tolerated with no grade 3+ toxicities, no perioperative mortality was recorded. Thirteen patients developed grade 3+ surgical complications. One patient (4%) died from treatment-related toxicity (empyema).

After a median follow-up of 23 months (range, 6–51), the cumulative 3-year survival reached 84% in epithelial subtypes compared with 13% in biphasic subtypes [68]. A subsequent report on 62 patients still confirmed very promising survival data, with median overall survival of 36 months. Patients with epithelioid MPM had a median overall and disease-free survival of 51 and 47 months. On the other side, toxicity rates were quite high, since the rate of complications grade 3 or greater was 39% [11]. As highlighted by ASCO experts, this high-risk strategy has not been validated by other institutions and should first be established at centers with significant expertise in the multimodality management of MPM before being used by a wider community. However, the survival rates are really encouraging, therefore research in the neoadjuvant setting should be advised. Indeed, these results are being tested in prospective studies (https://clinicaltrials.gov/ct2/show/NCT02613299, https://clinicaltrials.gov/ct2/show/NCT00797719).

A similar study with neoadjuvant IMRT followed by pleurectomy/decortication is ongoing (https://clinicaltrials.gov/ct2/show/NCT02672033).

A possible explanation for the good results of neoadjuvant IMRT is the activation of an immune response against the tumor after RT, on the basis of similar data in other kind of solid tumors. Therefore, also in MPM, there is an ongoing trial testing the possible benefit of combining RT and immunotherapy in stage IV patients (https://clinicaltrials.gov/ct2/show/NCT03399552).

14.9 Conclusion

The role of RT in MPM remains controversial in all the different scenarios and the future is unclear. Considering the trend toward a less complete surgical resection, it is predictable that adjuvant RT will become more and more necessary for improving locoregional control rates. It is undoubted that RT made dramatic progresses in recent years, due to a previously never seen technological improvement. How these changes will modify and improve RT results in MPM is still to be clarified, although initial clinical data are promising.

Considering the previous failure of almost all randomized trials in MPM due to slow accrual, it is required a major effort from the international community to deliver high quality, multicenter clinical trials, and/or to create large prospective database, in order to generate evidences in this challenging and unfavorable disease.

References

1. Häkkinenm AM, Laasonen A, Linnainmaa K, et al. Radiosensitivity of mesothelioma cell lines. Acta Oncol. 1996;35(4):451–6.
2. Arnold DT, Clive AO. Prophylactic radiotherapy for procedure tract metastases in mesothelioma: a review. Curr Opin Pulm Med. 2017;23(4):357–64.
3. Boutin C, Rey F, Viallat JR. Prevention of malignant seeding after invasive diagnostic procedures in patients with pleural mesothelioma. A randomized trial of local radiotherapy. Chest. 1995;108:754–8.
4. Bydder S, Phillips M, Joseph DJ, et al. A randomised trial of single-dose radiotherapy to prevent procedure tract metastasis by malignant mesothelioma. Br J Cancer. 2004;91:9–10.
5. O'Rourke N, Garcia JC, Paul J, et al. A randomised controlled trial of intervention site radiotherapy in malignant pleural mesothelioma. Radiother Oncol. 2007;84:18–22.
6. Lee C, Bayman N, Swindell R, Faivre-Finn C. Prophylactic radiotherapy to intervention sites in mesothelioma: a systematic review and survey of UK practice. Lung Cancer. 2009;66:150–6.
7. Nagendran M, Pallis A, Patel K, Scarci M. Should all patients who have mesothelioma diagnosed by video-assisted thoracoscopic surgery have their intervention sites irradiated? Interact Cardiovasc Thorac Surg. 2011;13:66–9.
8. Ung YC, Yu E, Falkson C, et al. The role of radiation therapy in malignant pleural mesothelioma: a systematic review. Radiother Oncol. 2006;80:13–8.
9. Clive AO, Taylor H, Dobson L, et al. Prophylactic radiotherapy for the prevention of procedure-tract metastases after surgical and large-bore pleural procedures in malignant pleural mesothelioma (SMART): a multicentre, open-label, phase 3, randomized controlled trial. Lancet Oncol. 2016;17:1094–104.

10. Bayman N, Appel W, Ashcroft L, et al. OA 02.03 prophylactic irradiation of tracts (PIT) in patients with pleural mesothelioma: results of a multicenter phase III trial. J Thorac Oncol. 2017;12(11 Suppl 2):S1747.
11. Kindler HL, Ismaila N, Armato SG III, et al. Treatment of malignant pleural mesothelioma: American society of clinical oncology clinical practice guideline. J Clin Oncol. 2018;36(13):1343–73.
12. Macleod N, Price A, O'Rourke N, et al. Radiotherapy for the treatment of pain in malignant pleural mesothelioma: a systematic review. Lung Cancer. 2014;83:133–8.
13. Bissett D, Macbeth FR, Cram I. The role of palliative radiotherapy in malignant mesothelioma. Clin Oncol (R Coll Radiol). 1991;3:315–7.
14. MacLeod N, Chalmers A, O'Rourke N, et al. Is radiotherapy useful for treating pain in mesothelioma?: a phase II trial. J Thorac Oncol. 2015;10:944–50.
15. Ashton M, O'Rourke N, MacLeod N, et al. SYSTEMS-2: a randomized phase II study of radiotherapy dose escalation for pain control in malignant pleural mesothelioma. Clin Transl Radiat Oncol. 2017;8:45–9.
16. Stahel RA, Weder W, Lievens Y, Felip E. Malignant pleural mesothelioma: ESMO clinical practice guidelines for diagnosis, treatment and follow-up. Ann Oncol. 2010;21:126–8.
17. Stewart DJ, Martin-Ucar A, Pilling JE, et al. The effect of extent of local resection on patterns of disease progression in malignant pleural mesothelioma. Ann Thorac Surg. 2004;78:245–52.
18. Yan TD, Tin M, Boyer M, et al. Treatment failure after extrapleural pneumonectomy for malignant pleural mesothelioma. J Thorac Dis. 2009;1:23–8.
19. Van Schil PE, Baas P, Gaafar R, et al. Trimodality therapy for malignant pleural mesothelioma: results from an EORTC phase II multicentre trial. Eur Respir J. 2010;36:1362–9.
20. Krug LM, Pass HI, Rusch VW. Multicenter phase II trial of neoadjuvant pemetrexed plus cisplatin followed by extrapleural pneumonectomy and radiation for malignant pleural mesothelioma. J Clin Oncol. 2009;27:3007–13.
21. Rusch VW, Rosenzweig K, Venkatraman E, et al. A phase II trial of surgical resection and adjuvant high-dose hemothoracic radiation for malignant pleural mesothelioma. J Thorac Cardiovasc Surg. 2001;122:788–95.
22. Yajnik S, Rosenzweig KE, Mychalczak B, et al. Hemithoracic radiation after extrapleural pneumonectomy for malignant pleural mesothelioma. Int J Radiat Oncol Biol Phys. 2003;56:1319–26.
23. Baldini EH, Recht A, Strauss GM, et al. Patterns of failure after trimodality therapy for malignant pleural mesothelioma. Ann Thorac Surg. 1997;63:334–8.
24. Hill-Kayser CE, Avery S, Mesina CF, et al. Hemithoracic radiotherapy after extrapleural pneumonectomy for malignant pleural mesothelioma: a dosimetric comparison of two well-described techniques. J Thorac Oncol. 2009;4:1431–7.
25. Krayenbuehl J, Oertel S, Davis JB, Ciernik IF. Combined photon and electron three-dimensional conformal versus intensity-modulated radiotherapy with integrated boost for adjuvant treatment of malignant pleural mesothelioma after pleuropneumonectomy. Int J Radiat Oncol Biol Phys. 2007;69:1593–9.
26. Ahamad A, Stevens CW, Smythe WR, et al. Promising early local control of malignant pleural mesothelioma following postoperative intensity modulated radiotherapy (IMRT) to the chest. Cancer J. 2003;9:476–84.
27. Allen AM, Czerminska M, Janne PA, et al. Fatal pneumonitis associated with intensity-modulated radiation therapy for mesothelioma. Int J Radiat Oncol Biol Phys. 2006;65:640–5.
28. Miles EF, Larrier NA, Kelsey CR, et al. Intensity-modulated radiotherapy for resected mesothelioma: the Duke experience. Int J Radiat Oncol Biol Phys. 2008;71:1143–50.
29. Rice DC, Smythe WR, Liao Z, et al. Dose-dependent pulmonary toxicity after postoperative intensity-modulated radiotherapy for malignant pleural mesothelioma. Int J Radiat Oncol Biol Phys. 2007;69:350–7.
30. Ashton M, O'Rourke N, Currie S, et al. The role of radical radiotherapy in the management of malignant pleural mesothelioma: a systematic review. Radiother Oncol. 2017;125(1):1–12.
31. de Perrot M, Feld R, Cho BC, et al. Trimodality therapy with induction chemotherapy followed by extrapleural pneumonectomy and adjuvant high-dose hemithoracic radiation for malignant pleural mesothelioma. J Clin Oncol. 2009;27:1413–8.
32. Thieke C, Nicolay NH, Sterzing F, et al. Long-term results in malignant pleural mesothelioma treated with neoadjuvant chemotherapy, extrapleural pneumonectomy and intensity-modulated radiotherapy. Radiat Oncol. 2015;10:267.
33. Gomez DR, Hong DS, Allen PK, et al. Patterns of failure, toxicity, and survival after extrapleural pneumonectomy and hemithoracic intensity-modulated radiation therapy for malignant pleural mesothelioma. J Thorac Oncol. 2013;8(2):238–45.
34. Rimner A, Zauderer MG, Gomez DR, et al. Phase II study of hemithoracic intensity-modulated pleural radiation therapy (IMPRINT) as part of lung sparing multimodality therapy in patients with malignant pleural mesothelioma. J Clin Oncol. 2016;34:2761–8.
35. Scorsetti M, Bignardi M, Clivio A, et al. Volumetric modulation arc radiotherapy compared with static gantry intensity-modulated radiotherapy for malignant pleural mesothelioma tumor: a feasibility study. Int J Radiat Oncol Biol Phys. 2010;77:942–9.
36. Kawashima M, Ozawa S, Haga A, et al. Comparison of total MU and segment areas in VMAT and step-and-shoot IMRT plans. Radiol Phys Technol. 2013;6:14–20.
37. Sterzing F, Sroka-Perez G, Schubert K, et al. Evaluating target coverage and normal tissue sparing in the adjuvant radiotherapy of malignant pleural mesothelioma: helical tomotherapy compared with step-and-shoot IMRT. Radiother Oncol. 2008;86:251–7.

38. Dumane V, Yorke ED, Rosenzweig KE. Volumetric-modulated arc therapy for malignant pleural mesothelioma after pleurectomy/decortication. Appl Radiat Oncol. 2016;5:28–37.
39. Kimura T, Doi Y, Nakashima T, et al. Clinical experience of volumetric modulated arc therapy for malignant pleural mesothelioma after extrapleural pneumonectomy. J Radiat Res. 2015;56:315–24.
40. Giraud P, Sylvestre A, Zefkili S, et al. Helical tomotherapy for resected malignant pleural mesothelioma: dosimetric evaluation and toxicity. Radiother Oncol. 2011;101:303–6.
41. Helou J, Clement-Colmou K, Sylvestre A, et al. Helical tomotherapy in the treatment of malignant pleural mesothelioma: the impact of low doses on pulmonary and oesophageal toxicity. Cancer Radiother. 2013;17:755–62.
42. Treasure T, Lang-Lazdunski L, Waller D, et al. Extra-pleural pneumonectomy versus no extrapleural pneumonectomy for patients with malignant pleural mesothelioma: clinical outcomes of the mesothelioma and radical surgery (MARS) randomized feasibility study. Lancet Oncol. 2011;12:763–72.
43. Taioli E, Wolf AS, Flores RM. Meta-analysis of survival after pleurectomy decortication versus extrapleural pneumonectomy in mesothelioma. Ann Thorac Surg. 2015;99:472–80.
44. Stahel RA, Riesterer O, Xyrafas A, et al. Neoadjuvant chemotherapy and extrapleural pneumonectomy of malignant pleural mesothelioma with or without hemithoracic radiotherapy (SAKK 17/04): a randomised, international, multicentre phase 2 trial. Lancet Oncol. 2015;16:1651–8.
45. Thomas R, Piccolo F, Miller D, et al. Intrapleural fibrinolysis for the treatment of indwelling pleural catheter-related symptomatic loculations: a multicenter observational study. Chest. 2015;148:746–51.
46. Novello S, Pinto C, Torri V, et al. The third Italian consensus conference for malignant pleural mesothelioma: state of the art and recommendations. Crit Rev Oncol Hematol. 2016;104:9–20.
47. Hiddinga BI, van Meerbeeck JP. Surgery in mesothelioma–where do we go after MARS? J Thorac Oncol. 2013;8:525–9.
48. Sugarbaker DJ, Wolf AS. Surgery for malignant pleural mesothelioma. Expert Rev Respir Med. 2010;4:363–72.
49. Maasilta P. Deterioration in lung function following hemithorax irradiation for pleural mesothelioma. Int J Radiat Oncol Biol Phys. 1991;20:433–8.
50. Gupta V, Mychalczak B, Krug L, et al. Hemithoracic radiation therapy after pleurectomy/decortication for malignant pleural mesothelioma. Int J Radiat Oncol Biol Phys. 2005;63:1045–52.
51. Rosenzweig KE, Zauderer MG, Laser B, et al. Pleural intensity-modulated radiotherapy for malignant pleural mesothelioma. Int J Radiat Oncol Biol Phys. 2012;83:1278–83.
52. Rimner A, Spratt DE, Zauderer MG, et al. Failure patterns after hemithoracic pleural intensity modulated radiation therapy for malignant pleural mesothelioma. Int J Radiat Oncol Biol Phys. 2014;90:394–401.
53. Shaikh F, Zauderer MG, von Reibnitz D, et al. Improved outcomes with modern lung-sparing trimodality therapy in patients with malignant pleural mesothelioma. J Thorac Oncol. 2017;12:993–1000.
54. Minatel E, Trovo M, Polesel J, et al. Tomotherapy after pleurectomy/ decortication or biopsy for malignant pleural mesothelioma allows the delivery of high dose of radiation in patients with intact lung. J Thorac Oncol. 2012;7:1862–6.
55. Dumane V, Yorke E, Rimner A, Rosenzweig GK. SU-E-T-595: comparison of volumetric modulated arc therapy (VMAT) and static intensity modulated radiotherapy (IMRT) for malignant pleural mesothelioma in patients with intact lungs/post pleurectomy. Med Phys. 2012;39:3842.
56. Yip K, James H, Lee V, Harden S. Hemi-thoracic irradiation post-cytoreductive surgery for mesothelioma: a theoretical planning study using tomotherapy and volumetric modulated arc therapy. Clin Oncol. 2011;23(3):S58.
57. Minatel E, Trovo M, Polesel J, et al. Radical pleurectomy/decortication followed by high dose of radiation therapy for malignant pleural mesothelioma. Final results with long-term follow-up. Lung Cancer. 2014;83:78–82.
58. Alberts AS, Falkson F, Goedhals L, et al. Malignant pleural mesothelioma: a disease unaffected by current therapeutic measures. J Clin Oncol. 1988;6:527–35.
59. Ball DL, Cruickshank DG. The treatment of malignant mesothelioma of the pleura: review of a 5-year experience, with special reference to radiotherapy. Am J Clin Oncol. 1990;13:4–9.
60. Munter MW, Christian T, Nikoghosyan A, et al. Inverse planned stereotactic intensity modulated radiotherapy (IMRT) in the palliative treatment of malignant mesothelioma of the pleura: the Heidelberg experience. Lung Cancer. 2005;49(S1):S83–6.
61. Weder W, Stahel RA, Bernhard J, et al. Multicenter trial of neo-adjuvant chemotherapy followed by extrapleural pneumonectomy in malignant pleural mesothelioma. Ann Oncol. 2007;18:1196–202.
62. Hasegawa S, Okada M, Tanaka F, et al. Trimodality strategy for treating malignant pleural mesothelioma: results of a feasibility study of induction pemetrexed plus cisplatin followed by extrapleural pneumonectomy and postoperative hemithoracic radiation (Japan Mesothelioma Interest Group 0601 Trial). Int J Clin Oncol. 2016;21:523–30.
63. Federico R, Adolfo F, Giuseppe M, et al. Phase II trial of neoadjuvant pemetrexed plus cisplatin followed by surgery and radiation in the treatment of pleural mesothelioma. BMC Cancer. 2013;13:22.
64. Pan HY, Jiang S, Sutton J, et al. Early experience with intensity modulated proton therapy for lung-intact mesothelioma: a case series. Pract Radiat Oncol. 2015;5(4):e345–53.
65. Lee H, Zeng J, Bowen SR, Rengan R. Proton therapy for malignant pleural mesothelioma: a three case series

describing the clinical and dosimetric advantages of proton-based therapy. Cureus. 2017;9(9):e1705.

66. Chang JY, Li H, Zhu XR, et al. Clinical implementation of intensity modulated proton therapy for thoracic malignancies. Int J Radiat Oncol Biol Phys. 2014;90:809–18.
67. Lorentini S, Amichetti M, Spiazzi L, et al. Adjuvant intensity-modulated proton therapy in malignant pleural mesothelioma. A comparison with intensity-modulated radiotherapy and a spot size variation assessment. Strahlenther Onkol. 2012;188:216–25.
68. de Perrot M, Feld R, Leighl NB, et al. Accelerated hemithoracic radiation followed by extrapleural pneumonectomy for malignant pleural mesothelioma. J Thorac Cardiovasc Surg. 2016;151:468–73.

Role of Chemotherapy in the Management of Malignant Pleural Mesothelioma

15

Letizia Gianoncelli, Maria Bonomi, and Giovanni Luca Ceresoli

15.1 Introduction

Malignant pleural mesothelioma (MPM) is a rare disease that typically arises from mesothelial surfaces of the pleural cavity, mostly related to previous occupational or environmental asbestos exposure. Its incidence has already peaked in the United States, whereas is still increasing in European countries, in which the incidence is expected to peak around 2020 [1, 2]. Due to its pattern of growth, MPM is generally diagnosed at a late stage and only a minority of patients can be suitable for radical surgery. Therefore, systemic treatments remain the standard of care for most patients [3].

Extensive research in mesothelioma therapeutics has been conducted in the last decades, especially focusing on antiangiogenic drugs and immunotherapies, but a number of small phase II studies and a few phase III trials with several targeted therapies have failed to improve patient outcome, with a median overall survival (mOS) ranging from 12 to 18 months after diagnosis. In particular, despite the recent results of the MAPS trial [4], the use of bevacizumab in addition to standard chemotherapy for the treatment of advanced MPM has not been approved in most countries. Therefore cytotoxic chemotherapy remains the only universally accepted therapeutic option with a proven survival benefit. Following the results of two large randomized phase III trials, doublets with cisplatin and antimetabolites (pemetrexed or raltitrexed) have been established as the standard of care for unresectable MPM [5, 6]. In patients unfit to receive cisplatin, several phase II studies [7, 8] and a large expanded access program [9] have shown that the association of carboplatin and pemetrexed can provide similar activity as compared to cisplatin and pemetrexed, with a simpler administration and perceived lower toxicity.

Unfortunately, almost all patients experience disease progression after initial chemotherapy, but no standard treatments are available in the second-line setting [10]. Therefore, the preferred option in second or further line should be patient enrollment in experimental trials, when available [11]. Alternatively, single-agent chemotherapy with vinorelbine or gemcitabine may be proposed, even though their activity is limited [12]. In the selected subset of patients achieving a prolonged benefit from first-line pemetrexed-platinum treatment, rechallenge with a pemetrexed-based regimen may be a reasonable option [13].

L. Gianoncelli
Division of Thoracic Oncology, European Institute of Oncology, Milan, Italy

Fondazione Buzzi Unicem, Casale Monferrato, Italy
e-mail: letizia.gianoncelli@ieo.it

M. Bonomi
Department of Oncology, Thoracic and GU Oncology Unit, Cliniche Humanitas Gavazzeni, Bergamo, Italy
e-mail: maria.bonomi@gavazzeni.it

G. L. Ceresoli (✉)

Fondazione Buzzi Unicem, Casale Monferrato, Italy

Department of Oncology, Thoracic and GU Oncology Unit, Cliniche Humanitas Gavazzeni, Bergamo, Italy
e-mail: giovanni_luca.ceresoli@gavazzeni.it

G. L. Ceresoli et al. (eds.), *Mesothelioma*, https://doi.org/10.1007/978-3-030-16884-1_15

15.2 Perioperative Chemotherapy

The role of perioperative chemotherapy for the management of MPM is controversial, considering that to date no prospective randomized phase III trial has established yet whether surgery itself, alone, or in combination with radiotherapy, leads to an improvement in survival [14]. Theoretically, as has been proved in other cancers, pre- and postoperative chemotherapy might reduce the risk of local and distant relapse also in MPM. There are no studies comparing neo-adjuvant versus adjuvant treatment in this setting. Most published studies regarding perioperative chemotherapy are small, single Institution trials; enrolled patients are therefore very heterogeneous as concerns stage, histology, chemotherapy regimens, and surgical techniques. Neo-adjuvant treatment has the potential to downstage the tumor and make radical surgical resection more feasible [15, 16]. Furthermore, induction treatment has the advantage of earlier treatment delivery and better compliance, and of "real time" identification of sensitive versus resistant disease [17]. This is particularly relevant, because offers the possibility to select for resection only patients not progressing during chemotherapy, avoiding unnecessary surgical procedures for those with rapidly evolving disease [18]. Finally, the availability of large surgical samples at the time of surgery gives the chance to study biological impact of therapy. On the other hand, the main disadvantages of induction chemotherapy are a potentially higher surgical mortality and morbidity and a delay of surgery [19, 20].

Several nonrandomized studies have evaluated a tri-modality treatment consisting of induction chemotherapy, followed by surgery and subsequent RT, with mOS ranging from 12.8 to 33.5 months and a median disease free survival (mDFS) ranging from 8.6 to 21.6 months [21, 22]. In an early trial, the combination of platinum and gemcitabine was identified as an active regimen in MPM [23] and this led to several small prospective trials using this regimen as neo-adjuvant therapy followed by surgery and radiotherapy [24–27]. Following the encouraging results of the phase III study of pemetrexed and cisplatin versus cisplatin alone in the first-line setting [5], this combination became the preferred induction regimen in prospective multimodality trials [18, 28–30]. In particular, Krug et al. performed a multicenter phase II trial of neo-adjuvant cisplatin plus pemetrexed followed by extra-pleural pneumonectomy (EPP) and adjuvant radiotherapy [18]. The reported mOS was 16.8 months in the overall population (95% CI, 13.6–23.2 months), and 29.1 months in patients completing all therapy. The radiologic response rate (RR) was 32.5% (95% CI, 22.2–44.1), and of note it was associated with an increased median OS [26.0 months compared with 13.9 months for patients with stable or progressive disease ($p = 0.05$)].

Despite the promising results of single arm phase II studies, the effectiveness of trimodality approach (specifically addressed in a dedicated chapter of this book), has not been confirmed in randomized trials. The Mesothelioma and Radical Surgery (MARS) trial randomized 50 patients to EPP following platinum-based chemotherapy, plus postoperative hemithoracic radiotherapy in selected cases, versus standard therapy alone (chemotherapy only) [31]. No survival nor quality of life benefit from EPP was shown; on the contrary, patients in the no-EPP group had a better outcome (HR adjusted for prognostic variables 2.75). Additionally, the SAKK 17/04 study, a randomized phase II trial investigating the role of high-dose hemithoracic radiotherapy after neo-adjuvant chemotherapy and EPP, reported no difference in mOS nor in loco-regional relapse-free survival (RFS) between the two groups, with a median loco-regional RFS from surgery of 9.4 months in the radiotherapy group and 7.6 months in the no radiotherapy group [32].

In conclusion, as highlighted in a recently published Cochrane systemic review [33], given the lack of evidence of multimodality treatment effectiveness, these interventions should currently be limited, and the use of perioperative chemotherapy outside clinical trials should be recommended for selected patients only, treated in centers with adequate expertise.

15.3 First-Line Chemotherapy

Several trials have demonstrated that first-line chemotherapy improves survival and quality of life in MPM patients; therefore guidelines strongly suggest to evaluate all patients for chemotherapy [34, 35]. Based on randomized phase III trials, combination of cisplatin, with either pemetrexed or raltitrexed, represent the standard up-front treatment (Table 15.1). Carboplatin is an acceptable alternative to cisplatin and may be better tolerated especially in the elderly population. Several phase II and III clinical trials are investigating the addition of novel agents to pemetrexed/cisplatin therapy, but to date no agent has proved an improvement upon the efficacy of standard chemotherapy.

15.3.1 Pemetrexed–Cisplatin

Despite extensive research into mesothelioma therapeutics, the nature of cytotoxic chemotherapy in clinical practice has remained unchanged since 2003, when the combination chemotherapy with cisplatin plus pemetrexed has become the standard first-line therapy worldwide [5].

The role of cisplatin–pemetrexed combination was initially assessed in a Phase I trial in which 11 MPM patients received pemetrexed plus cisplatin, at increasing doses. The results of the trial showed that the combination was safe and active with five patients (45%) experiencing a partial response [36].

Based on this background, the EMPHACIS phase III trial was designed to determine whether pemetrexed–cisplatin was associated with superior survival duration compared with cisplatin alone in the first-line treatment of MPM patients. From April 1999 to March 2001, 456 eligible patients were enrolled in the trial. Of them, 448 (226 receiving pemetrexed–cisplatin, and 222 receiving cisplatin alone) were assessable for efficacy and toxicity.

The mOS for patients treated with pemetrexed–cisplatin was longer than for patients receiving cisplatin alone: 12.1 months versus 9.3 months, with an HR 0.77. As with survival, the median time to progressive disease (mTTP) was significantly longer for patients who received the combination (5.7 months vs. 3.9 months; $p = 0.001$). All responses were partial responses (PRs): 41.3% for pemetrexed/cisplatin patients versus 16.7% for the control group. This study also analyzed the effect of vitamin supplementation with vitamin B12 and folic acid on those regimens. Patients receiving pemetrexed/cisplatin with vitamins had greater improvement in all efficacy parameters than those receiving the same regimen without vitamins. Supplementation enabled patients to receive more cycles of treatment, and this may explain the differences in outcomes.

Regarding quality of life, the previously validated Lung Cancer Symptom Scale for mesothelioma (LCSS-Meso) questionnaire [37, 38] was administered to patients in the EMPHACIS trial, with a 90% completion rate. The overall symptom score favored the combination arm after 6 cycles ($p = 0.004$). By week 12 (4 cycles), a statistically significant improvement in pain, cough, and dyspnea was noted in the pemetrexed plus cisplatin arm. Furthermore, improvements in global quality of life ($p = 0.025$) and fatigue ($p = 0.027$) were reported.

Table 15.1 First-line randomized phase III chemotherapy trials in MPM

Author (ref.)	Regimen	No. of pts	RR (%)	mPFS (m)	mOS (m)
Vogelzang et al. [5]	Cisplatin/pemetrexed	226	41.3	5.7	12.1
	vs.				
	Cisplatin	222	16.7	3.9	9.3
van Meerbeeck et al. [6]	Cisplatin/raltitrexed	126	23.6	5.5	11.4
	vs.				
	Cisplatin	124	13.6	4.0	8.8

Pts patients, *RR* response rate, *m* months, *mPFS* median progression free survival, *mOS* median overall survival

Regarding toxicity, in the pemetrexed/cisplatin arm, grade 3–4 neutropenia (27.9%) and grade 3–4 leukopenia (17.7%) were the most common hematologic toxicities. In both treatment groups, nausea, vomiting, and fatigue were the most commonly reported nonlaboratory toxicities, with 88% of events reported as grade 3.

15.3.2 Raltitrexed–Cisplatin

After promising phase II trials exploring the activity of raltitrexed, another antimetabolite, either as a single agent or in combination with a platinum agent, a Phase III randomized study promoted by the European Organization for the Research and Treatment of Cancer (EORTC) and the National Cancer Institute of Canada (NCI Canada) was performed [6]. A total of 250 patients were randomized to receive cisplatin 80 mg/m^2 with raltitrexed 3 mg/m^2 or cisplatin alone, both regimens administered every 3 weeks. In 213 patients with measurable disease, the combination of cisplatin and raltitrexed achieved a RR of 24% versus 11% in the control arm. A mOS of 11.4 versus 8.8 months and a 1-year survival rate of 46% versus 40% were reported in the experimental and in the control arm, respectively. These differences were of borderline statistical significance, probably because the study was underpowered. A separate analysis on quality of life pointed out that dyspnea was significantly improved in patients who received the combination [39].

To date no univocal data exist to prefer pemetrexed or raltitrexed in combination with cisplatin. Woods et al. [40] estimated the relative efficacy of raltitrexed plus cisplatin and pemetrexed plus cisplatin in an adjusted indirect comparison. A cost-effectiveness model was used to assess the lifetime costs and health outcomes associated with the two regimens. Raltitrexed plus cisplatin and pemetrexed plus cisplatin were not found to be statistically significantly different with respect to overall RR, PFS, or OS. The cost-effectiveness analysis found raltitrexed plus cisplatin to be cost-effective, offering marginally higher quality adjusted life years and life years at a substantially lower total cost. In another recently published paper [41], the efficacy and safety of the two combinations were compared using the model of the network meta-analysis of randomized clinical trials. Again, no significant differences emerged in an indirect comparison. However, although based on this evidence the combination of raltitrexed and cisplatin should be considered an active alternative to the pemetrexed regimen for patients with advanced MPM, it is not approved for this indication in many countries.

15.3.3 Pemetrexed–Carboplatin

Considering the toxicity profile of cisplatin and the great number of patient unfit to receive this drug, especially in a palliative setting, carboplatin is often used in clinical practice to reduce the risk of toxicity.

In a nonrandomized phase II trial [7], 102 MPM patients were treated with pemetrexed 500 mg/m^2 and carboplatin AUC5 every 21 days for a median of 6 cycles. All patients received vitamin B12 and folate supplementation. Two patients had complete responses (CR), and 17 had a PR, for a total RR of 18.6% (95% CI 11.6–27.5%). Stable disease (SD) was registered in 47% (95% CI 37.1–57.2%) of patients. mOS was 12.7 months, with mTTP of 6.5 months. Overall, 19.6% of patients developed grade 3–4 neutropenia, and 11.7% experienced grade 3–4 anemia. Treatment was generally well tolerated; in the 96 patients receiving over 2 cycles of pemetrexed and carboplatin, relative dose intensity was 97% for pemetrexed and 98% for carboplatin.

Another phase II study included 76 patients with measurable advanced MPM, treated with the same combination. A RR of 25% was reached (21% of PR and 4% of CR). Median TTP was 8 months and mOS was 14 months. Grade 3 hematological toxicity was observed in 36 (47.3%) patients; grade 4 hematological toxicity in 5 (6.5%) [8].

Furthermore, a large expanded access program collected data from 1704 chemotherapy-naive MPM patients, of whom 843 received pemetrexed plus cisplatin and 861 pemetrexed plus carboplatin AUC5 [9]. The analysis demonstrated similar

RR for carboplatin plus pemetrexed compared with cisplatin plus pemetrexed (21.7% vs. 26.3%), as well as similar mTTP (6.9 vs. 7 months) and 1-year OS rate (64% vs. 63.1%).

Considering the high rate of MPM diagnosis in elderly patients (≥70 years), a pooled retrospective analysis using individual patient data from the two previously described phase II trials [7, 8] was performed, in order to compare the efficacy, toxicity, and survival outcomes of carboplatin–pemetrexed in elderly versus younger patients. A total of 178 patients with an Eastern Cooperative Oncology Group performance status (ECOG PS) of ≤2 were included. Median age was 65 years (range 38–79), with 48 patients ≥70 years (27%). Grade 3–4 hematological toxicity was worse in ≥70 versus <70-year-old patients, with neutropenia observed in 25.0 versus 13.8% (p = 0.11), anemia in 20.8 versus 6.9% (p = 0.01), and thrombocytopenia in 14.6 versus 8.5% (p = 0.26). Nonhematological toxicity was mild and similar in the two groups. No significant difference was observed in terms of overall DCR (60.4 vs. 66.9%, p = 0.47), TTP (7.2 vs. 7.5 months, p = 0.42), and OS (10.7 vs. 13.9 months, p = 0.12) [42].

Based on these results, although not supported directly by a randomized comparison, carboplatin in combination with pemetrexed may be considered a valid alternative option if cisplatin toxicity represents a concern, as in elderly patients or patients with comorbidities [34, 35].

15.3.4 Other Combinations

Based on results of a preclinical study in murine mesothelioma models showing an additive antitumor effect of gemcitabine when administered with cisplatin [43], this combination was evaluated in several phase II trials. In the first single institution phase II study by Byrne et al., 10 of the 21 enrolled patients (47%) exhibited a partial response. Nine of the ten patients had epithelioid mesothelioma, and one patient had a mixed histology. The estimated mPFS was 25 weeks and the estimated mOS was 41 weeks (10 months) [23]. Subsequently, a multicenter phase II trial evaluated 53 patients with MPM. Seventeen of the 52 assessable patients (33%) achieved a PR and 31 (60%) exhibited a SD. The mTTP was 6.4 months, with a mOS of 11.2 months. Major toxicities were hematological, limiting the mean relative dose intensity of gemcitabine to 75% [44]. In both trials, patients were treated with cisplatin at 100 mg/m^2 i.v. day 1 and gemcitabine 1000 mg/m^2 i.v. days 1, 8, and 15 of a 28-day cycle, delivered for a maximum of 6 cycles.

Lower response rates were observed in other trials using this combination. In a study performed in the Netherlands, cisplatin was given at 80 mg/m^2 along with gemcitabine 1250 mg/m^2 every 21 days [45]. Four PRs were seen in 25 patients (16%). Median TTP was 6 months, with a mOS of 9.6 months. In an ECOG study in which cisplatin was administered at 75 mg/m^2 along with gemcitabine 1250 mg/m^2 on day 1 and 8, a PR was seen in nine patients (26%), with a mTTP of 8 months and a mOS of 13 months. An open-label phase II Southwest Oncology Group (SWOG) study enrolled 50 chemotherapy naïve MPM patients to receive gemcitabine 1000 mg/m^2 and cisplatin 30 mg/m^2 on days 1, 8, and 15 of a 28-day cycle, until progression of disease or 2 cycles beyond complete response. The RR was 12% and SD was seen in 50% of patients. Median OS was 10 months (95% CI 7–15 months), with a mPFS of 6 months. Sixteen patients experienced grade 4 toxicity, mainly hematological [46]. A modified schedule with divided dose of cisplatin combined with gemcitabine was also studied by Utkan et al. in 26 patients with epithelioid MPM or peritoneal mesothelioma, who received cisplatin 35 mg/m^2 and gemcitabine 800 mg/m^2 on days 1 and 8 of a 3-week cycle, up to maximum 6 cycles [47]. A PR was observed in 6 patients (23.1%) and 13 patients (50%) had SD. Median TTP and OS were 4 and 19.5 months, respectively. Toxicity was mild. Overall, divided dose of cisplatin and gemcitabine appeared to be an active and well-tolerated regimen. The use of carboplatin instead of cisplatin in association with gemcitabine was investigated in a multicenter phase II study that enrolled 50 patients. A PR was reported in 26% of patients. Median OS was 66 weeks with an mPFS of 40 weeks [48].

Cisplatin has also been tested in mesothelioma patients in combination with other older chemotherapeutic agents, such as anthracyclines, mitomycin, methotrexate, and vinblastine [49–53]. However, no possible advantage of these regimens, either in terms of activity or toxicity, was observed, as compared to the combinations of cisplatin with pemetrexed, raltitrexed, or gemcitabine.

15.4 Second-Line Chemotherapy

Unfortunately, nearly all MPM patients progress during or after first-line treatment. Second-line chemotherapy has been increasingly used in clinical practice, because patients frequently still have a good PS at the time of disease progression. Consequently, a number of clinical studies have been conducted to test different regimens in the salvage setting, but none of them provided definitive results to guide decisions regarding second-line therapy in MPM. Therefore, the role of systemic treatment in MPM patients progressing after the standard first-line regimens has yet to be proved, and the optimal regimens remain to be determined [11].

15.4.1 Pemetrexed Rechallenge

The role of pemetrexed in second-line setting was evaluated in a phase III trial where 243 pemetrexed-naive MPM patients were randomly assigned to receive pemetrexed 500 mg/m^2 plus best supportive care (BSC) every 21 days or BSC alone, after first-line treatment [54]. A statistical improvement in median PFS, TTP, and time to treatment failure (TTF) was seen in the pemetrexed arm. No statistically significant difference was detected in terms of mOS (8.4 vs. 9.7 months for pemetrexed vs. BSC, HR 0.95), probably because a higher percentage of patients in BSC arm received chemotherapy after discontinuation (51.7% vs. 28.5% in pemetrexed arm) and postdiscontinuation therapy was initiated earlier in BSC arm (4.3 vs. 15.7 months in pemetrexed arm).

For selected patients treated upfront with platinum-pemetrexed-based regimen, who have reached a prolonged TTF, retrospective analyses suggest a possible role for rechallenge with pemetrexed (Table 15.2). Razak et al. reported a case series of four patients pretreated with pemetrexed/carboplatin, with an extraordinarily prolonged PFS after first-line chemotherapy. With second-line pemetrexed combined with carboplatin or cisplatin, one of these patients achieved a new PR and three had prolonged SD [55]. In a retrospective analysis of 17 patients treated in a single center, a clinical benefit was observed in 65% of cases. All patients were pretreated with platinum/pemetrexed, five had also received a chemotherapy with platinum and gemcitabine before the availability of pemetrexed. Retreatment consisted mainly of carboplatin and pemetrexed or single-agent pemetrexed. Toxicity was mild [56]. Bearz et al.

Table 15.2 Retreatment with pemetrexed-based chemotherapy in MPM

Author (ref.)	Study type	Retreatment regimen	No. of pts	RR	DCR (%)	mTTP/PFS	mOS
Razak et al. [55]	Retrospective	Pem/plat	4	25%	100	NR	NR
Serke and Bauer [56]	Retrospective	Pem/plat	17	NR	65	NR	NR
Bearz et al. [57]	Retrospective	Pem	9	17%	67	5.1 m	13.6 m
		Pem/plat	21				
Ceresoli et al. [13]	Observational	Pem	15	19%	48	3.8 m	10.5 m
		Pem/plat	16				
Zucali et al. [58]	Retrospective	Pem	11	NR	71	6.2 m	10.6 m
		Pem/plat	31				

Pts patients, *RR* response rate, *DCR* disease control rate, *m* months, *mTTP* median time to progression, *mPFS* median progression free survival, *mOS* median overall survival, *Pem/plat* pemetrexed and platinum containing regimen, *Pem* single-agent pemetrexed

reported results of pemetrexed rechallenge in 30 patients from seven Italian centers in a retrospective study [57]. Mesothelioma histology was epithelioid in 28 cases and mixed in 2. All patients received first-line chemotherapy with pemetrexed plus a platinum compound (cisplatin 21 and carboplatin 9), achieving PR in 15 cases and SD in the remaining 15. Response duration was at least 6 months. The rechallenge chemotherapy was single-agent pemetrexed in nine patients and combination with platinum in the remaining (5 with cisplatin and 16 with carboplatin). Five patients (16.7%) obtained a PR, 15 a SD (50%), and 10 progressed on rechallenge. The mTTP was similar between single-agent pemetrexed (4 months) and the combination with platinum (5.7 months). The mOS was 13.6 months. In an observational study, Ceresoli et al. evaluated pemetrexed rechallenge in MPM patients that had progressed after at least 3 months from the end of first-line chemotherapy. First-line treatment was pemetrexed plus carboplatin in 27 cases or pemetrexed plus cisplatin in 4 patients [13]. Eighteen patients received pemetrexed rechallenge as second-line treatment, while the remaining were treated in subsequent lines, after therapy with vinorelbine or gemcitabine. Rechallenge was pemetrexed monotherapy in 15 and combination with platinum in 16 cases. One patient obtained a complete response and five a PR. Response rate was 19% in patients retreated with pemetrexed alone and 48% in patients receiving a rechallenge combination with platinum. Median PFS and OS were 3.8 months and 10.5 months, respectively. Significantly longer PFS and OS were observed in those patients who achieved a disease control longer than 12 months following first-line treatment. Finally, Zucali and colleagues reported results of a retrospective survey of second-line chemotherapy in 181 patients with MPM [58]. Among patients treated with a first-line pemetrexed-based chemotherapy, 42 received a pemetrexed rechallenge. Patients retreated with pemetrexed had a better disease control as compared to those treated at relapse with different chemotherapeutic agents (70.7% vs. 52%, respectively). Rechallenge was pemetrexed alone in 11 and the combination with a platinum compound in 31 patients. Median PFS (6.4 vs. 2.4 months; $p = 0.003$) and mOS (13.4 vs. 4.2 months; $p < 0.001$) were significantly longer in patients retreated with the combination of pemetrexed with platinum as compared to single-agent pemetrexed. However, the retrospective nature of this study does not allow any final conclusion since patients receiving combination were younger, with a better performance status and had obtained a better response to first-line chemotherapy.

Although retreatment with pemetrexed-based chemotherapy in selected MPM patients may be a valuable strategy, clinicians should be aware of the high incidence of hypersensitivity reactions to carboplatin in this setting. In a small study on 18 patients receiving retreatment with pemetrexed/carboplatin, 6 (33%) experienced a hypersensitivity reaction to carboplatin after a median of 9 cycles (range 8–13) and of 18.5 months (range 13–45) after first carboplatin administration [59]. All adverse reactions were classified as grade 2 and were easily managed with steroids and antihistaminics; carboplatin administration was omitted in subsequent cycles. In case of retreatment after first-line pemetrexed/carboplatin, single-agent pemetrexed should be considered. Alternatively, if patients are retreated with the same combination, premedication and desensitization strategies should be implemented.

15.4.2 Vinorelbine

Unfortunately, most patients progressing after pemetrexed/platinum are not candidate to pemetrexed rechallenge, and due to advanced age and comorbidity may be excluded from clinical trials of second or further-line therapy. In this contest, as reported in several guidelines and consensus papers on MPM, vinorelbine (as single agent or in combination with gemcitabine) may represent a therapeutic option in this setting (Table 15.3). Two different retrospective surveys, conducted in the phase III pemetrexed/cisplatin trial population [65] and in a "real-world" setting [58], reported the use of vinorelbine as second-line therapy in 9.5–10.5% of treated patients.

Table 15.3 Vinorelbine-based chemotherapy as second and beyond line therapy in MPM

Author (ref.)	Study design	Regimen	No. of pts	Setting	RR (%)	DCR	mTTP/ PFS	mOS (m)
Stebbing et al. [60]	Prospective, phase II	VNR i.v.	63	Second line	16	84%	NR	9.6
Zucali et al. [61]	Retrospective	VNR i.v.	59	58% second line	13	49%	2.3 m	6.2
				42% third line				
Zauderer et al. [12]	Retrospective	VNR i.v.	45	53% second line	0	25%	2.5 m	5
				46% third line				
Sørensen et al. [62]	Retrospective	VNR or	15	Second line	7	NR	2.3 m	2.5
Zucali et al. [63]	Prospective/ observational	GEM/VNR i.v.	30	Second line	10	43%	2.8 m	10.9
Toyokawa et al. [64]	Retrospective	GEM/VNR i.v.	17	82% second line	18	82%	6.0 m	11.2
				18% third line				

Pts patients, *RR* response rate, *DCR* disease control rate, *m* months, *TTP* time to progression, *mPFS* median progression free survival, *mOS* median overall survival, *VNR* vinorelbine, *GEM* gemcitabine, *i.v.* intravenous, *or* oral

Single-agent vinorelbine was found to be moderately active in a single center prospective phase II trial [60] and in several retrospective analyses [12, 61, 62], with RRs ranging between 0% and 18%, and a tolerable toxicity profile. In their prospective study, Stebbing et al. assessed the safety and efficacy of weekly vinorelbine (each cycle consisting of 30 mg/m^2 for 6 weeks) in 63 patients progressing during or after one previous line of chemotherapy, including pemetrexed and cisplatin. Most patients had ECOG PS of 0–1, and median age was 59 years. A PR was reported in 10 patients (16%) and SD in 43 (68%), with a mOS of 9.6 months (95% CIs 7.3–11.8). The median interval between the end of first-line chemotherapy and the start of second-line vinorelbine was 6 months. Grade 3–4 neutropenia was observed in 55% of patients; 17% experienced grade 3–4 anemia. Constipation and peripheral neuropathy occurred in 11% and 8% of the study population, respectively.

Zucali et al. retrospectively evaluated the activity and toxicity of vinorelbine in 59 consecutive pemetrexed-pretreated MPM patients, with predominantly epithelioid histology (89.9%) and a median age of 69 years (range 45–80) [61]. Vinorelbine, at a standard dose of 25 mg/m^2 i.v. on days 1, 8, and every 21 days, was administered in second (57.6%) or further line setting (42.4%), for a maximum of 6 cycles. Patients included in this analysis were generally good responders to first-line treatment, with a first-line PFS longer than 6 months in 56% of cases and ten patients only (16.9%) progressing during first line. With vinorelbine, a PR was achieved in 9 patients (15%) and SD was observed in 20 patients (34%), with an overall control rate of 49%. Median PFS and OS were 2.3 and 6.2 months, respectively. Of note, no difference was observed in terms of disease control rate, PFS, and OS according to gender, histology, age, line of vinorelbine therapy, and response to first-line treatment. Hematologic toxicity was mild, with grade 3 or 4 neutropenia observed in five patients (8.4%). No cases of febrile neutropenia were reported. Nonhematologic toxicity was generally mild, with grade 2 fatigue in 17 (28.8%) and constipation in 7 (11.8%) patients. Similarly, Zauderer and colleagues [12] conducted a retrospective analysis of 45 MPM pretreated patients who received vinorelbine, in second (53.3%), or further line (46.7%), at 25 mg/m^2 i.v. on days 1 and 8 in a 3-week cycle. Eighty percent of patients were previously treated with a combination of pemetrexed and a platinum compound, 47% underwent surgery, and 31% radiation therapy. Median age was 66 years (range 41–85) and histology was epithelioid in 67%, sarcomatoid in 18%, and biphasic in 16% of patients. Responses were evaluated according to modified RECIST criteria by a blinded radiologist, and no complete or partial response were reported; SD was achieved in 20 cases (43%). Median PFS and OS were 1.7 and 5.4 months, respectively. Consistently with other reported studies, the toxicity profile of this regimen was acceptable. Grade 3–4 neutropenia was reported in 16% and neutropenic fever in three patients (7%). Six patients (13%) discontinued vinorelbine due to toxicity.

Vinorelbine is also available as an oral compound, which may be more convenient in the palliative setting, mainly for pretreated and elderly patients. Oral vinorelbine in second-line treatment of MPM patient was evaluated in a small prospective study by Sørensen and colleagues [62]. Oral vinorelbine was administered at 80 mg/mq day 1 and 8 every 3 weeks in 15 patients with poor prognostic characteristics (nonepithelioid histology in 47% and ECOG PS 2 in 33% of patients) and a median age of 69 years (range 42–73). PR was achieved in one patient (7%), mPFS was 2.3 and mOS 4.5 months. Grade 4 leukopenia and thrombocytopenia were registered in 20% and 7% of patients, with three cases of febrile neutropenia. One toxic death was reported. A phase Ia/Ib trial, designed to confirm safety and evaluate efficacy of a metronomic oral vinorelbine schedule, was designed in a cohort of pretreated MPM patients, but no result has been reported so far [66].

15.4.3 Gemcitabine

Single-agent gemcitabine showed modest activity in chemonaïve MPM patients in early trials, with RRs ranging from 7 to 31% [67, 68]. Based on these results, a few studies have investigated the efficacy of second-line gemcitabine-based chemotherapy regimens.

In a retrospective multicenter survey in Italian MPM patients [58], single-agent gemcitabine was the most used second-line treatment in pemetrexed-pretreated cases (10.5%). A French retrospective study [69] reported a mOS of 12.2 months for second-line chemotherapy using gemcitabine alone or with oxaliplatin or pemetrexed in pemetrexed-pretreated patients with MPM. Xhantopoulos et al. reported a mOS of 24.3 weeks for the combination of gemcitabine plus oxaliplatin in the same population [70]. Furthermore, the efficacy of second-line gemcitabine plus docetaxel was evaluated in a single institution phase II trial with a mOS of 16.2 months [71]. In a study by Pasello and colleagues [72] patients were pretreated with cisplatin/pemetrexed or carboplatin/pemetrexed; most had been previously submitted to surgery in a multimodality treatment setting. Chemotherapy was gemcitabine associated with the alternative platinum compound with respect to first line, for 3–6 cycles. Response was assessable in 15 patients; 10 (67%) showed SD. Symptoms improved in 8 (53%) cases. In the intent-to-treat population mOS was 28 weeks and mTTF 15 weeks. Observed toxicities were grade 3–4 thrombocytopenia in 53%, grade 3 anemia in 20%, and grade 3 neutropenia in 40% of patients. Grade 3 nausea (14%) and asthenia (21%) were the main nonhematological adverse events. Finally, the result of a retrospective study investigating the efficacy of second-line gemcitabine-based chemotherapy in 73 MPM patients progressing after first-line pemetrexed-based combination were reported by Mutlu and colleagues [73]. Median OS values for patients treated with first-line pemetrexed-based regimens plus second-line gemcitabine, evaluated from initial diagnosis, was 20.8 months (17.5–24.1).

Therefore, based on these results and on the good toxicity profile of gemcitabine, despite the lack of solid literature data, single-agent gemcitabine may be considered as an alternative second-line chemotherapy in MPM patients progressing after platinum-pemetrexed.

15.4.4 Vinorelbine Plus Gemcitabine

Considering the results of vinorelbine in the first- and second-line setting of MPM patients, the modest but not negligible effect of gemcitabine in pretreated cases, and the good safety profile of both drugs, the doublet of gemcitabine and vinorelbine was explored.

In a prospective trial, 30 consecutive MPM patients pretreated with one chemotherapy regimen containing pemetrexed alone or combined with a platinum-derivative were enrolled [63]. Gemcitabine at the dose of 1000 mg/m^2 and vinorelbine at the dose of 25 mg/m^2 were administered i.v. on days 1, 8, and every 21 days, for a maximum of 6 cycles or until progression or unacceptable toxicity. Median patient age was 66 years (range 46–85 years). Most patients had an ECOG PS 1 (83%) and epithelioid subtype (70%). A PR was achieved in 3 patients (10%), and 10 patients (33%) had SD. Overall, disease control rate was 43%. The mTTP was 2.8 months (range, 0.6–12.1 months), and mOS was 10.9 months (range, 0.8–25.3 months). Hematologic toxicity was acceptable, with grade 3 or 4 neutropenia occurring in 11% of patients and thrombocytopenia in 4%; no case of febrile neutropenia was observed. Nonhematologic toxicity generally was mild. Disease progression during first-line therapy and a shorter interval from completion of first-line treatment were correlated to shorter TTP and OS after the study therapy. Toyokawa et al. retrospectively evaluated 17 consecutive Japanese patients pretreated with at least one regimen of platinum plus pemetrexed chemotherapy, receiving gemcitabine 1000 mg/m^2 plus vinorelbine 25 mg/m^2 on days 1 and 8 every 3 weeks as second or further line therapy [64]. PR and disease control rate were 18% and 82%, respectively. Median PFS was 6.0 months, whereas mOS was 11.2 months. Grade 3–4 neutropenia and anemia were observed in 41% and 29% of patients, respectively, and one patient experienced febrile neutropenia. Grade 3–4 nonhematologic toxicities included constipation (6%) and phlebitis (6%).

Based on these results, with the limitation of the small number of patients treated with this regimen, treatment with the combination of gemcitabine and vinorelbine does not seem to offer any potential advantage as compared to single-agent vinorelbine or gemcitabine, at the expense of increased toxicity, mainly hematological.

15.5 Conclusion

Cytotoxic chemotherapy represents the only therapeutic option with a proven survival benefit in patients with MPM. Following the results of two large phase III trial, the combination of cisplatin and antimetabolites (pemetrexed or raltitrexed) has been established as the standard of care for unresectable MPM. For elderly patient or for patients unfit to receive this doublet, schedules with carboplatin have been explored, with similar outcomes. Despite extensive efforts in the last decades, no standard treatment is available after progression on platinum-containing regimens. In second-line setting, if clinical trials are not available, single-agent therapy with vinorelbine or gemcitabine should be considered. Alternatively, patients achieving a prolonged benefit from first-line pemetrexed-platinum treatment should be candidate to rechallenge with pemetrexed.

References

1. Bianchi C, Bianchi T. Malignant mesothelioma: global incidence and relationship with asbestos. Ind Health. 2007;45:379–87.
2. Robinson BM. Malignant pleural mesothelioma: an epidemiological perspective. Ann Cardiothorac Surg. 2012;1:491–6.
3. Tsao AS, Wistuba I, Roth JA, Kindler HL. Malignant pleural mesothelioma. J Clin Oncol. 2009;27:2081–90.
4. Zalcman G, Mazieres J, Margery J, et al. Bevacizumab for newly diagnosed pleural mesothelioma in the mesothelioma avastin cisplatin pemetrexed study (MAPS): a randomised, controlled, open-label, phase 3 trial. Lancet. 2016;387:1405–14.
5. Vogelzang NJ, Rusthoven JJ, Symanowski J, et al. Phase III study of pemetrexed in combination with cisplatin versus cisplatin alone in patients with malignant pleural mesothelioma. J Clin Oncol. 2003;21:2636–44.
6. Van Meerbeeck JP, Gaafar R, Manegold C, et al. Randomized phase III study of cisplatin with or without raltitrexed in patients with malignant pleural mesothelioma: an intergroup study of the European Organisation for Research and Treatment of Cancer Lung Cancer Group and the National Cancer Institute of Canada. J Clin Oncol. 2005;23:6881–9.
7. Ceresoli GL, Zucali PA, Favaretto AG, et al. Phase II study of pemetrexed plus carboplatin in malignant pleural mesothelioma. J Clin Oncol. 2006;24:1443–8.

8. Castagneto B, Botta M, Aitini E, et al. Phase II study of pemetrexed in combination with carboplatin in patients with malignant pleural mesothelioma (MPM). Ann Oncol. 2008;19:370–3.
9. Santoro A, O'Brien ME, Stahel RA, et al. Pemetrexed plus cisplatin or pemetrexed plus carboplatin for chemonaïve patients with malignant pleural mesothelioma: results of the international expanded access program. J Thorac Oncol. 2008;3:756–63.
10. Ceresoli GL. Second line treatment in malignant pleural mesothelioma: translating the evidence into clinical practice. Lung Cancer Manag. 2014;3:263–71.
11. Buikhuisen WA, Hiddinga BI, Baas P, van Meerbeeck JP. Second-line therapy in malignant pleural mesothelioma. Lung Cancer. 2015;89:223–31.
12. Zauderer MG, Kass SL, Woo K, et al. Vinorelbine and gemcitabine as second or third-line therapy for malignant pleural mesothelioma. Lung Cancer. 2014;84:271–4.
13. Ceresoli GL, Zucali PA, De Vincenzo F, et al. Retreatment with pemetrexed-based chemotherapy in patients with malignant pleural mesothelioma. Lung Cancer. 2011;72:73–7.
14. Bueno R, Opitz I, IASLC Mesothelioma Taskforce. Surgery in malignant pleural mesothelioma. J Thorac Oncol. 2018;13:1638–54.
15. Weder W, Opitz I. Multimodality therapy for malignant pleural mesothelioma. Ann Cardiothorac Surg. 2012;1:502–7.
16. Cao C, Tian D, Manganas C, et al. Systematic review of trimodality therapy for patients with malignant pleural mesothelioma. Ann Cardiothorac Surg. 2012;1:428–37.
17. Bech C, Sorensen JB. Chemotherapy induced pathologic complete response in malignant pleural mesothelioma: a review and case report. J Thorac Oncol. 2010;5:735–40.
18. Krug LM, Pass HI, Rusch VW, et al. Multicenter phase II trial of neoadjuvant pemetrexed plus cisplatin followed by extrapleural pneumonectomy and radiation for malignant pleural mesothelioma. J Clin Oncol. 2009;27:3007–13.
19. Opitz I, Weder W. Induction therapy for mesothelioma. Semin Thorac Cardiovasc Surg. 2015;27:240–9.
20. Stamatis G. Risks of neoadjuvant chemotherapy and radiation therapy. Thorac Surg Clin. 2008;18:71–80.
21. Pasello G, Ceresoli GL, Favaretto A. An overview of neoadjuvant chemotherapy in the multimodality treatment of malignant pleural mesothelioma. Cancer Treat Rev. 2013;39:10–7.
22. Marulli G, Faccioli E, Bellini A, et al. Induction chemotherapy vs post-operative adjuvant therapy for malignant pleural mesothelioma. Expert Rev Respir Med. 2017;11:649–60.
23. Byrne MJ, Davidson JA, Musk AW, et al. Cisplatin and gemcitabine treatment for malignant mesothelioma: a phase II study. J Clin Oncol. 1999;17:25–30.
24. Weder W, Kestenholz P, Taverna C, et al. Neoadjuvant chemotherapy followed by extrapleural pneumonectomy in malignant pleural mesothelioma. J Clin Oncol. 2004;22:3451–7.
25. Flores RM, Krug LM, Rosenzweig KE, et al. Induction chemotherapy, extrapleural pneumonectomy, and postoperative high-dose radiotherapy for locally advanced malignant pleural mesothelioma: a phase II trial. J Thorac Oncol. 2006;1:289–95.
26. Rea F, Marulli G, Bortolotti L, et al. Induction chemotherapy, extrapleural pneumonectomy (EPP) and adjuvant hemi-thoracic radiation in malignant pleural mesothelioma (MPM): feasibility and results. Lung Cancer. 2007;57:89–95.
27. Weder W, Stahel RA, Bernhard J, et al. Multi-center trial of neo-adjuvant chemotherapy followed by extrapleural pneumonectomy in malignant pleural mesothelioma. Ann Oncol. 2007;18:1196–202.
28. Van Schil PE, Baas P, Gaafar R, et al. Trimodality therapy for malignant pleural mesothelioma: results from an EORTC phase II multicenter trial. Eur Respir J. 2010;36:1362–9.
29. Trousse DS, Avaro JP, D'Journo XB, et al. Is malignant pleural mesothelioma a surgical disease? A review of 83 consecutive extra-pleural pneumonectomies. Eur J Cardiothorac Surg. 2009;36:759–63.
30. Hasegawa S, Okada M, Tanaka F, et al. Trimodality strategy for treating malignant pleural mesothelioma: results of a feasibility study of induction pemetrexed plus cisplatin followed by extrapleural pneumonectomy and postoperative hemithoracic radiation (Japan Mesothelioma Interest Group 0601 Trial). Int J Clin Oncol. 2016;21:523–30.
31. Treasure T, Lang-Lazdunski L, Waller D, et al. Extrapleural pneumonectomy versus no extra-pleural pneumonectomy for patients with malignant pleural mesothelioma: clinical outcomes of the Mesothelioma and Radical Surgery (MARS) randomised feasibility study. Lancet Oncol. 2011;12:763–72.
32. Stahel RA, Riesterer O, Xyrafas A, et al. Neoadjuvant chemotherapy and extrapleural pneumonectomy of malignant pleural mesothelioma with or without emithoracic radiotherapy (SAKK 17/04): a randomised, international, multicentre phase II trial. Lancet Oncol. 2015;16:1651–8.
33. Abdel-Rahman O, Elsayed Z, Mohamed H, Eltobgy M. Radical multimodality therapy for malignant pleural mesothelioma. Cochrane Database Syst Rev. 2018;1:CD012605.
34. Baas P, Fennell D, Kerr KM, et al. Malignant pleural mesothelioma: ESMO clinical practice guidelines for diagnosis, treatment and follow-up. Ann Oncol. 2015;26:31–9.
35. Kindler HL, Ismaila N, Armato SG III, et al. Treatment of malignant pleural mesothelioma: American Society of Clinical Oncology clinical practice guideline. J Clin Oncol. 2018;36:1343–73.
36. Thödtmann R, Depenbrock H, Dumez H, et al. Clinical and pharmacokinetic phase I study of multitargeted antifolate (LY231514) in combination with cisplatin. J Clin Oncol. 1999;17:3009–16.

37. Hollen PJ, Gralla RJ, Liepa AM, et al. Adapting the lung cancer symptom scale (LCSS) to mesothelioma: using the LCSS-Meso conceptual model for validation. Cancer. 2004;101:587–95.
38. Gelhorn HL, Skalicky AM, Balantac Z, et al. Content validity and electronic PRO (ePRO) usability of the lung cancer symptom scale-mesothelioma (LCSS-Meso) in mesothelioma patients. Support Care Cancer. 2018;26:2229–38.
39. Bottomley A, Gaafar R, Manegold C, et al. Short-term treatment-related symptoms and quality of life: results from an international randomized phase III study of cisplatin with or without raltitrexed in patients with malignant pleural mesothelioma: an EORTC Lung-Cancer Group and National Cancer Institute, Canada, Intergroup Study. J Clin Oncol. 2006;24:1435–42.
40. Woods B, Paracha N, Scott DA, Thatcher N. Raltitrexed plus cisplatin is cost-effective compared with pemetrexed plus cisplatin in patients with malignant pleural mesothelioma. Lung Cancer. 2012;75:261–7.
41. Tassinari D, Cherubini C, Tamburini E, et al. Antimetabolites in the treatment of advanced pleural mesothelioma: a network meta-analysis of randomized clinical trials. J Chemother. 2017;29:365–71.
42. Ceresoli GL, Castagneto B, Zucali PA, et al. Pemetrexed plus carboplatin in elderly patients with malignant pleural mesothelioma: combined analysis of two phase II trials. Br J Cancer. 2008;99:51–6.
43. Davidson JA, Robinson BWS. Gemcitabine activity on murine and human malignant mesothelioma cell lines show additive activity in combination with cisplatin. Aust NZ J Med. 1997;27:213.
44. Nowak AK, Byrne MJ, Williamson R, et al. A multicenter phase II study of cisplatin and gemcitabine for malignant mesothelioma. Br J Cancer. 2002;87:491–6.
45. Van Haarst JMW, Baas P, Manegold C, et al. Multicentre phase II study of gemcitabine and cisplatin in malignant pleural mesothelioma. Br J Cancer. 2002;86:342–5.
46. Kalmadi SR, Rankin C, Kraut MJ, et al. Gemcitabine and cisplatin in unresectable malignant mesothelioma of the pleura: a phase II study of the Southwest Oncology Group (SWOG 9810). Lung Cancer. 2008;60:259–63.
47. Utkan G, Büyükçelik A, Yalçin B, et al. Divided dose of cisplatin combined with gemcitabine in malignant mesothelioma. Lung Cancer. 2006;53:367–74.
48. Favaretto AG, Aversa SM, Paccagnella A, et al. Gemcitabine combined with carboplatin in patients with malignant pleural mesothelioma. A multicentric phase II study. Cancer. 2003;97:2791–7.
49. Berghmans T, Lafitte JJ, Paesmans M, et al. A phase II study evaluating the cisplatin and epirubicin combination in patients with unresectable malignant pleural mesothelioma. Lung Cancer. 2005;50:75–82.
50. Chahinian AP, Antman K, Goutsou M, et al. Randomized phase II trial of cisplatin with mitomycin or doxorubicin for malignant mesothelioma by the Cancer and Leukemia Group B. J Clin Oncol. 1993;11:1559–65.
51. Ardizzoni A, Rosso R, Salvati F, et al. Activity of doxorubicin and cisplatin combination chemotherapy in patients with diffuse malignant pleural mesothelioma. An Italian Lung Cancer Task Force (FONICAP) Phase II study. Cancer. 1991;67:2984–7.
52. Hunt KJ, Longton G, Williams MA, et al. Treatment of malignant mesothelioma with methotrexate and vinblastine, with or without platinum chemotherapy. Chest. 1996;109:1239–42.
53. Middleton GW, Smith IE, O'Brien ME, et al. Good symptom relief with palliative MVP (mitomycin-C, vinblastine and cisplatin) chemotherapy in malignant mesothelioma. Ann Oncol. 1998;9:269–73.
54. Jassem J, Ramlau R, Santoro A, et al. Phase III trial of pemetrexed plus best supportive care compared with best supportive care in previously treated patients with advanced malignant pleural mesothelioma. J Clin Oncol. 2008;26:1698–704.
55. Razak AR, Chatten KJ, Hughes AN. Retreatment with pemetrexed-based chemotherapy in malignant pleural mesothelioma (MPM): a second line treatment option. Lung Cancer. 2008;60:294–7.
56. Serke M, Bauer T. Pemetrexed in second-line therapy in patients with malignant pleural mesotelioma. J Clin Oncol. 2007;25(18 Suppl):18198.
57. Bearz A, Talamini R, Rossoni G, et al. Re-challenge with pemetrexed in advanced mesothelioma: a multi-institutional experience. BMC Res Notes. 2012;5:482.
58. Zucali PA, Simonelli M, Michetti G, et al. Second-line chemotherapy in malignant pleural mesothelioma: results of a retrospective multicenter survey. Lung Cancer. 2012;75:360–7.
59. Stinco S, Ripa C, La Spina CM, et al. High incidence of hyper-sensitivity reactions in patients with malignant pleural mesothelioma re-treated with carboplatin/pemetrexed. Proceedings of IMIG Conference; 2012.
60. Stebbing J, Powles T, McPherson K, et al. The efficacy and safety of weekly vinorelbine in relapsed malignant pleural mesothelioma. Lung Cancer. 2009;63:94–7.
61. Zucali PA, Perrino M, Lorenzi E, et al. Vinorelbine in pemetrexed-pretreated patients with malignant pleural mesothelioma. Lung Cancer. 2014;84:265–70.
62. Sørensen JB, Urbanska E, Langer SW, Aamdal E. Second-line oral vinorelbine following first-line platinum and pemetrexed in malignant pleural mesothelioma. Eur J Clin Med Oncol. 2012;4:6–13.
63. Zucali PA, Ceresoli GL, Garassino I, et al. Gemcitabine and vinorelbine in pemetrexed-pretreated patients with malignant pleural mesothelioma. Cancer. 2008;112:1555–61.
64. Toyokawa G, Takenoyama M, Hirai F, et al. Gemcitabine and vinorelbine as second-line or beyond treatment in patients with malignant pleural mesothelioma pretreated with platinum plus pemetrexed chemotherapy. Int J Clin Oncol. 2014;19:601–6.

65. Manegold C, Symanowski J, Gatzemeier U, et al. Second-line (post-study) chemotherapy received by patients treated in the phase III trial of pemetrexed plus cisplatin versus cisplatin alone in malignant pleural mesothelioma. Ann Oncol. 2005;16:923–7.
66. Barlesi F, Imbs DC, Tomasini P, et al. Mathematical modeling for Phase I cancer trials: a study of metronomic vinorelbine for advanced non-small cell lung cancer (NSCLC) and mesothelioma patients. Oncotarget. 2017;8:47161–6.
67. Van Meerbeeck BP, Debruyne C, et al. A phase II study of gemcitabine in patients with malignant pleural mesothelioma. Cancer. 1999;85:2577–82.
68. Kindler HL, Millard F, Herndon JE II. Gemcitabine for malignant mesothelioma: a phase II trial by the Cancer and Leukemia Group B. Lung Cancer. 2001;31:311–7.
69. Margery J, Riviere F, Planchard D, et al. Second-line therapy in patients with malignant pleural mesothelioma. A French retrospective study (2005–2006). Rev Pneumol Clin. 2010;66:255–9.
70. Xanthopoulos A, Bauer TT, Blum TG, et al. Gemcitabine combined with oxaliplatin in pretreated patients with malignant pleural mesothelioma: an observational study. J Occup Med Toxicol. 2008;18:34.
71. Tourkantonis I, Makrilia N, Ralli M, et al. Phase II study of gemcitabine plus docetaxel as second-line treatment in malignant pleural mesothelioma: a single institution study. Am J Clin Oncol. 2011;34:38–42.
72. Pasello G, Nicotra S, Marulli G, et al. Platinum-based doublet chemotherapy in pre-treated malignant pleural mesothelioma (MPM) patients: a mono-institutional experience. Lung Cancer. 2011;73:351–5.
73. Mutlu H, Gündüz S, Karaca H, et al. Second-line gemcitabine-based chemotherapy regimens improve overall 3-year survival rate in patients with malignant pleural mesothelioma: a retrospective survey. Med Oncol. 2014;31:74.

16 Targeting Angiogenesis in Malignant Pleural Mesothelioma

Arnaud Scherpereel

16.1 Introduction

Malignant pleural mesothelioma (MPM) is an aggressive cancer issued from pleural mesothelial cells, usually associated with previous asbestos exposure. Although MPM is considered as a rare cancer, its incidence is still increasing in many Western countries, and it is not expected to peak before the 2020s. Moreover, asbestos is still not banned worldwide (Russia, Kazakhstan, India, China…) and a pandemic of asbestos-related cancers can be feared in the next decades, according to the 2013 WHO predictions [1–3].

The management of MPM is tricky due to the limited therapeutic options and the frequent failure or early relapse of patients under chemotherapy. Very few patients are potential candidates to "radical" surgery and multimodal treatment [4]. First-line chemotherapy by antifolate, pemetrexed, and platinum (cisplatin or carboplatin) (Cis/Pem or Carbo/Pem) has been already the international standard of care for the last 15 years [4–9]. However, based on phase III randomized trial data [10] and data later obtained from control arms in other trials, the median overall survival (mOS) with pemetrexed/platinum (P/P) does not exceed 16 months, with the best outcome in patients with epithelioïd MPM subtype. Finally, there is no recommended treatment after failure of frontline chemotherapy [4–6] even if anti-PD-1 ± anti-CTLA-4 antibodies were recently proposed following the exciting results of the IFCT MAPS-2 trial assessing Nivolumab ± Ipilimumab as the second of third-line treatment in this setting [11]. Usual second-line or beyond chemotherapy drugs, such as vinorelbine or gemcitabine, did very poorly in the literature [12] with mOS not exceeding 6 months. Thus, innovative treatments are urgently needed for MPM patients. After promising results in non-small cell lung cancer, strategies involving therapies targeting tumor angiogenesis were assessed in MPM [13].

Tumor (neo)angiogenesis, a process of formation and maintenance of (neo)vessels, is crucial for tumor growth and spreading, as suggested by Folkman in 1971 [14]. Its start (angiogenic switch) and its development are regulated by various signaling proteins including mainly vascular endothelial growth factor (VEGF), released by various cell types including tumor cells, interacting with its receptor (VEGFR). The VEGF family includes three receptors (VEGFR-1, VEGFR-2, and VEGFR-3) and five ligands (VEGF-A, VEGF-B, VEGF-C, VEGF-D, and placental growth factor). VEGFR-2 is the main regulator of angiogenesis and is activated by VEGF-A [15]. Hypoxia is the main stimulus of angiogenic switch, regulating angiogenesis by the hypoxia-inducible factor-1

A. Scherpereel (✉)
Pulmonary and Thoracic Oncology Department, Univ Lille, CHU Lille, Lille, France

French National Network of Clinical Expert Centers for Malignant Pleural Mesothelioma Management (MESOCLIN), Lille, France
e-mail: arnaud.scherpereel@chru-lille.fr

G. L. Ceresoli et al. (eds.), *Mesothelioma*, https://doi.org/10.1007/978-3-030-16884-1_16

(HIF-1). HIF-1 is induced by various signals and an adaptive response to the stress. In the light of recent major data of antitumor immunotherapies, it is of high importance to remind that hypoxia may be responsible for tumor angiogenesis but also for some immunosuppressive effects directly on effector T cells or indirectly on myeloid cells, and promoting PD-L1 expression on tumor cells [16, 17].

Angiogenesis plays an important role in malignant mesothelioma. In a mouse model, intraperitoneal injection of crocidolite asbestos fibers was found to be involved in peritoneal mesothelioma with the formation of neovessels surrounding asbestos fibers as soon as 2 weeks after their injection, underlining angiogenesis as one of the earliest events in mesothelioma pathogenesis. Moreover, malignant mesothelioma cell lines produce and release high amounts of proangiogenic factors (VEGF…) compared to the normal mesothelial cells and fibroblasts. MPM cells express VEGFR-1 and VEGFR-2 at their surface. The blockade of VEGFRs with monoclonal antibodies inhibits mesothelioma cell growth. Thus, VEGF promotes tumor angiogenesis, but is also an autocrine and paracrine growth factor for MPM cells. Tumor samples from MPM patients exhibited elevated expression of proangiogenic factors such as VEGF (as well as VEGF receptors), platelet-derived growth factor (PDGF), and fibrocyte growth factors (FGF)-1 and FGF-2 [18], correlated with increased intratumoral microvessel density and worse patient survival [18–21].

Different drugs have been proposed to target angiogenesis. The anti-VEGF-A monoclonal antibody, bevacizumab, was first approved in 2004 by the United States Food and Drug Administration (FDA). Several antiangiogenic molecules have been developed, including tyrosine kinase inhibitors (TKI, targeting VEGFR-2, and other pathways), such as sorafenib, sunitinib, pazopanib, axitinib, vandetanib, regorafenib, and lenvatinib [22], or even the VEGFR-2 inhibitor, cediranib.

The different mechanisms of VEGF inhibition are depicted in Fig. 16.1.

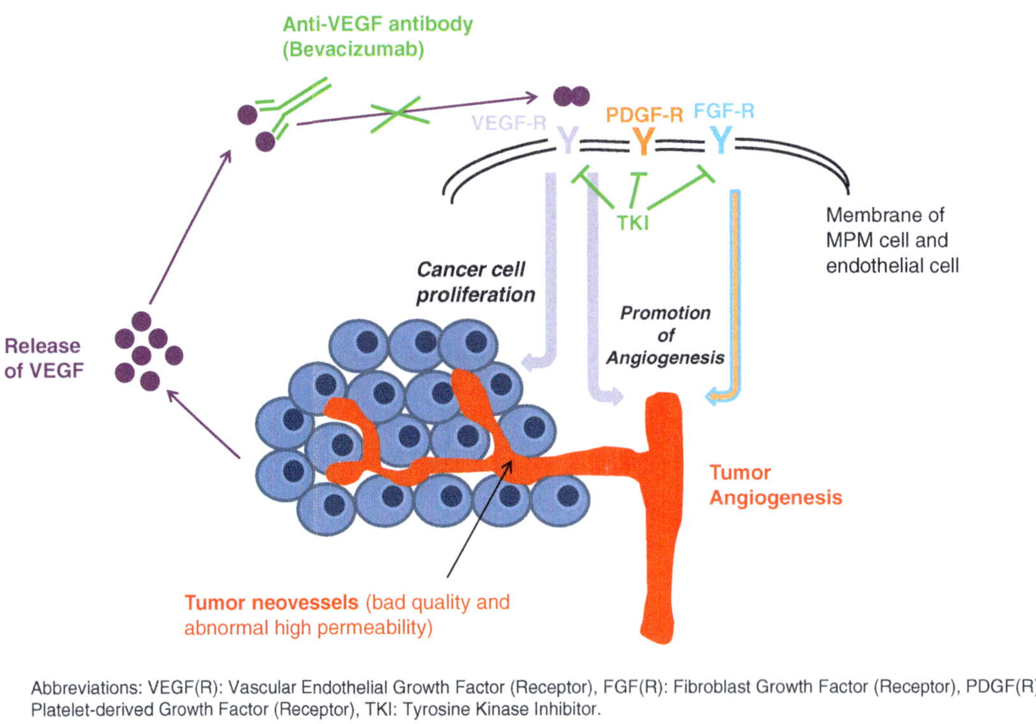

Fig. 16.1 Simplified scheme of antiangiogenic drugs (+ICI?) in malignant pleural mesothelioma. *VEGF(R)* vascular endothelial growth factor (receptor), *FGF(R)* fibroblast growth factor (receptor), *PDGF(R)* platelet-derived growth factor (receptor), *TKI* tyrosine kinase inhibitor

Thus, several antiangiogenic agents have been assessed in MPM patients, alone or in combination with standard first-line chemotherapy (Cis/Pem or Carbo/Pem), and/or as maintenance treatment. The main results of these drugs are summarized in Table 16.1 [15, 23].

16.1.1 Anti-VEGF Antibody/Bevacizumab

Bevacizumab is a recombinant humanized monoclonal immunoglobulin antibody against VEGF-A ligand. It is presently approved for use in different metastatic cancers, combined with chemotherapy, including cervical, colorectal, non-small cell lung cancer (nonsquamous histologic subtypes for NSCLC), ovarian, fallopian tube, primary peritoneal, and renal cell carcinomas. Bevacizumab is also approved as a monotherapy in the treatment of refractory glioblastoma.

Bevacizumab (15 mg/m^2 every 21 days) was initially assessed in a phase II trial in MPM patients, previously treated with systemic chemotherapy, in combination with erlotinib, an oral EGFR tyrosine kinase inhibitor (150 mg daily) [33]. The trial was negative with only half of the patients (12 out of 24) achieving stable disease (SD), without any objective response observed. The median time to progression (TTP) was 2.2 months, and the median OS was 5.8 months. The efficacy of bevacizumab-based combinations across trials in MPM is summarized in Table 16.1 [15, 23, 34].

Bevacizumab was tested in combination with first-line chemotherapy in a randomized, double-blind, placebo-controlled phase II trial [35]. Patients ($n = 115$) had gemcitabine (1250 mg/m^2; days 1 and 8) plus cisplatin (75 mg/m^2; day 1) with bevacizumab (15 mg/m^2; day 1) or placebo every 21 days. There was no benefit in bevacizumab arm vs. placebo arm in terms of response rate (RR; 24.5% vs. 21.8%), median progression-free survival (mPFS; 6.9 vs. 6.0 months, $p = 0.88$), or mOS (15.6 vs. 14.7 months, $p = 0.91$), respectively. Pretreatment plasma VEGF level had no predictive value but a prognostic value was found: higher baseline plasma VEGF levels were associated with a worse outcome (PFS and OS). However, a large number of patients received second-line pemetrexed in the placebo arm, likely decreasing the potential difference of mOS between the two arms. Moreover, gemcitabine/cisplatin is not currently the optimal standard first-line chemotherapy in MPM, nor the best combination with bevacizumab as already described in NSCLC [13, 36], and due to a potential negative interaction between gemcitabine and bevacizumab. In fact, preclinical studies have demonstrated that some chemotherapy drugs (such as paclitaxel, for example) induce angiogenesis by mobilization of circulating endothelial cells, enhancing bevacizumab effect [37].

Thus, bevacizumab was evaluated in combination with first-line Carbo/Pem in a non-comparative, phase II trial in unresectable MPM patients [38]. Patients were treated for a maximum of six cycles or until progressive disease (PD) and, in the absence of PD, were continued on maintenance bevacizumab for a maximum of 1 year. RR was 34.2% in the 76 evaluable patients; stable disease (SD) was observed in 57.9% of patients (disease control rate, DCR of 92.1%). The trial was negative with a short mPFS (6.9 months) and a quite deceptive mOS (15.3 months).

In another non-comparative, phase II trial, the combination of Cis/Pem and bevacizumab was tested in 53 patients with chemotherapy-naïve unresectable malignant pleural and peritoneal mesothelioma [39]. The tolerance was acceptable. PR and SD were noted in 40% and 35% of patients, respectively. This trial failed to meet its primary endpoint of a 33% improvement in the PFS rate at 6 months, as compared with the historical control of cisplatin and pemetrexed alone. In an unplanned post hoc analysis restricted to 44 patients with MPM, the PFS rate at 6 months was 52%, and an objective RR of 35% and an mOS of 14.1 months were found.

Finally, a large randomized phase III "IFCT MAPS" clinical trial tested the value of the combination of bevacizumab to Cis/Pem doublet (plus vitamins, up to six cycles) as first-line treatment, followed by maintenance by bevacizumab in nonprogressive patients versus chemotherapy

Table 16.1 A summary of the main targeted therapies previously or currently evaluated in malignant pleural mesothelioma (adapted from reference [23])

	Target(s)	Drug(s)	Trial design (development phase)	N (pts)	Primary Endpoint	Results Open studies status (clinicaltrials.gov) [ref]
Antiangiogenic therapies	VEGF	Bevacizumab	*(III)* In combination with Cis/Pem vs. Cis/Pem alone	448	OS	Positive (NCT00651456) [24]
	VEGF FGF	Thalidomide	*(III)* Maintenance therapy after frontline Cis/Pem	222	PFS	Negative (ISRCTN13632914) [25]
	VEGFR	Axitinib	*(I/II)* in combination with Cis/Pem	25	PFS	Negative (NCT01211275) [26]
	VEGFR PDGFR	Cediranib	*(II)* Cediranib	51	ORR	Negative (NCT01064648) [27]
			(II) Cediranib + Cis/Pem vs. Cis/Pem alone	116	PFS	Negative, not recruiting (NCT01064648) [28]
	VEGFR PDGFR FGFR	Nintedanib	*(II/III)* In combination with Cis/Pem followed by nintedanib vs. placebo vs. Cis/Pem followed by placebo (Epithelioïd subtype only in phase III)	87	PFS	Phase II: Positive [29]
				537	PFS/OS	Phase III (NCT01907100): Negative (WCLC 2018)
	VEGFR-2/ VEGFR-3 PDGFR Raf/c-kit	Sorafenib	*(II)* Sorafenib beyond the first line	53	6-months	Negative (NCT00794859) [30]
			(II) Sorafenib beyond the first line	51	PFS	Negative (NCT00107432) [31]
			(I) Sorafenib + Cis/Pem	16	ORR	Negative (NCT00703638)
	Bcr-abl c-kit PDGFR	Imatinib mesylate	*(I)* Imatinib + Cis/Pem	17	Safety, ORR	Negative (NCT00402766) [32]
			(II) Imatinib + Gemcitabin in Pemetrexed–pretreated patients	22	PFS	Active, not recruiting (NCT02303899)
Antiangiogenic therapies in combination with other drugs	VEGF + PD-L1	Bevacizumab + Atezolizumab	*(I)*			
	VEGFR PDGFR	Nintedanib	*(II)* PEMBIB trial			
	FGFR + PD-1	Pembrolizumab				
	EGFR + VEGF	Erlotinib + Bevacizumab	*(II)* previously treated mesothelioma	24	ORR	Negative (NCT00137826) [33]

VEGF(R) vascular endothelial growth factor (receptor), *FGF(R)* fibroblast growth factor (receptor), *EGFR* epidermal growth factor receptor, *PDGF(R)* platelet-derived growth factor (receptor), *FAK* focal adhesion kinase, *HDAC* histone deacetylase, *EZH2* enhancer of zeste homolog 2, *Cis* cisplatin, *Pem* pemetrexed, *pts* patients, *OS* overall survival, *PFS* progression-free survival, *ORR* overall response rate, *DCR* disease control rate

alone as control arm [24]. These 448 chemo-naïve patients were 18–77 years old, ECOG PS 0–2 without significant cardiovascular comorbidity and/or other usual chemotherapy or bevacizumab contraindications (uncontrolled HTA, gastrointestinal perforation…), with unresectable MPM, proved by pleural biopsies (thoracoscopy…), and with at least one evaluable or measurable lesion by CT scan. The primary endpoint, mOS, was significantly longer in the bevacizumab arm vs. the control arm: 18.82 vs. 16.07 months, respectively (HR = 0.67; 95% CI [0.61–0.94]; $p = 0.015$). Median PFS was also significantly increased by 2 months in favor of the bevacizumab arm: 9.59 vs. 7.48 months (HR = 0.61; 95% CI [0.50–0.75]; $p < 0.0001$). The patients had only a mild and manageable increase of toxicity and no negative impact on quality of life in the bevacizumab arm compared to the control arm [40]. Overall, 158 (71%) out of 222 patients given PCB and 139 (62%) out of 224 patients given PC had grade 3–4 adverse events. It was observed more grade 3 or higher hypertension (51 [23%] of 222 vs. 0) and thrombotic events (13 [6%] of 222 vs. 2 [1%] of 224) with PCB than with PC. Thus, this study suggested a new standard of care for unresectable MPM patients eligible for bevacizumab, as validated by some US [8, 9] and French guidelines for MPM management. However, to date, bevacizumab did not receive FDA or EMA approvals in MPM—the MAPS trial being not designed as a registration trial. It is still unclear why the MAPS trial succeeded where previous trials failed to show any survival benefit. Unfortunately, to date, there is no good predictive biomarker for antiangiogenic drugs in any cancer, which could help in selecting the good candidates, and to explain potential selection advantages. It is possible that the large size and the design of this phase III trial had the power to demonstrate the value of the combination of Cis/Pem and bevacizumab compared to previous smaller trials.

Several trials, summarized in Table 16.1, also evaluated different antiangiogenic TKI in MPM. Axitinib, an anti-VEGFR TKI, failed to improve mOS and PFS in combination with Cis/Pem vs. chemotherapy alone despite a positive signal for objective response rate (ORR) [26]. Similarly, all studies assessing sorafenib (targeting VEGFR2/3, PDGFR, and Raf/c-kit TKI) given combined with first-line chemotherapy or beyond first-line treatment [30, 31], or using imatinib mesylate (targeting Bcr-abl, c-kit, and PDGFR) [32] were negative.

Nintedanib is an antiangiogenic kinase inhibitor, targeting VEGFR 1–3, PDGFR α/β, FGFR (fibroblast growth factor receptor) 1–3, Src, and Abl kinases pathways. A randomized phase II trial [29] showed promising results in 87 patients treated by Cis/Pem combined with nintedanib or placebo for up to six cycles, followed by nintedanib or placebo in nonprogressive patients, till unacceptable toxicity or PD. The patients exhibited with manageable toxicity and a significant improvement in the nintedanib arm vs. placebo arm in mPFS (9.7 vs. 5.7 months, respectively) (HR = 0.54; 95% CI 0.33–0.87; $p = 0.010$) and in mOS (20.6 vs. 15.2 months, respectively) (HR = 0.77; 95% CI 0.46–1.29; $p = 0.319$). Therefore, nintedanib was assessed in a randomized phase III trial vs. placebo, again both in conjunction with first-line Cis/Pem, but in epithelioïd MPM patients ($n = 229 \times 2$) only as the most striking results were observed in epithelioïd MPM subtype. Unfortunately, the results of this trial recently presented by Scagliotti et al. at 2018 WCLC meeting were negative with no difference in mPFS between nintedanib and placebo arms: 6.8 vs. 7.0 months, respectively (HR = 1.01; 95% CI: 0.79–1.30; $p = 0.91$). In the interim OS analysis (28% of events), mOS was 14.4 vs. 16.1 months, respectively (HR = 1.12; 95% CI: 0.79–1.58; $p = 0.54$). There were no unexpected toxicities. It is not known yet if these negative results will stop the other trials in MPM including nintedanib such as the nintedanib as Maintenance Treatment of MPM (NEMO), a randomized double-blinded phase II trial of the EORTC Lung Cancer Group in nonprogressive patients after first-line platinum-pemetrexed chemotherapy for 4–6 cycles (NCT02863055) or a US phase II trial of nintedanib in recurrent MPM patients (NCT02568449).

In a phase I trial (SWOG 0905; $n = 20$), cediranib (a drug targeting VEGFR and PDGFR) was tested with Cis/Pem for safety [27]. This small early-phase trial found results consistent with those observed with bevacizumab or nintedanib trials: ORR 63%, mPFS of 8.6 months (95% CI: 6.1–10.9), and mOS of 16.2 months (95% CI: 10.5–28.7) [27]. At ASCO 2018 meeting, the investigators reported the results of a phase II randomized trial assessing the efficacy of Cis/Pem for six cycles with placebo or cediranib (20 mg daily) followed by cediranib or placebo maintenance in nonprogressive patients [28]. They recruited 92 eligible, unresectable, chemo-naïve MPM patients of different histologic subtypes (75% epithelioid and 25% biphasic or sarcomatoid histology). The tolerance in the cediranib arm was questionable with more grade 3–4 diarrhea, dehydration, hypertension, and weight loss compared to placebo arm. Moreover, the primary endpoint, mPFS by RECIST 1.1 criteria, was not improved in the cediranib arm vs. placebo arm (7.2 vs. 5.6 months, respectively; HR = 0.71, $p = 0.062$), or even assessed by modified RECIST 1.1 criteria (6.9 vs. 5.6 months, HR = 0.77, $p = 0.12$). Finally, the mOS was not significantly improved with cediranib vs. placebo arm (10 vs. 8.5 months, HR = 0.88; $p = 0.28$). In terms of efficacy, cediranib significantly increased RR by modified RECIST 1.1 criteria vs. placebo (50% vs. 20%, $p = 0.006$) but not by RECIST 1.1 criteria (26% vs. 15%, $p = 0.15$). In conclusion, the toxicity profile of cediranib and its nonsignificant survival benefit precludes further research in MPM.

Thalidomide was first developed in the 1950s to treat morning sickness in pregnant women, leading to a terrible man-made medical disaster with more than 10,000 children born with various severe and debilitating malformations [41]. Thus, thalidomide was withdrawn from the market as an antiemetic drug in the 1960s but then it has evolved to treat cutaneous manifestations of erythema nodosum leprosum and has shown antineoplastic properties by the inhibition of tumor angiogenesis and cell proliferation through immunomodulatory effects. Therefore, thalidomide was assessed in different cancers in clinical trials, leading to its approval for the treatment of multiple myeloma. In MPM, thalidomide was evaluated in clinical trials without prior preclinical significant data. Despite encouraging results in a phase II trial with 28% disease stabilization at 6 months observed with thalidomide as single agent in previously treated MPM patients [42], a phase III randomized trial did not find any survival benefit for thalidomide as maintenance therapy after first-line chemotherapy by Cis/Pem [25], with mOS of 10.6 months in the thalidomide arm vs. 12.9 months in the best supportive care (BSC) group (HR 1.2, $p = 0.21$).

Finally, there are three exciting trials of combinations of ICI with antiangiogenic drugs, based on the strong preclinical rationale that anti-VEGF (bevacizumab) or a drug targeting VEGFR, FGFR, and PDGFR such as nintedanib may have additional or synergistic effect when combined with anti-PD-L1 (Atezolizumab) or anti-PD-1 (Pembrolizumab) antibodies to stimulate antitumor immunity [43, 44]. Thus, there are two ongoing early-phase trials assessing the association of bevacizumab plus atezolizumab in the MD Anderson (USA) or of nintedanib plus pembrolizumab in France. Other trials are planned with bevacizumab plus atezolizumab alone in PD-L1+ relapsing mesothelioma in UK (Mesothelioma Stratified Therapy (MiST) trial; NCT03654833), or in combination with first-line Carbo/Pem (4–6 cycles) by the ETOP (randomized phase III BEAT-meso trial; EudraCT n° 2018–002180-25), similarly to the recent positive randomized phase III trial in NSCLC, IMpower 150 [45].

16.2 Conclusion

Before 2016, no significant improvement was observed with antiangiogenic drugs in the treatment of MPM patients. The MAPS trial established in different major guidelines the anti-VEGF bevacizumab as a standard first-line treatment in combination with Cis/Pem chemotherapy in unresectable MPM patients without contraindications for this drug. The rise of the immune checkpoint inhibitors (ICI) may challenge this new standard in the future. Or alternatively, ICI such as anti-PD-1 or anti-PD-L1 antibodies may have synergistic or additional effect when combined with anti-"angiogenic" molecules. In fact, these drugs targeting VEGF pathway and other growth factors pathways have potentially both antiangiogenic and pro-immunogenic effects against the tumors as already proved in NSCLC or kidney cancers. Thus, targeting angiogenesis is still promising in MPM patients despite several negative trials with several drugs of this class.

References

1. Robinson BM. Malignant pleural mesothelioma: an epidemiological perspective. Ann Cardiothorac Surg. 2012;1(4):491–6.
2. Robinson BW, Musk AW, Lake RA. Malignant mesothelioma. Lancet. 2005;366(9483):397–408.
3. Andujar P, Lacourt A, Brochard P, Pairon J-C, Jaurand M-C, Jean D. Five years update on relationships between malignant pleural mesothelioma and exposure to asbestos and other elongated mineral particles. J Toxicol Environ Health B Crit Rev. 2016;19(5–6):151–72.
4. Scherpereel A, Astoul P, Baas P, Berghmans T, Clayson H, de Vuyst P, et al. Guidelines of the European Respiratory Society and the European Society of Thoracic Surgeons for the management of malignant pleural mesothelioma. Eur Respir J. 2010;35(3):479–95.
5. Baas P, Fennell D, Kerr KM, Van Schil PE, Haas RL, Peters S. Malignant pleural mesothelioma: ESMO clinical practice guidelines for diagnosis, treatment and follow-up. Ann Oncol. 2015;26(Suppl 5):v31–9.
6. van Zandwijk N, Clarke C, Henderson D, Musk W, Fong K, Nowak AK, et al. Guidelines for the diagnosis and treatment of malignant pleural mesothelioma. J Thorac Dis. 2013;5(6):E254–307.
7. Woolhouse I, Bishop L, Darlison L, et al. British Thoracic Society guideline for the investigation and management of malignant pleural mesothelioma. Thorax. 2018;73:i1–i30.
8. Kindler HL, Ismaila N, Armato SG 3rd, et al. Treatment of malignant pleural mesothelioma: American Society of Clinical Oncology clinical practice guideline. J Clin Oncol. 2018;36:1343–73.
9. NCCN Malignant pleural mesothelioma guidelines. Version 2.2018 — February 26, 2018. https://www.nccn.org/professionals/physician_gls/pdf/mpm_blocks.pdf. Accessed 09 Sept 2018.
10. Vogelzang NJ, Rusthoven JJ, Symanowski J, Denham C, Kaukel E, Ruffie P, et al. Phase III study of pemetrexed in combination with cisplatin versus cisplatin alone in patients with malignant pleural mesothelioma. J Clin Oncol. 2003;21(14):2636–44.
11. Scherpereel A, Mazieres J, Greillier L, Gervais R, Bylicki O, Monnet I, et al. Second- or third-line nivolumab (Nivo) versus nivo plus ipilimumab (Ipi) in malignant pleural mesothelioma (MPM) patients: results of the IFCT-1501 MAPS2 randomized phase II trial. J Clin Oncol. 2017;35(18_suppl):LBA8507.
12. Zucali PA, Simonelli M, Michetti G, Tiseo M, Ceresoli GL, Collov E, et al. Second-line chemotherapy in malignant pleural mesothelioma: results of a retrospective multicenter survey. Lung Cancer. 2012;75(3):360–7.
13. Sandler A, Gray R, Perry MC, Brahmer J, Schiller JH, Dowlati A, Lilenbaum R, Johnson DH. Paclitaxel-carboplatin alone or with bevacizumab for non-small-cell lung cancer. N Engl J Med. 2006;355(24):2542–50.
14. Folkman J. Tumor angiogenesis: therapeutic implications. N Engl J Med. 1971;285(21):1182–6.
15. Levin PA, Dowell JE. Spotlight on bevacizumab and its potential in the treatment of malignant pleural mesothelioma: the evidence to date. Onco Targets Ther. 2017;10:2057–66.
16. Hendry SA, Farnsworth RH, Solomon B, et al. The role of the tumor vasculature in the host immune response: implications for therapeutic strategies targeting the tumor microenvironment. Front Immunol. 2016;7:621.
17. Li C, Liu T, Bazhin AV, Yang Y. The sabotaging role of myeloid cells in anti-angiogenic therapy: coordination of angiogenesis and immune suppression by hypoxia. J Cell Physiol. 2017;232(9):2312–22.
18. Kumar-Singh S, Weyler J, Martin MJ, Vermeulen PB, Van Marck E. Angiogenic cytokines in mesothelioma: a study of VEGF, FGF-1 and -2, and TGF beta expression. J Pathol. 1999;189(1):72–8.
19. Edwards JG, Cox G, Andi A, et al. Angiogenesis is an independent prognostic factor in malignant mesothelioma. Br J Cancer. 2001;85(6):863–8.
20. Ohta Y, Shridhar V, Bright RK, et al. VEGF and VEGF type C play an important role in angiogenesis and lymphangiogenesis in human malignant mesothelioma tumours. Br J Cancer. 1999;81(1):54–61.
21. Soini Y, Puhakka A, Kahlos K, et al. Endothelial nitric oxide synthase is strongly expressed in malignant mesothelioma but does not associate with vascular density or the expression of VEGF, FLK1 or FLT1. Histopathology. 2001;39(2):179–86.
22. Al-Husein B, Abdalla M, Trepte M, Deremer DL, Somanath PR. Antiangiogenic therapy for cancer: an update. Pharmacotherapy. 2012;32(12):1095–111.
23. Scherpereel A, Wallyn F, Albelda SM, Munck C. Novel therapies for malignant pleural mesothelioma. Lancet Oncol. 2018;19:e161–e72.
24. Zalcman G, Mazieres J, Margery J, Greillier L, Audigier-Valette C, Moro-Sibilot D, et al. Bevacizumab for newly diagnosed pleural mesothelioma in the mesothelioma avastin cisplatin pemetrexed study (MAPS): a randomised, controlled, open-label, phase 3 trial. Lancet. 2016;387(10026):1405–14.
25. Buikhuisen WA, Burgers JA, Vincent AD, Korse CM, van Klaveren RJ, Schramel FM, et al. Thalidomide versus active supportive care for maintenance in patients with malignant mesothelioma after first-line chemotherapy (NVALT 5): an open-label,

multicentre, randomised phase 3 study. Lancet Oncol. 2013;14(6):543–51.
26. Buikhuisen WA, Scharpfenecker M, Griffioen AW, Korse CM, van Tinteren H, Baas P. A randomized phase II study adding axitinib to pemetrexed-cisplatin in patients with malignant pleural mesothelioma: a single-center trial combining clinical and translational outcomes. J Thorac Oncol. 2016;11(5):758–68.
27. Tsao AS, Moon J, Wistuba I, Vogelzang NJ, Kalemkerian G, Redman M, et al. Phase I trial of cediranib in combination with cisplatin and pemetrexed in chemo naive patients with unresectable malignant pleural mesothelioma. J Thorac Oncol. 2017;12(8):1299–308.
28. Tsao AS, Miao J, Wistuba I, Vogelzang NJ, Heymach J, Fossella FV, Lu C, Velasco MR, Box-Noriega B, Hueftle JG, Gadgeel SM, Weber Redman M, Gandara DR, Kelly K. SWOG S0905: a randomized phase II study of cediranib versus placebo in combination with cisplatin and pemetrexed in chemonaive patients with malignant pleural mesothelioma. Abstract ASCO 2018. J Clin Oncol. 2018;36(suppl):abstr 8514.
29. Grosso F, Steele N, Novello S, Kowak AK, Popat S, Greillier L, et al. Nintedanib plus pemetrexed/cisplatin in patients with malignant pleural mesothelioma: phase II results from the randomized, placebo-controlled LUME-meso trial. J Clin Oncol. 2017;35:3591–600.
30. Papa S, Popat S, Shah R, Prevost AT, Lal R, McLennan B, et al. Phase 2 study of sorafenib in malignant mesothelioma previously treated with platinum-containing chemotherapy. J Thorac Oncol. 2013;8(6):783–7.
31. Dubey S, Jänne PA, Krug L, Pang H, Wang X, Heinze R, et al. A phase II study of sorafenib in malignant mesothelioma: results of cancer and leukemia group B 30307. J Thorac Oncol. 2010;5(10):1655–61.
32. Tsao AS, Harun N, Lee JJ, Heymach J, Pisters K, Hong WK, et al. Phase I trial of cisplatin, pemetrexed, and imatinib mesylate in chemonaive patients with unresectable malignant pleural mesothelioma. Clin Lung Cancer. 2014;15(3):197–201.
33. Jackman DM, Kindler HL, Yeap BY, et al. Erlotinib plus bevacizumab in previously treated patients with malignant pleural mesothelioma. Cancer. 2008;113(4):808–14.
34. Yap TA, Aerts JG, Popat S, Fennell DA. Novel insights into mesothelioma biology and implications for therapy. Nat Rev Cancer. 2017;17:475–88.
35. Kindler HL, Karrison TG, Gandara DR, et al. Multicenter, double-blind, placebo-controlled, randomized phase II trial of gemcitabine/cisplatin plus bevacizumab or placebo in patients with malignant mesothelioma. J Clin Oncol. 2012;30(20):2509–15.
36. Barlesi F, Scherpereel A, Rittmeyer A, Pazzola A, Ferrer Tur N, Kim JH, Ahn MJ, Aerts JG, Gorbunova V, Vikström A, Wong EK, Perez-Moreno P, Mitchell L, Groen HJ. Randomized phase III trial of maintenance bevacizumab with or without pemetrexed after first-line induction with bevacizumab, cisplatin, and pemetrexed in advanced nonsquamous non-small-cell lung cancer: AVAPERL (MO22089). J Clin Oncol. 2013;31(24):3004–11.
37. Shaked Y, Henke E, Roodhart JM, et al. Rapid chemotherapy-induced acute endothelial progenitor cell mobilization: implications for antiangiogenic drugs as chemosensitizing agents. Cancer Cell. 2008;14(3):263–73.
38. Ceresoli GL, Zucali PA, Mencoboni M, et al. Phase II study of pemetrexed and carboplatin plus bevacizumab as first-line therapy in malignant pleural mesothelioma. Br J Cancer. 2013;109(3):552–8.
39. Dowell JE, Dunphy FR, Taub RN, et al. A multicenter phase II study of cisplatin, pemetrexed, and bevacizumab in patients with advanced malignant mesothelioma. Lung Cancer. 2012;77(3):567–71.
40. Westeel V, Eberst G, Anota A, Scherpereel A, Mazieres J, Margery J, Greillier L, Audigier-Valette C, Moro-Sibilot D, Molinier O, Lena H, Rivière F, Monnet I, Gounant V, Janicot H, Gervais R, Locher C, Morin F, Zalcman G, French Cooperative Thoracic Intergroup (IFCT). Impact on health-related quality of life of the addition of bevacizumab to cisplatin-pemetrexed in malignant pleural mesothelioma in the MAPS phase III trial. J Clin Oncol. 2018;36(suppl):abstr 8505.
41. Boyer A, Pasquier E, Tomasini P, Ciccolini J, Greillier L, Andre N, Barlesi F, Mascaux C. Drug repurposing in malignant pleural mesothelioma: a breath of fresh air? Eur Respir Rev. 2018;27(147):170098.
42. Baas P, Boogerd W, Dalesio O, Haringhuizen A, Custers F, van Zandwijk N. Thalidomide in patients with malignant pleural mesothelioma. Lung Cancer. 2005;48:291–6.
43. Allen E, Jabouille A, Rivera LB, Lodewijckx I, Missiaen R, Steri V, et al. Combined antiangiogenic and anti–PD-L1 therapy stimulates tumor immunity through HEV formation. Sci Transl Med. 2017;9(385):eaak9679.
44. Voron T, Marcheteau E, Pernot S, et al. Control of the immune response by pro-angiogenic factors. Front Oncol. 2014;4:70.
45. Socinski MA, Jotte RM, Cappuzzo F, Orlandi F, Stroyakovskiy D, Nogami N, Rodríguez-Abreu D, Moro-Sibilot D, Thomas CA, Barlesi F, Finley G, Kelsch C, Lee A, Coleman S, Deng Y, Shen Y, Kowanetz M, Lopez-Chavez A, Sandler A, Reck M, IMpower150 Study Group. Atezolizumab for first-line treatment of metastatic nonsquamous NSCLC. N Engl J Med. 2018;378(24):2288–301.

17 Targeted Therapies in Mesothelioma

Loredana Urso and Giulia Pasello

17.1 Introduction

Malignant Pleural Mesothelioma (MPM) is fatal disease characterized by chemoresistance and poor prognosis [1]. Since 2003, when a platinum-based chemotherapy *plus* pemetrexed was introduced as standard first-line therapy [2], no significant improvements in MPM management have been done. To date, no indications for second-line therapies after first-line failure are available [3]. In the last years, many efforts have been directed to the identification of anticancer therapies able to target tumor-related molecular changes. Targeted therapies may improve cancer management in terms of both patients' prognosis and quality of life, because of the higher specificity and the lower toxicity profile compared to most cytotoxic drugs. The identification of key molecular targets in MPM represents a hard challenge because MPM pathogenesis is not completely known. This neoplasia is characterized by low mutational load, but recurrent somatic mutations in tumor suppressor genes [4]. Moreover, the three histologic subtypes are characterized by different biological and clinical behaviors, increasing the need to develop personalized therapeutic approaches. Here, we focus on potential molecular targets and specific targeted therapies under clinical investigation in MPM.

17.1.1 NF2/Merlin

NF2 is a tumor suppressor gene frequently altered in MPM [5–7]. Recent studies performed in a large series of MPM specimens using high-throughput technologies (whole-exome sequencing, RNA-seq) confirmed high frequency of *NF2* alteration including mutations and copy number variations [8–10]. Of note, sarcomatoid subtypes carried higher rate of *NF2* mutation compared to epithelioid ones [9].

NF2 gene encodes for merlin protein, a tumor suppressor blocking several signal transduction pathways involved in cell proliferation, survival, and metabolism. Wild-type merlin is regulated by post-translational modifications defining its conformational status and activity. It is inactivated through the phosphorylation at Serine 518 by cAMP-dependent kinase (PKA) and activated by the myosin phosphatase MYPT1-PP1 [11]. As a consequence, deregulation of merlin can occur in the absence of *NF2* gene mutation [12]. Indeed, mRNA overexpression of CPI-17 (phosphatase inhibitor of 17 kDa), a cellular inhibitor of MYPT1-PP1, has been detected in mesothelioma tumor samples carried wild-type *NF2*, suggesting that merlin is completely inactivated in MPM [13].

L. Urso
Department of Surgery, Oncology and Gastroenterology, University of Padova, Padova, Italy

G. Pasello (✉)
Medical Oncology 2, Istituto Oncologico Veneto IRCCS, Padova, Italy
e-mail: giulia.pasello@iov.veneto.it

G. L. Ceresoli et al. (eds.), *Mesothelioma*, https://doi.org/10.1007/978-3-030-16884-1_17

17.1.1.1 NF2/Merlin and Hippo Pathway

Merlin controls cell proliferation and viability through the regulation of the Hippo pathway, a signal transduction cascade including the proteins: MST1/2 Kinases (Mammalian STE20-like protein kinase 1/2), MST1/2 coactivator SAV1(Salvador1), LATS1/2 Kinases (Large Tumor Suppressor Kinases 1/2), and LATS1/2 coactivator MOB1 (Mps one-binder 1) [14]. Merlin-dependent activation of the Hippo pathway results in the phosphorylation and inactivation of YAP (Yes associated protein), a cofactor essential for TEAD (TEA domain family member) transcriptional activity. YAP/TEAD complex activates the transcription of genes involved in cell proliferation, cell growth, and inhibition of apoptosis [15] (Fig. 17.1). In MPM, Hippo pathway deregulation seems to be related mainly to merlin loss of function [16, 17], although concomitant mutations of *NF2* and *LATS2* genes have been reported [9, 18]. Immunohistochemistry analysis performed on MPM cell lines and tumor tissues revealed strong nuclear localization of YAP in a high percentage of samples [16, 19, 20] and YAP knockdown in MPM cells resulted in the inhibition of cell growth, motility, and invasive abilities [21]. Altogether, these observations highlight the strong link existing between YAP hyper-activation and MPM uncontrolled growth, suggesting that YAP may be a potential candidate for MPM-targeted therapies. A drug screening performed using the Johns Hopkins library identified the small-molecule Verteporfin (VP) (Visudyne, Novartis) as a YAP inhibitor [22]. VP is an FDA (Food and Drug Administration)-approved photosensitizer drug used for the treatment of neovascular macular degeneration. In addition to its photosensitizer properties, VP has light-independent ability in inducing YAP conformational change and in blocking YAP/TEAD interaction [23]. The potential of VP as anticancer drug is under investigation in phase I/II clinical trials in different human cancers, including

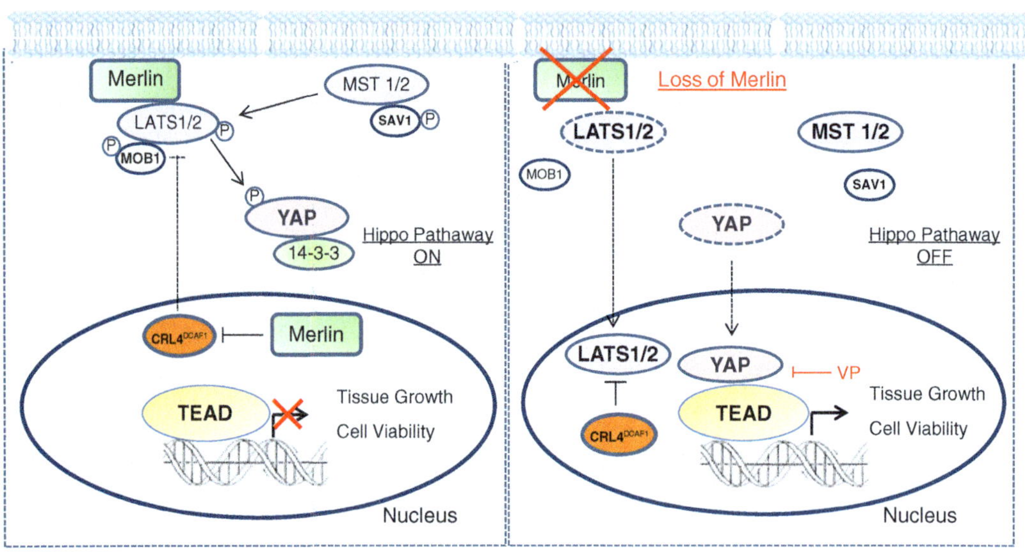

Fig. 17.1 *Merlin regulates Hippo pathway activation.* Merlin blocks TEAD transcriptional activity (left panel): following growth arrest signals, merlin recruits LATS1/2 and MOB1 in the cytoplasm at the membrane level. MST1/2 phosphorylates LATS1/2 and MOB1 activating LATS1/2 that, in turn, phosphorylates YAP; phospho-YAP binds 14-3-3 and is retained into the cytoplasm. Into the nucleus, merlin inhibits CRL4 ^{DCAF1}, the E3 ubiquitin ligase implied in LATS1/2 degradation. Loss of merlin (right panel) results in YAP/TEAD association and activation of transcription. Verteporfin induces YAP conformational change inhibiting YAP/TEAD interaction. *LATS* Large Tumor Suppressor Kinases 1/2, *MOB* Mps one-binder 1, *MST 1/2* Mammalian STE20-like protein kinase1/2, *SAV* salvador, *YAP* Yes-associated protein, *TEAD* TEA domain family member, *CRL4* cullin4A-RING E3 ubiquitin ligase, *DCAF1* DDB1- and CUL4-associated factor1, *VP* Verteporfin

breast and pancreatic cancers, brain tumors, and pleural malignancies (www.clinicaltrials.gov, NCT02939274, NCT03067051, NCT00002647; NCT02702700). As regard MPM, encouraging results have been obtained in in vitro studies demonstrating VP-dependent reduction of cell proliferation, cell viability, and cell invasion in MPM cell lines [18, 20].

17.1.1.2 NF2/Merlin and mTOR Pathway

PI3K-AKT-mTOR is a signal transduction pathway involved in cell proliferation, protein synthesis, glucose metabolism, apoptosis resistance, angiogenesis, and invasion. Activation of PI3K-AKT-mTOR passes through RTKs (Tyrosine Kinase Receptors) activation or G-Protein Coupled Receptors (GPCRs)-dependent RAS induction [24]. mTOR (mammalian target of rapamycin) is a serine/threonine kinase included in two protein complexes: the rapamycin-sensitive mTORC1 (mammalian target of rapamycin complex 1) and the rapamycin-insensitive mTORC2. mTORC1 induces mRNA translation, protein synthesis, and nucleotide production and negatively regulates autophagy and mTORC2 [25]; mTORC2 regulates protein kinases activity including AKT [26]. Physiological inhibitors of PI3K-AKT-mTOR pathway are the phosphatase and tensin homolog PTEN and merlin [27] (Fig. 17.2).

Aberrant activation of PI3K/AKT/mTOR pathway is a hallmark of many cancers including MPM [28, 29]. In MPM, recurrent *NF2* mutations [8–10], loss of PTEN [30], or gain of function mutations of PI3K or AKT [8] are reported to be responsible for mTOR pathway activation. In recent years, rapamycin or rapamycin-derived (rapalog) inhibitors have been used to inhibit mTORC1; among them, the most studied were sirolimus (rapamycin), temsirolimus (CCI-779), and everolimus (RAD001, Novartis Pharmaceuticals). Preclinical studies strongly encouraged the use of rapalogs in MPM. Indeed, Lopez-Lagos et al. [31] demonstrated that merlin null cells showed mTORC1 activation and higher sensitivity to rapamycin treatment compared to merlin-expressing cells. Moreover, Pignochino and coworkers observed anticancer activity of everolimus in MPM cell lines and mouse xenograft models. Of note, everolimus strongly synergized with sorafenib (a multi-kinase inhibitor) [32]. Unfortunately, phase II trials evaluating everolimus activity in unselected MPM patients (www.clinicaltrials.gov; NCT00770120; NCT01024946) showed no clinical efficacy [33]. Probably, the lack of efficacy of everolimus-based therapy in MPM was due to the wide spectrum of PI3K/AKT activities as well as the loss of mTORC1 negative regulation of mTORC2. To overcome low efficacy of mTORC1 inhibitors, the dual PI3K and mTORC1/2 inhibitor apitolisib (Genentech) was assessed in clinical trials. Although the promising response rate of MPM patients is in phase I trial (www.clinicaltrials.gov, NCT00854152; [34]), the drug revealed high toxicity profile in metastatic renal cell carcinoma phase II trials (www.clinicaltrials.gov, NCT01442090; [35] (Table 17.1). Encouraging results were obtained with another AKT inhibitor: Afuresertib (Novartis, Pharmaceuticals). In vitro preclinical study demonstrated that afuresertib strongly inhibited cell growth and clonogenic activity of MPM cell lines, induced cell cycle arrest, and acted in cooperation with cisplatin in inducing MPM apoptosis [36]. Of note, phase I clinical trial of Afuresertib in multiple myeloma showed promising results [37], encouraging further assessment of this drug for the treatment of other cancers including MPM.

17.1.1.3 NF2/Merlin and FAK

Cell anchorage to Extracellular Matrix (ECM) triggers signal transduction pathways involved in cell growth, survival, motility, and invasiveness [38]. A central role in transducing these signals is carried out by the Focal Adhesion Kinase (FAK). FAK is a non-receptor cytoplasmic tyrosine kinase consisting of four domains: N-terminal FERM domain (regulatory domain), catalytic domain, proline-rich domain, and C-terminal focal adhesion domain. It is activated by Integrin Receptors, Growth Factor and Cytokine Receptors [38] (Fig. 17.3). FAK overexpression and deregulation has been described in several types of cancers, and it was linked to uncontrolled

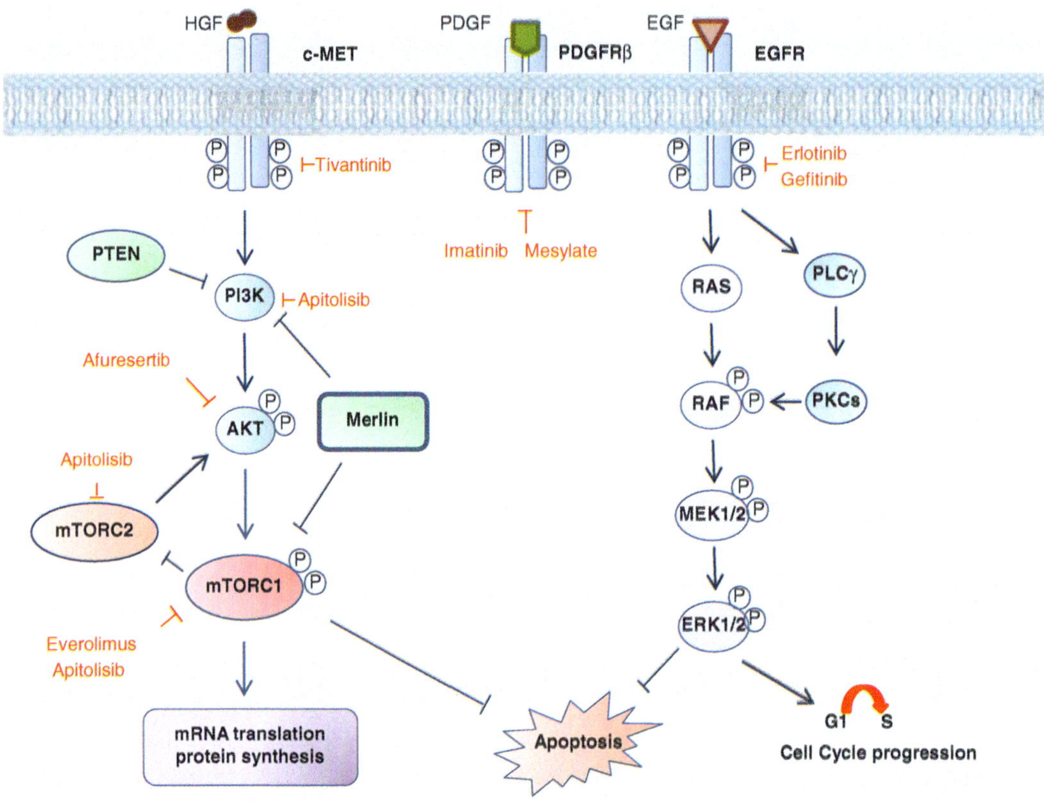

Fig. 17.2 *Schematic representation of TKRs-induced pathways*. Growth factors binding to their specific receptors induce intracytoplasmanic phosphorylation and activation of TKRs. TKRs transduce their signals mainly through PI3K-AKT-mTOR pathway and MAPK (Mitogen-Activated Protein Kinase) pathway and are mainly implicated in cell proliferation and survival. *PI3K-AKT-mTOR pathway*: activated PI3K induces AKT phosphorylation and activation. AKT activates mTORC1 that in turn induces mRNA translation and protein synthesis. mTORC1 inhibits mTORC2. Activated mTORC2 regulates the activity of several protein kinases including AKT. Merlin and PTEN are negative regulators of PI3K-AKT-mTOR pathway. Tivantinib inhibits the kinase domain of c-MET receptor; imatinib mesylate inhibits PDGFR; erlotinib and gefitinib inhibit EGFR. Everolimus inhibits mTORC1; apitolisib inhibits mTORC1, mTORC2, and PI3K; Afuresertib inhibits AKT. *HGF* Hepatocyte Growth Factor, *c-MET* mesenchymal–epithelial transition protein, *PGF* platelet-derived growth factor, *PDGFR* platelet-derived growth factor receptor, *EGF* epithermal growth factor, *EGFR* epithermal growth factor receptor, *PTEN* phosphatase and tensin homolog, *PI3K* phosphatidylinositide 3 kinase, *mTORC1/2* mammalian target of rapamycin complex 1/2, *RAS* rat sarcoma (small GTPase), *RAF* rapidly accelerated fibrosarcoma, *MEK* mitogen-activated protein kinase kinase, *ERK* extracellular signal-regulated kinase

tumor growth and metastasis [38]. FAK acts mainly at the membrane levels, but Nuclear Localization Sequence (NLS) in the FERM domain has also been described [39], supporting the hypothesis that FAK may have a role in genes regulation. Small-molecule FAK inhibitors were extensively used both in preclinical studies and in clinical trials. These drugs consist mainly of selective ATP-competitive inhibitors of FAK (e.g., VS-4718, GSK2256098), although some of them target both FAK and its homolog PYK2 (e.g., VS-6062, VS-6063). In vitro results obtained using VS-4718 (Verastem) and VS-6062 (Verastem) in several types of cancer showed a strong activity of FAK inhibitors in reducing cell growth, motility, invasiveness, and metastatic potential [40]. Moreover, VS-4718 was able to deplete tumor suppressive microenvironment [41], while VS-6062 blocked TGF-β-dependent epithelial-to-mesenchymal transition and showed

Table 17.1 Clinical trials with targeted therapies in MPM patients

Targets	Drugs	Phase	Setting	Biomarkers	Primary end points	Clinical trial ID	References
mTORC1	Everolimus	II	Second line		PFS	NCT00770120	[33]
	Everolimus	II	Second line	Merlin/NF2 loss	RR	NCT01024946	
PI3K; mTORC1/2	Apitolisib	I	First/ Second line		Safety, MTD, PK	NCT00854152	[34]
FAK	Defactinib	II	Second line	Merlin status	OS, PFS	NCT01870609	
	GSK2256098	I	First/ Second line	pFAK expression; merlin status	Safety, MTD	NCT01138033	[47]
	GSK2256098 *plus* Trametinib	I	First/ Second line	pFAK; pERK expression	Safety, MTD	NCT01938443	[48]
EGFR	Erlotinib	II	First line	pEGFR; pERK; pAKT; pmTOR; PTEN expression	RR, correlation with EGFR pathway activation	NCT00039182	[51]
	Erlotinib *plus* Bevacizumab	II	Second line		RR	NCT00137826	[103]
	Gefitinib	II	First line	EGFR expression	RR	NCT00025207	[49]
	Gefitinib	II	First line		RR, safety	NCT00787410	
c-MET	Tivantinib	II	Second line	MET status; HGF serum levels	RR	NCT01861301	[59]
	Tivantinib *plus* carbo/pem	I-Ib	First line	HGF, MET and VEGF serum levels, pMET, MET expression	DLT	NCT02049060	
PDGFR, c-Kit, BCR-ABL	Imatinib mesylate	II	First/ Second line		Effect on life-threatening rare diseases associated with imatinib mesylate-sensitive tyrosine kinases	NCT00154388	[61]
	Imatinib *plus* cis/ pem	I	First line	PDGFRα; PDGFRβ; pPDGFRβ expression	MTD	NCT00402766	[62]
	Imatinib *plus* Gemcitabine	II	Second line		PFS	NCT02303899	

(continued)

Table 17.1 (continued)

Targets	Drugs	Phase	Setting	Biomarkers	Primary end points	Clinical trial ID	References
EGFR, VEGFR, RET	Vandetanib	II	Second line		DC	NCT00597116	
PDGFR, BCR-ABL, Src family non-receptor TK	Dasatinib	II	Second line	EphA2 and PDGFRβ expression; plasma levels of VEGF and PDGFRβ	PFS	NCT00509041	[67]
	Dasatinib	I	First line	pSrc and pPDGFR expression	Modulation of pSrc	NCT00652574	[68]
HDACs	Vorinostat	III	Second line		OS, toxicity	NCT00128102	[78]
	Belinostat	II	Second line	Fetal hemoglobin	RR	NCT00365053	[79]
	Valproate *plus* Doxorubicin	II	Second line		Response rate	NCT00634205	[80]
Proteasome	Bortezomib	II	First/ Second line		RR	NCT00513877	[84]
	Bortezomib *plus* Cisplatin	II	First line		PFS	NCT00458913	[85]
microRNA	TargomiRs	I	Second/ Third line		MTD, DLT	NCT02369198	[89]
p16	Ribociclib	II	Second line	CDK4/6, CyclinD1/3, p16 status	Clinical benefit rate	NCT02187783	

PFS progression-free survival, *RR* response rate, *OS* overall survival, *MTD* maximum-tolerated dose, *DLT* dose-limiting toxicities, *PK* pharmacokinetic

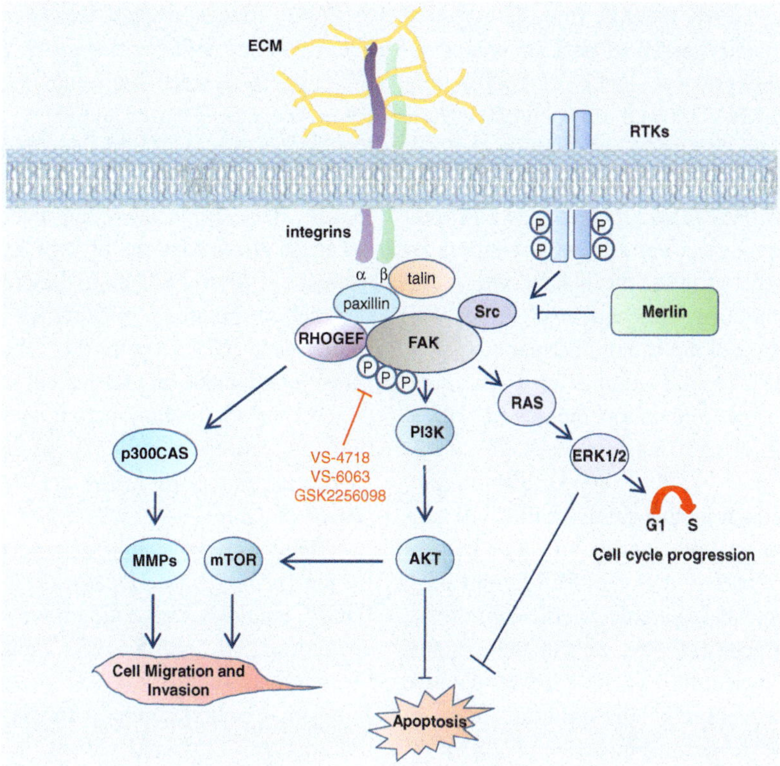

Fig. 17.3 *FAK pathway*: integrin or RTK-mediated activation of FAK involves recruitment of different proteins including talin, paxillin RHOGEF, and Src. Activated FAK induces cell cycle progression through RAS/ERK1/2 pathway, inhibits apoptosis through RAS/ERK1/2 and PI3K/AKT pathways, promotes cell migration and invasion through PI3K/AKT/mTOR pathway and activation of p300CAS. VS-4718, VS-6063, and GSK2256098 are ATP-competitive FAK inhibitors that block FAK autophosphorylation. *ECM* extracellular matrix, *RTKs* Tyrosine Kinase Receptors, *FAK* Focal Adhesion Kinase, *RHOGEF* Rho guanine nucleotide exchange factor, *ERK1/2* extracellular signal-regulated kinase 1/2, *PI3K* phosphatidylinositide 3 kinase, *mTOR* mammalian target of rapamycin, *p130Cas* p130 Crk-associated substrate, *MMPs* matrix metalloproteases

antiangiogenic effects [40]. As regard MPM, in vitro studies using FAK inhibitors revealed a link between merlin expression and anti-FAK therapy sensitivity. Indeed, MPM cell lines expressing merlin were more resistant to VS-4718 in respect of MPM cells characterized by loss of merlin. Shapiro et al. hypothesized that in merlin null cells, the loss of merlin-dependent signals derived from cell-to-cell contact may increase signals derived from cell-to-ECM contact, resulting in a hyper-activation of FAK [42]. In line with this hypothesis, reintroduction of merlin, in merlin null MPM cells, decreased FAK expression levels, FAK phosphorylation, and consequently cell invasiveness [43]. Although the strong preclinical evidence supporting the role of merlin as predictive biomarker for anti-FAK therapy, a phase II, double-blind, randomized, placebo-controlled trial aimed at determining the activity of VS-6063 (Defactinib, Verastem) in MPM, based on merlin status, showed no efficacy and was stopped (www.clinicaltrials.gov; COMMAND NCT01870609). A possible explanation of this failure was provided by Kato et al. that in their work identified E-cadherin as additional predictive biomarker for anti-FAK therapy in merlin null MPM. Using a large panel of MPM cell lines, they demonstrated that the expression levels of E-cadherin mRNA in merlin null cells significantly correlated with VS-4718 resistance, suggesting that evaluation of both markers may be useful for the selection of MPM patients suitable for anti-FAK therapy. Importantly, they also demonstrated that MPM patients characterized by low expression levels of merlin and E-cadherin mRNA showed the poorest overall survival [44]. An additional small-molecule FAK inhibitor tested in clinical trial was GSK2256098 (GlaxoSmithKline). GSK2256098 showed strong efficacy in reducing cell growth, anchorage-independent cell growth, survival, motility, and invasiveness both in vitro and in vivo [45, 46]. The first pharmacokinetic and pharmacodynamic study of GSK2256098 administered as single agent in advanced solid tumors included 29 MPM patients (46% of total patients enrolled) (www.clinicaltrials.gov, NCT01138033). Preliminary results showed a tolerable safety profile and antitumor activity in both merlin null and merlin-expressing MPM. Evaluation of PFS (progression free survival) revealed a greater efficacy in those patients characterized by merlin null status (23.4 weeks merlin null vs 10.9 merlin-positive patients), encouraging the stratification of patients based on merlin expression [47]. Finally, a clinical trial evaluating the efficacy of combined therapy using GSK2256098 and trametinib (a MAPK pathway inhibitor) in MPM is ongoing and preliminary results are promising (www.clinicaltrials.gov, NCT01938443) [48] (Table 17.1).

17.1.2 Tyrosine Kinase Receptors

Tyrosine Kinase Receptors (TKRs) are important class of transmembrane receptors transducing growth factor signals. The binding of growth factors with specific TKRs activates transduction pathways such as MAPKs (Mitogen Activated Protein Kinases), PI3K/AKT, Phospholipase Cγ (PLCγ), and Protein Kinases C (PKC), and regulates cell proliferation, survival, migration, invasion, and angiogenesis (Fig. 17.2). Oncogenic role of gain of function TKRs mutations or TKRs overexpression has been described in several types of cancers, and an important role in MPM carcinogenesis has been shown for c-MET (mesenchymal–epithelial transition protein), Platelet-Derived Growth Factor Receptor (PDGF), and Epidermal Growth Factor Receptors (EGFRs) (Fig. 17.2) [28].

EGFR overexpression has been detected in about 50% of MPM patients [49, 50]. Erlotinib (Tarceva, Genentech Inc.) and gefitinib (Iressa, Astra Zeneca Pharmaceuticals) are Tyrosine Kinase Inhibitors (TKIs) targeting specifically the intracytoplasmic catalytic domain of EGFR. These drugs have been successfully introduced in the treatment of NSCLC, where the response is strictly related to the presence of gain of function mutations in exons 19 and 21 of the EGFR gene [51]. Despite this, phase II clinical trials conducted in untreated mesothelioma patients failed to show activity with both erlotinib and gefitinib [50, 52], probably because EGFR mutations in MPM are infrequent [53] (Table 17.1).

c-MET is a tyrosine kinase receptor activated by the binding with Hepatocyte Growth Factor (HGF). HGF/MET signaling involved mainly the activation of PI3K/AKT pathway [54]. Overexpression of c-MET in mesothelioma tumors has been described, especially in epithelioid subtypes [55], and seemed to be related to mir-34 b/c silencing [56]. Moreover, mesothelioma patients expressed higher serum levels of HGF compared to healthy subjects [57]. These results encouraged the investigation of c-MET inhibitors in mesothelioma clinical trials. Tivantinib (ARQ 197), an orally bioavailable small-molecule c-MET inhibitor, was tested in phase II trial for the treatment of malignant mesothelioma previously treated (www.clinicaltrials.gov, NCT01861301). While in hepatocellular carcinoma the anticancer activity of tivantinib was related to c-MET overexpression [58], results of this trial showed disease control only in peritoneal mesothelioma group and no correlation with c-MET expression or mutation [59]. On the other hand, in MPM preclinical models, tivantinib showed low activity used as single agent, but synergistic antitumor activity in association with pemetrexed [60] or PI3K/mTOR inhibitors [61]. To date, phase I-Ib trial testing the efficacy of tivantinib plus carboplatin/pemetrexed as first-line therapy for malignant pleural mesothelioma and non-small cell lung cancer is ongoing (www.clinicaltrials.gov, NCT02049060) and results are awaited (Table 17.1).

PDGF is a growth factor inducing proliferation of mesothelioma cells. Its receptor is expressed in two different isoforms (PDGFRα and PDGFRβ). Normal mesothelial cells express PDGFRα, while mesothelioma tumors express high levels of PDGFRβ [51]. Imatinib mesylate (STU 571, Gleevec, Novartis), an inhibitor of tyrosine kinase associated with PDGFR, c-Kit and BCR-ABL fusion protein, was tested in several trials both as single-agent and combined therapies. Phase II trials showed no results when imatinib was administered as single agent [62, 63]; in a phase I study designed to determine the maximum-tolerated dose of imatinib mesylate in association to cisplatin and pemetrexed on 17 MPM patients, the combination was not well tolerated discouraging further examination [64]; finally, phase II trial aimed at assessing the antitumoral activity of a combination of imatinib mesylate and gemcitabine in patients with unresectable malignant mesothelioma expressing either PDGFR or c-Kit is ongoing (www.clinicaltrials.gov, NCT02303899) (Table 17.1).

Failure of TKIs in MPM treatment can be caused by the concomitant activation of different TKRs (MET; EGFR; PDGFR). For example, high percentage of MPM tumors and cell lines (70%) showed simultaneous overexpression of c-MET and EGFR and preclinical models revealed a synergistic antitumor activity using crizotinib (c-MET kinase inhibitor) and afatinib (EGFR inhibitor) [65]. Multi-targeted TKIs have been developed. Vandetanib (ZD6474, Zactima, Astra Zeneca Pharmaceuticals), an oral inhibitor of EGFR, VEGFR and RET tyrosine kinases, showed strong anticancer activity in MPM cell lines acting both inhibiting RET-dependent cell survival and VEGFR-dependent angiogenesis [66], and strongly enhancing carboplatin/pemetrexed cytotoxicity [67]. Despite this, its efficacy as single agent in vandetanib versus vinorelbine randomized phase II trial in 25 patients with inoperable or relapsed malignant mesothelioma showed disappointing results (www.clinicaltrials.gov;NCT00597116). Dasatinib (BMS354825, Sprycel, Bristol-Myers) targets BCR-ABL fusion protein and inhibits signals derived from PDGFR and Src family of non-receptor tyrosine kinase [68]. Single-agent dasatinib assessed in second-line or neoadjuvant setting showed high toxicity profile without anticancer efficacy [69, 70] (Table 17.1). These negative results highlight the need to test further TKI combinations and to identify reliable predictive biomarkers to select those patients suitable for specific therapies.

17.1.3 Apoptosis Dysregulation

Dysregulation of apoptotic pathway is a feature of MPM. O'kane et al., analyzing 54 MPM tumor samples that consist of both sarcomatoid and epithelioid subtypes, revealed overexpression of the antiapoptotic proteins BCL-2, BCL-XL, and Mcl-1 and downregulation of the proapoptotic Bad, Bax, and Bid. Most important, percentage of patients overexpressing BCL-XL and under-expressing Bad and Bid was significantly higher in sarcomatoid than in epithelioid subtypes [71]. Overexpression of caspase inhibitors XIAP (X-Linked Inhibitor Of Apoptosis) and survivin in MPM specimens has also been reported [72].

17.1.3.1 Apoptosis Dysregulation and HDAC Inhibitors

Histone deacetylases are 18 different enzymes divided into four classes based on functional criteria [73]. They control a plethora of cellular function including cell cycle arrest, apoptosis, angiogenesis, and immunomodulation regulating the activity of both histones and nonhistone proteins, such as p53, NF-kB, HSP90, and HIF-1alpha [74]. HDAC inhibitors include a wide spectrum of natural and synthetic compounds [75], and are classified as pan-deacetylase inhibitors, including vorinostat (Suberoylanilide Hydroxamic Acid-SAHA: Zolinza, Merck), panobinostat (LBH589; Farydak, Novartis), belinostat (PXD101; Beleodaq, Spectrum Pharmaceuticals), and trichostatin A, and class-specific inhibitors such as butyrate and valproate (inhibit class I and IIa HDACs) and SBHA (suberohydroxamic acid) (inhibits HADC 1 and 3) [73]. In MPM cell lines, downregulation of BCL-XL was implicated in butyrate-induced apoptosis [76], and in SBHA sensitization to TNF-Related

Apoptosis-Inducing Ligand (TRAIL) [77]. Sensitization to TRAIL treatment was also obtained with panobinostat that acted inhibiting the expression of XIAP and increasing caspases' activation [78]. Vandermeers et al. demonstrated increased apoptosis induction combining cisplatinum and pemetrexed treatment with both valproate and SAHA. Anticancer efficacy of valproate *plus* cisplatinum/pemetrexed therapy was also validated in an epithelioid in vivo model [79]. In MPM, HDAC inhibitors have been tested in clinical trials both as single agent and combined therapy (Table 17.1). Oral vorinostat, an FDA-approved drug for the treatment of cutaneous T-cell lymphoma, was tested in a phase III, double-blind, randomized, placebo-controlled trial (www.clinicaltrials.gov; NCT00128102). Six hundred and sixty-one mesothelioma patients progressed after platinum *plus* pemetrexed treatment were included in the study. Results of this phase III study showed no improvement in Overall Survival (OS) in vorinostat versus placebo-treated group [80]. Negative results were also obtained with belinostat in a phase II study in which 13 MPM patients were included for second-line treatment and received intravenous infusion of the drug. The study was stopped for lack of efficacy [81]. On the contrary, a phase II trial aimed at evaluating oral valproate administration plus doxorubicin for refractory or recurrent mesothelioma after platinum-based first-line therapy showed encouraging response rate (16%) and disease control (36%). Among 45 MPM patients enrolled into the study, the best response was observed in those patients with good performance status at the time of protocol inclusion [82].

17.1.3.2 Apoptosis Dysregulation and Proteasome Inhibitors

Proteasome is a multiprotein complex responsible for proteins degradation and homeostasis. Bortezomib (Velcade) is a potent proteasome inhibitor, approved by FDA for multiple myeloma treatments. It is able to activate intrinsic apoptosis mainly blocking the degradation of IKB (Inhibitor KB) and consequently the activation of the pro-survival NF-kB (nuclear factor kappa-light-chain-enhancer of activated B cells) pathway [83].

In MPM preclinical studies, the ability of bortezomib to induce apoptosis was confirmed [84]. Of note, a strong synergizing activity was reported when bortezomib was administrated in combination with carboplatin/pemetrexed therapy [85]. Despite this, clinical evaluation of bortezomib in MPM patients failed to reach satisfactory results. Phase II trial designed to evaluate the efficacy of bortezomib as single agent in first- and second-line setting showed no activity, discouraging further evaluations [86]; phase II study aimed at evaluating the efficacy of first-line therapy combining cisplatin and bortezomib did not fulfill the primary endpoint (progression-free survival rate at 18 weeks >67.5%) and showed higher toxicity than cisplatin/pemetrexed (or raltitrexed) therapy [87] (Table 17.1).

17.1.3.3 Apoptosis Dysregulation and MicroRNAs

MicroRNAs (miRNAs) are short, noncoding, RNAs that targeting sequence-specific mRNAs are implied in post-transcriptional regulation of genes expression. Based on their target mRNAs, microRNAs can act as oncogenes or tumor suppressor genes. Dysregulation of miRNAs expression has been described in many malignancies, including cancers. In MPM mir-34b/c, mir-16 and mir-193a-3p are downregulated. These miRNAs are implied in the regulation of pro-survival and antiapoptotic pathways [56, 88–90]. TargomiRs are minicells loaded with specific microRNAs (EDVs—EnGeneIC Dream Vector) representing a reliable delivery system for in vivo administration. Mir-16 mimic encapsulated in an EGFR-targeted EDVs was successfully tested in MPM xenograft model [89] paving the way for clinical assessment. Van Zandwijk et al. conducted a phase I, open-label, dose-escalation study aimed at testing safety and activity of mir-16-loaded minicells in patients with recurrent pleural mesothelioma previously treated (Table 17.1). Twenty-six MPM patients were enrolled into the study. 5×10^9 TargomiRs per week were well tolerated and revealed early signs of antitumor activity detected by CT and PET-CT (5% of patients had partial response and 68% of patients had stable disease). However, Targomir activity could not be clearly attributed to mir-16 targeting because the evaluation of mir-16 silencing on post-treatment biopsies has not been performed [91]. Nevertheless, results of the study are encouraging and warrant further clinical investigations.

17.1.4 Cell Cycle Regulation

Molecular pathogenesis of MPM is characterized by frequent deletion of CDKN2A gene. CDKN2A encodes p14/ARF and p16/INK4A proteins. p16/INK4a plays an important role in the regulation of the G1/S cell cycle checkpoint; it inhibits the activity of Cyclin-Dependent Kinases (CDKs) 4/6 preventing the phosphorylation of RB (Retinoblastoma protein) and thus G1/S cell cycle progression [51] (Fig. 17.4). Low expression of p16/INK4a significantly correlated with chemotherapy resistance and worse survival of MPM patients [92], suggesting that MPM patients carrying p16 deletion may benefit from CDK inhibitor-based therapy. CDK4/6 inhibitors

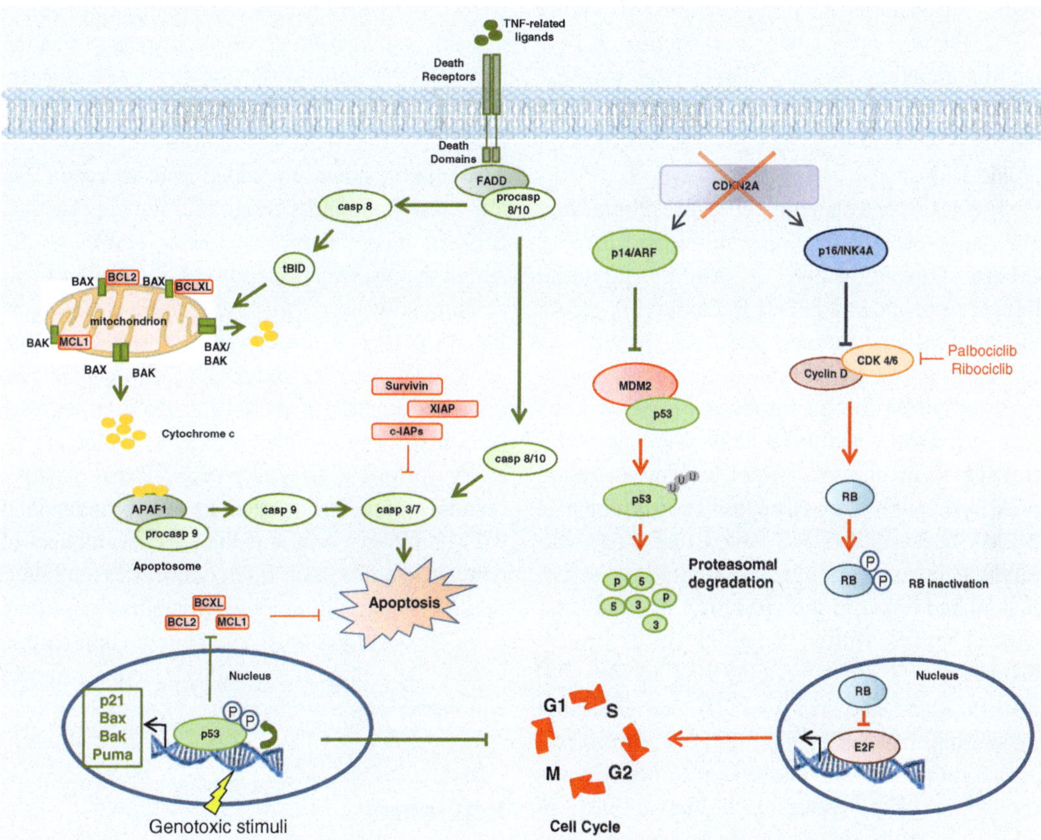

Fig. 17.4 *Apoptotic pathways are represented on the left.* TNF (Tumor Necrosis Factor)-related ligands trigger extrinsic apoptosis. Genotoxic agents induce mitochondrial intrinsic apoptosis through p53 phosphorylation and activation. Proapoptotic proteins are represented in green. Antiapoptotic proteins are represented in red. *The role of p14ARF and p16INK4a proteins in the cell cycle regulation is represented on the right.* p14ARF inhibits MDM2 and subsequently induces p53 accumulation and activation. p16INK4a inactivates cyclinD/CDK4/6 complex preventing the phosphorylation and inactivation of Rb, thus inducing G1/S cell cycle arrest. Palbociclib and ribociclib inhibit CDK4/6. *FADD* Fas-associated protein death domain, *procasp/casp* procaspase/caspase, *BCL2* B-cell lymphoma 2, *BCLXL* B-cell lymphoma extra-large, *MCL1* myeloid cell leukemia 1, *BAX* BCL2-associated X protein, *BAK* BCL2 Antagonist Killer, *APAF1* apoptotic protease activating factor-1, *c-IAP* cellular inhibitor of apoptosis, *XIAP* X-linked inhibitor of apoptosis, *MDM2* mouse double minute 2, *CDK4/6* cyclin-dependent kinase 4/6, *RB* retinoblastoma protein

(such as palbociclib and ribociclib) are under investigation in several tumors. These drugs mimic p16 activity preventing RB phosphorylation [93]. Palbociclib (PD-033299; Pfizer) is an oral available, potent CDK4/6 inhibitor characterized by a mild toxicity profile. It was approved by FDA for the treatment of estrogen-positive metastatic breast cancer. Of note, palbociclib showed efficacy in MPM cell lines when associated with PI3K inhibitors [94], but clinical trials aimed at testing its efficacy in MPM patients has not been performed yet.

The efficacy of ribociclib (LEE01; Novartis) is under evaluation in solid tumor, including MPM. Phase II open-label, nonrandomized clinical trial including patients characterized by aberrant expression of CDK4/6, cyclin D1/3, or p16 is ongoing (www.clinicaltrials.gov; NCT02187783) (Table 17.1).

p14/ARF controls both cell cycle progression and apoptosis activation inhibiting MDM2 (Mouse Double Minute 2), the E3 ubiquitin ligase responsible for p53 degradation (Fig. 17.4). In p53 wild-type tumors, p14/ARF activity can be bypassed using small-molecule p53 activators such as Nutlin 3a, an inhibitor of MDM2-p53 interaction [95]. Nutlin 3a showed greater activity in those tumor characterized by over-activation of MDM2 [96]. This is of particular interest in MPM because MDM2 overexpression was reported in tumor samples, especially in sarcomatoid and biphasic subtypes [97]. In MPM preclinical studies, Nutlin 3a caused p53-dependent G1/S cell cycle arrest inducing p21 increase [98] also in ZL34 and MSTO-211H cell lines not expressing p14/ARF [92, 99]. Moreover, p53 activation was able to decrease the antiapoptotic protein survivin. However, in the absence of strong apoptotic stimuli, Nutlin 3a did not induce MPM cell death but strongly synergized with rhTRAIL-dependent apoptosis [98]. Clinical trial aimed at testing the activity of RG7112 (Roche), a Nutlin 3a analog optimized for clinical use, showed promising activity in leukemias [100] but modest responses and high toxicity in solid tumors [101]. A more potent nutlin analog, RG7388 (Roche) (idasanutlin) [102], is in phase III trial in relapsed/refractory AML (Acute Myeloblastic Leukemia) (www.clinicaltrials.gov; NCT02545283) encouraging future assessment in MPM both as single agent and combined therapy.

17.2 Conclusions

Although clinical evaluation of targeted therapies in MPM found a strong rationale in several molecular alterations characterizing this neoplasia, clinical trials aimed at evaluating the efficacy of biologic agents targeting key oncogenic pathways did not achieve the expected results [28]. A possible explanation of this failure may lie in the lack of driver mutations, which instead characterize other types of cancers. Indeed, while TKIs are ineffective in MPM, EGFR-mutated NSCLC is particularly suited to anti-EGFR therapies, so that these treatments entered in clinical practice. Loss of tumor suppressor genes results in the simultaneous dysregulation of different downstream pathways. For example, loss of *NF2*/merlin triggers cell proliferation through Hippo, PI3K-ATK-mTOR, and FAK pathways. In this context, targeting a single transduction pathway has shown to be ineffective to abrogate the proliferative pressure of cancer cells. These negative results highlight the need to better understand MPM biology. A comprehensive evaluation of cellular features, their interconnections, and their relationships with tumor microenvironment may help to develop novel therapeutic approaches aimed at targeting multiple key signals simultaneously.

References

1. Tsao AS, Wistuba I, Roth JA, Kindler HL. Malignant pleural mesothelioma. J Clin Oncol Off J Am Soc Clin Oncol. 2009;27(12):2081–90. Epub 2009/03/04.
2. Vogelzang NJ, Rusthoven JJ, Symanowski J, Denham C, Kaukel E, Ruffie P, et al. Phase III study of pemetrexed in combination with cisplatin versus cisplatin alone in patients with malignant pleural mesothelioma. J Clin Oncol Off J Am Soc Clin Oncol. 2003;21(14):2636–44. Epub 2003/07/16.
3. Kindler HL, Ismaila N, Armato SG 3rd, Bueno R, Hesdorffer M, Jahan T, et al. Treatment of malignant

pleural mesothelioma: American Society of Clinical Oncology clinical practice guideline. J Clin Oncol Off J Am Soc Clin Oncol. 2018;36(13):1343–73. Epub 2018/01/19.

4. Sekido Y. Genomic abnormalities and signal transduction dysregulation in malignant mesothelioma cells. Cancer Sci. 2010;101(1):1–6. Epub 2009/10/02.
5. Sekido Y, Pass HI, Bader S, Mew DJ, Christman MF, Gazdar AF, et al. Neurofibromatosis type 2 (NF2) gene is somatically mutated in mesothelioma but not in lung cancer. Cancer Res. 1995;55(6):1227–31. Epub 1995/03/15.
6. Cheng JQ, Lee WC, Klein MA, Cheng GZ, Jhanwar SC, Testa JR. Frequent mutations of NF2 and allelic loss from chromosome band 22q12 in malignant mesothelioma: evidence for a two-hit mechanism of NF2 inactivation. Genes Chromosomes Cancer. 1999;24(3):238–42. Epub 1999/08/19.
7. Baser ME, De Rienzo A, Altomare D, Balsara BR, Hedrick NM, Gutmann DH, et al. Neurofibromatosis 2 and malignant mesothelioma. Neurology. 2002;59(2):290–1. Epub 2002/07/24.
8. Lo Iacono M, Monica V, Righi L, Grosso F, Libener R, Vatrano S, et al. Targeted next-generation sequencing of cancer genes in advanced stage malignant pleural mesothelioma: a retrospective study. J Thorac Oncol. 2015;10(3):492–9. Epub 2014/12/17.
9. Bueno R, Stawiski EW, Goldstein LD, Durinck S, De Rienzo A, Modrusan Z, et al. Comprehensive genomic analysis of malignant pleural mesothelioma identifies recurrent mutations, gene fusions and splicing alterations. Nat Genet. 2016;48(4):407–16. Epub 2016/03/02.
10. Hylebos M, Van Camp G, Vandeweyer G, Fransen E, Beyens M, Cornelissen R, et al. Large-scale copy number analysis reveals variations in genes not previously associated with malignant pleural mesothelioma. Oncotarget. 2017;8(69):113673–86. Epub 2018/01/27.
11. Petrilli AM, Fernandez-Valle C. Role of Merlin/NF2 inactivation in tumor biology. Oncogene. 2016;35(5):537–48. Epub 2015/04/22.
12. Sato T, Sekido Y. NF2/Merlin inactivation and potential therapeutic targets in mesothelioma. Int J Mol Sci. 2018;19(4):988. Epub 2018/03/29.
13. Thurneysen C, Opitz I, Kurtz S, Weder W, Stahel RA, Felley-Bosco E. Functional inactivation of NF2/merlin in human mesothelioma. Lung Cancer. 2009;64(2):140–7. Epub 2008/10/07.
14. Yu FX, Zhao B, Guan KL. Hippo pathway in organ size control, tissue homeostasis, and cancer. Cell. 2015;163(4):811–28. Epub 2015/11/07.
15. Felley-Bosco E, Stahel R. Hippo/YAP pathway for targeted therapy. Translational Lung Cancer Res. 2014;3(2):75–83. Epub 2015/03/26.
16. Murakami H, Mizuno T, Taniguchi T, Fujii M, Ishiguro F, Fukui T, et al. LATS2 is a tumor suppressor gene of malignant mesothelioma. Cancer Res. 2011;71(3):873–83. Epub 2011/01/20.
17. Sekido Y. Inactivation of Merlin in malignant mesothelioma cells and the Hippo signaling cascade dysregulation. Pathol Int. 2011;61(6):331–44. Epub 2011/05/28.
18. Tranchant R, Quetel L, Tallet A, Meiller C, Renier A, de Koning L, et al. Co-occurring mutations of tumor suppressor genes, LATS2 and NF2, in malignant pleural mesothelioma. Clin Cancer Res. 2017;23(12):3191–202. Epub 2016/12/23.
19. Meerang M, Berard K, Friess M, Bitanihirwe BK, Soltermann A, Vrugt B, et al. Low Merlin expression and high Survivin labeling index are indicators for poor prognosis in patients with malignant pleural mesothelioma. Mol Oncol. 2016;10(8):1255–65. Epub 2016/07/06.
20. Zhang WQ, Dai YY, Hsu PC, Wang H, Cheng L, Yang YL, et al. Targeting YAP in malignant pleural mesothelioma. J Cell Mol Med. 2017;21(11):2663–76. Epub 2017/05/05.
21. Mizuno T, Murakami H, Fujii M, Ishiguro F, Tanaka I, Kondo Y, et al. YAP induces malignant mesothelioma cell proliferation by upregulating transcription of cell cycle-promoting genes. Oncogene. 2012;31(49):5117–22. Epub 2012/01/31.
22. Liu-Chittenden Y, Huang B, Shim JS, Chen Q, Lee SJ, Anders RA, et al. Genetic and pharmacological disruption of the TEAD-YAP complex suppresses the oncogenic activity of YAP. Genes Dev. 2012;26(12):1300–5. Epub 2012/06/09.
23. Gibault F, Corvaisier M, Bailly F, Huet G, Melnyk P, Cotelle P. Non-Photoinduced biological properties of Verteporfin. Curr Med Chem. 2016;23(11):1171–84. Epub 2016/03/17.
24. Vanhaesebroeck B, Guillermet-Guibert J, Graupera M, Bilanges B. The emerging mechanisms of isoform-specific PI3K signalling. Nat Rev Mol Cell Biol. 2010;11(5):329–41. Epub 2010/04/10.
25. Julien LA, Carriere A, Moreau J, Roux PP. mTORC1-activated S6K1 phosphorylates Rictor on threonine 1135 and regulates mTORC2 signaling. Mol Cell Biol. 2010;30(4):908–21. Epub 2009/12/10.
26. Janku F, Yap TA, Meric-Bernstam F. Targeting the PI3K pathway in cancer: are we making headway? Nat Rev Clin Oncol. 2018;15(5):273–91. Epub 2018/03/07.
27. Li W, Cooper J, Karajannis MA, Giancotti FG. Merlin: a tumour suppressor with functions at the cell cortex and in the nucleus. EMBO Rep. 2012;13(3):204–15. Epub 2012/04/07.
28. Stahel RA, Weder W, Felley-Bosco E, Petrausch U, Curioni-Fontecedro A, Schmitt-Opitz I, et al. Searching for targets for the systemic therapy of mesothelioma. Ann Oncol. 2015;26(8):1649–60. Epub 2015/02/28.
29. Cedres S, Ponce-Aix S, Pardo-Aranda N, Navarro-Mendivil A, Martinez-Marti A, Zugazagoitia J, et al. Analysis of expression of PTEN/PI3K pathway and programmed cell death ligand 1 (PD-L1) in malignant pleural mesothelioma (MPM). Lung Cancer. 2016;96:1–6. Epub 2016/05/03.

30. Agarwal V, Campbell A, Beaumont KL, Cawkwell L, Lind MJ. PTEN protein expression in malignant pleural mesothelioma. Tumour Biol. 2013;34(2):847–51. Epub 2012/12/18.
31. Lopez-Lago MA, Okada T, Murillo MM, Socci N, Giancotti FG. Loss of the tumor suppressor gene NF2, encoding merlin, constitutively activates integrin-dependent mTORC1 signaling. Mol Cell Biol. 2009;29(15):4235–49. Epub 2009/05/20.
32. Pignochino Y, Dell'Aglio C, Inghilleri S, Zorzetto M, Basirico M, Capozzi F, et al. The combination of sorafenib and everolimus shows antitumor activity in preclinical models of malignant pleural mesothelioma. BMC Cancer. 2015;15:374. Epub 2015/05/09.
33. Ou SH, Moon J, Garland LL, Mack PC, Testa JR, Tsao AS, et al. SWOG S0722: phase II study of mTOR inhibitor everolimus (RAD001) in advanced malignant pleural mesothelioma (MPM). J Thorac Oncol. 2015;10(2):387–91. Epub 2015/01/23.
34. Dolly SO, Wagner AJ, Bendell JC, Kindler HL, Krug LM, Seiwert TY, et al. Phase I study of Apitolisib (GDC-0980), dual Phosphatidylinositol-3-kinase and mammalian target of Rapamycin kinase inhibitor, in patients with advanced solid Tumors. Clin Cancer Res. 2016;22(12):2874–84. Epub 2016/01/21.
35. Powles T, Lackner MR, Oudard S, Escudier B, Ralph C, Brown JE, et al. Randomized open-label phase II trial of Apitolisib (GDC-0980), a novel inhibitor of the PI3K/mammalian target of Rapamycin pathway, versus Everolimus in patients with metastatic renal cell carcinoma. J Clin Oncol Off J Am Soc Clin Oncol. 2016;34(14):1660–8. Epub 2016/03/10.
36. Yamaji M, Ota A, Wahiduzzaman M, Karnan S, Hyodo T, Konishi H, et al. Novel ATP-competitive Akt inhibitor afuresertib suppresses the proliferation of malignant pleural mesothelioma cells. Cancer Med. 2017;6(11):2646–59. Epub 2017/09/30.
37. Spencer A, Yoon SS, Harrison SJ, Morris SR, Smith DA, Brigandi RA, et al. The novel AKT inhibitor afuresertib shows favorable safety, pharmacokinetics, and clinical activity in multiple myeloma. Blood. 2014;124(14):2190–5. Epub 2014/07/31.
38. Sulzmaier FJ, Jean C, Schlaepfer DD. FAK in cancer: mechanistic findings and clinical applications. Nat Rev Cancer. 2014;14(9):598–610. Epub 2014/08/08.
39. Lim ST, Mikolon D, Stupack DG, Schlaepfer DD. FERM control of FAK function: implications for cancer therapy. Cell Cycle. 2008;7(15):2306–14. Epub 2008/08/05.
40. Roy-Luzarraga M, Hodivala-Dilke K. Molecular pathways: endothelial cell FAK-A target for cancer treatment. Clin Cancer Res. 2016;22(15):3718–24. Epub 2016/06/05.
41. Serrels A, Lund T, Serrels B, Byron A, McPherson RC, von Kriegsheim A, et al. Nuclear FAK controls chemokine transcription, Tregs, and evasion of anti-tumor immunity. Cell. 2015;163(1):160–73. Epub 2015/09/26.
42. Shapiro IM, Kolev VN, Vidal CM, Kadariya Y, Ring JE, Wright Q, et al. Merlin deficiency predicts FAK inhibitor sensitivity: a synthetic lethal relationship. Sci Transl Med. 2014;6(237):237ra68. Epub 2014/05/23.
43. Poulikakos PI, Xiao GH, Gallagher R, Jablonski S, Jhanwar SC, Testa JR. Re-expression of the tumor suppressor NF2/merlin inhibits invasiveness in mesothelioma cells and negatively regulates FAK. Oncogene. 2006;25(44):5960–8. Epub 2006/05/03.
44. Kato T, Sato T, Yokoi K, Sekido Y. E-cadherin expression is correlated with focal adhesion kinase inhibitor resistance in Merlin-negative malignant mesothelioma cells. Oncogene. 2017;36(39):5522–31. Epub 2017/05/30.
45. Zhang J, He DH, Zajac-Kaye M, Hochwald SN. A small molecule FAK kinase inhibitor, GSK2256098, inhibits growth and survival of pancreatic ductal adenocarcinoma cells. Cell Cycle. 2014;13(19):3143–9. Epub 2014/12/09.
46. Thanapprapasr D, Previs RA, Hu W, Ivan C, Armaiz-Pena GN, Dorniak PL, et al. PTEN expression as a predictor of response to focal adhesion kinase inhibition in uterine cancer. Mol Cancer Ther. 2015;14(6):1466–75. Epub 2015/04/03.
47. Soria JC, Gan HK, Blagden SP, Plummer R, Arkenau HT, Ranson M, et al. A phase I, pharmacokinetic and pharmacodynamic study of GSK2256098, a focal adhesion kinase inhibitor, in patients with advanced solid tumors. Ann Oncol. 2016;27(12):2268–74. Epub 2016/10/14.
48. Arkenau H-T, Gazzah A, Plummer R, Blagden SP, Mak G, Soria J-C, et al. A phase Ib dose-escalation study of GSK2256098 (FAKi) plus trametinib (MEKi) in patients with selected advanced solid tumors. J Clin Oncol. 2015;33(15_suppl):2593.
49. Dazzi H, Hasleton PS, Thatcher N, Wilkes S, Swindell R, Chatterjee AK. Malignant pleural mesothelioma and epidermal growth factor receptor (EGF-R). Relationship of EGF-R with histology and survival using fixed paraffin embedded tissue and the F4, monoclonal antibody. Br J Cancer. 1990;61(6):924–6. Epub 1990/06/01.
50. Govindan R, Kratzke RA, Herndon JE 2nd, Niehans GA, Vollmer R, Watson D, et al. Gefitinib in patients with malignant mesothelioma: a phase II study by the cancer and Leukemia group B. Clin Cancer Res. 2005;11(6):2300–4. Epub 2005/03/25.
51. Pasello G, Favaretto A. Molecular targets in malignant pleural mesothelioma treatment. Curr Drug Targets. 2009;10(12):1235–44. Epub 2009/11/17.
52. Garland LL, Rankin C, Gandara DR, Rivkin SE, Scott KM, Nagle RB, et al. Phase II study of erlotinib in patients with malignant pleural mesothelioma: a southwest oncology group study. J Clin Oncol Off J Am Soc Clin Oncol. 2007;25(17):2406–13. Epub 2007/06/15.
53. Mezzapelle R, Miglio U, Rena O, Paganotti A, Allegrini S, Antona J, et al. Mutation analysis of the EGFR gene and downstream signalling pathway in histologic samples of malignant pleural mesothelioma. Br J Cancer. 2013;108(8):1743–9. Epub 2013/04/06.

54. Gaudino G, Yang H, Carbone M. HGF/met Signaling is a key player in malignant mesothelioma carcinogenesis. Biomedicine. 2014;2(4):327–44. Epub 2014/11/14.
55. Bois MC, Mansfield AS, Sukov WR, Jenkins SM, Moser JC, Sattler CA, et al. c-Met expression and MET amplification in malignant pleural mesothelioma. Ann Diagn Pathol. 2016;23:1–7. Epub 2016/07/13.
56. Kubo T, Toyooka S, Tsukuda K, Sakaguchi M, Fukazawa T, Soh J, et al. Epigenetic silencing of microRNA-34b/c plays an important role in the pathogenesis of malignant pleural mesothelioma. Clin Cancer Res. 2011;17(15):4965–74. Epub 2011/06/16.
57. Jagadeeswaran R, Ma PC, Seiwert TY, Jagadeeswaran S, Zumba O, Nallasura V, et al. Functional analysis of c-Met/hepatocyte growth factor pathway in malignant pleural mesothelioma. Cancer Res. 2006;66(1):352–61. Epub 2006/01/07.
58. Santoro A, Rimassa L, Borbath I, Daniele B, Salvagni S, Van Laethem JL, et al. Tivantinib for second-line treatment of advanced hepatocellular carcinoma: a randomised, placebo-controlled phase 2 study. Lancet Oncol. 2013;14(1):55–63. Epub 2012/11/28.
59. Maron SB, Karrison T, Kanteti R, Rao KA, Gandara DR, Koczywas M, et al. ARQ 197 in patients with previously-treated malignant mesothelioma (MM): a phase II trial from the University of Chicago phase II consortium. J Clin Oncol. 2015;33(15_suppl):7511.
60. Leon LG, Gemelli M, Sciarrillo R, Avan A, Funel N, Giovannetti E. Synergistic activity of the c-Met and tubulin inhibitor tivantinib (ARQ197) with pemetrexed in mesothelioma cells. Curr Drug Targets. 2014;15(14):1331–40. Epub 2014/12/09.
61. Kanteti R, Dhanasingh I, Kawada I, Lennon FE, Arif Q, Bueno R, et al. MET and PI3K/mTOR as a potential combinatorial therapeutic target in malignant pleural mesothelioma. PLoS One. 2014;9(9):e105919. Epub 2014/09/16.
62. Porta C, Mutti L, Tassi G. Negative results of an Italian Group for Mesothelioma (G.I.Me.) pilot study of single-agent imatinib mesylate in malignant pleural mesothelioma. Cancer Chemother Pharmacol. 2007;59(1):149–50. Epub 2006/04/26.
63. Mathy A, Baas P, Dalesio O, van Zandwijk N. Limited efficacy of imatinib mesylate in malignant mesothelioma: a phase II trial. Lung Cancer. 2005;50(1):83–6. Epub 2005/06/14.
64. Tsao AS, Harun N, Lee JJ, Heymach J, Pisters K, Hong WK, et al. Phase I trial of cisplatin, pemetrexed, and imatinib mesylate in chemonaive patients with unresectable malignant pleural mesothelioma. Clin Lung Cancer. 2014;15(3):197–201. Epub 2014/02/05.
65. Huang L, Cai M, Zhang X, Wang F, Chen L, Xu M, et al. Combinational therapy of crizotinib and afatinib for malignant pleural mesothelioma. Am J Cancer Res. 2017;7(2):203–17. Epub 2017/03/25.
66. Ogino H, Yano S, Kakiuchi S, Yamada T, Ikuta K, Nakataki E, et al. Novel dual targeting strategy with vandetanib induces tumor cell apoptosis and inhibits angiogenesis in malignant pleural mesothelioma cells expressing RET oncogenic rearrangement. Cancer Lett. 2008;265(1):55–66. Epub 2008/03/28.
67. Giovannetti E, Zucali PA, Assaraf YG, Leon LG, Smid K, Alecci C, et al. Preclinical emergence of vandetanib as a potent antitumour agent in mesothelioma: molecular mechanisms underlying its synergistic interaction with pemetrexed and carboplatin. Br J Cancer. 2011;105(10):1542–53. Epub 2011/10/06.
68. Tsao AS, He D, Saigal B, Liu S, Lee JJ, Bakkannagari S, et al. Inhibition of c-Src expression and activation in malignant pleural mesothelioma tissues leads to apoptosis, cell cycle arrest, and decreased migration and invasion. Mol Cancer Ther. 2007;6(7):1962–72. Epub 2007/07/11.
69. Dudek AZ, Pang H, Kratzke RA, Otterson GA, Hodgson L, Vokes EE, et al. Phase II study of dasatinib in patients with previously treated malignant mesothelioma (cancer and leukemia group B 30601): a brief report. J Thorac Oncol. 2012;7(4):755–9. Epub 2012/03/20.
70. Tsao AS, Lin H, Carter BW, Lee JJ, Rice D, Vaporcyan A, et al. Biomarker-integrated Neoadjuvant Dasatinib trial in Resectable malignant pleural mesothelioma. J Thorac Oncol. 2018;13(2):246–57. Epub 2018/01/10.
71. O'Kane SL, Pound RJ, Campbell A, Chaudhuri N, Lind MJ, Cawkwell L. Expression of bcl-2 family members in malignant pleural mesothelioma. Acta Oncol. 2006;45(4):449–53. Epub 2006/06/09.
72. Kleinberg L, Lie AK, Florenes VA, Nesland JM, Davidson B. Expression of inhibitor-of-apoptosis protein family members in malignant mesothelioma. Hum Pathol. 2007;38(7):986–94. Epub 2007/03/14.
73. Khan O, La Thangue NB. HDAC inhibitors in cancer biology: emerging mechanisms and clinical applications. Immunol Cell Biol. 2012;90(1):85–94. Epub 2011/11/30.
74. Paik PK, Krug LM. Histone deacetylase inhibitors in malignant pleural mesothelioma: preclinical rationale and clinical trials. J Thorac Oncol. 2010;5(2):275–9. Epub 2009/12/26.
75. Bolden JE, Peart MJ, Johnstone RW. Anticancer activities of histone deacetylase inhibitors. Nat Rev Drug Discov. 2006;5(9):769–84. Epub 2006/09/07.
76. Cao XX, Mohuiddin I, Ece F, McConkey DJ, Smythe WR. Histone deacetylase inhibitor downregulation of bcl-xl gene expression leads to apoptotic cell death in mesothelioma. Am J Respir Cell Mol Biol. 2001;25(5):562–8. Epub 2001/11/20.
77. Neuzil J, Swettenham E, Gellert N. Sensitization of mesothelioma to TRAIL apoptosis by inhibition of histone deacetylase: role of Bcl-xL down-regulation. Biochem Biophys Res Commun. 2004;314(1):186–91. Epub 2004/01/13.
78. Symanowski J, Vogelzang N, Zawel L, Atadja P, Pass H, Sharma S. A histone deacetylase inhibitor LBH589 downregulates XIAP in mesothelioma cell lines which is likely responsible for increased apoptosis with TRAIL. J Thorac Oncol. 2009;4(2):149–60. Epub 2009/01/31.

79. Vandermeers F, Hubert P, Delvenne P, Mascaux C, Grigoriu B, Burny A, et al. Valproate, in combination with pemetrexed and cisplatin, provides additional efficacy to the treatment of malignant mesothelioma. Clin Cancer Res. 2009;15(8):2818–28. Epub 2009/04/09.
80. Krug LM, Kindler HL, Calvert H, Manegold C, Tsao AS, Fennell D, et al. Vorinostat in patients with advanced malignant pleural mesothelioma who have progressed on previous chemotherapy (VANTAGE-014): a phase 3, double-blind, randomised, placebo-controlled trial. Lancet Oncol. 2015;16(4):447–56. Epub 2015/03/25.
81. Ramalingam SS, Belani CP, Ruel C, Frankel P, Gitlitz B, Koczywas M, et al. Phase II study of belinostat (PXD101), a histone deacetylase inhibitor, for second line therapy of advanced malignant pleural mesothelioma. J Thorac Oncol. 2009;4(1):97–101. Epub 2008/12/20.
82. Scherpereel A, Berghmans T, Lafitte JJ, Colinet B, Richez M, Bonduelle Y, et al. Valproate-doxorubicin: promising therapy for progressing mesothelioma. A phase II study. Eur Respir J. 2011;37(1):129–35. Epub 2010/06/10.
83. Fennell DA, Chacko A, Mutti L. BCL-2 family regulation by the 20S proteasome inhibitor bortezomib. Oncogene. 2008;27(9):1189–97. Epub 2007/09/11.
84. Sartore-Bianchi A, Gasparri F, Galvani A, Nici L, Darnowski JW, Barbone D, et al. Bortezomib inhibits nuclear factor-kappaB dependent survival and has potent in vivo activity in mesothelioma. Clin Cancer Res. 2007;13(19):5942–51. Epub 2007/10/03.
85. Gordon GJ, Mani M, Maulik G, Mukhopadhyay L, Yeap BY, Kindler HL, et al. Preclinical studies of the proteasome inhibitor bortezomib in malignant pleural mesothelioma. Cancer Chemother Pharmacol. 2008;61(4):549–58. Epub 2007/05/25.
86. Fennell DA, McDowell C, Busacca S, Webb G, Moulton B, Cakana A, et al. Phase II clinical trial of first or second-line treatment with bortezomib in patients with malignant pleural mesothelioma. J Thorac Oncol. 2012;7(9):1466–70. Epub 2012/08/17.
87. O'Brien ME, Gaafar RM, Popat S, Grossi F, Price A, Talbot DC, et al. Phase II study of first-line bortezomib and cisplatin in malignant pleural mesothelioma and prospective validation of progression free survival rate as a primary end-point for mesothelioma clinical trials (European Organisation for Research and Treatment of Cancer 08052). Eur J Cancer. 2013;49(13):2815–22. Epub 2013/06/25.
88. Williams M, Kirschner MB, Cheng YY, Hanh J, Weiss J, Mugridge N, et al. miR-193a-3p is a potential tumor suppressor in malignant pleural mesothelioma. Oncotarget. 2015;6(27):23480–95. Epub 2015/07/01.
89. Reid G, Pel ME, Kirschner MB, Cheng YY, Mugridge N, Weiss J, et al. Restoring expression of miR-16: a novel approach to therapy for malignant pleural mesothelioma. Ann Oncol. 2013;24(12):3128–35. Epub 2013/10/24.
90. Truini A, Coco S, Genova C, Mora M, Dal Bello MG, Vanni I, et al. Prognostic and therapeutic implications of MicroRNA in malignant pleural mesothelioma. MicroRNA. 2016;5(1):12–8. Epub 2016/01/29.
91. van Zandwijk N, Pavlakis N, Kao SC, Linton A, Boyer MJ, Clarke S, et al. Safety and activity of microRNA-loaded minicells in patients with recurrent malignant pleural mesothelioma: a first-in-man, phase 1, open-label, dose-escalation study. Lancet Oncol. 2017;18(10):1386–96. Epub 2017/09/06.
92. Jennings CJ, Murer B, O'Grady A, Hearn LM, Harvey BJ, Kay EW, et al. Differential p16/INK4A cyclin-dependent kinase inhibitor expression correlates with chemotherapy efficacy in a cohort of 88 malignant pleural mesothelioma patients. Br J Cancer. 2015;113(1):69–75. Epub 2015/06/10.
93. O'Leary B, Finn RS, Turner NC. Treating cancer with selective CDK4/6 inhibitors. Nat Rev Clin Oncol. 2016;13(7):417–30. Epub 2016/04/01.
94. Bonelli MA, Digiacomo G, Fumarola C, Alfieri R, Quaini F, Falco A, et al. Combined inhibition of CDK4/6 and PI3K/AKT/mTOR pathways induces a synergistic anti-tumor effect in malignant pleural mesothelioma cells. Neoplasia. 2017;19(8):637–48. Epub 2017/07/14.
95. Urso L, Calabrese F, Favaretto A, Conte P, Pasello G. Critical review about MDM2 in cancer: possible role in malignant mesothelioma and implications for treatment. Crit Rev Oncol Hematol. 2016;97:220–30. Epub 2015/09/12.
96. Tovar C, Graves B, Packman K, Filipovic Z, Higgins B, Xia M, et al. MDM2 small-molecule antagonist RG7112 activates p53 signaling and regresses human tumors in preclinical cancer models. Cancer Res. 2013;73(8):2587–97. Epub 2013/02/13.
97. Pasello G, Urso L, Mencoboni M, Grosso F, Ceresoli GL, Lunardi F, et al. MDM2 and HIF1alpha expression levels in different histologic subtypes of malignant pleural mesothelioma: correlation with pathological and clinical data. Oncotarget. 2015;6(39):42053–66. Epub 2015/11/07.
98. Urso L, Cavallari I, Silic-Benussi M, Biasini L, Zago G, Calabrese F, et al. Synergistic targeting of malignant pleural mesothelioma cells by MDM2 inhibitors and TRAIL agonists. Oncotarget. 2017;8(27):44232–41. Epub 2017/06/01.
99. Hopkins-Donaldson S, Belyanskaya LL, Simoes-Wust AP, Sigrist B, Kurtz S, Zangemeister-Wittke U, et al. p53-induced apoptosis occurs in the absence of p14(ARF) in malignant pleural mesothelioma. Neoplasia. 2006;8(7):551–9. Epub 2006/07/27.
100. Andreeff M, Kelly KR, Yee K, Assouline S, Strair R, Popplewell L, et al. Results of the phase I trial of RG7112, a small-molecule MDM2 antagonist

in leukemia. Clin Cancer Res. 2016;22(4):868–76. Epub 2015/10/16.
101. Burgess A, Chia KM, Haupt S, Thomas D, Haupt Y, Lim E. Clinical overview of MDM2/X-targeted therapies. Front Oncol. 2016;6:7. Epub 2016/02/10.
102. Ding Q, Zhang Z, Liu JJ, Jiang N, Zhang J, Ross TM, et al. Discovery of RG7388, a potent and selective p53-MDM2 inhibitor in clinical development. J Med Chem. 2013;56(14):5979–83. Epub 2013/07/03.
103. Jackman DM, Kindler HL, Yeap BY, Fidias P, Salgia R, Lucca J, et al. Erlotinib plus bevacizumab in previously treated patients with malignant pleural mesothelioma. Cancer. 2008;113(4):808–14.

18 Mesothelin-Targeted Agents in Mesothelioma

Loredana Urso and Giulia Pasello

18.1 Introduction

Mesothelin (MSLN) is a cell surface glycoprotein expressed by mesothelial cells of the pleural, peritoneum, and pericardium. It is synthesized as a precursor protein of about 70 KD and then processed by the Furin protease to form the mature form of Mesothelin, a glycosylated membrane-bound protein of about 40 KD, and the soluble Megakariocyte Potentiating Factor (MPF) of about 30 KD [1]. Mesothelin functions are not yet completely understood. Nonetheless, it acquired a great interest in oncology because of its overexpression in several types of cancers, particularly in Malignant Mesothelioma, Ovarian Cancer and Pancreatic Cancer [1]. Since it was discovered in the 1990s by Pastan and Willingham, several studies have been conducted to demonstrate the potential role of Mesothelin as a biomarker for cancer diagnosis and as a suitable target for cancer immunotherapy. In Malignant Mesothelioma, which is characterized by late diagnosis and few therapeutic options, Mesothelin may represent a promising treatment option for affected patients.

L. Urso
Department of Surgery, Oncology and Gastroenterology, University of Padova, Padova, Italy

G. Pasello (✉)
Medical Oncology 2, Istituto Oncologico Veneto IRCCS, Padova, Italy
e-mail: giulia.pasello@iov.veneto.it

18.1.1 Role of Mesothelin in Malignant Mesothelioma

The physiological role of Mesothelin has not been clarified yet, but several reports investigating its function in tumor cells suggested an important role in the different aspect of cancer progression. Mesothelin has high binding affinity for MUC16 (CA125), a typical marker of ovarian cancer, thus promoting heterotypic cell adhesion responsible for ovarian cancer spread across peritoneum [2–4]. In pancreatic cancer cells, mesothelin promotes cell proliferation by inducing IL-6 expression [5, 6] and has an antiapoptotic role in TNF-alpha-induced apoptosis by promoting AKT phosphorylation and subsequent inhibition of pro-apoptotic proteins (BAX and Bad) [7]. Mesothelin overexpression increases anchorage-independent growth of breast cancer cells [8], and high levels of Mesothelin correlate with poor prognosis and resistance to chemotherapy in epithelial ovarian carcinoma patients [9]. Mesothelin is overexpressed in 95% of epithelioid malignant pleural mesothelioma (MPM) and epithelioid component of biphasic MPM tissues [10]. High level of soluble mesothelin detected in the serum of affected patients was associated with worse prognosis, while its change during chemotherapy treatment correlated with radiological response [11]. Preclinical studies demonstrated that Mesothelin may be implicated in mesothelioma invasiveness. Servais et al. demonstrated in an orthotopic mouse model that mesothelin-expressing MPM showed

G. L. Ceresoli et al. (eds.), *Mesothelioma*, https://doi.org/10.1007/978-3-030-16884-1_18

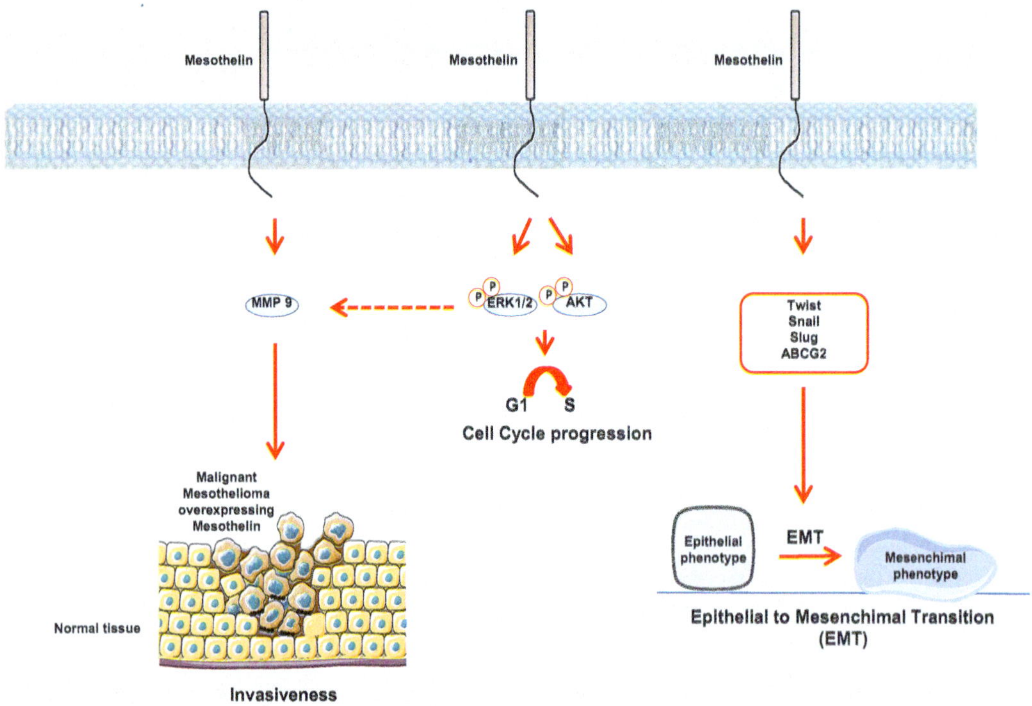

Fig. 18.1 Role of Mesothelin in MPM. Mesothelin overexpression in MPM seems to be involved in: MPM invasiveness promoting the activation of metalloprotease 9 (MMP9) [12]; MPM cell proliferation promoting the activation of Extracellular Signal-regulated Kinase 1/2 (ERK1/2) and Protein Kinase B (AKT/PKB) [14]; promotion of the epithelial to mesenchymal transition by inducing the expression of EMT markers such as Twist, Snail, Slug, ABCG2 [13]. The Figure was created with Smart Servier Medical Art

a more aggressive phenotype characterized by increased local tumor invasion and metalloprotease 9 (MMP9) expression at the invasive edge compared to Mesothelin negative MPM. This aggressive phenotype was significantly associated with reduced survival of mice with Mesothelin-positive tumors. Of note, a strong correlation between Mesothelin and MMP9 expression was observed in surgically resected epithelioid MPM specimens [12]. Mesothelin seems to be involved in epithelial-to-mesenchymal transition (EMT) as demonstrated by the downregulation of EMT markers (twist, snail, slug, and ABCG2) following mesothelin silencing [13]. Conflicting results have been reported regarding mesothelin-induced cell proliferation in MPM. Indeed, MSTO-211H cell lines transduced with mesothelin showed no changes in cell proliferation [12], while mesothelioma cell lines characterized by high mesothelin expression, Mero 14 and H2052, demonstrated a decreased proliferation rate, colony formation, and tumor sphere formation after protein silencing [13, 14]. To reinforce the existing link between Mesothelin and cell proliferation, Melaiu and coworkers showed that, in Mero 14 cells, Mesothelin silencing downregulated AKT and ERK phosphorylation (two proteins generally implicated in proliferative pathways) [14] (Fig. 18.1).

More efforts are needed in order to clarify the role of mesothelin in MPM. A deep knowledge of its pro-tumorigenic function may help in developing new therapeutic strategies able to counteract MPM progression.

18.1.2 Mesothelin as a Therapeutic Target in Malignant Mesothelioma

Mesothelin is considered a good target for cancer immunotherapy because of its limited expression in normal tissues and overexpression in cancers. Overexpression of mesothelin in MPM, especially in the epithelioid subgroup [15], makes this tumor particularly suited for mesothelin-based immunotherapy approaches.

18.1.2.1 Immunotoxins

In 1998, Chowdhury et al. realized the recombinant immunotoxin-targeting mesothelin-expressing cells, called SS1P. It consists of a variable fragment of murine anti-mesothelin antibody conjugated with domain 2 and 3 of the pseudomonas exotoxin A [16]. SS1P internalization following antibody/mesothelin binding carries the exotoxin into mesothelin-expressing cells. Once internalized, the exotoxin inhibits protein synthesis by blocking EEF2 (eukaryotic elongation factor 2) and induces apoptosis. Highly selective antibody/mesothelin binding renders SS1P a specific system to kill cancer cells with marginal effects on normal cells [16]. Two phase I dose escalation studies were conducted to test the safety of SS1P. The first study, enrolling 34 patients, 20 of which were mesothelioma patients (7 pleural mesothelioma), administered SS1P in endovenous bolus as second-line treatment. In the second one, the drug was administered by 10 days continuous infusion in patients not eligible for surgery after first-line treatment. Of 20 patients included, 9 were MPM. In both studies, mesothelin IHC positivity in more than 30% of tumor cells was an inclusion criterium. Exclusion criteria included antibody-related serum neutralizing activity for SS1P higher than 75%. These studies demonstrated an acceptable safety profile of SS1P at the dose level of 45 ug/kg and 25 ug/kg for bolus and continuous infusion, respectively. Pleural pain, probably due to the inflammatory response of mesothelin-expressing mesothelial cells, represented the major adverse event, but it was managed by prednisone co-administration. However, antitumor activity was modest and the majority of patients had no more than one cycle of therapy because neutralizing antibodies were produced. Indeed, after the first cycle, most patients developed serum neutralizing activity for SS1P > 75% [17, 18]. Based on preclinical studies demonstrating a synergistic anticancer activity of SS1P associated with standard chemotherapy in tumor xenografts models [19], a phase I dose escalation study of SS1P in combination with standard doses of Cisplatin and Pemetrexed in Mesothelioma patients was designed. The primary endpoint of the study was to assess the recommended dose of SS1P in combination with chemotherapy; secondary endpoints were the evaluation of the anticancer activity and the evaluation of the role of serum Mesothelin, MPF and CA125 as biomarkers of tumor response [20]. The study demonstrated a potential improvement of anticancer activity of the combination and biomarkers assessment seemed to be predictive of response. However, chemotherapy not influenced anti-SS1P antibodies production, so that patients developed serum neutralizing activity after the first cycle of treatment [20]. Because serum immunization was the major limit of SS1P activity, delaying host immunity response seemed to be the way to improve immunotoxin efficacy. Depletion of B and T cells during SS1P treatment by pentostatin and cyclophosphamide administration was tested in a pilot study [21] showing promising clinical benefit, while the use of new-generation immunotoxin with reduced immunogenicity is under active investigation. LMB-100 (RG7787) consists in a humanized anti-mesothelin Fab fragment linked to a modified domain 3 of pseudomonas exotoxin A. Modifications include amino acids substitution which silences B-cell epitopes in the toxin domain and reduces immunogenicity [22]. LMB-100 showed low anticancer activity in patient-derived mesothelioma xenograft models when tested as a single agent. However, its combination with Nab-paclitaxel (albumin bound paclitaxel) induced strong tumor regression [23]. To date, LMB-100 is under evaluation in clinical trials aimed at evaluating its activity as a single agent or in combination with nab-Paclitaxel (NCT02798536), pembrolizumab (NCT03644550), or SEL-110 (NCT03436732) for the treatment of epithelioid and biphasic mesothelioma patients (Table 18.1).

18.1.2.2 Anti-mesothelin Monoclonal Antibodies

Amatuximab (MORAb-009) is a chimeric (mouse/human) monoclonal IgG1/k antibody specifically targeting mesothelin-expressing cells.

Table 18.1 Clinical trials with mesothelin-targeted therapies in MPM patients

Mesothelin targeted drug	Additional drugs	Phase	Setting	Primary end points	ClinicalTrial ID	Status	References
SS1P		I	Second line	MTD	NCT00066651	Completed	[17]
		I	Second line	MTD	NCT00006981	Completed	[18]
	Cisplatin plus Pemetrexed	I	First line	Safety and MTD	NCT01445392	Terminated	[20]
	Pentostatine plus cyclophosphamide	Pilot	Second or + lines	RR, SS1P antibody formation, AE	NCT01362790	Active, not recruiting	[21]
LMB-100	Nab-paclitaxel	I	Second or + lines	Safety, MTD	NCT02798536	Active, not recruiting	
	Pembrolizumab	II	Second line	RR	NCT03644550	Not yet recruiting	
	SEL-110	I	Second or + lines	Safety and tolerability	NCT03436732	Recruiting	
MORAb-009 (Amatuximab)		I		Dose escalation safety and tolerability	NCT00325494	Completed	[26]
		I		MTD	NCT01018784	Completed	[27]
	Cisplatin plus Pemetrexed	II	First line	PFS	NCT00738582	Completed	[28]
	Cisplatin plus Pemetrexed	II	First line	OS	NCT02357147	Active, not recruiting	
Indium-radiolabeled MORAb-009 (Amatuximab)		I		Biodistribution of radiolabeled amatuximab in tumor and non tumor tissues	NCT01413451/ NCT01521325	Terminated	
BAY94-9343 (Anetumab Ravtasine)		I	First line	Safety, tolerability and PK	NCT01439152	Completed	[31]
	Vinorelbine	II	Second line	PFS	NCT02610140	Active, not recruiting	
	Cisplatin plus pemetrexed	I		Safety, tolerability, MTD	NCT02639091	Active, not recruiting	[32]
CART meso		I	First or further lines	Adverse Events	NCT01355965	Completed	[35]
	Cyclophosphamide	I	Second or + line	AE	NCT02159716	Completed	
	Cyclophosphamide fludarabine Aldesleukin	I/II	Second line	Safety, tumor regression	NCT01583686	Recruiting	
	Cyclophosphamide	I	Second or + line	Safety and feasibility	NCT03054298	Active, not recruiting	
	Cyclophosphamide	I	Second or + line	Measure of severity and number of AE	NCT02414269	Recruiting	

Mesothelin targeted drug	Additional drugs	Phase	Setting	Primary end points	ClinicalTrial ID	Status	References
CRS-207		I	First line	DLT	NCT00585845	Terminated	[39]
	Cisplatin plus pemetrexed w/ wo cyclophosphamide	Ib	First line	AE, induction of immune response	NCT01675765	Active, not recruiting	[40]
	Pembrolizumab	II	Second or + line	RR	NCT03175172	Active, not recruiting	

PFS progression-free survival, *RR* response rate, *OS* overall survival, *MTD* maximum tolerated dose, *DLT* dose-limiting toxicities, *PK* pharmacokinetic, *AE* adverse event

Potential anticancer activity of amatuximab was demonstrated in in vitro studies where amatuximab was able to kill mesothelin-expressing cells by activating human peripheral blood mononuclear cell (PBMC) immune effectors (antibody-dependent cellular cytotoxicity: ADC). Amatuximab was also able to inhibit mesothelin/CA125 binding [24]. In preclinical mouse model amatuximab showed moderate antitumor activity when used as a single agent but induced a long-term inhibition of tumor growth when combined with gemcitabine, and complete tumor regression in a high percentage of treated mice when combined with taxol [24]. Of note, amatuximab specifically localized in tumor sites as demonstrated by a study of ^{111}In-amatuximab biodistribution detected by SPECT-CT imaging in mesothelioma patients [25]. Phase I clinical trials established that amatuximab at the MTD (200 mg/m^2 once a week) was well tolerated, thereby some patients experienced low-grade drug-related hypersensitivity [26, 27]. Based on these results, two phase II trials aimed at testing the efficacy of amatuximab plus cisplatin/pemetrexed as first line therapy in MPM patients with unresectable epithelioid or biphasic MPM were conducted. The first study was a multicenter, single arm, non-randomized trial (NCT00738582), in which 89 MPM patients were enrolled. Treatment with amatuximab plus cisplatin/pemetrexed did not achieve the primary endpoint (6 month PFS response rate of 62%), although interesting OS data and no overlapping toxicities were observed [28]. Thus, OS was set as the primary endpoint of the second multicenter, randomized, double-blind, placebo-controlled phase II study ARTEMIS; this clinical trial was initiated to determine if amatuximab combined with the standard of care chemotherapy improves the overall survival of unresectable, previously untreated, MPM patients. Induction treatment of 4–6 cycles was followed by maintenance with amatuximab or placebo, in the experimental and control arms respectively. Secondary objectives include evaluating progression-free survival, objective response rate, duration of response, disease control and performance status maintenance, disease control rate, health-related quality of life, and safety (NCT02357147) (Table 18.1).

18.1.2.3 Anti-mesothelin Antibody Drug Conjugates

More specific ADC can be achieved using antibody–drug conjugates such as BAY94-9343 (anetumab-ravtansine). BAY94-9343 consists of a human anti-mesothelin antibody bound through a disulfide linkage to DM4 toxophore. BAY94-9343 showed good ADC properties because of its high binding affinity to human mesothelin (Kd 10 nmol/L), and its ability to internalize into target cells, delivering the toxophore inside. Once internalized, the disulfide linker is degraded in lysosomes and DM4 released into the cells. DM4 is a microtubule inhibitor able to induce cell death particularly in active proliferating cells, sparing normal mesothelial cells. Importantly, free DM4 is a cell-permeable molecule that can spread into neighboring cells eliciting bystander cytotoxic activity [29, 30]. BAY94-9343 showed high potent and selective cytotoxicity on mesothelin-expressing cells. In patient-derived xenograft tumor models, characterized by high heterogeneity in mesothelin expression, BAY94-9343 showed specific antitumor activity in pancreatic, ovarian, and mesothelioma models. In MPM, BAY94-9343 treatment resulted in higher efficacy when compared with cisplatin or pemetrexed treatments, and similar activity of vinorelbine [29]. Similarly, although patients with advanced mesothelioma showed durable partial response in phase I trial [31], clinical evaluation of anetumab ravtansine in phase II trial showed no advantage in terms of PFS compared with vinorelbine treatment in locally advanced or metastatic MPM patients (NCT02639091) [32]. The combination of BAY 94-9343 with pemetrexed and cisplatin is currently under evaluation in a phase I trial (NCT02639091) (Table 18.1).

18.1.2.4 CAR-T Cell Therapy

Recently, great advances have been made in the field of targeted cancer immunotherapy. In this contest, CAR (chimeric antigen receptor)-T cells therapy represents a promising strategy to activate a selective and persistent immune response, redirecting T cells toward tumor-specific antigen.

CARs are engineered receptors composed of an antigen-specific extracellular domain (an antibody-derived single-chain Fragment variant (scFv)), a linking transmembrane domain and an intracellular T-cell activation domain (CD3ζ) [33]. In the second-generation CARs costimolatory signaling domains (e.g. CD28 and 4-1BB) have been included. This structure allows a full and persistent T-cell activation increasing T-cell proliferation and cytokines production [34]. T cells isolated from patients' derived PBMC can be transduced to express CARs, expanded and reinfused to the patient. Anti-mesothelin CAR-T cell therapies are currently ongoing in different early phase (I/II) clinical trials (Table 18.1) aimed at testing safety and feasibility of CARTmeso therapy in chemotherapy refractory or recurred malignancies [35].

Systemic administration of CARTmeso therapy may delay CAR-T cell homing in the microenvironment of locally invasive tumors, limiting its efficacy. To overcome this limit, intrapleural administration of anti-meso CAR-T is under investigation in phase I dose escalation study in Malignant Pleural Disease (NCT02414269). The rationale of the study derived from preclinical experiments conducted in an orthotopic MPM mouse model shows higher activity of intrapleural administration of CARTmeso cells compared with intravenous infusion [36], probably due to an earlier CD4 CAR-T activation. CARTmeso cells used in this trial are also equipped with a safety switch system: the concomitant transduction of the inducible-caspase 9 gene. If needed, the gene can be activated through AP1903 administration inducing a rapid suicide of engineered T cells [37], thus increasing the safety of therapy.

18.1.2.5 Anti-mesothelin Vaccine

Stimulation of mesothelin-specific T-cell response is also the primary goal of anti-mesothelin vaccine therapy. To address this objective, a live-attenuated, double-deleted *Listeria monocytogenes* was engineered to secrete mesothelin in the cytosol of infected antigen-presenting cells (CRS-207) [38]. When tested in phase I trial (NCT00585845), CRS-207 showed the ability to induce mesothelin-specific T-cell response associated with a good toxicity profile [39]. These favorable results encouraged the evaluation of anticancer activity of CRS-207 in combined therapy. CRS207 associated with cisplatin/pemetrexed is being evaluated in phase Ib trial (NCT01675765) in chemo naïve, unresectable MPM patients. Sixty patients have been enrolled and treated with CRS-207 before and after chemotherapy cycles (up to 6). CRS-207 maintenance treatment in responder subjects was also administered. A preliminary evaluation on 38 patients showed that the treatment was well tolerated and induced partial response in 59% of 34 evaluable patients [40].

The association of CRS 207 with the PD-1 immune checkpoint inhibitor pembrolizumab is currently under investigation in phase II trial aimed at evaluating objective response rate of the combined therapy in previously treated MPM (NCT03175172) (Table 18.1).

18.2 Conclusion

Mesothelin seems a promising target for malignant pleural mesothelioma treatment, although multicenter clinical trials with monoclonal antibodies or antibody–drug conjugates showed disappointing results or are currently ongoing to confirm their antitumor activity in larger series. New mesothelin-targeted strategies such as CAR-T cells or vaccines seem promising, but the scientific community should wait for early phase trial results in order to plan a translation to clinical practice.

References

1. Pastan I, Hassan R. Discovery of mesothelin and exploiting it as a target for immunotherapy. Cancer Res. 2014;74(11):2907–12.
2. Rump A, Morikawa Y, Tanaka M, Minami S, Umesaki N, Takeuchi M, et al. Binding of ovarian cancer antigen CA125/MUC16 to mesothelin mediates cell adhesion. J Biol Chem. 2004;279(10):9190–8.
3. Gubbels JA, Belisle J, Onda M, Rancourt C, Migneault M, Ho M, et al. Mesothelin-MUC16 binding is a high affinity, N-glycan dependent interaction that facilitates peritoneal metastasis of ovarian tumors. Mol Cancer. 2006;5(1):50.

4. Tang Z, Qian M, Ho M. The role of mesothelin in tumor progression and targeted therapy. Anti Cancer Agents Med Chem. 2013;13(2):276–80.
5. Bharadwaj U, Marin-Muller C, Li M, Chen C, Yao Q. Mesothelin overexpression promotes autocrine IL-6/sIL-6R trans-signaling to stimulate pancreatic cancer cell proliferation. Carcinogenesis. 2011;32(7):1013–24.
6. Bharadwaj U, Li M, Chen C, Yao Q. Mesothelin-induced pancreatic cancer cell proliferation involves alteration of cyclin E via activation of signal transducer and activator of transcription protein 3. Mol Cancer Res. 2008;6(11):1755–65.
7. Bharadwaj U, Marin-Muller C, Li M, Chen C, Yao Q. Mesothelin confers pancreatic cancer cell resistance to TNF-alpha-induced apoptosis through Akt/PI3K/NF-kappaB activation and IL-6/Mcl-1 overexpression. Mol Cancer. 2011;10:106.
8. Uehara N, Matsuoka Y, Tsubura A. Mesothelin promotes anchorage-independent growth and prevents anoikis via extracellular signal-regulated kinase signaling pathway in human breast cancer cells. Mol Cancer Res. 2008;6(2):186–93.
9. Cheng WF, Huang CY, Chang MC, Hu YH, Chiang YC, Chen YL, et al. High mesothelin correlates with chemoresistance and poor survival in epithelial ovarian carcinoma. Br J Cancer. 2009;100(7):1144–53.
10. Baldo P, Cecco S. Amatuximab and novel agents targeting mesothelin for solid tumors. OncoTargets Ther. 2017;10:5337–53.
11. Creaney J, Francis RJ, Dick IM, Musk AW, Robinson BW, Byrne MJ, et al. Serum soluble mesothelin concentrations in malignant pleural mesothelioma: relationship to tumor volume, clinical stage and changes in tumor burden. Clin Cancer Res. 2011;17(5):1181–9.
12. Servais EL, Colovos C, Rodriguez L, Bograd AJ, Nitadori J, Sima C, et al. Mesothelin overexpression promotes mesothelioma cell invasion and MMP-9 secretion in an orthotopic mouse model and in epithelioid pleural mesothelioma patients. Clin Cancer Res. 2012;18(9):2478–89.
13. He X, Wang L, Riedel H, Wang K, Yang Y, Dinu CZ, et al. Mesothelin promotes epithelial-to-mesenchymal transition and tumorigenicity of human lung cancer and mesothelioma cells. Mol Cancer. 2017;16(1):63.
14. Melaiu O, Stebbing J, Lombardo Y, Bracci E, Uehara N, Bonotti A, et al. MSLN gene silencing has an anti-malignant effect on cell lines overexpressing mesothelin deriving from malignant pleural mesothelioma. PLoS One. 2014;9(1):e85935.
15. Forest F, Patoir A, Dal Col P, Sulaiman A, Camy F, Laville D, et al. Nuclear grading, BAP1, mesothelin and PD-L1 expression in malignant pleural mesothelioma: prognostic implications. Pathology. 2018;50(6):635–41.
16. Chowdhury PS, Viner JL, Beers R, Pastan I. Isolation of a high-affinity stable single-chain Fv specific for mesothelin from DNA-immunized mice by phage display and construction of a recombinant immunotoxin with anti-tumor activity. Proc Natl Acad Sci U S A. 1998;95(2):669–74.
17. Hassan R, Bullock S, Premkumar A, Kreitman RJ, Kindler H, Willingham MC, et al. Phase I study of SS1P, a recombinant anti-mesothelin immunotoxin given as a bolus I.V. infusion to patients with mesothelin-expressing mesothelioma, ovarian, and pancreatic cancers. Clin Cancer Res. 2007;13(17):5144–9.
18. Kreitman RJ, Hassan R, Fitzgerald DJ, Pastan I. Phase I trial of continuous infusion anti-mesothelin recombinant immunotoxin SS1P. Clin Cancer Res. 2009;15(16):5274–9.
19. Zhang Y, Xiang L, Hassan R, Paik CH, Carrasquillo JA, Jang BS, et al. Synergistic antitumor activity of taxol and immunotoxin SS1P in tumor-bearing mice. Clin Cancer Res. 2006;12(15):4695–701.
20. Hassan R, Sharon E, Thomas A, Zhang J, Ling A, Miettinen M, et al. Phase 1 study of the antimesothelin immunotoxin SS1P in combination with pemetrexed and cisplatin for front-line therapy of pleural mesothelioma and correlation of tumor response with serum mesothelin, megakaryocyte potentiating factor, and cancer antigen 125. Cancer. 2014;120(21):3311–9.
21. Hassan R, Miller AC, Sharon E, Thomas A, Reynolds JC, Ling A, et al. Major cancer regressions in mesothelioma after treatment with an anti-mesothelin immunotoxin and immune suppression. Sci Transl Med. 2013;5(208):208ra147.
22. Liu W, Onda M, Lee B, Kreitman RJ, Hassan R, Xiang L, et al. Recombinant immunotoxin engineered for low immunogenicity and antigenicity by identifying and silencing human B-cell epitopes. Proc Natl Acad Sci U S A. 2012;109(29):11782–7.
23. Zhang J, Khanna S, Jiang Q, Alewine C, Miettinen M, Pastan I, et al. Efficacy of anti-mesothelin immunotoxin RG7787 plus nab-paclitaxel against mesothelioma patient-derived xenografts and mesothelin as a biomarker of tumor response. Clin Cancer Res. 2017;23(6):1564–74.
24. Hassan R, Ebel W, Routhier EL, Patel R, Kline JB, Zhang J, et al. Preclinical evaluation of MORAb-009, a chimeric antibody targeting tumor-associated mesothelin. Cancer Immun. 2007;7:20.
25. Lindenberg L, Thomas A, Adler S, Mena E, Kurdziel K, Maltzman J, et al. Safety and biodistribution of 111In-amatuximab in patients with mesothelin expressing cancers using single photon emission computed tomography-computed tomography (SPECT-CT) imaging. Oncotarget. 2015;6(6):4496–504.
26. Hassan R, Cohen SJ, Phillips M, Pastan I, Sharon E, Kelly RJ, et al. Phase I clinical trial of the chimeric anti-mesothelin monoclonal antibody MORAb-009 in patients with mesothelin-expressing cancers. Clin Cancer Res. 2010;16(24):6132–8.
27. Fujisaka Y, Kurata T, Tanaka K, Kudo T, Okamoto K, Tsurutani J, et al. Phase I study of amatuximab, a novel monoclonal antibody to mesothelin, in Japanese

patients with advanced solid tumors. Investig New Drugs. 2015;33(2):380–8.
28. Hassan R, Kindler HL, Jahan T, Bazhenova L, Reck M, Thomas A, et al. Phase II clinical trial of amatuximab, a chimeric antimesothelin antibody with pemetrexed and cisplatin in advanced unresectable pleural mesothelioma. Clin Cancer Res. 2014;20(23):5927–36.
29. Golfier S, Kopitz C, Kahnert A, Heisler I, Schatz CA, Stelte-Ludwig B, et al. Anetumab ravtansine: a novel mesothelin-targeting antibody-drug conjugate cures tumors with heterogeneous target expression favored by bystander effect. Mol Cancer Ther. 2014;13(6):1537–48.
30. Kovtun YV, Audette CA, Ye Y, Xie H, Ruberti MF, Phinney SJ, et al. Antibody-drug conjugates designed to eradicate tumors with homogeneous and heterogeneous expression of the target antigen. Cancer Res. 2006;66(6):3214–21.
31. Blumenschein GR, Hassan R, Moore KN, Santin A, Kindler HL, Nemunaitis JJ, et al. Phase I study of anti-mesothelin antibody drug conjugate anetumab ravtansine (AR). J Clin Oncol. 2016;34(15_suppl):2509.
32. Kindler HL, Novello S, Fennell D, Blumenschein G, Bearz A, Ceresoli G, et al. OA 02.01 randomized phase II study of anetumab ravtansine or vinorelbine in patients with metastatic pleural mesothelioma. J Thorac Oncol. 2017;12(11):S1746.
33. Zhang C, Liu J, Zhong JF, Zhang X. Engineering CAR-T cells. Biomarker Res. 2017;5:22.
34. Morello A, Sadelain M, Adusumilli PS. Mesothelin-targeted CARs: driving T cells to solid tumors. Cancer Discov. 2016;6(2):133–46.
35. Beatty GL, Haas AR, Maus MV, Torigian DA, Soulen MC, Plesa G, et al. Mesothelin-specific chimeric antigen receptor mRNA-engineered T cells induce anti-tumor activity in solid malignancies. Cancer Immunol Res. 2014;2(2):112–20.
36. Adusumilli PS, Cherkassky L, Villena-Vargas J, Colovos C, Servais E, Plotkin J, et al. Regional delivery of mesothelin-targeted CAR T cell therapy generates potent and long-lasting CD4-dependent tumor immunity. Sci Transl Med. 2014;6(261):261ra151.
37. Di Stasi A, Tey SK, Dotti G, Fujita Y, Kennedy-Nasser A, Martinez C, et al. Inducible apoptosis as a safety switch for adoptive cell therapy. N Engl J Med. 2011;365(18):1673–83.
38. Brockstedt DG, Giedlin MA, Leong ML, Bahjat KS, Gao Y, Luckett W, et al. Listeria-based cancer vaccines that segregate immunogenicity from toxicity. Proc Natl Acad Sci U S A. 2004;101(38):13832–7.
39. Le DT, Brockstedt DG, Nir-Paz R, Hampl J, Mathur S, Nemunaitis J, et al. A live-attenuated Listeria vaccine (ANZ-100) and a live-attenuated Listeria vaccine expressing mesothelin (CRS-207) for advanced cancers: phase I studies of safety and immune induction. Clin Cancer Res. 2012;18(3):858–68.
40. Jahan T, Hassan R, Alley E, Kindler H, Antonia S, Whiting C, et al. 208O_PR: CRS-207 with chemotherapy (chemo) in malignant pleural mesothelioma (MPM): results from a phase 1b trial. J Thorac Oncol. 2016;11(4):S156.

19 Immunotherapy of Mesothelioma: Vaccines and Cell Therapy

A Focus on Dendritic Cell Therapy

R. A. Belderbos, R. Cornelissen, and J. G. J. V. Aerts

19.1 Introduction

Malignant pleural mesothelioma is an aggressive, deadly cancer and its pathological origin lies in the mesothelial cells that are present in the visceral and parietal pleura, which is the tissue lining surrounding the lungs. Mesothelioma can also occur in the peritoneum, pericardium, and tunica vaginalis, but less frequently. Approximately 70–80% of mesotheliomas occur in the pleura. Evidence shows that there is a direct causal connection between patients with malignant pleural mesothelioma (MPM) and asbestos exposure [1]. Moreover, 10% of people who have had prolonged exposure to asbestos develop MPM. Asbestos has been used extensively in construction and other industries. The latency period depends on the amount of exposure with a median time from exposure to diagnosis of 30–50 years [2]. This is the reason for a relative late ban of workplace usage of asbestos in the United States and Western European countries in the 1980s. Furthermore, countries such as China, India, and Russia are still producing asbestosis in large amounts and in Turkey environmental exposure is still a hazard. Altogether, the incidence worldwide has not yet reached its peak and a future epidemic awaits countries mass-producing asbestos [1–3].

The exact etiology of MPM is still under debate. The best-known theory hypothesizes chronic pleural irritation as instigator of inflammation with subsequent DNA damage, and eventually development of MPM. Histologically three phenotypes are described: epithelioid, sarcomatoid, and biphasic. The epithelioid variant accounts for approximately 60% of all mesotheliomas and is associated with favorable prognosis compared to the other two types [1].

In general MPM responds minimally to medical treatment. Current first-line treatment consists of antifolate and platinum combination chemotherapy which leads to an overall survival benefit of 3 months compared to single platinum-based chemotherapy [4]. Response rates to first-line treatment are 40% and result in an overall survival of 9–12 months. Unfortunately, not all patients are fit enough to receive chemotherapy. Surgery is only viable in a very early stage of the disease, which is seldom the case at the time of diagnosis, and even in these patients the benefit is doubted. A large randomized trial comparing extrapleural pneumonectomy to best supportive care showed no evidence for implicating extrapleural pneumonectomy for MPM [5, 6]. Because of a great demand for effective treatment options in MPM, randomized trials with varying therapeutic targets

R. A. Belderbos · R. Cornelissen · J. G. J. V. Aerts (✉)
Department of Pulmonary Medicine,
Erasmus MC Rotterdam, Rotterdam, The Netherlands

Erasmus MC Cancer Institute,
Erasmus MC Rotterdam, Rotterdam, The Netherlands
e-mail: r.belderbos@erasmusmc.nl;
r.cornelissen@erasmusmc.nl; j.aerts@erasmusmc.nl

G. L. Ceresoli et al. (eds.), *Mesothelioma*, https://doi.org/10.1007/978-3-030-16884-1_19

have been conducted. The majority of these trials failed to show efficacy for several therapies, such as tremelimumab (CTLA-4 checkpoint inhibitor), vorinostat (histone deacetylase (HDAC) inhibitor), and defactinib (focal adhesion kinase (FAK) inhibitor) [1, 7]. However, the Mesothelioma Avastin Cisplatin Pemetrexed Study (MAPS) trial showed that concurrent treatment of bevacizumab, a monoclonal anti-VEGF antibody, to first-line treatment results in a significant survival benefit of 2 months [8]. Subsequently, France approved this combination as standard treatment for MPM. Nintedanib, a multitargeted tyrosine kinase inhibitor, is currently being tested (LUME-Meso trial), but unfortunately it has been disclosed that the primary endpoint (PFS) was not met [9]. Checkpoint inhibition of the programmed death receptor (PD-1) and programmed death ligand 1 (PD-L1) in MPM showed response rates between 9 and 25% in phase I/II trials. Results of a phase III trial for nivolumab (PD-1 inhibitor) in MPM patients, the CONFIRM-trial, are awaited [10]. There is an urgent need for new treatment modalities that drastically improve survival and response rates in MPM patients.

Checkpoint inhibitors (CIs) reinvigorate antitumor immunity by blocking inhibitory signaling of tumor and suppressive immune cells. Not surprisingly, the pre-treatment presence of tumor-infiltrating T cells (TILs) correlates to efficacy and response to CIs. Cancer vaccines, Dendritic cell (DC) therapy, and CAR T cell therapy are capable of inducing tumor (antigen)-specific T cells. Especially in MPM, a tumor with low mutational burden and low number of TILs, vaccination which induces tumor infiltration of tumor-specific T cells could be an effective treatment modality, possibly enhancing response to CIs. These cell therapies are currently upcoming in the cancer immunology field and will be discussed separately.

19.2 Antigen

One of the key aspects in the efficacy of vaccination and cellular therapy is the choice of the antigen. This choice of antigen is one of great debate; the ideal target for cancer immunotherapy would be a tumor-associated antigen (TAA) that is exclusively expressed on all tumor cells, but not at all in normal tissues in order to avoid potential induction of autoimmunity. Also, the TAA should be essential for the malignant cell's growth and survival, so that downregulation to escape the immunotherapeutic effect of the vaccine is impossible. In mesothelioma, Wilm's tumor suppressor gene 1 (WT-1), mesothelin, calretinin, fibroblast activation protein (FAP), telomerase and different cancer testis antigens (CTA) such as melanoma-associated antigen (MAGE), cancer/testis antigen cancer-associated gene (GAGE), and synovial sarcoma X (SSX) gene families have been described as TAA [11–16], and have been used in different vaccination studies.

Currently, it is uncertain which antigen is the best target for immunotherapeutic treatment. In addition, most TAAs are self-derived proteins and thus in vivo poorly immunogenic.

Also, data do exist that targeting a single TAA has several possible drawbacks: These proteins are not expressed on the membranes of all MPM tumor cells. The efficacy of vaccination against a single or a few TAA is limited by peptide restriction to a given human leukocyte antigen (HLA) type and the induction of CTL. Furthermore, the propensity of tumors to downregulate antigens, and so escape immunological detection, is a major disadvantage when using the single target approach. This process is called immunoediting. Therefore, it has now been described that preferably multiple antigens need to be targeted to obtain a long-lasting effective tumor-specific T cell response. This strategy decreases the possibility of tumor escape by eliciting a broader immune response.

Polyvalent therapeutic strategies, aimed at targeting many antigens at once, may overcome these problems. One such strategy is to use tumor cell lysates, either from autologous or allogeneic background. The tumor cell lysates can be injected directly as vaccination or combined with dendritic cells. This can even be done without further defining the antigens. Tumor cells, by definition, express all relevant candidate TAAs, and this rich source of antigens contains epitopes of both CD8$^+$ T cells and CD4$^+$ T cells. Tumor lysates might be advantageous in providing the full antigenic repertoire of the tumor and, particularly, unique tumor antigens, which will theoretically decrease the ability of tumors to evade the immune response by downregulation of a single antigen. Therefore, it diminishes the chance of tumor escape compared to using single epitope vaccines.

To generate an autologous whole tumor lysate a number of logistic challenges exist. This is hampered by the need of sufficient autologous tumor material, both in quality and in quantity to either directly load the dendritic cells or derive cell lines from. This is only the case in a small proportion of patients screened.

The use of allogeneic lysate to inject directly or pulse DC has many advantages: access to a sustained and virtually limitless source of TAA, it allows standardization and large-scale production with constant quality and composition of the vaccines and reliable comparative analysis of clinical outcome facilitated. In addition, the production process is less laborious, with simple logistics and increased cost-effectiveness.

A method of allogeneic lysate loading of DCs was first demonstrated in MPM from pre-clinic to clinic by our group [17]. It showed that this method was feasible and safe. In addition, radiological responses were seen in patients, warranting further study.

19.3 Cancer Vaccine for Mesothelioma

Since Rudolf Virchow discovered leukocytes to be present in cancerous tumor material in the nineteenth century, inflammation and carcinogenesis have been linked to each other. The protective role of the immune system in cancer development has only recently been revealed. This process is called immunosurveillance, whereby immune cells eliminate tumor cells upon recognition.

During carcinogenesis numerous genetic mutations cause a loss of normal cellular metabolic processes. These changes are necessary for tumor development and rapid proliferation of cancer cells and cause upregulation of tumor-associated antigens (TAAs) such as neo-antigens, differentiation antigens, or cancer testis antigens on the cell surface (see former paragraph). Upon cancer cell death, calreticulin (CRT) is expressed on the cell surface and works as an engulfment signal for DCs. Secretion of ATP and high mobility group box 1 (HGMB-1) during apoptosis enhance DC migration and antigen presentation to T cells. This process of apoptosis is referred to as immunogenic cell death (ICD). DCs are the most effective antigen-presenting cells and capable of cross-presentation of antigen, which is a mechanism where engulfed proteins are presented in major histocompatibility complex class I (MHC I) in stead of MHC II. In this way DCs can present antigen in MHC class I as well as II, thereby activating both CD4$^+$ T cells and CD8$^+$ T cells. After phagocytosis of TAAs, DCs mature and migrate to the lymph node to present TAAs to naïve CD4$^+$ and CD8$^+$ T cells. During this process of antigen presentation three signals have to be given by a DC to a T cell in order to activate the T cell. These signals are: presentation of the antigen (signal 1), co-stimulation through surface molecules (i.e. CD 40, CD 80, CD 86) (signal 2) and secretion of pro-inflammatory cytokines (i.e. IFN-y, IL-12) (signal 3). Antigen presentation without signal 2 and 3 will lead to tolerance. After being activated, tumor-specific T cells migrate to the tumor and elicit their cytotoxic effect upon antigen recognition on tumor cells [18, 19].

This whole process of immunosurveillance leading to anti-tumor immunity can be hampered at every step by the tumor. During the first step, the TME can cause cancer cell death to be tolerogenic instead of immunogenic. This is achieved by inducing tolerogenic phagocytosis through secretion of immunosuppressive cytokines leading to immature DCs and antigen presentation destitute of signal 2 and 3. Furthermore, cancer cells can downregulate their antigen presentation on the cell surface making them invisible to tumor-specific T cells. To overcome this mechanism of immune evasion by tumor cells, cancer vaccines aim to induce antitumor responses *in vivo*. Cancer vaccines can contain autologous tumor lysates, allogeneic tumor cell lysates, single or multiple peptides. DC maturating stimuli can be given simultaneously to support the initiation of an immune response. Peptides used in cancer vaccines can vary in length to fit onto MHC I and MHC II molecules enabling $CD4^+$ and $CD8^+$ T cell activation. In 98% of MPM tumors, immunohistochemical staining shows expression of Wilms' tumor 1 (WT1) antigen. WT1 gene, first cloned in pediatric kidney cancer, is overexpressed in multiple hematological and solid tumors and has been defined as the most important cancer antigen [20].

A cancer vaccine called Galinpepimut-S, consisting of four WT1 peptides of different lengths, has been used in MPM patients [21]. In this phase II trial patients received either Galinpepimut-S with adjuvant granulocyte-macrophage colony-stimulating factor (GM-CSF) and Montanide or GM-CSF and Montanide without Galinpepimut-S. Patients were eligible for participation if they had received multimodality therapy consisting of combination chemotherapy and/or radiotherapy and pleurectomy/decortication or extrapleural pneumonectomy. There was not enough power in this study to objectively compare efficacy between these two different treatment strategies. Additionally, the study closed early because of futility in the non-vaccinated arm. Despite all this, a non-significant improvement of PFS and OS was seen of 36% and 25%, respectively. Immunological analysis was done on less than half of the patients. In the vaccine-treated arm 4 out of 8 patients tested positive for a $CD4^+$ T cell proliferation assay. Two out of 3 patients were eligible for tetramer analysis and tested positive for both IFN-y ELISPOT assay and the tetramer assay. These results were inconclusive and did not correlate to clinical outcome. The clinical results were not supported by immunological analysis and still have to be confirmed by a phase III randomized controlled trial, which is currently approved by the FDA and is pending. Galinpepimut-S uses one specific antigen (WT1) for priming the anti-tumor immune response. As stated before, most of the MPM tumors express WT1 antigen on the cell surface. However, studies have shown that MPM is a very heterogeneous tumor and antigen expression varies a lot between different histological types and also the level of expression is highly variable, ranging from >50% to 1% for WT-1 [20]. Response to therapy with vaccination against WT1 antigen can therefore vary in effectivity. Moreover, tumor cells can escape the initial immune response by a process called immunoediting. Immunoediting can be divided into three phases: Elimination, Equilibrium, and Escape [22]. The elimination phase essentially is comparable to normal immunosurveillance, where the anti-tumor immune response kills tumor cells. During the equilibrium phase, cancer cells with a non-immunogenic (i.e. non-WT1 expressing) phenotype get positively selected. This process of selecting non-immunogenic, immune-escaping cells can take long time. In the last phase (Escape), control on the tumor cells is lost and unlimited proliferation takes place. The cancer cells have *escaped* the anti-tumor immunity. This whole process of immunoediting is easier when there is only one specific antigen immune response to escape from.

Another reason for impaired efficacy of cancer vaccines in MPM encompasses the DCs themselves. All major DC subtypes (cDC1, cDC2, and pDC) are lower in numbers and functionality in MPM patients compared to healthy controls. DCs do not upregulate their activation and co-stimulatory markers in response to maturation stimuli. This means that administration of concurrent maturation stimuli next to cancer vaccination does not lead to maturation and subsequently could lead to antigen presentation in the absence of signal 2 and 3 and thus induce tolerance. Tumor-induced immunosuppresion could be the cause for the impaired functionality of DCs. The amount of tumor load is associated with a higher level of immunosuppppresion. Reduction of tumor load with surgery could benefit DC function in MPM patients. In the Galinpepimut-S trial patients were selected that received surgery. However, most MPM patients get diagnosed in a late stage and are not eligible for surgery, making tumor reduction and therefore reducing immunosuppression not possible. Moreover, implementing the treatment sequence of the Galinpepimut trial in everyday practice is not feasible for the majority of MPM paitents.

Concluding, MPM is a treatment-resistant cancer with a heterogenous histology. Current attempts targeting the immune system with cancer vaccines have not yet proven to be effective. This could be due to immunoediting of the tumor, the use of single peptide vaccines and reduced numbers and functionality of DCs in MPM.

19.4 DC Therapy

A comprehensive understanding of the role of DCs in the immune system and the exact process of antigen processing and presentation helped researchers develop new vaccination therapies. Therapies improving DC function can obviate the problem of low numbers and less functional DCs in MPM which hampered cancer vaccine efficacy. Moreover, a meta-analysis in patients with NSCLC showed a significant benefit of cellular therapies (dendritic cell-based immunotherapy and chimeric antigen receptor T cell therapy) over peptide cancer vaccination [23].

Different forms of DC therapy do exist ranging from *in vivo* activation of DCs to *ex vivo* generation and loading of DCs. Live-attenuated *Listeria monocytogenes* (Lm) can target DCs *in vivo* and Lm vaccines loaded with TAAs showed efficacy in animal models and promising clinical results in human trials. Mesothelin has been used as a TAA in Lm vaccines because of its high expression on several solid tumors, such as pancreatic carcinoma, mesothelioma, and ovarian cancer. One specific mesothelin-targeted Lm vaccine, CRS-207, has been tested in a phase I clinical trial where 63% of patients had a partial response and 29% had stable disease with an median PFS of 7.4 months (https://www.ejcancer.com/article/S0959-8049(16)30316-1/abstract). Another way of targeting DCs *in vivo* is with GM-CSF-secreting allogeneic tumor cells (GVAX). In the above mentioned and discussed Galinpepimut-S trial, GM-CSF was added to the cancer vaccine to create the same effect. GVAX followed by CRS-207 treatment led to increased overall survival in pancreatic cancer patients suggesting possible synergy between these immunotherapies. Phase II and III trials have been instigated with CRS-207 in combination with other treatment modalities (checkpoint inhibitors, GVAX, chemotherapy) (NCT 01675765, NCT03175172, NCT02243371). However, all of these trials are still not recruiting.

Ex vivo DC therapy is another way to generate functional DCs that can be loaded with TAAs. An advantage of *ex vivo* DC generation is that it circumvents the immunosuppressive effect of the tumor on DCs. DCs for DC therapy can be genreated from monocytes that are cultured with GM-CSF and interleukin (IL)-4. These DCS are reffered to as monocyte derived DCs (moDC). However, with the recent development of immunomagnetic isolation, naturally occuring DCs (nDC) can be directly selected from the apheresis product resulting in a shorter maturation process and possibly increased immunological and migratory potential than in moDC therapy. In a phase 1 trial in 14 melanoma patients, nDC therapy resulted in promising PFS and anti-tumor specific immune responses which warrants further research in large randomized trials [24]. In mesothelioma nDC therapy has not yet been evaluated.

moDC therapy involves isolation of monocytes from the peripheral blood and pulsing them with antigen followed by addition of maturation stimuli providing signal 2 and 3. Reinjection of already activated and matured DCs will circumvent the barrier of immunosuppressed and low functioning DCs. During culture a wide array of methods can be used to pulse DCs such as synthetic peptides coding for TAAs, autologous or allogeneic whole tumor lysates, RNA or DNA electroporation and immunogenic cell death (ICD)-based lysates. Autologous WT1 messenger (m)RNA-loaded DCs showed promising results in uterine, ovarian and endometrial cancer, MPM and acute myeloid leukemia. Seven out of 10 MPM patients treated with this DC therapy had stable disease with an overall survival from start of chemotherapy of 35.7 months [25]. As WT1 is highly expressed in MPM, a clinical single arm phase I/II trial (MESODECtrial) evaluating the effect of Wilms' Tumor protein 1 (WT1)-targeted DC therapy has started and is currently recruiting (NCT02649829). In this trial, DC therapy will be used in conjunction with first-line chemotherapy and hopefully provide safety and feasibility for the use of DC therapy next to chemotherapy in MPM. In mRNA-pulsed DC therapy multiple naturally processed peptides are presented in both MHC class I and II which broadens the repertoire of responding lymphocytes compared to peptide loaded DC therapy. However, using only one TAA, such as WT1, to load DCs leads to a single antigen-specific anti-tumor immune response which can be eveded by tumor cells through immunoediting.

Apart from WT1 mRNA pulsed DC therapy, tumor lysate-pulsed DC therapy is upcoming in MPM. Pulsing DCs with tumor lysate leads to a broad spectrum of antigens that are potentially presented to naïve T cells, which induces a broad anti-tumor response possibly troubling the immune escape of tumor cells. Autologous tumor lysate-pulsed DC therapy was safe and effective in murine models. Autologous tumor lysate-pulsed DC therapy showed promising efficacy, radiological responses, and ongoing survival up to 6 years after diagnosis in MPM patients [17, 26, 27]. Safety and feasibility were also established. Pleural effusions, tumor biopsies or surgical tumor resections were used to generate autologous tumor lysate. This was well tolerated but the varying quality and amount of available tumor material made treatment of some patients impossible and averted upscaling this DC therapy to a larger scale. Allogeneic tumor lysate could be an "off-the-shelf" source of TAA with a broad spectrum of antigens that enables upscaling of production. This allogenic tumor lysate was prepared from tumor cell lines derived from malignant cells in pleural effusions of 5 MPM patients. Allogeneic tumor lysate-pulsed DC therapy proved to be just as effective in murine models as autologous tumor lysate-pulsed DCs. Furthermore, safety and feasibility were established in humans in a phase I trial that also showed radiological responses and ongoing survival of 45 months in 3 out of 9 patients [28]. To prove efficacy, a multicenter phase III randomized trial (DENIM-trial) has started (NCT03610360). Patients with MPM without progression after 4–6 cycles of first line chemotherapy are randomized to receive either DC immunotherapy plus Best Supportive Care (BSC) or BSC according to the discretion of the local investigator. In this study the efficacy of allogeneic DC immunotherapy will be evaluated.

In conclusion, DC therapy instigates a potent and broad anti-tumor immune response that can circumvent the immunosuppressive influence of MPM on DCs. Phase I/II/III clinical trials are being conducted to determine optimal vaccination strategy, dosing, and antigen loading.

19.5 CAR T Cells

T cells are the effectors of the anti-tumor immune response. They hunt down and kill abnormal cells, including cancer cells. Apart from eliciting an immune response through targeting DCs, directly targeting T cells could also be an option for anti-cancer immunotherapy. This T cell therapy was shown to be effective in hematological malignancies.

Adoptive T cell therapy is limited in efficacy since a number of cancer cells are not recognized by T cells. This can be due to various mechanisms such as the limited availability of tumor-specific T cells, deficiencies in antigen processing or major histocompatibility complex (MHC) expression of cancer cells. Chimeric antigen receptors (CAR) are fused receptors engineered to provide antigen specificity to T cells against TAAs on the cell surface of target cells. Patient's T cells are engineered *ex vivo* with pre-defined specificity by a recombinant CAR. The specificity of CAR-mediated T cell recognition is defined by the antibody domain, is independent of MHC presentation, and can be extended to any target for which an antibody is available [29].

Currently, there are three generations of CARs: First-generation CARs consisted of an extracellular domain that bound the tumor antigen via a single-chain variable antibody fragment that was fused to a CD3ζ intracellular activating domain. The effectivity of this first generation of

CARs was hampered by the inability of the CD3ζ chain to adequately activate resting T cells. Therefore, second-generation CARs were developed with a co-stimulatory intracellular signaling domain in tandem with the CD3ζ chain. This improved anti-tumor efficacy *in vivo*. The third-generation CARs incorporated a CD3ζ domain, and two co-stimulatory domains within their cytoplasmic tail. These third-generation CARs have demonstrated superior antitumor efficacy compared with second-generation CARs.

CARs are transduced into autologous T cells using viral or non-viral gene transfer systems to achieve permanent CAR expression or using messenger RNA electroporation to achieve transient expression for assessment [30]. Following transduction, these CAR T cells can be expanded *ex vivo* in specialized facilities and re-infused to the patient, either systemically or regionally.

CARs targeting the B-cell antigen CD19 have good results in clinical trials for a number of non-solid malignancies, such as non-Hodgkin lymphoma and acute lymphoblastic leukemia [31, 32]. The results have pushed the development for CARs in solid tumors, including MPM.

As stated above, CARs need a specific and highly expressed antigen in mesothelioma. The drawbacks of using a single antigen are discussed earlier in this chapter. In clinical trials treating MPM patients with CARs, two such candidate target TAAs are currently being investigated in clinical trials: mesothelin, which is overexpressed on the tumor cells, and fibroblast activation protein (FAP) that is overexpressed on tumor stromal cells.

19.5.1 Mesothelin CARs

Multiple phase I clinical trials using mesothelin CARs have been performed or are currently recruiting (NCT01355965, NCT01583686, NCT02159716, NCT02414269, and NCT02580747). Mesothelin CAR appeared feasible and safe in most patients. Although in one patient, an immediate serious anaphylactic reaction was noted during the third mesothelin CAR T cell infusion. The anaphylactic reaction was attributed to the immunogenicity of the murine SS1 antibody related single-chain variable fragment (scFv) used in the CAR construct. In all trials reported so far no clinical responses were seen. The trafficking of T cells to the tumor is regarded as the main obstacle for lack of efficacy in solid tumors. Therefore, intrapleural delivery is used by investigators at the Memorial Sloan Kettering (NCT02414269) in an attempt to overcome this drawback of CARs.

19.5.2 FAP CARs

Targeting the stroma in MPM patients could also be beneficial; targeting these stromal cells can modify the tumor microenvironment (TME) and improve the efficacy of other systemic therapies. Stromal cells are more genetically stable than tumor cells and therefore less likely to lose antigen expression. FAP, a transmembrane serine protease, is highly expressed in all MPM subtypes, therefore making it a logical target. Currently, a phase I clinical trial is ongoing, also using intrapleural administration (NCT01722149).

19.6 Combination Therapies with DC Therapy

Overall response rates to DC therapy lie around 15% in all solid tumors including MPM [33]. This is hypothesized to have several reasons or explanations. An underestimation of the clinical response due to the use of. Response Evaluation Criteria in Solid Tumor (RECIST) criteria for solid tumors could explain the response rates to DC therapy. For MPM these criteria do not comply with the circular growth pattern across the outer linings of the lung. Modified RECIST criteria should compensate to a certain extent for the peculiar growth pattern of MPM. However, this evaluation method has a great inter-observer variability and thus is not perfect either. Additionally, RECIST criteria underestimate the response to immunotherapy (checkpoint inhibitors (CIs)) with approximately 15% [18, 34]. This could be due to "delayed response" because immune activation takes time, but also due to a phenomenon called "pseudoprogression" where the tumor volume increases after infiltration of T cells. Immune-related response criteria (irRC) give a more accurate representation of response to immunotherapy, especially CIs. Another important reason for the relatively low response rates to DC therapy probably is the immunosuppressive influence of the tumor and TME on the anti-tumor immune reponse. As stated earlier, in every step of the process of an anti-tumor response, the tumor can interfere with the immunological response. Tumor cells create their "own" TME through secretion of cytokines and chemokines leading to migration of certain immunosuppresive immune cells to the tumor. Furthermore, immune cells that are originally inflammatory can be suppressed or skewed into an immunosuppressive phenotype by tumor cells. The main immunosuppressive cells present in the TME are regulatory T cells (Treg), myeloid-derived suppressor cells (MDSC), and tumor-associated macrophages (TAM).

Tregs can induce immune suppression directly through cell–cell contact (i.e. inhibitory receptors PD-1, CTLA-4) or indirectly through secretion of immunosuppressive cytokines (IL-10, TGF-b) or pore-forming proteins (granzyme, perforin). Increased levels of Tregs are correlated to poor clinical outcome in multiple solid tumors, such as lung, head and neck, gastrointestinal and pancreatic malignancies and melanoma and glioblastoma. Depletion or suppression of Tregs can be established by several therapies such as low-dose chemotherapy, anti-CD25 mAb, and CI. In a phase I trial MPM patients received DC therapy with concurrent low-dose cyclophosphamide, which resulted in radiological responses and long-lasting survival with ongoing survival up to 8 years after diagnose [17].

MDSCs can exert their immunosuppressive function by inducing Tregs or inhibition of tumor-specific T cells. High levels of MDSCs at baseline correlate to poorer overall survival time in several cancer types. MDSCs can be depleted by (low-dose) gemcitabine and 5-fluorouracil (5-FU). The functionality can be influenced by cyclooxygenase-2 (COX-2) inhibition. In a MPM murine model, COX-2 inhibition combined with DC therapy led to refinement of DC therapy and decrease of numbers of MDSCs and a change from an immunosuppressive phenotype to a mor inflammatory phenotype [35].

TAMs can be categorized into two main phenotypes. The M1 phenotype causes inflammatory signaling by secretion of pro-inflammatory cytokines, interleukins, and tumor necrosis factor-a (TNF-a). The M2 phenotype is linked to T-helper 2 cell responses and is responsible for tissue remodeling and associated with tumor progression. TAMs can be depleted by CSF1R blockade or skewed into a more favorable M1 phenotype by CD-40 agonistic antibodies. In pancreatic cancer models, depletion of TAMs led to enhancement of CI efficacy [36].

In conclusion, influencing different immune cell subsets in the TME with conventional treatments, such as chemotherapy, could lead to off the shelf immune modulating agents with the potential of enhancing DC therapy, CAR T cell therapy, or cancer vaccines.

Additionally, inhibitory surface molecules (PD-(L)1, CTLA4, TIM-3 LAG-3) present on tumor cells and immune cells can hamper anti-tumor immunity. CIs restore tumor-specific T cell activity by blocking inhibitory signaling of tumor cells or other immunosuppressive cells in the TME or lymph nodes. Great results have been booked in the development of immunotherapy that led to the registration of anti-CTLA-4 (durvalumab), anti PD-L1 (atezolizumab, durvalumab, and avelumab), and anti PD-1 (nivolumab and pembrolizumab) monoclonal antibodies (mAB). These registrations are in tumors with a high mutational burden, such as melanoma and non-small cell lung cancer (NSCLC), that have a higher level of TILs and subsequently relative high response rates of 57% are reported. Phase II trials did not prove efficacy of these treatment modalities in MPM. Response rates for CI in MPM vary between 9% and 25% [37]. CTLA-4 and PD-1 are both inhibitory molecules with different regulatory mechanisms. CTLA-4 regulates T cell proliferation primarily in the lymph node at the antigen presenting side. Whilst PD-1 inhibits the tumor-specific T cells mainly at the tumor site in the peripheral tissues. Concurrent treatment with these modalities could be beneficial and showed promising results in a phase II trial (NIBIT-MESO-1). Furthermore, the CheckMate 743 trial (NCT02899299) will compare current first-line treatment to nivolumab and ipilimumab combined, it has completed the recruitment of 600 patients, making it the largest trial on immunotherapy in mesothelioma and results are eagerly awaited. Combining CIs often leads to increased immune-related toxicity. Thus, combining one of these treatments with cellular therapy, which has a favorable side-effect profile, could lead to less toxicity. To summarize, cellular therapy can be hampered by inhibitory molecules and the efficacy of CIs correlates with high numbers of tumor-infiltrating lymphocytes. As cellular therapy induces tumor-specific T cell activation and migration to the tumor, this rationalizes a two-sided synergy between these treatment modalities.

19.7 Conclusion

Immunotherapy has revolutionized cancer treatment in a number of malignancies. Most breakthroughs have been derived from antibodies targeting PD-1/PD-L1. In mesothelioma, promising clinical results with these antibodies have been shown, but only in a minority of patients and responses are not durable.

This seems related to the absence of an activated T cell response to the tumor. DC therapy, T cell therapy or cancer vaccines may increase the number of tumor-directed T cells and in this way activate the immune system toward the tumor. Elaborate studies among which numerous randomized trials, are currently underway and more are planned to investigate the efficacy of these novel treatments.

References

1. Yap TA, Aerts JG, Popat S, Fennell DA. Novel insights into mesothelioma biology and implications for therapy. Nat Rev Cancer. 2017;17:475–88.
2. Baas P, Fennell D, Kerr KM, et al. Malignant pleural mesothelioma: ESMO clinical practice guidelines for diagnosis, treatment and follow-up. Ann Oncol. 2015;26:v31–9.
3. Robinson BWS, Musk AW, Lake RA. Malignant mesothelioma. Lancet. 2005;366:397–408.
4. Vogelzang NJ, Rusthoven JJ, Symanowski J, et al. Phase III study of pemetrexed in combination with cisplatin versus cisplatin alone in patients with malignant pleural mesothelioma. J Clin Oncol Off J Am Soc Clin Oncol. 2003;21:2636–44.
5. Ricciardi S, Cardillo G, Zirafa C, et al. Surgery for malignant pleural mesothelioma: an international guidelines review. J Thorac Dis. 2018;10:S285.
6. Treasure T, Lang-Lazdunski L, Waller D, et al. Extra-pleural pneumonectomy versus no extra-pleural pneumonectomy for patients with malignant pleural mesothelioma: clinical outcomes of the Mesothelioma and Radical Surgery (MARS) randomised feasibility study. Lancet Oncol. 2011;12:763–72.
7. Bronte G, Incorvaia L, Rizzo S, et al. The resistance related to targeted therapy in malignant pleural mesothelioma: why has not the target been hit yet? Crit Rev Oncol Hematol. 2016;107:20–32.
8. Zalcman G, Mazieres J, Margery J, et al. Bevacizumab for newly diagnosed pleural mesothelioma in the Mesothelioma Avastin Cisplatin Pemetrexed Study (MAPS): a randomised, controlled, open-label, phase 3 trial. Lancet. 2016;387:1405–14.
9. Scagliotti GV, Gaafar R, Nowak AK, et al. LUME-Meso: design and rationale of the phase III part of a placebo-controlled study of Nintedanib and Pemetrexed/Cisplatin followed by maintenance Nintedanib in patients with unresectable malignant pleural mesothelioma. Clin Lung Cancer. 2017;18:589–93.
10. Fennell DA, Kirkpatrick E, Cozens K, et al. CONFIRM: a double-blind, placebo-controlled phase III clinical trial investigating the effect of nivolumab in patients with relapsed mesothelioma: study protocol for a randomised controlled trial. Trials. 2018;19:233.
11. Hassan R, Bullock S, Premkumar A, et al. Phase I study of SS1P, a recombinant anti-mesothelin immunotoxin given as a bolus I.V. infusion to patients with mesothelin-expressing mesothelioma, ovarian, and pancreatic cancers. Clin Cancer Res. 2007;13:5144–9.
12. Kreitman RJ, Hassan R, Fitzgerald DJ, Pastan I. Phase I trial of continuous infusion anti-mesothelin recombinant immunotoxin SS1P. Clin Cancer Res. 2009;15:5274–9.
13. Krug LM, Dao T, Brown AB, et al. WT1 peptide vaccinations induce CD4 and CD8 T cell immune responses in patients with mesothelioma and non-small cell lung cancer. Cancer Immunol Immunother. 2010;59:1467–79.
14. Petrausch U, Schuberth PC, Hagedorn C, et al. Re-directed T cells for the treatment of fibroblast activation protein (FAP)-positive malignant pleural mesothelioma (FAPME-1). BMC Cancer. 2012;12:615.
15. Sigalotti L, Coral S, Altomonte M, et al. Cancer testis antigens expression in mesothelioma: role of DNA methylation and bioimmunotherapeutic implications. Br J Cancer. 2002;86:979–82.

16. Watanabe Y, Kojima T, Kagawa S, et al. A novel translational approach for human malignant pleural mesothelioma: heparanase-assisted dual virotherapy. Oncogene. 2010;29:1145–54.
17. Cornelissen R, Hegmans J, Maat A, et al. Extended tumor control after dendritic cell vaccination with low-dose cyclophosphamide as adjuvant treatment in patients with malignant pleural mesothelioma. Am J Respir Crit Care Med. 2016;193:1023–31.
18. Garg AD, Coulie PG, Van den Eynde BJ, Agostinis P. Integrating next-generation dendritic cell vaccines into the current cancer immunotherapy landscape. Trends Immunol. 2017;38:577–93.
19. Garg AD, Vara Perez M, Schaaf M, et al. Trial watch: dendritic cell-based anticancer immunotherapy. Oncoimmunology. 2017;6:e1328341.
20. Eguchi T, Kadota K, Mayor M, et al. Cancer antigen profiling for malignant pleural mesothelioma immunotherapy: expression and coexpression of mesothelin, cancer antigen 125, and Wilms tumor 1. Oncotarget. 2017;8:77872–82.
21. Zauderer MG, Tsao AS, Dao T, et al. A randomized phase II trial of adjuvant Galinpepimut-S, WT-1 Analog peptide vaccine, after multimodality therapy for patients with malignant pleural mesothelioma. Clin Cancer Res. 2017;23:7483–9.
22. Claesson MH. Why current peptide-based cancer vaccines fail: lessons from the three Es. Immunotherapy. 2009;1:513–6.
23. Dammeijer F, Lievense LA, Veerman GD, et al. Efficacy of tumor vaccines and cellular immunotherapies in non-small-cell lung cancer: a systematic review and meta-analysis. J Clin Oncol Off J Am Soc Clin Oncol. 2016;34:3204–12.
24. Schreibelt G, Bol KF, Westdorp H, et al. Effective clinical responses in metastatic melanoma patients after vaccination with primary myeloid dendritic cells. Clin Cancer Res. 2016;22:2155–66.
25. Berneman Z, Van de Velde A, Anguille S, et al. Vaccination with Wilms' tumor antigen (<em>WT1)</em> mRNA-Electroporated dendritic cells as an adjuvant treatment in 60 cancer patients: report of clinical effects and increased survival in acute myeloid Leukemia, metastatic breast cancer, glioblastoma and mesothelioma. Cytotherapy. 2016;18:S13–4.
26. Hegmans JP, Veltman JD, Lambers ME, et al. Consolidative dendritic cell-based immunotherapy elicits cytotoxicity against malignant mesothelioma. Am J Respir Crit Care Med. 2010;181:1383–90.
27. Hegmans JPJJ, Hemmes A, Aerts JG, Hoogsteden HC, Lambrecht BN. Immunotherapy of murine malignant mesothelioma using tumor lysate–pulsed dendritic cells. Am J Respir Crit Care Med. 2005;171:1168–77.
28. Aerts JG, Goeje P, Cornelissen R, et al. Autologous dendritic cells pulsed with allogeneic tumor cell lysate in mesothelioma: from mouse to human. Clin Cancer Res. 2017;24:766–76.
29. Chmielewski M, Hombach AA, Abken H. Antigen-specific T-cell activation independently of the MHC: chimeric antigen receptor-redirected T cells. Front Immunol. 2013;4:371.
30. Klampatsa A, Haas AR, Moon EK, Albelda SM. Chimeric antigen receptor (CAR) T cell therapy for malignant pleural mesothelioma (MPM). Cancers. 2017;9:115.
31. Davila ML, Riviere I, Wang X, et al. Efficacy and toxicity management of 19-28z CAR T cell therapy in B cell acute lymphoblastic leukemia. Sci Transl Med. 2014;6:224ra25.
32. Kochenderfer JN, Rosenberg SA. Treating B-cell cancer with T cells expressing anti-CD19 chimeric antigen receptors. Nat Rev Clin Oncol. 2013;10:267–76.
33. Anguille S, Smits EL, Lion E, van Tendeloo VF, Berneman ZN. Clinical use of dendritic cells for cancer therapy. Lancet Oncol. 2014;15:e257–67.
34. Byrne MJ, Nowak AK. Modified RECIST criteria for assessment of response in malignant pleural mesothelioma. Ann Oncol. 2004;15:257–60.
35. Veltman JD, Lambers MEH, van Nimwegen M, et al. COX-2 inhibition improves immunotherapy and is associated with decreased numbers of myeloid-derived suppressor cells in mesothelioma. Celecoxib influences MDSC function. BMC Cancer. 2010;10:1–13.
36. Dammeijer F, Lau SP, Eijck C, Burg S, Aerts JGJV. Rationally combining immunotherapies to improve efficacy of immune checkpoint blockade in solid tumors. Cytokine Growth Factor Rev. 2017;36:5–15.
37. Steendam CMJ, Dammeijer F, Aerts JGJV, Cornelissen R. Immunotherapeutic strategies in non-small-cell lung cancer: the present and the future. Immunotherapy. 2017;9:507–20.

Immunotherapy, the Promise for Future of Mesothelioma Treatment?

20

S. Brosseau, V. Gounant, and G. Zalcman

20.1 Introduction

Understanding the interplay between cancer, cancer-associated fibroblasts (CAFs) and immune cells (T-cells, monocyte-macrophages, pre-dendritic, and dendritic cells) within the malignant pleural mesothelioma (MPM) microenvironment is important in developing novel therapies for MPM patients [1] (see Fig. 20.1). Through chronic inflammation due to asbestosis fibers deposit in pleural space or deep lung, the immune system has been suspected to play a major role in MPM pathogenesis although yet imperfectly understood. Improved outcome was reported to correlate with higher intra-tumor infiltration by cytotoxic T CD8+ cells [2]. Conversely, we will see in the current review that high tumor expression of programmed cell death-ligand 1 (PD-L1), inhibiting T cell function *via* binding the programmed cell death-1 (PD-1) protein at the T-cell surface, has been associated with poor prognosis in mesothelioma patients. Among the different immunotherapies evaluated so far to restore anti-tumor immune response in cancer, immune checkpoint inhibitors (ICI) have generated the most attention based on their clinical efficacy, particularly in melanoma and non-small cell lung cancer (NSCLC) [3]. Cytotoxic T lymphocyte-associated protein (CTLA-4) is one of these checkpoint inhibitor proteins, expressed at cell surface of naïve T-cells, which interacts with B7 protein expressed by antigen presenting cells (APC), such as dendritic cells, this interaction impairing T-cell activation by APC, early in the immune response, at the so-called "priming" phase, presumably in regional lymph nodes close to cancer sites. The PD-1/PD-L1 pathway is generally thought to play a role within the tumor microenvironment itself, at the effector phase of immune response to cancer [3] (see Fig. 20.2). In fact, such a dichotomization is probably simplistic, since CTLA-4 proteins are also expressed by

S. Brosseau
Thoracic Oncology Department and Early Phase Unit CIC1425, University Hospital Bichat-Claude Bernard, Paris, France

Faulty of Medicine, University Paris-Diderot, Paris, France
e-mail: solenn.brosseau@aphp.fr

V. Gounant
Thoracic Oncology Department and Early Phase Unit CIC1425, University Hospital Bichat-Claude Bernard, Paris, France
e-mail: valerie.gounant@aphp.fr

G. Zalcman (✉)
Thoracic Oncology Department and Early Phase Unit CIC1425, University Hospital Bichat-Claude Bernard, Paris, France

Faulty of Medicine, University Paris-Diderot, Paris, France

Institut National de la Santé et de la Recherche Médicale (INSERM) U830, "Genetics and Biology of Cancers" Institut Curie Research Center, Paris, France
e-mail: gerard.zalcman@aphp.fr

G. L. Ceresoli et al. (eds.), *Mesothelioma*, https://doi.org/10.1007/978-3-030-16884-1_20

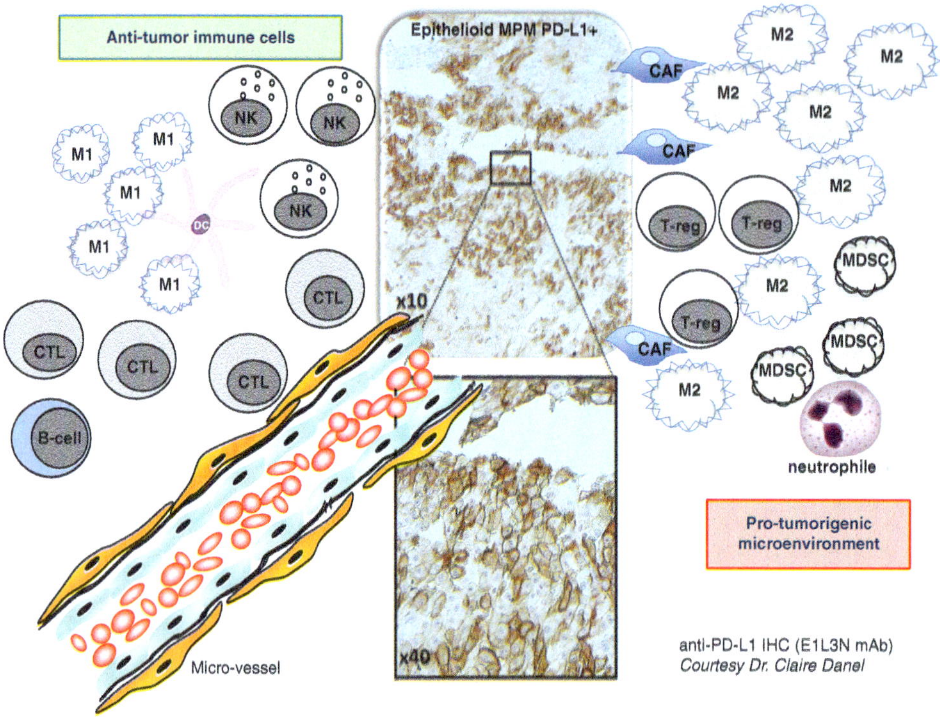

Fig. 20.1 A schematic representation of MPM microenvironment. Green: Anti-tumor immune cells (*NK* natural killer cells (CD16+, KIR+, and granzyme+), *DC* mature dendritic cells (IL12+, CD1c+, CD141+, and CD86+), *M1* macrophage type 1 (IL12+ and CD86+), *CTL* cytotoxic T-lymphocyte (CD8+, CD28+ and granzyme+), *B-cell* B lymphocyte). Red: Pro-tumorigenic cells (*M2* Macrophage type 2 (IL10+, TGFb+, CD163+, and CD23+), *CAF* cancer associated fibroblast, *T-reg* regulatory T-cell (FoxP3+, CD8+, and CD4+), *MDSC* myeloid-derived-suppressor cell (CD11b+, CD33+, CD14+, and CXRC2+), Neutrophile). *PD-L1* Programmed-cell Death receptor Ligand-1

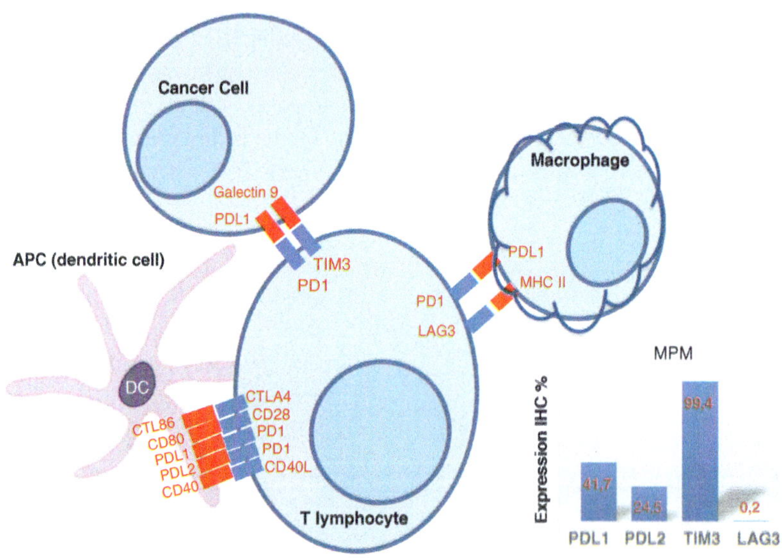

Fig. 20.2 Co-expression of immune checkpoints in micro-environment cells from MPM

T-cells infiltrating the tumor tissue, and since PD-L1 protein is expressed by both immune and tumor cells. However, in contrast with historical studies using systemic or local, intra-pleural interleukin 2 or vaccines which will not be developed here, several studies assessing ICI targeting the PD-1/PD-L1 pathway generated promising results that will be the main topic of this chapter.

20.2 Biological Background

Yamada et al. revealed that lymphocyte infiltration was correlated with an improved clinical outcome and might play a pivotal role in the anti-tumor immune response against MPMs [2]. However, host immune response against cancer cells was shown to be tightly and negatively regulated by the complex Programmed Death-1 (PD-1) and its main ligand PD-L1. The current view is that cancer cells expressing PD-L1 inhibit CD4+ and CD8+ T-cell activation in vitro or lead to T-cell apoptosis, allowing tumor growing without any anti-tumor response in vivo.

While clinical efficacy of ICI, leading to registrations of such drugs, has been claimed to correlate with high tumor mutational burden such as in melanoma or NSCLC patients, mesothelioma was consistently reported to harbor low numbers of mutations per megabase of genomic DNA [4], and thus should not have exhibited exquisite sensitivity to ICI targeting PD-1/PD-L1. It was probably a too simplistic interpretation of first biological-clinical correlations, since rather than mutational burden by itself, it is probably the type of mutated genes that drive the effect of mutational burden and plays a major role. Indeed, in colorectal cancer, mutations or expression of the genes responsible for micro-satellite instability are clearly associated with response to ICI, probably generating a higher content of tumor neo-antigens. In the same way, the major gene driving the effect of mutational burden in NSCLC was shown to be p53 [5], possibly both by its high intrinsic immunogenicity when mutated, and by its role on DNA stability and repair, p53 alterations being associated with higher genetic instability. Which genes could then drive potential efficacy in MPM remains unclear, since p53 mutation rate is much lower than in other tumor types. p16 and BAP-1 could possibly drive such effect as they could both regulate cell cycle arrest and DNA repair or chromatin remodeling. Hippo genes pathway alterations (RASSF1A and NF2, but also MST1/hippo or LATS2) [4], by governing Yes-Associated Protein (YAP) transcriptional co-activator activity state, could also influence anti-tumor immune response, YAP controlling transcription of multiple immune genes such as the cytokine CXLC5, able to attract CXRC2-expressing myeloid-derived suppressor cells (MDSC) [6], while cross-talks between Hippo/YAP pathway and TGF-β or JAK-STAT pathways involved in immune response regulation have been extensively described [7]. But still, MPM was not initially anticipated to be particularly responsive to ICI on the basis of its genetic background. However, the rich inflammatory stromal component of these tumors, especially in the sarcomatoid or biphasic subtypes led to the commune view of a so-called "hot" tumor, with tumor stromal infiltration by mono-macrophage cells, T-lymphocytes, or even neutrophils (see Fig. 20.1). Two retrospective studies actually showed that PD-L1 tumor expression was related to worse outcome in MPM patients [8, 9].

Mansfield et al., using the anti-PD-L1 clone 5H1-A3 antibody and reported a 40% positivity rate in 106 patients, when both cytoplasmic and membranous staining were considered with a 5% cutoff [9]. When their analysis was restricted to exclusive membranous staining, which seems to be more relevant and specific, only 24% of their specimens were scored as positive. Cedrés et al. found 20% positivity in their 77 specimens out of a 119 retrospective series, with E1L3N monoclonal antibody from Cell Signaling technology™, and a generally admitted 1% positivity cutoff [8]. Again, both cytoplasmic and membranous tumor cells staining were considered, in a series comprising a large majority of epithelioid MPM.

More recently, an Australian group [1] used tissue microarrays and E1L3N clone, from 311 specimens (of which 30% non-epithelioid subtypes), the largest series of MPM patients analyzed in the literature to date. While PD-L1 membranous expression in 5% or more tumor cells, regardless of intensity, was shown in 42% of patients, only 9.6% had high PD-L1 positivity, of moderate to high intensity in at least 50% tumor cells, which correlated with non-epithelioid histology (double number of PD-L1 highly expressing tumors as compared with epithelioid tumors). In this large series of patients, PD-L1 tumor expression was reported to correlate with a significantly worse overall survival (OS) (5.33 months of median survival *vs.* 11.33 and 13.5, in patients with highly positive, positive, and negative PD-L1 staining, respectively, HR = 2.37). This poorer prognosis was maintained when both histological categories (epithelioid and non-epithelioid) were analyzed separately and in multivariate analysis. By contrast, CD4-positive, CD8-positive, or FOXP3-positive (T-reg) infiltration (see Fig. 20.1), as evaluated by a semi-automated image quantification method, expressed as the number of T-cells per 10,000 tumor cells, and then dichotomized by the median, did not correlate with survival, although high infiltrations of each of these three cell T-cell subsets was significantly associated to high expression of PD-L1 staining. The role of mono-macrophage or dendritic cells infiltration was not studied while both anti-tumor macrophages type 1 (M1) and pro-tumorigenic macrophages type 2 (M2) are found in the MPM tumor microenvironment (see Fig. 20.1) [10]. The major caveat of such study was the use of therapeutic monoclonal antibody (TMA), which could not have assessed the huge tissue heterogeneity of MPM specimens, some parts of the tumors expressing high content of PD-L1+ cells, while others being totally devoid of such cells.

In an Australian cohort of 46 MPM patients treated off-label by the anti-PD-1 pembrolizumab (n = 45) or the anti-PD-L1, BGB-A317, mainly in second- or more line setting (43/46 = 93%), PD-L1 expression was assessed with the E1L3N antibody, with 5% of tumor cells membranous staining as a cut-off for positivity [11]. They had predominantly epithelioid (n = 32/46; 70%). PD-L1 testing was performed in 14 samples, with PD-L1+ in 5 (36%) and PD-L1 high (over 50% of tumor cells stained) in 4 (29%). PD-L1$^{\text{high} > 50\%}$ subjects exhibited 50% overall response rate (ORR) *vs.* 22% in PDL1-negative patients and 40% in PD-L1+ patients. progression-free survival (PFS) and OS were greater in both PD-L1+ (PFS HR: 0.26) and PD-L1^{hi} (PFS HR: 0.17), although not significantly because of the low numbers. PD-L1+ positivity remained a borderline predictor of improved survival on multivariate analysis (p = 0.06), suggesting here a possible positive predictive value in these immunotherapy-treated patients.

In the MAPS phase 3 study [12], using E1L3N clone in diagnostic specimens from 214 patients accrued with remaining available tissue, a cut-off set at 1% of membranous staining regardless of intensity, only 36% of patients were scored as positive, again with a significantly higher rate of positivity in sarcomatoid or biphasic tumors (68% of positive specimens as compared 29.6% in epithelioid, with p < 0.001) (G. Zalcman, S. Brosseau, personal unpublished data). With this 1% cut-off, there was no impact of PD-L1 tumor positivity on OS in multivariate analysis including stratification prognostic variables of the randomized trial, even if median OS was 12.3 months in patients with PD-L1 positive tumors, *vs.* 22.2 in patients with PD-L1 negative patients, suggesting a possible lack of power.

Raffit Hassan's group studied tumor samples from 65 patients, as malignant effusions from patients with pleural and peritoneal mesothelioma, for PD-L1 expression, both on tumors cells and infiltrating lymphocytes [13]. They found 41 (63%) were PD-L1-positive (with a 5% cut-off for positivity, but they did not detail the antibody used), and exhibited a poorer OS (although not statistically significantly: median 23.0 *vs.* 33.3 months). More interestingly, in nine mesothelioma effusion samples evaluated, the investigators were able to show that there was a fraction of floating cells expressing PD-L1 ranging from 12% to 83%. In seven patients with paired malignant effusion and peripheral blood mononuclear cell (PBMC) samples, PD-L1 expression was significantly higher on CD3-positive T cells identified in malignant effusions, as compared with PBMCs (p = 0.016). The numbers of CD14-

positive PD-1-positive cells were also increased in malignant effusions compared with PBMCs (p = 0.03). Accordingly, the lymphocytes contained in malignant effusions recognized autologous tumor cells as shown by induced interferon-γ-mediated PD-L1 expression on the tumor cell surface. These experiments showed there actually was an anti-tumor immune response elicited by T-cells within pleural cavity, leading to an attempt of tumor cells to limit this anti-tumor T-cell action by expressing PD-L1 at their surface, these observations supporting the rationale for anti PD-1/PD-L1 drug's efficacy in mesothelioma.

Lastly, a series of primary diffuse pleural mesotheliomas including the epithelioid (n = 148), biphasic (n = 15), and sarcomatoid (n = 12) histotypes, were recently evaluated immunohistochemically for cancer stem cell markers and for PD-L1, with the E1LN3 antibody [10]. Thirty-three percent of the analyzed tumors (57/175) contained PD-L1–positive cells (membranous and/or cytoplasmic staining, again using a 5% cut-off), with a decreased OS in the 66 patients with available survival data (median OS = 6.0 months *vs.* 18.0 months for patients with PD-L1 negative tumors, $p < 0.01$). Expression of PD-L1 in tumor-associated immune cells (TAIs, mostly macrophages) was also evaluated and detected in 35 cases (20%). The cancer stem cell marker ALCAM (CD166) was co-expressed with PD-L1 in 20 tumors, with some correlation between expression of both markers (p = 0.04), and these patients showed the shortest survival (median OS = 4 months *vs.* 36.0 months without ALCAM or PD-L1; $p < 0.01$). It is of interest that CD166 was reported to act upstream Hippo/YAP pathway to regulate EMT, a feature of tumor aggressiveness in MPM, in which such pathway is frequently altered.

Thus, malignant pleural mesothelioma tumors were reported to express PD-L1 in 30–63% of cases, in archival paraffin-embedded specimens, according to different retrospective studies and authors, with series of various size, the use of whole slides or TMA, different diagnostic monoclonal antibodies, different scoring systems (cancer cells and immune cells, membranous and cytoplasmic staining), and various immunohistochemistry platforms. However, in all these studies PD-L1 expression was shown to be substantially higher in sarcomatoid or biphasic MPM, and to correlate with a shorter overall survival in most series, even if the PD-L1 expression prognostic impact is difficult to discriminate from the major prognostic impact of these histological sub-types, in such retrospective series, even though using multivariate analyses.

20.3 Available Data from Currently Presented Clinical Trials

20.3.1 Second-Line Trials Using Single Therapy with Anti-CTLA-4 Monoclonal Antibodies (Table 20.1)

Cytotoxic T lymphocyte-associated protein (CTLA-4) is the first checkpoint inhibitors targeted in clinical trials dedicated to MPM, probably because of the availability of anti-CTLA-4 antibodies and their efficacy in melanoma, while anti-PD-1 or PD-L1 antibodies were evaluated in more frequent tumors at that time. First results, considered as encouraging were reported in patients with chemotherapy-resistant advanced malignant mesothelioma, using tremelimumab, a selective human immunoglobulin G2 monoclonal antibody against CTLA-4 that promotes T-cell activity, but claimed to not deplete regulatory T, in an academic, open-label, and single-arm phase 2 trial (MESOTTREM-2008) [14]. Performance status (PS) 0–2 patients with MPM or peritoneal (only one case, as understood from the first table of the paper describing the study population), and measurable lesions received tremelimumab 15 mg/kg intravenously once every 90 days until progressive disease or severe toxicity. The primary endpoint of this trial was overall response rate (ORR) as assessed by modified response evaluation criteria in solid tumors (RECIST) for pleural malignant mesothelioma, but without independent central assessment of response. A classical Simon's optimal two-stage

Table 20.1 Clinical trials assessing monotherapy anti-CTLA-4 monoclonal antibody in Mesothelioma patients

Trial	Line of therapy	Drug	Site	Phase	nb patients	DCR (mRECIST) (%)	PFS (mo)	OS (mo)	Ref.
MESOTTREM- 2008 (NCT01649024)	Second	Tremelimumab	Pleural + peritoneal	2	29	31	6.2	10.7	[14]
MESOTTREM- 2012 (NCT01655888)	Second	Tremelimumab	Pleural + peritoneal	2	29	37.9	6.2	11.3	[15]
DETERMINE (NCT01843374)	Second	Tremelimumab	Pleural + peritoneal	2b R	571 (382 Treme 189 placebo)	27 *vs.* 21.7	2.8 *vs.* 2.7	7.7 *vs.* 7.3	[16]

NA Not Available, *mo* months, *DCR* Disease Control Rate, *PFS* Progression-Free Survival, *OS* overall Survival

design was used, leading to the accrual of 29 patients in a relatively long period of time (30 months), with a target response rate of 17% considered as indicative of the drug activity in that setting, which would have needed 4 objective responses in 29 patients to reach this endpoint. A majority of these patients (25/29, 86%) did receive a standard first-line treatment with platinum combined with pemetrexed. Of 29 patients, 23 (79%) had documented disease progression within 6 months from first-line platinum-based chemotherapy, of whom 15 (68%) progressed during chemotherapy. Thus, one-fifth of these patients (21%) had indolent disease progressing beyond 6 months post platinum-based first line treatment, which must lead to caution in interpreting the meaning of the rate of stable disease patients. The median time from the end of the first platinum containing regimen to documented progressive disease was 2.1 months, with a further median time of 1.3 months (3.4 months median time, in total) from documented progressive disease to the beginning of treatment with anti-CTLA4, again indicative of relatively indolent tumors (a classical bias of such single arm, phase 2 trials).

Only two responses were observed, and this trial should have been thus considered as negative, with seven patients more with stable disease, leading to a 31% of disease control rate (DCR), considered by the authors as encouraging, despite the recruitment of patients with potential slowly growing tumors. Median duration of disease control was estimated to 12.4 months. Of note, the two responder patients showed long-lasting response over 6 months, which obviously grabbed investigator's attention. Median PFS of the whole cohort of the study was 6.2 months, which also could be interpreted in two ways: either effect of the drug or accrual of patients with indolent tumors. Median OS was 10.7 months with a 37% 2-year survival that could be interpreted in the same way, taking into account for the relative inefficacy of second or third-line treatments in MPM, with the exception of pemetrexed re-challenge for patients who did not receive pemetrexed within the previous 6–12 months [15]. Unfortunately, no data on subsequent therapies were shown. Safety profile of tremelimumab was favorable with no toxic death and only 14% of patients with grade 3–4 events. Seventy two percent of grade 1–2 events observed resolved spontaneously or with symptomatic treatments of short steroid course. Two patients experienced microscopic colitis with diarrhea, a commune immune-related adverse event, and frequent with anti-CTLA-4 drugs. The most interesting data of this seminal study was the blood lymphocyte monitoring data, in 28 out of 29 accrued patients. CD4+/ICOS+ circulating T-cells rate, as assessed by surface expression of selected markers by direct immunofluorescence and flow cytometry at day 30 of the first cycle was associated with longer overall survival, while T-cells sub-types counts at baseline did not help to predict longer survival upon tremelimumab. Such observation suggested that some readouts of tremelimumab efficacy could be observed as soon as after 1 month of treatment, yet with a costly fluorescence-activated cell sorting (FACS) technology.

The same investigators reported a second academic open-label, single-arm phase 2 study, (MESOTTREM-2012) [16], with an "intensified" schedule of tremelimumab, at 10 mg/kg every 4 weeks for six doses, and every 12 weeks thereafter, until progression or toxicity. The primary endpoint again was the ORR, but using iRECIST, and then determining the proportion of patients achieving an immune-related objective response (complete or partial), provided they received at least one dose of the study drug. Inclusion criteria were substantially the same as the previous trial, with again only one peritoneal mesothelioma patient. In this trial, patients with evidence of progressive disease at the first tumor assessment were allowed to continue to receive tremelimumab if they did not have clinical signs or symptoms of progression. Unless the patient was deteriorating rapidly, disease progression was confirmed by two CT scans at least 6 weeks apart, although, again, not centrally assessed. As the in the previous trial, using a Simon's optimal 2-stage design the target response rate of 17% was chosen to consider the study drug clinically active, leading, with a 70% power, to a 29 patients accrual target, which was here obtained within one year. A pre-specified interim safety analysis was successful since no clinically relevant toxic effects were recorded in the first phase among the initial 11 patients treated. Four patients had an immune-related partial response: one at the first tumor assessment (after about 12 weeks) and three at the second tumor assessment (about 24 weeks), leading to only 13.8% iRECIST ORR, thus not clearly indicating a significant activity. More puzzling, when the classical mRECIST for mesothelioma was used, only one partial response was found. The proportion of patients with disease control was 51.7% (15 of 29 patients), with iRECIST, with a consistent median duration of disease control of 10.9 months, but DCR was only 37.9% with mRECIST. Median immune-related progression-free survival was 6.2 months, median overall survival was 11.3 months and 1-year survival was 48.3%, all values being strictly comparable with the previous trial. However, the seven patients with biphasic or sarcomatoid malignant mesothelioma had a median overall survival of 15.8 months which compared favorably with what was observed in the seminal pemetrexed registrations trial, in such subset known to have a worse prognosis and resistance to chemotherapy, suggesting this subtype could specifically take advantage from immunotherapy, as it was suspected by immune content pathological analyses and PD-L1 expression data, reported above. However, the limited size of this subset was claimed to explain why no significant correlation with iORR, iPFS, or OS was observed, while PS or European Organization for Research and Treatment of Cancer (EORTC) score did significantly associate with iPFS or OS. Again, safety profile was favorable with no toxic death reported and very few and not unexpected grade 3–4 adverse events (AE). Patients with a ratio of circulating neutrophils to CD4-positive, ICOS-positive T cells below the median on day 14 of the second cycle, but not at earlier time-points investigated, had significantly better overall survival than those with a ratio equal to or greater than the median, reminiscent of previous observations, although expressed differently, and measured at a different time-point (44 days *vs.* 30 post the first cycle), possibly by lack of reproducibility or stability of this prognostic/predictive variable. Lastly, that authors were to be congratulated since this study was one of the rare studies which had included a pharmacokinetics analysis, performed on the 14 first patients, and showing that most of patients maintained concentrations of tremelimumab at or above the target of 30 μg/mL, during the entire dosing interval, thus supporting the new schedule and dosing, chosen in this study.

Based in these data, although, as mentioned, some caveats could have obscured the interpretation of both trials, tremelimumab was tested alone *vs.* placebo in second- or third-line treatment in MPM in the DETERMINE large randomized Phase IIb trial [17]. PS 0–1 patients with unresectable pleural or peritoneal malignant mesothelioma and measurable disease, who had progressed after one or two previous systemic treatments for advanced disease, were eligible. Patient randomization was stratified by EORTC status (low risk *vs.* high risk), line of therapy (second line *vs.* third line), and anatomic site (pleural *vs.* peritoneal). However, the time elapsed between last-line therapy including pemetrexed was not included as a stratification variable and thus an unbalance in the accrual of indolent tumors between the two arms could not be controlled with such stratification policy. Intravenous tremelimumab was given at 10 mg/kg, or placebo, every 4 weeks for seven doses and every 12 weeks thereafter, until progression or toxicity. Accrual was particularly fast, since in 18 months, 571 patients were randomly assigned (2:1) to receive tremelimumab or placebo in 105 study centers worldwide. Since this trial was placebo-controlled, since classical mRECIST for meso was used, and since OS was the primary endpoint, there was no central assessment of response in this company-sponsored trial (AstraZeneca). The possibility was offered to investigators to continue treatment despite mRECIST progression if they felt that patient derived a clinical benefit, to take into account a so-called pseudo-progression, particularly frequent in melanoma patients, but of which incidence is currently unknown in MPM patients. However, if the tumor burden at the confirmatory scan was more than 20% larger than the tumor burden at the initial scan showing progressive disease, the patient was considered to have progressive disease and was to be discontinued from study treatment. The trial initially designed to accrue 180 patients based on a superiority design, à 80% power and a two-sided α-risk of 20%, was amended after 107 patients were randomized, before any un-blinding, according to the analysis of the two phase 2 trials described above. Overall, 382 patients were assigned to receive tremelimumab, 189 to placebo, median age 66.0 years. 95.5% had pleural mesothelioma, 16.4% had non-epithelioid histological subtype mesothelioma, one-third had received previously two lines of therapy, of which 99% had received first-line pemetrexed-based therapy, 58% had low-risk EORTC score, and 95% had stage IIIB/IV mesothelioma. Patients received a median number of three cycles. Unfortunately, no survival gain was obtained in tremelimumab group, compared to placebo (median OS: 7.7 *vs.* 7.3 months, respectively; HR = 0.92; $p = 0.408$) and not a single subset of patients did significantly benefit from tremelimumab, although non-significant trends were observed in the group of sarcomatoid MPM (HR = 0.68) and in the group of earlier stages (≤III). With high maturity (#80% of patients had died at the time of analysis), long-term survivals did no differ either, survival curves remaining desperately superimposed, while no difference in subsequent therapies was observed, no patients in either group receiving further anti-PD-1 or anti-PD-L1 drugs. Only eight patients exhibited confirmed partial response, supporting the total lack of efficacy of tremelimumab single-therapy, even if 27% of patients had stable disease (≥6 weeks post-randomization), the placebo arm patients doing similarly at 22%, showing how stable disease should be considered cautiously in MPM, and supporting the use of a control arm in MPM trials, even in phase 2 trials to avoid the bias of indolent pleural tumors. These results could have torpedoed further trials with ICI, if anti-PD-1/PD-L1 drugs had not given rapid and striking results of which amplitude clearly appeared, as compared with DETERMINE historical yet recent data.

20.3.2 Second-Line Trials Using Single Therapy with Anti-PD-1 or PD-L1 Monoclonal Antibodies (Table 20.2)

Several studies assessing ICI targeting the PD-1/PD-L1 pathway indeed generated promising results, all presented in oral session of last international meetings most of them deserving definitive publication.

The first data came from a Phase Ib large multicenter, non-randomized, open-label, and multi-cohort "basket" trial (Keynote 028), with a stratum dedicated to MPM, including 25 patients with PD-L1-expressing MPM, treated with the anti-PD-1 antibody pembrolizumab from Merck, 10 mg/kg IV every 2 weeks [18]. They had to be PS 0-1, to have measurable disease, histological diagnosis of MPM, to have failed to standard therapy or to be considered as "unable to receive chemotherapy". PD-L1 expression was assessed with the use of the 22C3 antibody (Merck, Kenilworth, NJ, USA) assay, with a cut-off set at ≥1% of tumor cells *or associated inflammatory cells,* with membranous staining, regardless of intensity. Upon 83 patients with evaluable histological specimen, 45.7% ($n = 38$) had positive results, of which 25 were found eligible for the protocol. Although highly selected for such a phase I trial (two third were PS = 1), patients did not fundamentally differ from a MPM standard population, as expected in that setting, with median age 65.0 years, two-third men, 72% with epithelioid histology, one-third with two or more previous lines (but two naive of any treatment), 84% who had previously received pemetrexed and 88% exposed to a platinum salt. Primary endpoint was shared in all strata, to show an ORR exceeding 10% at an overall one-sided 8% α-level. Twenty-two patients had to be recruited to give an 80% power. Actually, 25 patients were accrued and received at least one dose of pembrolizumab. Safety was found as manageable, with classical immune-related adverse events (IRAEs) in 12% of patients, a dose reduction needed in only one patient, grade 3 AEs in only 20% of patients, but not grade 4 or 5.

Table 20.2 Clinical trials assessing monotherapy anti-PD-1 or PD-L1 monoclonal antibody in Mesothelioma patients

Trial	Line of therapy	Drug	Site	Phase	n patients	DCR (mRECIST)	PFS	OS	Ref.
KEYNOTE 028 (NCT0205480)	Second	Anti-PD-1 pembrolizumab	Pleural + peritoneal	1b	25	72%	5.4 mo	18 mo	[18]
KEYNOTE-139 Chicago University/NCI (NCT02399371)	Second/ third	Anti-PD1 pembrolizumab	Pleural + peritoneal	2	65	63%	4 mo	11 mo	[19]
Swiss national registry	Second or further lines	Anti-PD1 pembrolizumab	Pleural + peritoneal		48	52%	3.6 mo	7.2 mo	[20]
NIVOMES (NCT02497508)	Second or further lines	Anti-PD-1 nivolumab	Pleural + peritoneal	2	34	29% at 6 mo	3.6 mo	11.8 mo	[21]
MERIT (ONO-4538-41/Japic CTI-No.163247)	Second/ third	Anti-PD-1 nivolumab	Pleural + peritoneal	2	29	67.6% at 6 mo	6.1 mo	17.3	[22]
JAVELIN	Second or further lines	Anti- PD-L1 avelumab	Pleural + peritoneal	1b	53	58.5%	4.1 mo	10.9 mo	[23]
ETOP 9-14 PROMISE-Meso (NCT02991482)	Second/ third	Anti-PD-1 pembrolizumab *vs.* gemcitabine or vinorelbine	Pleural + peritoneal	3	144	NA	NA	NA	http://www. etop-eu
CONFIRM (University of Southampton) (UK trial number CRUK 16/022)	Second	Anti-PD-1 nivolumab *vs.* placebo	Pleural + peritoneal	3	336 (2:1 random)	NA	NA	NA	https://www. southampton. ac.uk/
KEYNOTE-158[a] (NCT02628067)	Second or further lines	Anti-PD1 pembrolizumab	Pleural + peritoneal	2 basket	1350 (total all cancers)	NA	NA	NA	https:// clinicaltrials.gov

NA not available, *mo* months, *DCR* disease control rate, *PFS* progression-free survival, *OS* overall Survival, *NR* not reached

[a]Keynote-158 is a large basket trial in which the number of MPM patients is unknown, among other cancer sites

The results turned out to be encouraging with 20% ORR and 52% of patients exhibiting stable disease (SD). More convincing was the durability of responses, since the median duration of response (DOR) was 12 months (95%CI: 3.7-not reached [NR]), while the durability of stable disease (5.6 months) was in accordance with the duration observed in the DETERMINE placebo arm. The time to response was short (median 1.9 months (1.7–3.8)) and the median PFS was not fantastic at 5.4 months. However, median OS was 18 months and 62.6% of patients were alive at 1 year, two patients having received the maximal length of 24 months treatment, while two other responders were still under treatment at 22 months. More strikingly, four patients exhibited more than 70% decrease of their tumor burden, clearly supporting an activity of the drug, a feature not reported in previous anti-CTLA-4 trials.

Final results from a U.S. phase 2 single-arm trial assessing the activity of a fixed-dose of pembrolizumab (200 mg every 3 weeks) in second-line setting (KEYNOTE-139, NCT02399371) confirmed the activity and the tolerability of such anti-PD-1 drug in pre-treated MPM patients [19]. Sixty-five MPM patients, PS = 0–1, with disease progression after 1 or 2 prior regimens of which one included pemetrexed-platinum doublet, and measurable disease were treated with pembrolizumab 200 mg IV q21 days with first CT-scan evaluation at 9 weeks. Median age was 68 years, 53% were PS = 0, 77% had epithelioid histology, 12% had peritoneal disease, and 61% had received only one prior treatment. Partial response according to mRECIST was observed in 14 patients (22%), while 26 more had stable disease at 9 weeks (56%) giving a 63% DCR at 9 weeks. While toxicity was estimated manageable (4.5% of grade 2–3 pneumonitis, 4.5% of grade 3 adrenal insufficiency, 1.5% grade 3 colitis and 3% grade 3–5 hepatitis), one patient had grade 5 autoimmune hepatitis, another died from an unknown cause. With a centrally-assessed 22C3 antibody-based immunohistochemistry assay (Qualtek laboratory), PDL1 expression was available in 62 patients: 45% were found negative (<1%), 32% had low PD-L1 expression (1–49%), while 23% had high expression (≥50%). When used as a continuous marker, higher PD-L1 expression was associated with a higher response rate (ROC area under the curve = 0.69; 95%CI: 0.53–0.84). ORR was higher and PFS longer in patients with high PD-L1 expression as compared with no and low PD-L1 expression (0.021 and 0.034 respectively), but OS was not influenced by PD-L1 tumor content. 1-year PFS was 40.2% in patients with high PD-L1 expression *vs.* 9.3% in the others ($p = 0.019$).

Lastly, a Swiss registry analysis of 48 MPM patients, PS 0-2, who progressed after a single line of pemetrexed-based treatment, and were treated on an off label basis by pembrolizumab, was presented at ESMO 2017 meeting [20]. An investigator-based analysis of responses according mRECIST found a 25% ORR and a 53% DCR (11% for PS2 patients *vs.* 42% for the 19 PS 0–1 patients and 33 *vs.* 72% for ORR and DCR respectively). Median PFS was 3.6 months in the whole cohort, with a 7.2 months median OS. PS 0–1 patients had a 10.2 months OS. Of course such retrospective data, without central assessment of response, should be considered cautiously, even if such "real-life" data could support the phase I–II data of activity of second-line pembrolizumab. In this series, PD-L1 assessment showed a clear correlation between activity of pembrolizumab and increasing PD-L1 tumor cell expression, all four patients with more than 50% tumor cell expression exhibiting disease control, *vs.* 32% for PD-L1 negative patients (with <1% of PD-L1 stained tumor cells), with a significant 0.27HR for PFS.

Convinced by these preliminary data, another group, ETOP, also launched the well-designed ETOP 9-14 PROMISE-meso trial, which aims to compare, after one previous line of chemotherapy, pembrolizumab 200 mg fixed dose i.v., day 1 of each 3-week cycle, until progressive disease by iRECIST, for maximum 2 years, with second-line chemotherapy by institutional choice either Gemcitabine 1000 mg/m^2 d1/d8, q3w i.v., or Vinorelbine 30 mg/m^2 d1/d8, q3w i.v., or Vinorelbine 60 mg/m^2 d1/d8 q3w p.o. with a cross-over allowed at progression. This phase 3 trial aims to increase progression-free survival based on an independent review, from 3 to 6 months (HR = 0.58), needing 142 patients to accrue.

Another anti-PD-1 antibody, nivolumab (Nivo), has been evaluated in second- or third-line setting by the Dutch group, in the NivoMes study presented orally at IMIG 2016 and WCLC 2017 meetings by Dr. Paul Baas [21]. Patients should have progressed after ≥1 line, histological specimens were to be available at baseline, the tumor being accessible for new biopsies, with FACS studies on peripheral blood mononuclear cells baseline sampling. Primary endpoint was DCR at 12 weeks, with the aim to increase DCR from 20 to 40%, leading with an 80% power at 5% α-level to the accrual of 33 patients, according to a Simon minimax plan, needing to observe five OR in the first 18 accrued patients. Patients received Nivolumab IV infusion, 3 mg/kg, q2 weeks and were to have re-biopsy and PBMC sampling at 6 weeks. Accrual was fast, with 34 (28 epithelioid/6 sarcomatoid/biphasic) enrolled in less than 1 year. Patients have classical epidemiological features with median age 68 years, 28 male, but only one patient having received more one previous line. Only 9/34 (26.5%) patients had mesothelioma sample with 1% or more PD-L1-stained tumor cells, and three with 50% or more stained cells, using 28.8 DAKO assay. The trial was clearly positive since DCR was 29% at 6 months (of which two cases of pseudo-progression), with a 23.5% of ORR (n = 8) and a median PFS of 110 days (3.6 months). Six patients were still treated at 40 weeks at the time of the last presentation, with 33% DCR at 6 months (including four patients with SD), showing again a convincing duration of the treatment effect. There was not unexpected safety profile with 26% grade 3–4 IRAEs, but one treatment-related death due to pneumonitis. Responses were seen in all groups irrespective of PDL1 expression, although small numbers precluded any definitive conclusion.

A Japanese multicenter trial, MERIT (ONO-4538-41/JapicCTI-No.163247), was presented at 2018 WCLC meeting, by Nakano et al., in second or third line advanced or metastatic MPM, resistant or intolerant to platinum-based combination therapy with Pemetrexed (n = 34) [22]. Primary endpoint was ORR and Nivolumab was used with a 240 mg flat dose q2 weeks. The expected response rate was 19.2% giving an 80% power at 5% α-level. Median age was 68.0 years, 29.4% of patients received two previous lines of treatment, 79.4% had epithelioid MPM, and 61% had PS = 1. The trial was positive since ORR reached 29.4% and DCR at 6 months was 67.6% without unexpected safety concerns. With a median follow-up of 16.8 months, median PFS was 6.1 months, median OS was 17.3 months. PD-L1 status determined using the Dako PD-L1 IHC 28-8 pharmDx test clearly influenced survival with median PFS of 7.2 months in patients with PD-L1 tumor expression >1% *vs.* 2.9 months for the others, and median OS being 17.3 months in PD-L1-positive patients *vs.* 11.6 for the PD-L1-negative patients. Grade 3 interstitial pneumonia or pneumonitis occurred three of the 20 PD-L1-positive patients (15%). Based on the results of the MERIT study, nivolumab was approved on Aug 21st in Japan for unresectable advanced or recurrent MPM patients, who have progressed after chemotherapy.

Finally, results from the strata dedicated to MPM of the multicenter non-randomized, open-label, and multicohort "basket" trial phase Ib "JAVELIN" (NCT01772004), assessing the anti-PDL-1 fully humanized IgG1 avelumab in about 2200 patients with more than 15 types of cancer, were presented as a poster at ASCO meeting 2018 [23]. Fifty-three patients with unresectable pleural or peritoneal mesothelioma, whose disease had progressed after platinum and pemetrexed therapy, were treated by avelumab, 10 mg/kg IV Q2W until progression, unacceptable toxicity, or withdrawal. Patients had previously received 1 (n = 18), 2 (n = 15) or ≥ 3 (n = 20) prior lines of therapy. After a median follow-up of 24.8 months, confirmed was only 9.4% of ORR, with 15.2 months median duration of response, contrasting with previous data although more patients were highly pretreated in this series. DCR was 58.5%, which is also modest, median PFS was 4.1 months and median OS was only 10.9 months. However, in evaluable patients with PD-L1+ (n = 16) tumors (≥5% tumor cell cutoff), ORR was 18.8% although 6-months PFS did not differ from the whole series. Safety profile was acceptable with no treatment-related deaths occurring.

20.3.3 Trials Using Combination Therapy with Anti-PD-1 or PD-L1 and Anti-CTLA-4 Monoclonal Antibodies (Table 20.3)

With this background in mind, IFCT 1501 MAPS2 trial (NCT 02716272) was launched as a randomized, non-comparative phase 2 trial, which assessed in MPM patients the value of anti-PD-1 mAb Nivolumab as a single therapy, or in combination with the anti-CTLA-4 mAb ipilimumab (Ipi), from BMS, in second- or third-line setting [24]. PS 0–1 patients, with histological diagnosis of pleural unresectable mesothelioma, measurable disease according to central assessment by an independent radiological panel using mRECIST criteria, with documented progression (all CT-scanners were centrally reviewed), were randomized 1:1 between nivolumab (nivo) 3 mg/kg, q2 weeks and nivo 3 mg/kg, q2 weeks plus ipilimumab (ipi) at 1 g/kg q6 weeks, and treated until progression or unacceptable toxicity for up to two years. A non-comparative phase 2, one-step Fleming design analyzing each arm independently was used, with DCR at 12 weeks as primary endpoint, assuming a target DCR ≥40%, with a one-sided α error of 0·05, leading to 54 eligible patients to be recruited in each arm, and with the assumption of a 5% of ineligibility rate, 57 patients in each arm in total. Patients were stratified according to histology (epithelioid *vs.* non-epithelioid), line of treatment (second *vs.* third line) and a readout for previous line chemosensitivity (progression ≥3 months after the chemo completion *vs.* <3 months). Sixteen failure-free patients had to be observed at 12 weeks to conclude to activity in either arm. Results of this trial were presented at ASCO and ESMO 2017 meetings. The accrual, supported by investigators' enthusiasm for immunotherapy and previous results, was impressively fast since 125 patients were recruited in less than 5 months in 25 French centers, 11 being registered the last day! 63 were allocated to nivo, 62 to the combination, 63 and 61 receiving the allocating treatment, and all analyses being performed in intent-to-treat (ITT). Median age was slightly older than in the previous studies (72.3 and 71.1 years), probably reflecting less patient selection than in previous small-sized studies. Overall, 84% had epithelioid histology, two-third were PS = 1, there was slightly more male in the combo arm (85 *vs.* 75%, respectively, not significant), and more patients having progressed beyond 3 months after last chemotherapy completion (66 *vs.* 59%, respectively, not significant). Roughly 70% were second-line patients. 86.4% had stage III–IV tumors, and prognostic biological characteristics such as leukocytes, platelets count, or hemoglobin concentration (variables from the EORTC prognostic), were similar in both groups. PD-L1 tumor cell expression was centrally assessed with both 28.8 Dako PharmDX™ assay in 99 available specimens and SP-263 Ventana™ assay in 104 specimens, with ≥1% cut-off, as previously described by the French pathological panel (Mesopath), which reviewed all pathological diagnoses. 41.4% and 45.2% of specimens were scored as positive with 28.8 and SP-263 assays respectively, with a surprisingly low concordance kappa index ($\kappa = 0.56$) by the very same pathologists for both assays. Drug delivery was good, but better in the single-therapy arm since 49.2% and 38.7% of patients received at least 10 injections, with 100% of the drug dose being delivered during all infusions. The safety profile again was not unexpected with slightly more toxicity in the combo arm compared with the nivo arm, showing 26.2 grade 3–4 AEs *vs.* 12.7%. Three toxic deaths were observed, including a fulminant hepatitis and one encephalitis, all in the combo arm, and all observed, within the first 5 months of the trial, with no further toxic death in the last period, possibly because the investigators got trained with more accuracy to early diagnose and manage immune-related toxicities in these patients. Despite such toxicities, patients reported outcomes (PROs), which were not different at baseline, did not significantly differ at 12 weeks, using LCSS questionnaires in the two

Table 20.3 Clinical trials assessing combination therapy of anti-PD-1 or PD-L1 plus anti-CTLA-4 monoclonal antibody or chemotherapy in Mesothelioma patients

Trial	Line of therapy	Drug	Site	Phase	n patients	DCR (mRECIST)	PFS	OS	Ref
INITIATE (NCT03048474)	Second	Anti-PD-1 nivolumab+ Anti-CTLA-4 ipilimumab	Pleural + peritoneal	2	33	75%	4.8 mo	NA	[26]
IFCT 1501 MAPS2 (NCT 02716272)	Second	Anti-PD-1 nivolumab+ Anti-CTLA-4 ipilimumab or Anti-PD-1 nivolumab	Pleural	2R not comparative		51.6% 39.7%	5.6 mo 4.0 mo	15.9 mo 11.9 mo	[25]
NIBIT-meso-1 (NCT022588131)	Second	Anti-PD-L1 durvalumab + anti-CTLA-4 tremelimumab	Pleural + peritoneal	2	40	63%	5.7 mo	16.6 mo	[27]
DREAM (ALTG15003) (NCT03075527)	First	Anti-PD-L1 durvalumab+ pemetrexed-platinum doublet	–	2	54	85%	6.2 mo	NR	[29]
CheckMate-743 (NCT02899299)	First	Anti-PD-1 nivolumab+ Anti-CTLA-4 ipilimumab *vs.* pemetrexed-platinum doublet	–	3	600	NA	NA	NA	https://clinicaltrials.gov/
CANADIAN CANCER TRIALS GROUP (CCTG 1227) (NCT02784171)	First	pembrolizumab *vs.* nivolumab+ pemetrexed-cisplatin	–	2/3	390	NA	NA	NA	https://www.ctg.queensu.ca/

NA not available, *NR* not reached, *mo* months, *DCR* disease control rate, *PFS* progression-free survival, *OS* overall survival

groups of patients. The trial met its primary endpoint in both arms, with 44.4% DCR in the nivo arm in the first 54 eligible patients, and 39.7% in the ITT group of 63 patients, while DCR was 50.0% in the combo arm in the first 54 eligible patients and 51.6% in the ITT group of 62 patients, as evaluated by an independent panel of three radiologists expert in MPM and blinded to the treatment group. Objective response rates were 18.5% ($n = 10$) and 27.8% ($n = 15$) in Nivo and Nivo+Ipi, respectively. ORR was significantly increased in the PD-L1 positive subset, with both assays used, despite the observed low correlation ($p = 0.003$ for 28.8 assay), while both ORR and DCR were significantly increased in patients with histological high PD-L1 expression (cut-off ≥25% of membranous tumor cell staining), this cut-off giving seven positive specimens with 28.8 assay and 16 positive specimens with SP-263 assay, which thus proved to be more sensitive. Strikingly, waterfall plots of percentage change from baseline in tumor size at 12 weeks, clearly confirmed a major activity with respectively 3 and 10 patients exhibiting tumor shrinking of more than 60%, in the nivo and the combo group, irrespective of the histological subset [25]. Conversely, 12 and 5 patients showed more than 60% of tumor size increase, with major and rapid tumor burden progression of more than 80% was observed in few patients (six and two respectively), suggesting hyper-progression in a quite indolent disease like MPM, with no obvious correlation with the histological subtype. With a median follow-up exceeding 20 months, median duration of response was 7.4 months in the nivo group *vs.* 8.3 months in the combo group. Median PFSs were 4.0 months and 5.6 months in Nivo and Nivo+Ipi, respectively, with 90 and 85 events respectively. More strikingly, 1-year PFS were 15.9% and 22.6% and mOS was 11.9 months and 15.9 months in Nivo and Nivo+Ipi, respectively, with 65 and 50% of events observed, supporting the maturity of the trial. One-year survivals were 49.2 and 58.1% in Nivo and Nivo+Ipi respectively, with no imbalance in the post-discontinuation treatments received by patients detected between both arms. Such results supported a clear activity of Nivo and Nivo+Ipi in relapsing MPM patients with good general condition, at the cost of a higher toxicity in the combo arm, but with OS comparing favorably with the historical first-line OS observed in the seminal pemetrexed phase 3 registration trial, 15 years ago. Patients in this trial were clearly selected and fit, although the randomized design did limit this classical bias for phase 2 trials. Interestingly, an exploratory analysis gives some hypothesis-generating data, to choose between single or combination therapy, showing for instance that patients with PD-L1 positive tumors did survive longer than patients with PD-L1 negative tumors when treated by Nivolumab (adj. HR = 0.53), while the combination therapy was equally effective in patients with PD-L1 negative or positive tumors. In the same way, the combination did profit to patients with non-epithelioid tumor as compared with patients having epithelioid subtype mesothelioma (adj. HR = 0.46), while patients with tumors containing a sarcomatoid cell contingent had poorer OS with nivolumab single therapy compared to patients with pure epithelioid (adj. HR = 1.48) tumors. And finally, patients with chemo-sensitive tumors (having progressed more than 3 months after completion of the last chemo line) did significantly better with nivolumab than patients with chemo-resistant tumors (adj. HR = 0.35, $p = 0.002$), while the combination therapy did equally well in patients with chemo-resistant or -sensitive tumors (adj. HR = 0.76).

Another smaller, yet non-randomized trial ("INITIATE", NCT03048474) by Baas et al., with the very same design as NIVOMES trial, was recently presented at the 2017 WCLC and the 2018 international Mesothelioma interest group (IMIG) meetings, similarly assessing in 35 patients the value of Nivo (1 mg/kg/3 weeks *vs.* /2 weeks as in MAPS-2) plus Ipi (1 mg/kg/6 weeks) as second-/third-line treatment in MPM (85% of patients) [26]. Similar trends were observed with treatment benefits at 12 weeks since ORR and DCR were 30% and 75% respectively with a 4.8 months PFS but still immature OS data.

All these data prone to the second/third line nivolumab versus placebo phase III academic UK trial "CONFIRM" (*Cancer Research UK* trial number CRUK/16/022), the placebo arm being debatable and raising some ethical issues taking into account for the results of the French trial.

MAPS2 results showed that checkpoint antibody combination trials represent another area of great interest. Indeed, combined 1 mg/kg tremelimumab and 20 mg/kg durvalumab given in four intravenous doses every 4 weeks, followed by maintenance durvalumab at the same dose and schedule for nine dosings, was tested in a single-arm Phase II trial ("NIBIT-MESO-1"; NCT02588131) as first- or second-line treatment for unresectable malignant mesothelioma patients [27]. This trial met its primary endpoint with 11/40 (27.5%) patients exhibiting immune-related (ir)-partial response (median DOS: 16.1 months), and 25/40 (65%) ir-disease control, leading to median ir-progression free survival (PFS) of 8 months (mPFS = 5.7 months) and mOS of 16.6 months (95%CI, 13.1–20.1). In this specific trial, baseline tumor PD-L1 expression had no predictive or prognostic value.

A phase Ib trial published in 2015, with no further results of any phase 2 trial, first reported in 15 PS = 0–1 patients with unresectable MPM, the safety results of the association of pemetrexed-cisplatin doublet with a fully humanized agonist antibody against CD40L, CP-870,893 given at D8 of 21-days cycles for a maximum of six cycles [28]. CD40 agonist monoclonal antibody CP-870,893 binds to CD40 on a variety of immune cell types, triggering the cellular proliferation and activation of antigen-presenting cells (APCs), activating B cells and T cells, and enhancing the immune response. Indeed, MTD was rapidly reached with a cytokine release syndrome as the main adverse event. It was observed six objective responses (40%) and nine stable diseases (53%) as best response, with 6.3 months PFS, in line with what is usually observed with first-line pemetrexed-cisplatin doublet. Three patients survived beyond 30 months which is not unusual for some indolent MPM, with a median OS of 16.5 months as observed in the control pemetrexed-cisplatin arm of MAPS trial. Biological markers of actual CD40 signaling stimulation were reported such as increase of activated memory B-cells, compared to baseline. However, no signal of any unusual activity or synergy could be ascertained, while toxicity was increased although manageable. No further development of such combinations with this CD40 agonist is currently on-going in MPM patients although.

Immunotherapy-based combinations are currently evaluated as first-line treatment in on-going trials. Thus, a large randomized Phase III trial sponsored by BMS ("CheckMate CA209-743"; NCT 02899299; $n = 600$) assessing the benefit of Nivo+Ipi *vs.* standard frontline chemotherapy (platinum + pemetrexed × six cycles maximum) with OS as primary endpoint as completed its inclusions with results expecting for ASCO 2019 meeting.

A phase 2–3 active-comparator trial (NCT02784171) was initiated by the Canadian Cancer Trials Group, currently exploring the efficacy of first-line therapy with pembrolizumab *versus* either cisplatin and pemetrexed, or the pembrolizumab-cisplatin-pemetrexed combination, the phase 3 part beginning by Fall 2018, with the triplet arm compared with the chemotherapy standard arm.

Lastly, two single-arm Phase II trials are assessing durvalumab anti-PD-L1 monoclonal antibody form AstraZeneca combined with the cisplatin-pemetrexed doublet in the USA (NCT 02899195; $n = 55$, results still pending), and Australia ("DREAM" trial; $n = 54$). The final results for the 54 patients of this latest trial were just presented at WCLC meeting 2018 by Dr. Anna Nowak. First-line MPM patients, PS = 0–1, received cisplatin-pemetrexed at standard dosing, with durvalumab 1125 mg q3 weeks, for six cycles as induction therapy, and in case of disease control, up to 17 cycles of maintenance durvalumab 1125 mg q3 weeks, until progression or toxicity [29]. The primary endpoint was PFS at 6 months, using mRECIST and a Simon-2 stage design. Again, accrual runs very fast with 54 patients enrolled in 10 sites within 10 months, showing the unmet need for efficient systemic treatment in MPM patients. Median age was 68 years, 60% of patients had PS = 0, 83% had epithelioid histotype. Dose-intensity of both chemotherapy and durvalumab was excellent since 97% of patients received six doses of platinum with only 13 patients (24%) for whom cisplatin was converted to carboplatin and with a median number of 11.5 durvalumab doses (94% dose-intensity). Confirmed ORR was 48% with 37% more with stable disease, when mRECIST was used for evaluation, with two patients more experiencing a pseudo-progression (giving a 58% iRECIST ORR). Overall, a remarkable 85% disease control rate was thus obtained, with six patients having major tumor shrinkage of 80% or more. Median PFS was 6.2 months and 6-months PFS was 57%. Median OS was not reached after 14.4 months of median follow-up, 1-year OS estimate being 64.5% (52.9, 78.7). Ten percent of patients experienced immune-related adverse events, while 66% of patients experienced grade 3–5 adverse events, including five patient deaths during study treatment, (with one tumor progression), with no death adjudicated to durvalumab. If confirmed these preliminary results will warrant a randomized phase 3 trial, using the best control arm available which should be the bevacizumab-pemetrexed-cisplatin triplet in accordance with the results of MAPS phase 3 trial.

20.4 Conclusions

Although MPM is low mutational burden tumor, although PD-L1 expression level is moderate in MPM tissue samples, data are now accumulating supporting the use of modern immunotherapy in MPM patients, based on anti-PD-1, or anti-PD-L1 antibodies, with or without an anti-CTLA-4 antibody (but not on an anti-CTLA-4 antibody single therapy). Available data actually support the adverse prognostic effect of PD-L1 expression in MPM, while more and more data are accumulating, suggesting a favorable predictive effect of such PD-L1 tumor expression, in MPM patients treated with anti-PD-1 or PD-L1 antibodies.

Phase 2 results seem concordant with pembrolizumab or nivolumab-based therapy, in fit pretreated MPM patients, since over 300 patients have been treated now in such trials, with remarkable progression-free and long-term survival data, never observed in literature to date, with previously available drugs, which rarely gave over 25% ORR and significant PFS over 3 months. Knowing that there is no currently recommended second-line treatment in these patients, it remains debatable, from the ethical point of view, to wait for eventual randomized phase 3 trials with a placebo arm, or even a low-efficacy, not recommended treatment, such as vinorelbine single therapy.

In particular, MAPS2 phase 2 randomized trial, although not comparative, could be considered as having given sufficient data on their tolerability and efficacy, to justify nivolumab single therapy, or nivolumab plus ipilimumab doublet, as second or third line therapy in PS 0-1 MPM patients. Based on this reasoning, particularly sound in such an orphan-disease like MPM, last version of NCCN guidelines has integrated this possible second-line therapeutic option without waiting for putative phase 3 results.

Conversely, results of first-line combination of anti-PD-1 and anti-CTLA-4 antibodies are awaited, the first results of the company-sponsored phase 3 trial assessing such combo as compared with standard pemetrexed-platinum-based doublet being expected within the next 12 months. Early results of phase 2 trials assessing the combination of anti-PD-L1 antibody with the chemotherapy standard doublet, support a manageable safety profile, with very encouraging efficacy results, clearly deserving first-line trials with such combinations. Design of such trials should be the same as the trials recently presented in advanced NSCLC patients, leading to rapid registration because a dramatic increase of survivals, whatever is the level of PD-L1 expression. However, the control arm of such trials is still debatable, and should probably consist of the triplet bevacizumab-pemetrexed-cisplatin, in patients eligible for bevacizumab, knowing that the next step could be to assess a 4-drug combination with bevacizumab, anti-PD-1, or anti-PDL1 antibody, pemetrexed and platinum, such combo recently being proved to be efficient in NSCLC patients, with a biological rationale supporting the synergy between anti-VEGF therapy and immuno-therapeutics. Further clinical trials are thus needed, but future years will clearly see a major improvement in the care of MPM patients after years of stagnation and therapeutic failures.

References

1. Thapa B, Salcedo A, Lin X, Walkiewicz M, Murone C, Ameratunga M, et al. The immune microenvironment, genome-wide copy number aberrations, and survival in mesothelioma. J Thorac Oncol. 2017;12(5):850–9.
2. Yamada N, Oizumi S, Kikuchi E, Shinagawa N, Konishi-Sakakibara J, Ishimine A, et al. CD8+ tumor-infiltrating lymphocytes predict favorable prognosis in malignant pleural mesothelioma after resection. Cancer Immunol Immunother. 2010;59(10):1543–9.
3. Sharpe A, Pauken K. The diverse functions of the PD1inhibitory pathway. Nat Rev Immunol. 2018;18:153–67.
4. Bueno R, Stawiski E, Goldstein L, Durinck S, De Rienzo A, Modrusan Z, et al. Comprehensive genomic analysis of malignant pleural mesothelioma identifies recurrent mutations, gene fusions and splicing alterations. Nat Genet. 2016;48(4):407–16.
5. Hellmann MD, Callahan MK, Awad MM, Calvo E, Ascierto PA, Atmaca A, et al. Tumor mutational burden and efficacy of Nivolumab Monotherapy and in combination with Ipilimumab in small-cell lung cancer. Cancer Cell. 2018;33(5):853–61 e4.
6. Wang G, Lu X, Dey P, Deng P, Wu CC, Jiang S, et al. Targeting YAP-dependent MDSC infiltration impairs tumor progression. Cancer Discov. 2016;6(1):80–95.
7. Rehrauer H, Wu L, Blum W, Pecze L, Henzi T, Serre-Beinier V, et al. How asbestos drives the tissue towards tumors: YAP activation, macrophage and mesothelial precursor recruitment, RNA editing, and somatic mutations. Oncogene. 2018;37(20):2645–59.
8. Cedres S, Ponce-Aix S, Zugazagoitia J, Sansano I, Enguita A, Navarro-Mendivil A, et al. Analysis of expression of programmed cell death 1 ligand 1 (PD-L1) in malignant pleural mesothelioma (MPM). PLoS One. 2015;10(3):e0121071.
9. Mansfield AS, Roden AC, Peikert T, Sheinin YM, Harrington SM, Krco CJ, et al. B7-H1 expression in malignant pleural mesothelioma is associated with sarcomatoid histology and poor prognosis. J Thorac Oncol. 2014;9(7):1036–40.
10. Inaguma S, Lasota J, Wang Z, Czapiewski P, Langfort R, Janusz Rys J, et al. Expression of ALCAM (CD166) and PD-L1 (CD274) independently predicts shorter survival in malignant pleural mesothelioma. Hum Pathol. 2018;71:1–7.
11. Rivalland G, Kao S, Pavlakis N, Gordon B, Hughes M, Thapa B, et al. Outcomes of anti-PD-1 therapy in mesothelioma and correlation with PD-L1 expression. J Clin Oncol. 2017;35(15_suppl):8514.
12. Zalcman G, Mazieres J, Margery J, Greillier L, Audigier-Valette C, Moro-Sibilot D, et al. Bevacizumab for newly diagnosed pleural mesothelioma in the Mesothelioma Avastin Cisplatin Pemetrexed Study (MAPS): a randomised, controlled, open-label, phase 3 trial. Lancet. 2016;387(10026):1405–14.
13. Khanna S, Thomas A, Abate-Daga D, Zhang J, Morrow B, Steinberg S, et al. Malignant mesothelioma effusions are infiltrated by CD3þ T cells highly expressing PD-L1 and the PD-L1þ tumor cells within these effusions are susceptible to ADCC by the anti–PD-L1 antibody Avelumab. J Thorac Oncol. 2016;11(11):1993–2005.
14. Calabro L, Morra A, Fonsatti E, Cutaia O, Amato G, Giannarelli D, et al. Tremelimumab for patients with chemotherapy-resistant advanced malignant mesothelioma: an open-label, single-arm, phase 2 trial. Lancet Oncol. 2013;14(11):1104–11.
15. Ceresoli GL, Zucali PA, De Vincenzo F, Gianoncelli L, Simonelli M, Lorenzi E, et al. Retreatment with pemetrexed-based chemotherapy in patients with malignant pleural mesothelioma. Lung Cancer. 2011;72(1):73–7.
16. Calabro L, Morra A, Fonsatti E, Cutaia O, Fazio C, Annesi D, et al. Efficacy and safety of an intensified schedule of tremelimumab for chemotherapy-resistant malignant mesothelioma: an open-label, single-arm, phase 2 study. Lancet Respir Med. 2015;3(4):301–9.
17. Maio M, Scherpereel A, Calabro L, Aerts J, Perez SC, Bearz A, et al. Tremelimumab as second-line or third-line treatment in relapsed malignant mesothelioma (DETERMINE): a multicentre, international, randomised, double-blind, placebo-controlled phase 2b trial. Lancet Oncol. 2017;18(9):1261–73.
18. Alley EW, Lopez J, Santoro A, Morosky A, Saraf S, Piperdi B, et al. Clinical safety and activity of pembrolizumab in patients with malignant pleural mesothelioma (KEYNOTE-028): preliminary results from a non-randomised, open-label, phase 1b trial. Lancet Oncol. 2017;18(5):623–30.
19. Desai A, Karrison T, Rose B, Pemberton E, Hill B, Mendoza A, et al. Phase II trial of Pembrolizumab (NCT02399371) in previously treated malignant mesothelioma: final analysis. J Thorac Oncol. 2018;13(10):S339. IASLC 19th World Conference on Lung Cancer; OA 08-03.
20. Mauti L, Klingbiel D, Schmid S, Bouchaab H, Bartnick T, Gautschi O, Rothschild S, et al. Pembrolizumab as second or further line treatment in relapsed malignant pleural mesothelioma: a Swiss registry study. Ann Oncol. 2017;28(suppl_5):v568–72. abstr. 1615O.
21. Quispel-Janssen J, Zago G, Schouten R, et al. A phase II study of nivolumab in malignant pleural mesothelioma (NivoMes): with translational research (TR) biopies. J Thorac Oncol. 2017;12(1):S292–S93. abstr. OA 13.01.
22. Nakano T, Okada M, Kijima T, Aoe K, Kato T, Fujimoto N, et al. Long-term efficacy and safety of nivolumab in second- or third-line Japanese malignant pleural mesothelioma patients (phase II: MERIT study). J Thorac Oncol. 2018;13(10):S338. IASLC 19th World Conference on Lung Cancer; OA 08-01.

23. Hassan R, Thomas A, Nemunaitis J, Patel M, Bennouna J, Chen F, et al. Phase 1b study of avelumab in advanced previously treated mesothelioma: long-term follow-up from JAVELIN solid tumor. J Clin Oncol. 2018;36(15_suppl):abstr 8563.
24. Scherpereel A, Mazieres J, Greillier L, Dô P, Bylicki O, Monnet I, et al. Second- or third-line nivolumab (Nivo) versus nivo plus ipilimumab (Ipi) in malignant pleural mesothelioma (MPM) patients: results of the IFCT-1501 MAPS2 randomized phase II trial. J Clin Oncol. 2017;35(suppl):abstr LBA8507.
25. Zalcman G, Mazieres J, Greillier L, Do P, Bylicki O, Monnet O, et al. Second or 3rd line Nivolumab (Nivo) versus Nivo plus Ipilimumab (Ipi) in Malignant Pleural Mesothelioma (MPM) patients: up-dated results of the IFCT-1501 MAPS2 randomized phase 2 trial. Ann Oncol. 2017;28(suppl):Abstract LBA58_PR.
26. Baas P, Disselhorst M, Harms E, Quispel J, K M, Burgers S. Phase II trial of Nivolumab and Ipilimumab in patients with malignant mesothelioma. J Thorac Oncol. 2017;12(11, suppl.2):S292–S93. OA 9389.
27. Calabro L, Morra A, Giannarelli D, Amato G, D'Incecco A, Covre A, et al. Tremelimumab combined with durvalumab in patients with mesothelioma (NIBIT-MESO-1): an open-label, non-randomised, phase 2 study. Lancet Respir Med. 2018;6(6):451–60.
28. Nowak A, Cook A, McDonnell A, Millward M, Creaney J, Francis R, et al. A phase 1b clinical trial of the CD40-activating antibody CP-870,893 in combination with cisplatin and pemetrexed in malignant pleural mesothelioma. Ann Oncol. 2015;12:2483–90.
29. Nowak AK, Kok PS, Lesterhuis WJ, Hughes BGM, Brown C, Chuan-Hao Kao S, et al. DREAM: final results of a phase 2 trial of DuRvalumab with first line chEmotherApy in mesothelioma. J Thorac Oncol. 2018;13(10):S338–9. IASLC 19th World Conference on Lung Cancer; OA 08-02.

Dr. Brosseau has no potential conflict of interest to disclose.

Dr. Gounant received reimbursements for attendance to ASCO annual meetings 2016 from Roche and is the co-PI or the SAVIMMUNE phase 2 trial with durvalumab, sponsored by the French Intergroup (IFCT) with the support of Astra-Zeneca.

Dr. Zalcman participated in advisory boards for Roche, Bristol-Myers-Squibb (BMS), Merck & Co, Boehringer Ingelheim, and Astra-Zeneca, and received reimbursements for attendance to ASCO annual meetings 2016 and 2017 from Roche, ASCO annual meeting 2018 from Abbvie, ESMO annual meeting 2017 from Astra-Zeneca, and WCLC meeting 2016 from BMS. He is the co-PI of the MAPS2 trial with nivolumab and ipilimumab, sponsored by the French Intergroup (IFCT) with the support of BMS. His research group received a research grant by Roche for a PhD student funding.

Peritoneal Mesothelioma: Diagnosis and Management

21

Marcello Deraco, Shigeki Kusamura, Marcello Guaglio, Antonello Cabras, Eran Nizri, and Dario Baratti

21.1 Introduction

Mesothelioma is an uncommon tumor arising from the mesothelial cells lining the pleura, peritoneum, pericardium, and tunica vaginalis layer of testis [1]. Peritoneal mesothelioma (PM) represents about one-fifth to one-third of all forms of mesothelioma. The definition of PM includes a constellation of disease entities with different clinical presentation, biological behavior, and prognosis. Localized PM is uncommon and generally benign. On the contrary, diffuse malignant peritoneal mesothelioma (DMPM) is the commonest and more aggressive variant. Well-differentiated papillary peritoneal mesothelioma (WDPPM) and multicystic peritoneal mesothelioma are exceedingly rare and borderline malignant conditions. In its malignant forms, the disease has been traditionally considered as an end-stage disseminated condition and treated with debulking (DBK) and/or palliative systemic chemotherapy (sCT). Treatment options were mainly palliative and minimally effective. The interest in this disease on part of biological and clinical researchers was poor. Only in recent years, an increasing number of patients with PM have been treated with cytoreductive surgery (CRS) and hyperthermic intraperitoneal chemotherapy (HIPEC), resulting in remarkable survival improvements and increased interest in this disease. This chapter reviews several relevant issues regarding the surgical and local-regional management of DMPM and the borderline PM sub-variants.

21.2 Epidemiology of Peritoneal Mesothelioma

Age-adjusted incidence rates in the Surveillance, Epidemiology, and End Results (SEER) database (1973–2003) for DMPM were 1.2 per 1,000,000

M. Deraco (✉) · S. Kusamura · M. Guaglio
D. Baratti
Peritoneal Surface Malignancy Unit, Department of Surgery, Fondazione IRCCS Istituto Nazionale dei Tumori Via Venezian, Milan, Italy
e-mail: marcello.deraco@istitutotumori.mi.it; shigeki.kusamura@istitutotumori.mi.it; marcello.guaglio@istitutotumori.mi.it; dario.baratti@istitutotumori.mi.it

A. Cabras
Department of Pathology, Fondazione IRCCS Istituto Nazionale dei Tumori Via Venezian, Milan, Italy
e-mail: antonello.cabras@istitutotumori.mi.it

E. Nizri
Peritoneal Surface Malignancy Unit, Department of Surgery, Fondazione IRCCS Istituto Nazionale dei Tumori Via Venezian, Milan, Italy

Department of Pathology, Fondazione IRCCS Istituto Nazionale dei Tumori Via Venezian, Milan, Italy

Division of Surgery, Department of Surgery A, Tel-Aviv Sourasky Medical Center and Sackler Faculty of Medicine, Tel Aviv, Israel
e-mail: eran.nizri@mail.huji.ac.il

G. L. Ceresoli et al. (eds.), *Mesothelioma*, https://doi.org/10.1007/978-3-030-16884-1_21

person-year in men and 0.8 per 1,000,000 person-year in women. In Europe, crude incidence based on the RARECARE database (1995–2002) for both genders combined was 1.3 per 1,000,000 person-year [2]. In 2008 in Italy, the incidence of DMPM in men and women were 2.6 and 1.2 per 1,000,000 person-year, respectively, with wide variations within the country. Higher rates are reported in smaller areas with widespread past use of asbestos, such as the harbor city of Genoa or Casale Monferrato (age-standardized incidence in men in 1995 was 5.5/1,000,000) (www.ispesl.it\renam\index.asp). An increase of 5–10% in the annual mortality rate will be observed worldwide at least until 2020. The disease has likely already reached its incidence peak in the USA. On the contrary, in Europe and Australia, the peak is expected during this decade [3]. The role of asbestos exposure in DMPM has not been clearly established as in the pleural forms. It is estimated that 58% of men and only 20% of women with DMPM had past asbestos exposure [4]. Therefore, it has been suggested that etiology of DMPM may differ between men and women. Since no asbestos exposure is documented in about 20–40% of DMPM, it has been suggested that other factors may be the determinants. Simian Virus 40 (SV40) is a possible co-factor in mesothelioma oncogenesis, and the hypothesis of a genetic susceptibility with an autosomal dominant pattern is based on observations gathered in Cappadocia [5, 6].

21.3 Molecular Biology

The molecular and cellular mechanisms underlying the proliferative potential and resistance to therapy of DMPM are still poorly understood. The biology of this disease has been thoroughly investigated by clinical and basic science researchers in our institution during the last decade. It has been demonstrated that p16 expression is frequently absent or reduced in DMPM, and EGFR over-expression is more common in peritoneal than pleural forms. However, no correlation with prognosis of over-expression of EGFR, matrix metalloprotease-2 (MMP-2), and MMP-9 was found in patients treated in our center [7, 8].

The Ki-67 is a nuclear antigen expressed during all cellular cycle, except the quiescent (G0) phase. The Ki-67 is an excellent marker of cellular proliferation and tumor aggressiveness. Our group and other groups have shown low Ki-67 expression in DMPM, with a median of 0.6–10% positive cells, but higher expression has been demonstrated to be a strong prognostic factor [8–12]. Analogously, mitotic count is generally low in DMPM, but higher proliferative activity predicts poor prognosis [8].

On the other side, over-expression of cytoprotective factors, such as telomerase activity (TA) and anti-apoptotic mechanisms has been demonstrated in DMPM. TA is expressed in the majority of DMPM and negatively impact prognosis [13]. In DMPM specimens from 38 patients undergoing various therapies; we assessed TA using the telomeric repeat amplification protocol. The alternative lengthening of telomeres (ALT) mechanisms was studied by assaying ALT-associated promyelocytic leukemia nuclear bodies. ALT or TA alone was found in 18.2 and 63.6% of cases, respectively; both ALT and TA were positive in two cases. In the overall series, TA expression was significantly associated with disease relapse (p = 0.018) and cancer-related death (p = 0.045). ALT was not associated with outcome. The prognostic relevance of TA was confirmed in patients uniformly treated by CRS/HIPEC.

Over-expression of cytoprotective factors, including survivin and members of the Inhibitors of apoptosis protein (IAP) family was recently demonstrated by Zaffaroni et al. [14]. The authors have analyzed DMPM proliferative and apoptotic features and tested a survivin knockdown approach in a human DMPM cell line. DMPM cells were transfected with small-interfering RNA (siRNA) targeting survivin mRNA. Survivin expression, growth rate, and ability to undergo spontaneous and drug-induced apoptosis were measured, showing low proliferation rates and poor apoptotic activity in DMPM cells. Survivin was expressed in 91% of cases, and the other IAPs in 69–100%. Transfection of DMPM cells with survivin siRNA resulted in survivin inhibition, decrease in cell growth, and enhancement of spontaneous and drug-induced apoptosis, suggesting that survivin may be a potential target for biological treatments of DMPM.

The above biological features contribute to the lack of effective treatment options in DMPM. We explored novel immunotherapy approaches in an attempt to improve DMPM patients' survival [15]. We tested CpG-oligodeoxynucleotides (CpG-ODN), synthetic DNA sequences recognized by Toll-like receptor 9 and able to induce innate/adaptive immune response, in two DMPM orthotopic xenografts established in our center, namely MesoII and STO, which properly recapitulate the dissemination pattern of DPMP. Several combined immunodeficiency mice carrying DMPM xenografts were treated at different stages of tumor development with intraperitoneally delivered CpG-ODN1826 for 4 weeks. CpG-ODN1826-induced modulation in the composition of peritoneal immune infiltrate was assessed by flow cytometry. When administered to early-stage tumors (i.e., 4 days after i.p. DMPM cell injection in mice), the agent completely inhibited tumor growth and ascites development (no evidence of tumor masses and ascites in 6/6 mice at necropsy), and also impaired STO tumor uptake and growth (4/6 tumor-free mice; i.p. tumor masses reduced by 94% in the two remaining mice, $p = 0.00005$). Interestingly, when tested against late-stage STO tumors (i.e., 11 days after i.p. DMPM cell injection in mice), CpG-ODN1826 was still able to reduce the growth of i.p. tumor masses by 66% ($p = 0.0009$). Peritoneal washings of tumor-bearing mice revealed a strong increase of macrophage infiltration together with a decrease in the presence of B-1 cells and a reduced IgM concentration after CpG-ODN1826 treatment. These data suggest that locally administered CpG-ODN1826 is able to markedly affect the growth of both early- and late-stage DMPM orthotopic xenografts in the absence of severe side effects, and suggest a possible clinical role for the agent in the therapy of DMPM.

An additional line of research has involved the expression of tyrosine kinases receptors (TKRs) [16]. In surgical samples from 20 DMPM patients undergoing CRS/HIPEC in our center, Perrone analyzed TKRs and TKRs downstream pathways, with mTOR and its effectors S6 and 4EBP1, through biochemical and mutational analysis and fluorescent in situ hybridization (FISH). Activation/phosphorylation was shown in 90% of cases for EGFR, in 75% of cases for PDGFRB, and 45% of cases for PDGFRA by immunoprecipitation/Western blot technique. In 100% of cases, no EGFR, PDGFRA, and PDGFRB mutation and gene amplification were demonstrated. AKT, ERK1/2 mTOR, S6, and 4EBP1 were most highly expressed and activated. No mutations of PI3KCA, PTEN, KRAS, and BRAF were seen. The ligand and heterodimerization-dependent activation/expression of EGFR and PDGFRB were demonstrated. Taken together, these findings strongly suggest the potential of TKR receptors and their downstream effectors as targets for molecularly tailored treatments. Based on the concurrent activation of TKR and their downstream effectors, we have designed a clinical-biological study to test the combination TKRs and mTOR inhibitors. In a further analysis, we evaluated the EGFR inhibitor gefinitib, the mTOR inhibitor RAD001, and the multiple TKR inhibitor sorafenib in a DMPM cell line: gefitinib and RAD001 alone showed poor cytotoxic activity; sorafenib had a stronger effect on cellular proliferation and sequential treatment with RAD001 followed by sorafenib-induced a marked synergistic effects in DMPM cells [16].

21.4 Pathology of Peritoneal Mesothelioma

The correct pathological diagnosis of PM is necessary as a variety of other abdominal and pelvic malignancies may present with peritoneal seeding. For example, the majority of patients with papillary serous ovarian cancer do have peritoneal seeding. A high index of suspicion is needed on the part of the pathologist to properly integrate clinical, morphological, and immunostaining findings in order to recognize PM.

Table 21.1 Classification of peritoneal mesothelioma

Clinical presentation	Biological behavior	Histological subtype	Histological pattern	Prevalence %
Localized	Benign	Adenomatoid tumor		Uncommon
		Solitary fibrous tumor		Uncommon
Diffuse	Borderline	Multicystic		Uncommon
		Papillary well-differentiated		Uncommon
	Malignant	Epithelial	Tubulopapillary	75–80%
			Solid	
			Small cells	
			Adenomatoid	
			Acinar	
			Clear-cells	
			Signet-ring cells	
			Deciduoid	
			Rhabdoid	
		Biphasic (mixed)		10–15%
		Sarcomatoid	Desmoplastic	4–6%
			Limpho-histiocytoid	
			Anaplastic	
			Giant-cell	

Tumors arising from the mesothelial cells lining the abdominal cavity demonstrate a wide spectrum of biological aggressiveness [17]. Adenomatoid tumor and solitary fibrous tumor are truly benign lesions that very unlikely recur after simple excision. The former is a solitary asymptomatic lesion which most often involves genital region peritoneum in reproductive-aged women. Solitary fibrous tumor affects primarily men in their sixth decade [18]. The multicystic variant of PM (MCPM) and well-differentiated papillary variant of PM (WDPPM) are uncommon entities with uncertain malignant potential. At the other extreme, DMPM is a rapidly lethal malignancy, with a median survival of only 1 year when treated with standard therapies. Borderline mesotheliomas and DMPM attract more interest on the part of the medical community and pose substantial problems in the clinical practice.

Classification of PM according to clinical presentation, biological behavior, and pathological features is shown in Table 21.1.

21.4.1 Diffuse Malignant Peritoneal Mesothelioma

DMPM is macroscopically characterized by multiple variably sized grey-white nodules throughout the abdominal cavity. As the disease progresses, the nodules become confluent to form plaques, masses, bowel encasement, or uniformly cover the peritoneal surfaces. Abundant effusion is often present.

Similar to its more frequent pleural counterpart, DMPM is classified as epithelial, sarcomatoid, or biphasic (mixed) [19]. However, the incidence of biphasic tumors is lower than in pleural disease, and pure sarcomatoid DMPM is rare. Epithelial DMPM is composed of polygonal, oval, or cuboidal cells exhibiting cytonuclear features and architectural formations ranging from well-differentiated to anaplastic/pleomorphic appearance. Sarcomatoid tumors and the sarcomatoid component of biphasic DMPM consist of spindle cells arranged in fascicle or storiform pattern [20, 21].

Epithelial DMPM can be further categorized according to the patterns of the epithelial component. The tubulopapillary pattern is one of the most common patterns. It consists of a mixture of small tubules and papillary structures with fibro-vascular cores lined by bland flat, cuboidal, or polygonal cells. The solid pattern consists of nests, cords, or sheets of round, oval, or polygonal cells with abundant eosinophilic cytoplasm and round, vesicular nuclei with prominent nucleoli. The adenomatoid (micro-glandular), acinar, clear-cell, deciduoid, signet-ring cell, small-cell, and rhabdoid patterns are rare [18–21].

Sarcomatoid DMPM may demonstrate anaplastic, giant-cell, and desmoplastic features, or osteosarcomatous/chondrosarcomatous areas. Atypical histiocytoid-appearing cells within an intense lymphoplasmacytic infiltrate can be seen.

Lymph-node metastases within and outside the abdominal cavity can occur even at the initial manifestation of DMPM. Node involvement has been reported in 7–14% of patients undergoing extensive cytoreductive surgery. By contrast, metastatic disease outside the abdominal cavity is uncommon, except for direct invasion of pleural spaces through the diaphragm [22].

21.4.2 Multicystic and Well-Differentiated Papillary Peritoneal Mesothelioma

Both of these rare disease entities generally affect reproductive-aged women with no history of asbestos exposure and show indolent clinical behaviors. MCPM is often associated with previous abdominal surgery, inflammation, or endometriosis. However, early recurrences requiring multiple surgical interventions, transformation into truly malignant disease, lymph-node involvement, and even death have been described. This, along with the reported clear evidence of diffuse disease distribution throughout the peritoneum and invasion into peritoneal surfaces, suggest that MCPM and WDPPM should be considered as borderline or low-malignant potential conditions, rather than benign tumors [23, 24].

At macroscopic examination, MCPM forms multiple variably sized thin-walled cysts involving primarily the pelvis, but often spreading throughout the abdominal cavity. Microscopically, these cysts are separated by fibrous/adipose septa, and lined by single layers of flattened to cuboidal cells with no or little atypia. WDPPM is characterized by multiple small nodules and, at microscopic level, by well-developed papillary structures with fibrovascular core. The papillae are covered by bland cuboidal cells. Mitoses and atypia are rarely present. The differential diagnosis of WDPPM from the histologically similar but more aggressive tubulopapillary epithelial DMPM is important [25].

21.4.3 Diagnosis and Pathologic Assessment

According to the consensus of expert pathologists from the International Mesothelioma Interest Group (Chicago, IL, October 2006), the diagnosis of DMPM must always be based on an adequate biopsy in the context of appropriate clinical, radiological, and surgical findings [18]. Cytology still plays a limited role in the primary diagnosis, despite the increased accuracy of immunohistochemical and ultrastructural techniques.

The objectives of the pathological workup are:

- Separating benign from malignant mesothelial proliferations.
- Differentiating DMPM from other metastatic or primary peritoneal malignancies.
- Defining the histological sub-variant and other relevant prognostic determinants.

The first step for the diagnosis is hematoxylin–eosin staining. Demonstration of stromal invasion into visceral or parietal peritoneum (or beyond) is the key feature in the differential diagnosis with reactive mesothelial proliferations. However, invasion must be carefully differentiated from entrapment, and the distinction between the rare desmoplastic DMPM and reactive fibrosis may be difficult [25, 26].

Any gastrointestinal carcinoma and, in women, ovarian, primary peritoneal, and, more rarely, lobular breast carcinoma should be considered for the differential diagnosis of epithelial DMPM. The differential diagnosis for sarcomatoid DMPM includes sarcoma and other spindle cells neoplasms, such as sarcomatoid renal carcinoma and, particularly for biphasic DMPM, synovial sarcoma [18]. Since no immunohistochemical marker is entirely specific and sensitive for mesothelioma, the standard is to use panels of positive and negative markers. Mesothelioma is characterized by positive staining for EMA, calretinin, Wilms tumor-1 antigen,

Table 21.2 Immunostains of adenocarcinoma and peritoneal mesothelioma. The data summarize the percent positive staining to be expected

	Gastrointestinal adenocarcinoma	Mesothelioma
VIMENTIN	0–6	40
CEA	90–100	0–10
EMA	83	80–100
PAN-cytokeratin	100	100
B72.3	81	0–5
BER-EP4	90–100	0–11
CD15 (LEU-MI)	58–100	0–10
PLAP	50	0
Calretinin	6–9	42–100
S-100	31	0–11
CA125	90	14–94
P53	43–53	45

cytokeratin 5/6, HBME-1, podoplanin, and mesothelin. Depending on the tumor being considered in the differential diagnosis, CEA, Leu-M1, Ber-Ep4, claudine, B72.3, Bg8, and MOC-31 can be used as negative marker (see Table 21.2) [18–22]. Electron microscopy may help in difficult cases [27].

To date, PM lacks of a grading system. However, histomorphologic parameters can be used to estimate survival. Biphasic/sarcomatoid histology and MCPM/WDPPM have poorer and better prognosis, respectively, than epithelial DMPM. However, the low incidence of biphasic/sarcomatoid and borderline mesotheliomas restricts the clinical utility of this variable.

An exhaustive clinicopathological analysis of 62 patients undergoing comprehensive treatment at the Washington Cancer Institute revealed that nuclear and nucleolar size (rated by a four-tiered score) correlated with survival [28]. Clinical data from our Institution demonstrated that both pathologically involved lymph nodes and inadequate nodal sampling correlate with poor prognosis. Accordingly, careful examination of lymph nodes that drain the visceral and parietal peritoneum is recommended, including bilateral iliac, right gastroepiploic, and ileocolic nodes [22]. Proliferative activity has been reported to be useful for prognostic stratification. It may be quantified either by means of mitotic count or immunohistochemical staining with Ki-67 antigen, an excellent marker of cellular proliferation. Proliferative activity is generally low in PM, but higher rates correlate with poor outcome [7–11].

21.5 Diagnosis of Peritoneal Mesothelioma

DMPM growth is characterized by peritoneal seeding, eventually leading to death due to bowel encasement, obstruction, and intractable ascites. Patients are usually diagnosed at an advanced disease stage.

21.5.1 Clinical Presentation

The initial symptoms of DMPM were prospectively recorded in 51 patients treated at the Washington Cancer Institute [4]. Patients were categorized into three groups: about one-third of them presented with abdominal distention, another one-third with abdominal pain, and the remaining with combined symptoms of distention, pain, and other findings. The investigators designated these three types as a "wet type" presenting with symptoms of malignant ascites causing an increase in abdominal girth, a "dry-painful type" presenting with a focal mass seen at computed tomography (CT) scan usually causing pain, and a "combined type" characterized by both pain and ascites.

In a more recent series of 81 DMPM Italian patients, ascites, abdominal pain, and asthenia were the most frequent symptoms, followed by weight loss, anorexia, abdominal mass, fever, diarrhea, and vomiting; 13% of patients presented with abdominal hernia. Systemic symptoms, such as thrombocytosis and anemia were present in 73% of cases. About 25% of female patients came to medical attention due to non-specific gynecological symptoms [29].

21.5.2 Circulating Tumor Markers

Circulating tumor markers that could be used as an adjunct to clinical and radiological assessment would be valuable tools in the initial evaluation of peritoneal dissemination of unknown origin. Literature data on serum markers of DMPM are scarce. In 2006, our group reported CA125 above normal limits in 53.3% and CA15.3 in 48.5% of 60 patients undergoing CRS/HIPEC. On the contrary, CEA and CA19.9 were mostly normal. Also, serial CA125 measurements paralleled with tumor growth or regression after CRS/HIPEC, and preoperative CA125 showed borderline prognostic significance only among patients not previously treated with sCT [30]. More recently, we have assessed the diagnostic and prognostic role of mesothelin and osteopontin (which are markers currently used in pleural mesothelioma) [31]. Mean mesothelin levels were 7.84 ng/dl (SD = 5.14) in DMPM group and 3.00 ng/dl (SD = 1.25) in control group ($p = 0.001$). Mean CA19.9 levels were 5.3 ng/dl (SD = 4.7) and 61.96 ng/dl (SD = 112.5) in the two groups ($p = 0.008$). No statistical difference was seen for osteopontin ($p = 0.738$), CEA ($p = 0.081$), CA125 ($p = 0.600$), and CA15.3 ($p = 0.365$). The area under the receiver operating characteristic (AUC-ROC) curves was 0.836 for CA19.9, 0.812 for mesothelin, 0.793 for CEA, and lower for CA125 (0.652), osteopontin (0.531), and CA15.3 (0.481). Using diagnostic cut-offs selected by ROC methodology, mesothelin attained 100% specificity and 100% positive predictive value in the differential diagnosis of DMPM and peritoneal disseminations of unknown origin. These data suggest that serum mesothelin, in combination with negative CEA and CA19.9, would be especially useful during the early assessment, in order to shorten the current diagnostic delay of DMPM. Additionally, osteopontin correlated with survival at multivariate analysis (hazard rate 6.46; 95% CI 1.81–23.05; $p = 0.004$), suggesting that it might be a prognostic marker to select DMPM patients for aggressive treatment approaches.

21.5.3 Imaging Studies

Contrast-enhanced CT scan is currently the preferred diagnostic radiological tools for DMPM. CT features of PM have been defined as "dry" and "wet," with the dry appearance consisting of peritoneal-based lesions and the wet appearance consisting of ascites, irregular, or nodular peritoneum thickening and an omental mass that may scallop or directly invade adjacent abdominal viscera (see Fig. 21.1) [32, 33]. The two clinical types, wet or dry-painful type, correspond well to these different CT appearances. In the wet type, there is little or no evidence of solid tumor. The CT/radiologic presentation of the dry-painful type may disclose several mass lesions, but often there is a dominant mass isolated to one part of the abdomen.

Yan examined the CT imaging of a series of 33 patients with PM and described the presence of pleural abnormalities in 8 out of 33 patients

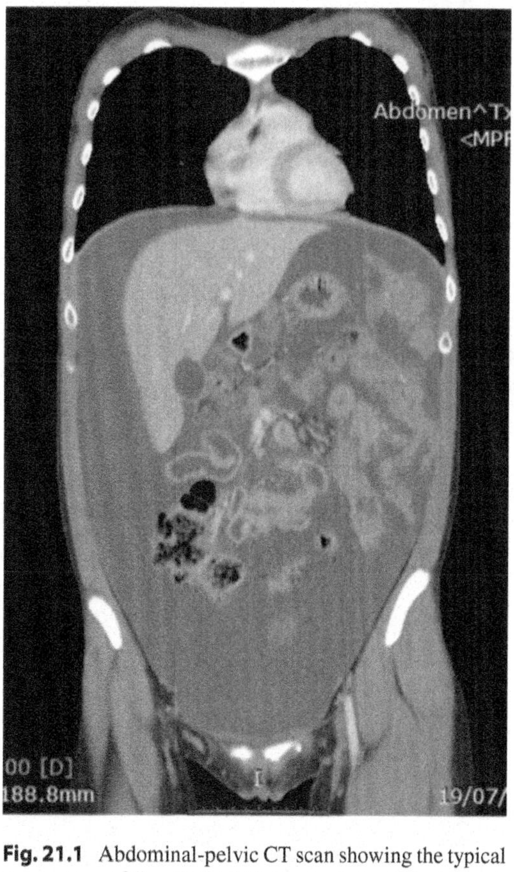

Fig. 21.1 Abdominal-pelvic CT scan showing the typical appearance of "wet" DMPM. The radiological picture is characterized by abundant ascites in all the abdominal-pelvic quadrants, with relatively limited peritoneal solid nodules

(24%), 91% of patients having involvement of the greater omentum, 97% of patients having pelvic involvement, and 66% of patients having ascites. This predominant central abdominal and pelvic disease burden observed may be the characteristic pattern of disease presentation [34].

The CT appearance of cystic PM can be a contrast to the CT appearance of DMPM. Despite a severe distortion of the abdominal and pelvic space by fluid-filled cysts and ascites, there is no disruption of intestinal function or segmental bowel obstruction. Small bowel compartmentalization may be seen [34].

CT scan is also useful in patient selection for a comprehensive surgical approach. Thirty-nine CT scan parameters were statistically analyzed to determine their association with the likelihood to perform an adequate surgical cytoreduction (residual lesions ≤ 2.5 cm), that is a predominant prognostic variable. Seven patients (64%) undergoing suboptimal cytoreduction and two patients (11%) undergoing adequate cytoreduction had a tumor mass > 5 cm in the epigastric region ($p = 0.004$). In 9 patients (82%) of the suboptimal group and 2 (11%) of the adequate cytoreductive surgery group, CT scans showed loss of normal architecture of the small bowel and its mesentery ($p < 0.001$) (see Fig. 21.2). In a composite analysis, none of the patients with tumor mass >5 cm in the epigastric region and loss of normal architecture of the small bowel and its mesentery had adequate cytoreduction. Patients who lacked these two preoperative CT scan findings had a 94% probability of an adequate cytoreduction [35].

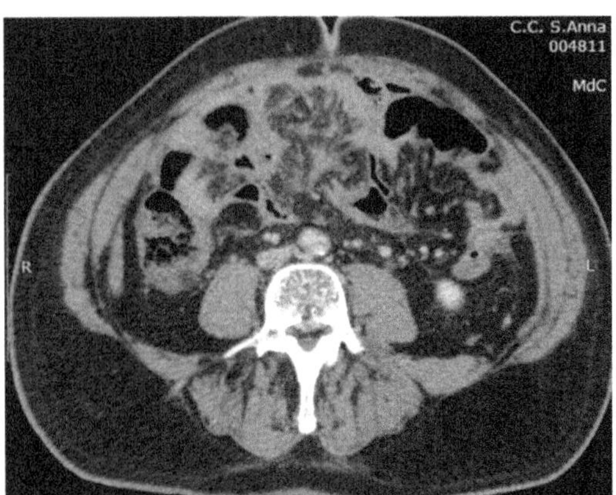

Fig. 21.2 Contrast-enhanced abdominal- pelvic CT scan showing massive disease involvement of the small bowel and its mesentery, with loss of the normal anatomical architecture. This radiological picture is associated with a very low probability to obtain an adequate surgical cytoreduction. This patient is a poor surgical candidate

The role of fluorine-18 fluorodeoxyglucose (18F-FDG)-PET has been recently tested in 9 patients with MCPM and 14 with Epithelioid PM. PET scan showed mild focal uptake in 1 of 8 cases of MCPM, and was positive in 12 of 14 cases of Epithelioid PM. Sensitivity, specificity, and accuracy were 86%, 89%, and 87%, respectively ($p = 0.002$). Multicystic histology was significantly associated with lower SUV ($p = 0.006$). SUV was significantly associated with PFS in epithelioid PM ($p = 0.028$) [36].

21.5.4 Laparoscopy

Esophagogastroduodenoscopy and colonoscopy may exclude a primary gastrointestinal malignancy. A diagnostic laparoscopy is a tool to perform biopsies, especially when there is no tumor deposit amenable to imaging-guided percutaneous biopsy, due to the unfavorable anatomic sites or small volume disseminated disease. Diagnostic laparoscopy can also provide an opportunity to evaluate the peritoneal disease burden and to assess the feasibility of optimal cytoreductive surgery. However, an important caveat accompanies the recommendation for laparoscopy in the diagnosis of PM. In outpatient follow-up, port site recurrence is frequently observed at trocar sites. It is recommended to limit the trocar sites along the linea alba.

In a series of 33 patients with DMPM who underwent CRS/HIPEC, we assessed laparoscopy effectiveness in predicting complete cytoreduction (residual tumor nodules ≤2.5 mm). At preliminary laparoscopy, peritoneal disease was considered amenable for complete CRS in 30 of 33 patients (91%). In this group, cytoreduction was complete in 29 patients and incomplete in one patient. Cytoreduction was grossly incomplete in the remaining three patients who were deemed not amenable for complete CRS. Our data suggest that laparoscopy can integrate clinical and radiological information in the selection process of patients with DMPM for combined treatment [37].

21.6 Treatment of Peritoneal Mesothelioma

Historically, PM has been treated by palliative or debulking surgery. Systemic/intraperitoneal chemotherapy and abdominal irradiation have been used in malignant variants. These treatments were disappointing, resulting in a median survival of about 12 months (Table 21.3). In the last two decades, the approach to PM radically changed with the introduction of a surgical treatment with curative intent. PM remains confined within the peritoneal surfaces of the abdominal cavity for most of its history. Lymph node and extra-abdominal metastases appear to develop later in the course of disease progression. This is the rationale base supporting a comprehensive local-regional approach to treat DMPM with CRS and intraeritoneal administration of chemotherapic drugs including the most commonly used methodology named hyperthermic intraperitoneal chemotherapy (HIPEC) direct targeting the disease, achieving peritoneal disease control, and prolonged disease-free survival. CRS may be seen as a tool to maximize response to intraperitoneal chemotherapy, because the penetration depth in tumor tissue of locally delivered drugs is only 2–3 mm [47]. On the other side, the role of local-regional chemotherapy is to preserve the macroscopically complete surgical response by eradicating microscopic residual disease.

21.6.1 Systemic Therapies

Due to its rarity and inherent difficulties of radiologic assessment, few studies of sCT have been conducted in DMPM. A variety of systemic drugs has been extrapolated from pleural mesothelioma treatment. The most commonly used agents were cisplatin, gemcitabine, doxorubicin, and pemetrexed. Historical Dana-Farber Cancer Institute and Brigham and Women's Hospital's series of 180 mesothelioma patients (37 with PM) reported a median survival of 15 months following various palliative sCT [48]. A randomized cancer and leukemia group B (CALGB) trial comparing cisplatin and mitomycin with cisplatin and doxorubicin in 79 patients with pleural or PM reported an overall response rate of 26% with median time-to-failure of 3.6–8.8 months according to different schedules [49]. More recent studies have demonstrated improved outcomes with pemetrexed in combination with cisplatin/carboplatin. In the expanded access program, 109 patients with DMPM were treated with pemetrexed or pemetrexed-containing sCT. Response rates for the combination of cisplatin/carboplatin with pemetrexed appeared to be higher than pemetrexed alone (24.1% versus 12.5%). One-year survival was 57.4% versus 41.5% [50]. Pemetrexed is a multi-targeted antifolate that inhibits thymidylate synthase (TS), dihydrofolate reductase (DHFR), and glycinamide ribonucleotide formyltransferase (GARFT) was

Table 21.3 Selected historical series of palliative/debulking surgery and/or systemic/intraperitoneal chemotherapy

Authors	Year	Pts (n.)	Treatment	Median surv. (months)
Rogoff [38]	1973	12	Debulking, RT, ip 32P	13
Jones [39]	1979	7	Syst. CT	6
Chahinian [40]	1982	12	Syst. CT, RT	7
Antman [41]	1988	16	Debulking, ip cisplatin + doxorubicin, RT	16.4
Kirmani [42]	1988	19	Ip cisplatin	12
Van Gelder [43]	1989	19	Surgery, syst. CT	6
Markmann [44]	1992	19	Ip cisplatin, ip mitomycin-C	9
Neumann [45]	1999	74	Not stated	12 (mean)
Etabbakh [46]	1999	15	Debulking, syst. CT, ip CT	12.5
De Pangher [29]	2009	81	CRS + HIPEC ($n = 7$), debulking ($n = 23$), syst. CT	13

approved for use in pleural mesothelioma based on results of a phase III trial [51]. Activity of pemetrexed in PM was observed in two expanded access programs (EAPs) which allowed access to pemetrexed for eligible patients prior to its regulatory approval in pleural mesothelioma, suggesting a role for pemetrexed-based combinations in DMPM [50, 52].

In the international EAP, 109 patients with chemo-naïve or previously treated surgically unresectable DMPM received pemetrexed alone or with cisplatin or carboplatin. Response rate and 1-year survival rate were 18.7 and 47.4%, respectively. Combination chemotherapy was well-tolerated [50]. In the USA EAP, 73 patients with chemo-naïve or previously treated surgically unresectable PM received 6 cycles of pemetrexed alone or combined with cisplatin. Response rates were 26, 19.2, and 29.8% in the overall population, pemetrexed and pemetrexed/cisplatin groups, respectively. Median survival was 13.1 months for patients who received pemetrexed with cisplatin and 8.7 months for pemetrexed alone [52]. In a phase II study, 6 cycles of pemetrexed (500 mg/m^2 on day 8) plus gemcitabine (1250 mg/m^2 on days 1 and 8) were evaluated in 20 chemo-naïve patients. Response rate was 15%, median time to disease progression was 10.4 months, and median overall survival (OS) was 26.8 months. However, toxicity from this treatment was significant, including one treatment-related death. Grade 3–4 neutropenia and febrile neutropenia were observed in 60 and 10% of patients, respectively [53].

There are isolated reports of the role of whole-abdominal radiation. However, this treatment such a treatment is highly associated with morbidity. Nonetheless a series of patients treated with surgery, HIPEC, and whole abdominal radiation was reported to achieve improved disease-free survival [54].

Limited data are available to guide the use of sCT in combination with CRS/HIPEC in the adjuvant or neoadjuvant setting. Since CRS/HIPEC does not achieve complete cytoreduction in all patients and recurrence is common even after complete cytoreduction [55], sCT is given in combination with intraperitoneal chemotherapy by several groups. We have retrospectively analyzed data from our institutional prospective database regarding 116 DMPMs treated with CRS/HIPEC from 1995 to 2011. Sixty cases had preoperative sCT, 30 had postoperative sCT, and 26 had no sCT. Platinum and pemetrexed were given to 55 cases. Preoperative sCT was not associated with complete cytoreduction or severe morbidity. There was no significant difference in survival among preoperative, postoperative, and no sCT groups, suggesting that operative and long-term outcomes were not influenced by perioperative CT. Only a weak correlation was seen between use of perioperative platinum and pemetrexed and improved survival. However, the potential bias associated with the retrospective study design has to be taken into account [56].

In a recent study, 126 DMPM patients undergoing CRS/HIPEC from 1991 to 2014, at 20 French tertiary centers were divided into four groups: (1) preoperative sCT; (2) postoperative sCT; (3) perioperative (both pre and postoperative sCT; (4) no sCT. At multivariate analysis, preoperative sCT was associated with worse survival (HR = 2.30; 95% CI = 1.07–4.94; $p = 0.033$), with no impact on treatment toxicity [57]. In summary, sCT with pemetrexed and cisplatin should be considered in patients with surgically unresectable DMPM. Carboplatin may be a reasonable alternative to cisplatin in elderly patients and those with poor performance, given its better safety profile. No conclusive data are available regarding perioperative sCT in patients undergoing CRS/HIPEC.

21.7 Cytoreductive Surgery and Intraperitoneal Chemotherapy

CRS for peritoneal tumors was developed by Sugarbaker who described six peritonectomy procedures to surgically remove all of the peritoneal linings of the abdominopelvic cavity [47]. The loose attachment of parietal peritoneum allows for stripping of the serosal layers by means of bilateral diaphragmatic, anterior abdominal wall, pelvic peritonectomy, and plus

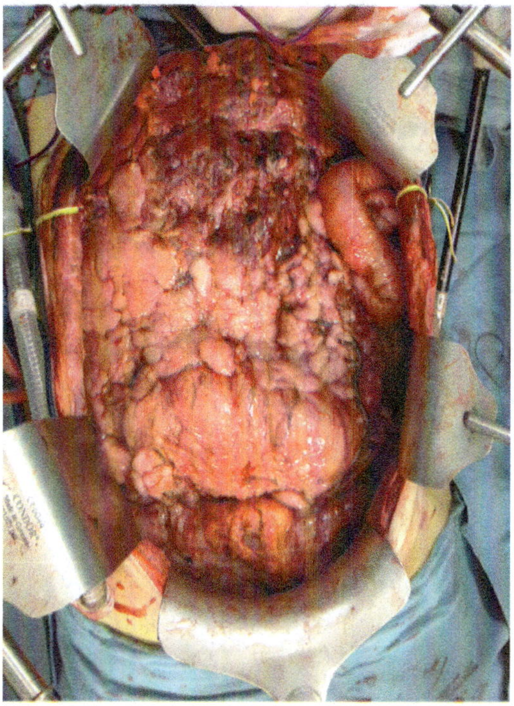

Fig. 21.3 Clinical appearance of a typical case of advanced DMPM at surgical exploration. A massive omental-cake is covering the central and lower abdominal quadrants. The anatomical structures in the upper abdomen are extensively involved by the disease

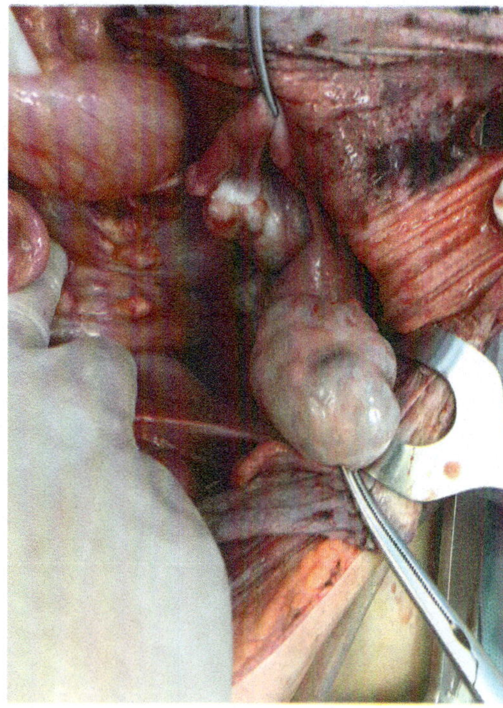

Fig. 21.4 Intraoperative picture of the same patient as in Fig. 21.3, showing large disease massively involving the pelvic peritoneum, uterus, sigmoid colon, and both ovaries

omental bursa stripping. Greater and lesser omentectomy are usually performed for both oncologic reasons and to facilitate intra-abdominal drug circulation. Because visceral peritoneum is more intimately attached to underlying structures, tumor implants on visceral surfaces require organ resections, except for liver and pancreatic capsulectomy. Figure 21.3 shows the amount of disease as it can be seen during the early phase of the CRS procedure in a typical case of high-volume DMPM. Figure 21.4 is an intraoperative picture of the same patient showing large disease involving pelvic peritoneum, uterus, sigmoid colon, and both ovaries. Massive disease involving the sub-hepatic/perigastric region is displayed in Fig. 21.5.

The adaptation of the original technique to DMPM is still a challenge, and several modifications have been undertaken. In the next paragraphs, CRS procedures performed in our center are described (see Table 21.4), with a focus on the modifications emerged during a 20-year experience, and a special attention on the most debated issues.

21.7.1 Importance of Complete Cytoreduction

The current literature consistently supports the notion that CRS must be aimed at removing all visible tumors. The completeness of cytoreduction (CCR) is classified at the end of the surgical phase according to Sugarbaker, as CCR-0 (macroscopically complete); CCR-1 (residual disease ≤2.5 mm in any region); CCR-2 (residual disease >2.5 mm and ≤25 mm), and CCR-3 (residual disease >25 mm) [58]. Numerous studies have stratified survival on the basis of this surgical endpoint, and CCR is the major prognostic factor in all PSM [59]. Near complete cytoreduction, leaving behind millimetric residual tumor may be pursued only

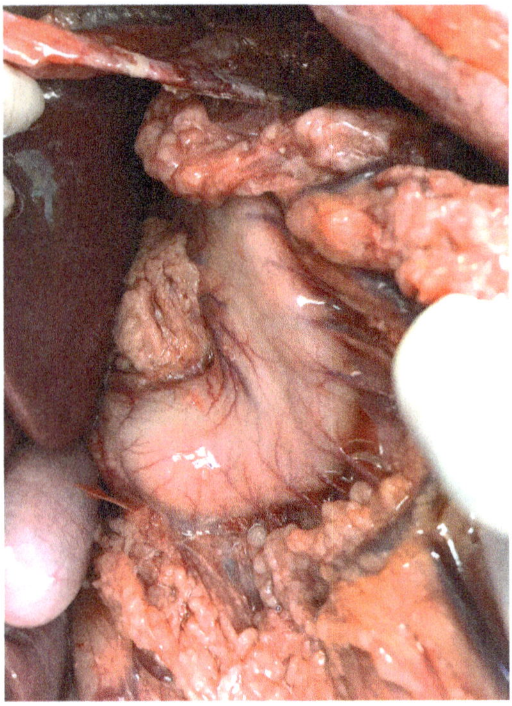

Fig. 21.5 Massive disease involving the sub-hepatic/perigastric region. Confluent disease localizations involve massively the lesser omentum close to the vascular arcade along the lesser gastric curvature, and the pyloric area. An impressive omental-cake is seen

when complete cytoreduction is not feasible, in order to preserve organ functions postoperatively. We have demonstrated the survival advantage of macroscopically complete cytoreduction, over minimal residual disease in 70 patients with DMPM undergoing CCR-0 or CCR-1 and HIPEC by analyzing clinicopathological factors correlating to disease progression in 13 abdominopelvic regions [55]. Residual tumor ≤ 2.5 mm (versus non-visible tumor) was the only independent risk factor for disease progression in epigastric region ($p = 0.047$), upper ileum ($p = 0.029$), upper jejunum ($p = 0.034$), and lower jejunum ($p = 0.002$). Before our study, the definition of optimal cytoreduction for DMPM was controversial as other authors suggested that a residual disease up to 25 mm could be adequate. On the contrary, we demonstrated that minimal residual disease, compared with macroscopically complete cytoreduction, correlated to failure in critical anatomical areas, and supporting the need for maximal cytoreductive surgical efforts. The final results of macroscopically complete CRS are shown in Fig. 21.6. The results of complete CRS in the sub-hepatic region and pelvis are shown in Figs. 21.7 and 21.8.

Table 21.4 Cytoreductive surgical procedures commonly performed at the National Cancer Institute, Milan (Italy)

Abdominal regions	Peritonectomies	Visceral resections
1. Right upper	Right sub-phrenic peritonectomy Resection of round, falciform and triangular liver ligaments	Glisson's capsule dissection
2. Left upper/anterior	Left sub-phrenic peritonectomy Greater omentectomy	Splenectomy Distal pancreatectomy
3. Right-lateral	Stripping of right paracolic gutter	Appendectomy Right colectomy
4. Sub-hepatic	Lesser omentectomy Stripping of the omental bursa Dissection of the duodenal-hepatic ligament	Gastric antrectomy Total gastrectomy Cholecystectomy
5. Pelvis	Pelvic peritonectomy Stripping of left paracolic gutter	Sigmoidectomy Hysterectomy Bilateral adnexectomy
6. Small bowel/mesentery	Mesenteric peritonectomy	Small bowel resection(s)
7. Other		Transverse, subtotal/total colectomy Retroperitoneal and pelvic lymphadenectomy Diaphragmatic muscle resection(s) Liver resection(s) Previous scar or port site resections

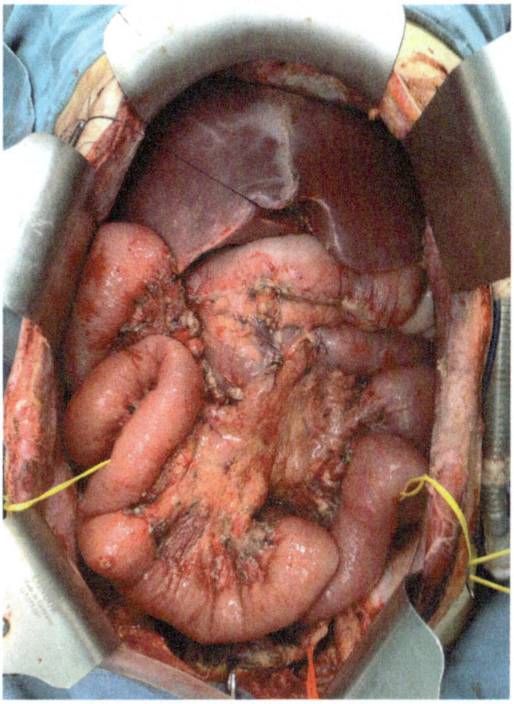

Fig. 21.6 Final results at the end of the surgical cytoreduction. All the macroscopic disease has been completely resected. The entire parietal peritoneum has been removed. Complete peritonectomy of both aspects of the mesentery has been performed, together with radical greater omentectomy and round and falciform liver ligament resection

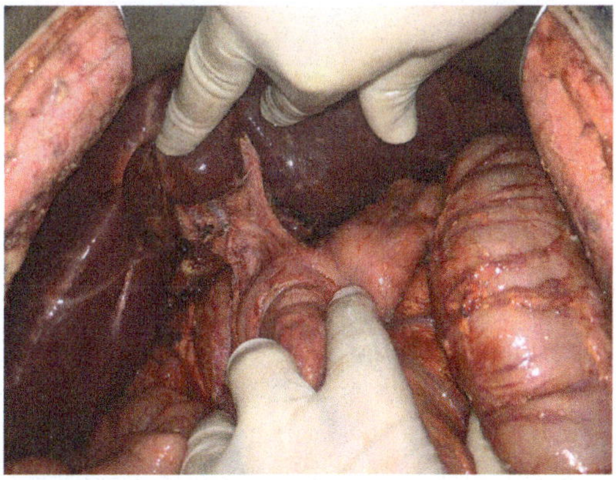

Fig. 21.7 Sub-hepatic region after macroscopically complete surgical cytoreduction in the same patient as Fig. 21.5. Both the greater and lesser gastric curvature have been made clear of tumor, sparing the blood supply through the left gastric artery. The gall bladder has been removed and the serosal layer covering the hepatoduodenal ligament has been dissected

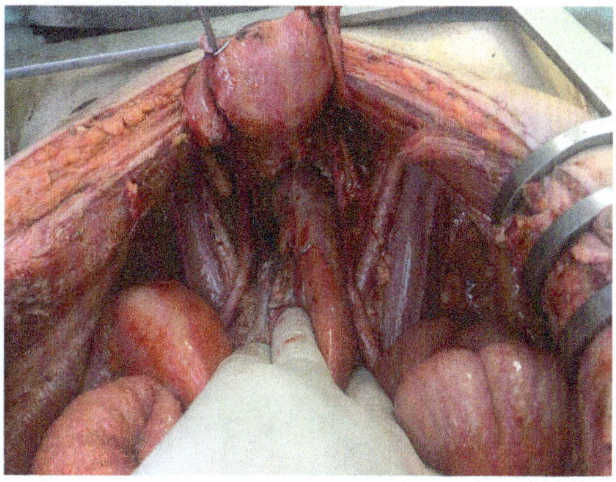

Fig. 21.8 Complete surgical cytoreduction in the pelvic region. The peritoneum has been surgically removed from the anterior aspect of the bladder, and lateral and posterior pelvic walls. The bladder is suspended to show the sigmoid colon, proximal rectum, and vaginal stump. No sigmoid colon resection has been performed in this case. The peritoneum of the Douglas pouch has been surgically removed. Both ureters, iliac arteries, and veins have been dissected and preserved. Bilateral iliac and obturatory lymphnodes have been removed

21.7.2 Complete Versus Selective Parietal Peritonectomy

Parietal peritonectomy is generally limited to surfaces involved by visible tumor, as well as organ resections, to preserve sufficient postoperative function. We have reported that systematic complete parietal peritonectomy (including both macroscopically involved and normal surfaces) regardless of disease distribution is associated with better survival in DMPM because of its biological characteristics and dissemination pattern with frequent microscopic (not visible) peritoneal disease. In a retrospective matched case-control study, we compared 30 patients with DMPM undergoing selective parietal peritonectomy with 30 matched controls undergoing routine complete parietal peritonectomy. Median overall survival was 29.6 months in the selective peritonectomy group and not reached in the complete peritonectomy group; 5-year overall survival was 40.0% and 63.9%, respectively ($p = 0.027$). At multivariate analysis, complete versus selective peritonectomy was recognized as an independent prognostic factor, along with complete cytoreduction, negative lymph nodes, epithelial histology, and lower MIB-1 labeling index. Morbidity rates were not different between groups. Furthermore, pathologic examination detected disease involvement on parietal surfaces with no evident tumor at surgical exploration in 12 of 24 patients undergoing complete parietal peritonectomy [60].

21.7.3 Lymph Node Assessment

The importance of nodal sampling and its impact on outcome has been shown to be important in DMPM. In our experience, negative lymph nodes are independent predictor of improved survival, after adjustment for other prognostic variables. In our study, negative nodes, as compared to positive or non-assessed nodes, were associated with increased survival. Since then, we use to perform careful nodal sampling during CRS for DMPM. Although node positivity ultimately bears a poorer outcome and is unlikely to be modified through extended lymphadenectomy, an approach to standardized lymph node sampling would assist in disease staging [22].

21.7.4 Small-Bowel Mesentery Cytoreduction

The involvement of the small-bowel mesentery by neoplastic cells is regulated by factors, such as cell biological aggressiveness and peritoneal features, such as the presence of a relatively low density of lymphatic lacunae, stomata, and milky spots [59]. With low or moderately aggressive malignancies, this typically results in sparing of small bowel surfaces or isolated small tumor implants, that can be locally resected. Conversely, high-grade malignant tumors may massively involve small bowel and its mesentery, thus hampering an adequate cytoreduction. In intermediate-grade tumors, small-to-medium-sized nodules and plaques are observed on the mesentery surface up to the transition line between the mesentery and the small bowel, with minimal deep tissue invasion. In these circumstances, we perform a partial or a complete peritonectomy on both sides of the mesentery. The serosal layer may be stripped up to the limits of bowel wall by either blunt or sharp dissection. It is important to avoid any vascular injury (especially close to the small bowel), as it could result in disruption to the blood supply. This procedure is made easier by finding the space between the serosal layer and the mesenteric fat tissue; it is possible at that time to use the fingers to perform a complete mesenteric peritonectomy by blunt dissection. In our experience, no major surgical complication appeared to be related to the mesenteric peritonectomy, except for a moderate prolongation of postoperative ileus [61]. In Fig. 21.6, the final results of complete parietal peritonectomy with complete mesentery peritonectomy are shown.

21.7.5 Intraperitoneal Perioperative Chemotherapy

Local-regional chemotherapy is performed either as intra-operative hyperthermic intraperitoneal chemotherapy (HIPEC), or normothermic early intraperitoneal chemotherapy (EPIC) [59]. The pharmacological advantage of intraperitoneal administration consists in higher local-regional drug concentration with minimal systemic toxicity. Intra-operative or early postoperative time settings allow optimal distribution of chemotherapeutic agents before the development of postoperative adhesions and tumor cell entrapment in scar tissue, which can contribute to disease recurrence. Additionally, mild hyperthermia (41–43 °C) has a direct cytotoxic effect, increases the efficacy of antiblastic agents, such as mitomycin-C and platinum compounds, as well as their penetration into tumor tissue.

HIPEC techniques vary widely among centers, in terms of closed versus open abdomen technique, drug(s), drug dosage, target temperature, duration, flow rate, type, and volume of carrier solutions. However, no technical variation has demonstrated an advantage in comparative trials. The choice of drugs is based on their clinical efficacy and pharmacokinetics variables, such as hydrophilic properties, high molecular weight to limit passage through the peritoneal-plasma barrier, high plasma clearance, and mechanisms of action potentiated by hyperthermia. Also, only cell cycle phase non-specific agents are indicated for this single-shot treatment. Currently, cisplatin alone or cisplatin in combination with doxorubicin are often used to treat DMPM.

When performing EPIC, the administration of normothermic antiblastic agents is started immediately after surgery using a peritoneal Tenckhoff catheter or a subcutaneous port, and continued for 1–5 days. Generally, 2–4 closed suction drains placed at surgery are maintained closed for 23 h and opened for 1 h a day, to take out the perfusate solution. Drugs with a high rate of hepatic extraction and no significant heat enhancement may be used for EPIC, such as 5-fluoruracil, doxorubicin, or taxanes [61].

A treatment protocol of adjuvant bidirectional chemotherapy with intraperitoneal pemetrexed combined with intravenous cisplatin has been developed at the Washington Cancer Institute. Peritoneal ports are placed at the time of CRS/HIPEC. The treatment consists of pemetrexed 500 mg/m^2 given intraperitoneally and cisplatin 50 mg/m^2 given intravenously simultaneously on day 1 of every 21-day cycle for 6 cycles. Nine of 10 patients were reported to be able to complete all 6 cycles of therapy without delays or dose modifications. One patient developed a catheter infection after 3 cycles and required catheter removal. He was switched to intravenous pemetrexed and cisplatin for 1 cycle, then a new peritoneal catheter was placed and the remaining 2 cycles were completed. Mild fatigue, nausea, and abdominal pain were observed [62].

21.8 Results of Treatment and Prognostic Factors

Treatment results of DMPM have been reported by a small number of referral centers only in recent years, but this disease has become a classical CRS/HIPEC indication. The most relevant literature series are reported in Table 21.5. Median survival ranged from 30 to 92 months and it appears to improve with growing experience, as the most recent updates report median survival of 4–5 year and more. One French, one American, and one International multi-institutional series have been published, collecting 249, 211, and 405

Table 21.5 Selected literature series of CRS/HIPEC for peritoneal mesothelioma

Centre (ref.)	Pts n.	HIPEC	EPIC	F.up	Median OS	5-year OS
Winston-Salem, NC [63]	34	CDDP *or* MMC	–	72	41	17%
Bethesda, MD [12]	49	CDDP	5FU +taxol	28	92	59%
Turin, It [64]	42	CDDP + DX	–	72	65	44%
New York, NY [8]	54	CDDP + MMC	–	48	55	50%
Washington, DC [28]	62	CDDP + DX	Taxol	37	79	50%
Villejuif, Fr [65]	26	OX ± IRI	–	54	NS	68%
Sydney, Au [66]	20	CDDP + DX	–	18	30	
Basingstoke, UK [67]	76[a]	CDDP + DX	CDDP + DX	NS	98	NS
Milan, It [11]	108	CDDP + DX	–	49	63	52%
International [68]	401	Various	Various	33	53	47%
Bethesda, Pittsburgh, Baltimore [69]	211	CDDP or MMC	5FU +taxol	NS	38	26%
Lyon, FR [70]	28	CDDP + MMC	–	34	37	NE
Pittsburgh, PA [71]	65	CDDP + MMC	–	37	46	39%
Washington, DC [72]	205	CDDP + DX	Taxol	31	77	52%
RENAPE [73]	249	Various	–	24	NR	80%[b]

CDDP cisplatin, *DX* doxorubicin, *MMC* mitomycin-C, *OX* oxaliplatin, *IRI* irinotecan, *NS* not stated, *NR* not reached, *5FU* 5 fluorouracil, *OS* overall survival, *HIPEC* hyperthermic intraperitoneal chemotherapy, *EPIC* early postoperative intraperitoneal chemotherapy

[a]Thirty-nine patients were affected by multicystic or papillary well-differentiated mesothelioma

[b]Three year survival

patients, respectively [68, 69, 73]. The International study was sponsored by the Peritoneal Surface Oncology Group International (PSOGI) and included patients treated in eight centers from 1989 to 2009. Major operative morbidity of 46%, mortality of 2%, median survival of 53 months, and 5-year survival of 47% were reported [68].

We reported operative long-term outcomes for 108 patients treated with complete CRS/HIPEC (post-cytoreductin residual disease ≤2.5 mm). Treatment-related morbidity and mortality were 38.9% and 1.9%, respectively. Median survival was 63.2 months. Interestingly, there were 19 (43.6%) actual survivors of the 39 patients with potential follow-up >7 years, suggesting that patients surviving >7 years may be cured. On multivariate analysis, epithelioid histology and negative lymph node correlated with both overall survival and progression-free survival [11].

Several predictive factors for overall survival in patients with DMPM have been identified. Consistently with the notion that HIPEC penetration depth in residual tumor tissue is only a few millimeters, complete cytoreduction is mandatory for successful treatment [47]. Achievement of CCR-0/1 cytoreduction is highly dependent on the extent of peritoneal disease, involvement of crucial anatomic regions, and tumor aggressiveness [30]. Outcomes from numerous studies have supported this finding: disease stage based on percutaneous coronary interventions (PCI) was identified as a prognostic factor by Yan [74], Schaub et al. created a nomogram to predict survival that was partly based on PCI [75]. Magge found similar finding with lower PCI being predictive of increased survival [71]. Male sex and older age have been also associated with poorer prognosis [69, 71, 76].

Significant pathological and biological prognostic factors reported in the literature are summarized in Table 21.6. One of the most consistent factors is the histological type. Significantly, worse outcomes have been reported for sarcomatoid and biphasic DMPM than the epithelioid subtype [11, 68, 75]. Both Schaub and Alexander further sub-categorized the epithelioid subtype into tumors with significant solid component as a marker for worse outcomes, as compared with epithelioid DMPM with a tubule-papillary pattern [69, 75]. Magge showed that there may be no benefit from CRS-HIPEC in the sarcomatoid and biphasic groups, with a median survival of 10.5 versus 51.5 months for epithelioid DMPM [71]. On the contrary, a recent PSOGI registry study reported better results, with a median survival of

Table 21.6 Significant prognostic factors of peritoneal mesothelioma

Author (ref)	Pts	Factors	HR (95% CI)	*p* Value (Cox)
Feldman [12]	49	Deep invasion	4.24 (1.06–16.9)	0.041
Borczuk [8]	54	P16 Mitotic count	3.65 (1.3-10.2) 3.07 (1.05-9.0)	0.014 0.04
Deraco [7]	49	Mitotic count	10.46 (1.98–5.23)	0.01
Villa [13]	38	Telomerase	3.30 (1.23–8.86)	0.018
Cerruto [28]	62	Histology Nuclear size	NA NA	0.01 0.01
Yan [68]	402	Histology Node status	7.54 (2.91–10.36) 3.93 (1.75–6.02)	0.001 0.001
Baratti [11]	110	Histology Node status Ki67	3.70 (1.69–7.69) 2.10 (1.08–4.09) 2.94 (1.38–6.24)	0.001 0.003 0.005
Alexander [69]	211	Histology	2.14 (1.17–3.91)	0.01
Hommell-Fontaine [70]	28	GLUT-1	21.5 (2.7–171.4)	0.004
Pillai [84]	28	Ki-67	4.8 (1.2–14.2)	0.016
Magge [71]	65	Histology	5.4 (2.1–14.0)	0.001
Ihemelandu [72]	205	Histology	6.1 (2.7–14.0)	0.001

HR hazard rates, *NA* not assessed

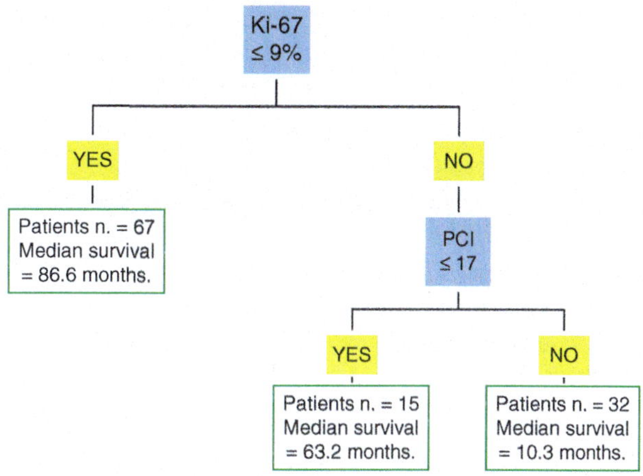

Fig. 21.9 Conditional inference tree method. Three prognostic groups are identified, based on Ki-67 and peritoneal Cancer Index (PCI): (I) Ki-67 ≤ 9%; (II) Ki-67 > 9% and PCI ≤ 17; and (III) Ki-67 > 9% and PCI > 17. The median OS for the three group was, 86.6, 63.2, and 10.3 months, respectively

7.8 years in patients with biphasic histology undergoing CCR-0 cytoreduction, thus suggesting that biphasic DMPM should not be considered as an absolute contraindication [78].

The prognostic impact of lymph-node metastases has been reported in both single center and multi-institutional series [11, 68, 74]. Individual studies have also identified mitotic rate [8, 11, 79], GLUT-1 expression [80], preoperative CA-125 [30, 75], telomere maintenance mechanisms [13], estrogen receptors [81], BCL2 [77], MUC-1 [82], BAP1, NF2, CDKN2A [83], PD-L1 [80], and preoperative thrombocytosis [84] as predictors of survival.

We recently developed an algorithm by means of conditional inference tree model [9]. This model relies on pre-cytoreduction PCI and tumor proliferative index measured by Ki-67 using immunohistochemistry. Three prognostic subsets were defined: (I) Ki-67 ≤ 9%; (II) Ki-67 > 9% and PCI 17; and (III) Ki-67 > 9% and PCI > 17. The median OS for subsets I, II, and III were, 86.6, 63.2, and 10.3 months, respectively. The model had an acceptable discriminant capacity with a bootstrap-corrected Harrell c-index of 0.74 (see Fig. 21.9).

21.8.1 Low-Grade Peritoneal Mesotelioma

MCPM and WDPM are rare variants of mesothelioma. In a few centers, these disease entities have been treated by CRS/HIPEC due to their tendencies to give multiple local-regional recurrences and reported potential to evolve into truly malignant DMPM. In 2007, we reported a series of four women with MPM and eight with WDPPM undergoing cytoreduction and close-abdomen HIPEC with cisplatin and doxorubicin. Seven of them were treated for recurrent disease after previous debulking. After a median follow-up of 27 months (range 6–94), 5-year overall and progression-free survival were 90.0% and 79.7%, respectively. Transition of typical WDPPM to malignant biphasic mesothelioma was documented in one patient who died of disease progression following incomplete cytoreduction and HIPEC. We were able to calculate median progression-free survival of 24 months (range 2–87) following previous debulking surgery in 7 patients (one operation in five patients, two operations in one, and four operations in one), that was statistically worse than the corresponding figure after CRS/HIPEC in the same patients ($p = 0.0156$) [24].

Outcomes of MPM were also studied as a subgroup analysis from the PSOGI registry. There were 26 patients (6.4%) with a large preponderance of females ($n = 20$). Following a median follow up of 54 months (range 5–129), all patients treated were alive and free of disease [85]. In our most recent institutional update, we reviewed 19 patients with MCPM who underwent 20 CRS/HIPEC procedures in our center between August 1997 and October 2017. The majority of the patients were females (n = 17, 89%), and mean age was 42. Mean PCI was 15.5 ± 9.9 and total number of procedures performed 6.7 ± 2.6. Major complications occurred in 3 (15%) patients, with no perioperative mortality. After a median of follow-up of 69 months (range 4–220) all patients were alive and four patients had recurrence (21%). Patients with high PCI (defined by median PCI) had shorter recurrence-free survival (106.4 ± 6.6 months versus 125.6 ± 34.1; $p = 0.03$) [86].

21.8.2 Staging of Peritoneal Mesothelioma

No staging system exists for DMPM, because of its rarity and unique clinical presentation with diffuse disease dissemination throughout the peritoneum, and no primary lesion. As a curative-intent treatment has become available, the international PSOGI registry collecting 292 DMPM patients undergoing CRS/HIPEC has been used to formulate a new tumor-node-metastasis (TNM) staging system [74].

Yan assessed tumor (T) category according to the extent of peritoneal involvement, as scored intraoperatively by PCI. PCI was categorized into T1 (PCI 1–10), T2 (PCI 11–20), T3 (PCI 21–30), and T4 (PCI 30–39). Node (N) and metastasis (M) factors were defined according to the presence versus absence of positive intra-abdominal lymph nodes and hepatic or extra-abdominal involvement. The T1, N0, M0 defined stage 1. T2-3, N0, M0 defined stage 2. T4, N0, M0, and N1 or M1 with any T, defined stage 3. Five-year survival associated with stage I, II, and III was 87, 53, and 29%, respectively. The proposed TNM staging was associated with survival in the multivariate analysis, together with histological subtype, and complete cytoreduction.

Based on the evidence that prognosis of DMPM is predominantly dependent on pathological and biological features, such as histological subtype and proliferative activity, we hypothesized that the prognostic stratification of the recently proposed TNM could be improved by the incorporation of a pathological grading system. We defined pathological grading as follows:

- Grade 1: mitotic count (MC) ≤ 5/10 high power fields (HPF), *or* Ki-67 index ≤ 5% (percentage of positive cells among 2000 tumor cells).
- Grade 2: MC 5–25/10 HPF *or* Ki-67 index > 5%.
- Grade 3: MC > 25/10 HPF *or* Ki-67 index > 25% *or* presence of any spindle cell component.

Stage grouping was revised as follows: T1-3, N0, M0, G1 defined stage I; T4, N0, M0, G1, *or* T1-3, N0, M0, G2 defined stage II. Stage III was defined by any of the following: (1) G3; (2) N1; (3) M1; (4) T4, N0, M0, G2.

For stage I, median overall survival was not reached (71.6% at 5-year). For stage II and III, median survival was 39.5 months (95% CI = 34.6–44.4) and 12.6 months (95% CI = 6.8–18.5), respectively. In a Cox multivariable model, modified TNM (hazard ratio (HR) = 2.3, 95% CI = 1.7–3.3; $p < 0.001$), completeness of cytoreduction (HR = 2.0; 95% CI = 1.4–2.9; $p < 0.001$), and major complications (HR = 1.7; 95% CI = 1.1–2.8; $p = 0.030$) independently correlated with survival. The previously proposed TNM was not significant ($p = 0.507$) [87].

By means of 25 demographic, laboratory, operative, and histopathological variables, Schaub developed a nomogram using machine-learned Bayesian belief networks with stepwise training, testing, and cross-validation to predict prognosis of DMPM patients who underwent CRS/HIPEC. Among 104 patients treated at the National Cancer Institute/NIH, Bethesda, MD, mean PCI was 15, 66% of patients had a CCR-0/1 cytoreduction, and 87% of patients had epithelioid histology. Median follow-up was 49 months (1–195), and 3- and 5-year survival rates were 58 and 46%, respectively. Histological subtype, PCI, and preoperative serum CA-125 had the greatest impact on survival and were included in the nomogram. The mean areas under the ROC curve for the ten-fold cross-validation of the 3- and 5-year models were 0.77 and 0.74, respectively.

This nomogram may potentially individualize patient care and prevent CRS in patients unlikely to achieve favorable outcomes [75].

21.9 Conclusion

Even in the absence of controlled data, the current evidence suggests that the comprehensive approach of CRS/HIPEC is now the benchmark against which other treatments have to be evaluated. The optimization of several important clinical issues is still ongoing, including patient selection for treatment, adaptation of CRS techniques to this peculiar disease, and role of integrated systemic and local-regional therapies in the individual patients. CRS/HIPEC and sCT should be applied according to histology, tumor biology, disease stage, and patient condition as follows:

- CRS/HIPEC is recommended for low-grade PM (WDPM and MCPM) with no need of further treatment.
- Patients with not resectable or metastatic DMPM, and/or poor general status not allowing major abdominal surgery, should be considered for sCT.
- Patients with DMPM confined to the peritoneum and not fit for major abdominal surgery or with disease not fully resectable or resectable with extensive surgery conditioning higher risk of postoperative morbidity should be proposed for neoadjuvant sCT. In these patients, CRS/HIPEC should be considered after sCT in case of important response.
- Patients with DMPM confined to the peritoneum fit for major abdominal surgery, and with disease amenable to complete resection. This is the group of patients in whom CRS HIPEC is indicated as first-line treatment.

We believe that the rarity of this disease entity and complexity of its treatment approaches would make it necessary to be treated these patients in highly qualified referral centers. Novel systemic combination chemotherapy warrants further assessments as an adjunct to intraperitoneally delivered drugs. Basic science research is rapidly evolving and future developments may come from integrating innovative molecular and cellular approaches into comprehensive treatment strategies.

References

1. Robinson BWS, Lake RA. Advanced in malignant mesothelioma. N Engl J Med. 2005;353:1591–603.
2. Conti S, Minelli G, Ascoli V, Marinaccio A, Bonafede M, Manno V, Crialesi R, Straif K. Peritoneal mesothelioma in Italy: trends and geography of mortality and incidence. Am J Ind Med. 2015;58:1050–8.
3. Boffetta P. Epidemiology of peritoneal mesothelioma: a review. Ann Oncol. 2007;18:985–90.
4. Sugarbaker PH, Welch LS, Mohamed F, Glehen O. A review of peritoneal mesothelioma at the Washington Cancer Institute. Surg Oncol Clin N Am. 2003;12:605–21.
5. Gazdar AF, Carbone M. Molecular pathogenesis of mesotheliom and its relationship to Simian virus 40. Clin Lung Cancer. 2003;5:177–81.
6. Roushdy-Hammady I, Siegel J, Emri S, et al. Genetic-susceptibility factor and malignant mesothelioma in the Cappadocian region of Turkey. Lancet. 2001;357:444–5.
7. Nonaka D, Kusamura S, Baratti D, et al. Diffuse malignant mesothelioma of the peritoneum: a clinicopathological study of 35 patients treated locoregionally at a single institution. Cancer. 2005;104:2181–8.
8. Borczuk AC, Taub RN, Hesdorffer M, et al. P16 loss and mitotic activity predict poor survival in patients with peritoneal malignant mesothelioma. Clin Cancer Res. 2005;11:3303–8.
9. Kusamura S, Torres Mesa PA, Cabras A, Baratti D, Deraco M. The role of Ki-67 and pre-cytoreduction parameters in selecting diffuse malignant peritoneal mesothelioma (DMPM) patients for Cytoreductive surgery (CRS) and Hyperthermic Intraperitoneal Chemotherapy (HIPEC). Ann Surg Oncol. 2016;23:1468–73.
10. Deraco M, Cabras A, Baratti D, Kusamura S. Immunohistochemical evaluation of Minichromosome maintenance protein 7 (MCM7), topoisomerase IIα, and Ki-67 in diffuse malignant peritoneal mesothelioma patients using tissue microarray. Ann Surg Oncol. 2015;22:4344–51.
11. Baratti D, Kusamura S, Cabras AD, Bertulli R, Hutanu I, Deraco M. Diffuse malignant peritoneal mesothelioma: long-term survival with complete cytoreductive surgery followed by hyperthermic intraperitoneal chemotherapy (HIPEC). Eur J Cancer. 2013;49:3140–8. 8A.L.
12. Feldman AL, Libutti SK, Pingpank JF, et al. Analysis of factors associated with outcome in patients with

malignant peritoneal mesothelioma undergoing surgical debulking and intraperitoneal chemotherapy. J Clin Oncol. 2003;21:4560–7.

13. Villa R, Daidone MG, Motta R, Venturini L, De Marco C, Vannelli A, Kusamura S, Baratti D, Deraco M, Costa A, Reddel RR, Zaffaroni N. Multiple mechanisms of telomere maintenance exist and differentially affect clinical outcome in diffuse malignant peritoneal mesothelioma. Clin Cancer Res. 2008;14:4134–40.
14. Zaffaroni N, Costa A, Pennati M, De Marco C, Affini E, Madeo M, Erdas R, Cabras A, Kusamura S, Baratti D, Deraco M, Daidone MG. Survivin is highly expressed and promotes cell survival in malignant peritoneal mesothelioma. Cell Oncol. 2007;29:453–66.
15. De Cesare M, Sfondrini L, Pennati M, De Marco C, Motta V, Tagliabue E, Dera M, Balsari A, Zaffaroni N. CpG-oligodeoxynucleotides exert remarkable antitumor activity against diffuse malignant peritoneal mesothelioma orthotopic xenografts. J Transl Med. 2016;14:25.
16. Perrone F, Jocollè G, Pennati M, Deraco M, Baratti D, Brich S, Orsenigo M, Tarantino E, De Marco C, Bertan C, Cabras A, Bertulli R, Pierotti MA, Zaffaroni N, Pilotti S. Receptor tyrosine kinase and downstream signalling analysis in diffuse malignant peritoneal mesothelioma. Eur J Cancer. 2010;46:2837–48.
17. Churg A, Roggli VL, Galateau-Salle F, et al. Tumours of the pleura: Mesothelial tumours. In: Travis WD, Brambilla E, Harris CC, Muller-Hermelink HK, editors. Pathology and genetics of tumours of the lung, pleura, thymus and heart. Lyon: IARC Press; 2004.
18. Husain AN, Colby TV, Ordóñez NG, et al. Guidelines for pathologic diagnosis of malignant mesothelioma: 2017 update of the consensus statement from the international mesothelioma interest group. Arch Pathol Lab Med. 2018;142:89–108.
19. Battifora H, McCaughey WTE. Tumours and pseudotumours of the serosal membranes. In: Atlas of tumour pathology 3rd series, fascicle 15. Washington, DC: Armed Forces Institute of Pathology; 1995. p. 15–88.
20. Roggli VL, Cagle PT. Pleura, pericardium and peritoneum. In: Silverberg SG, DeLellis RA, Frable WJ, LiVolsi VA, Wick MR, editors. Silverberg's principles and practice of surgical pathology. 4th ed. New York: Churchill-Livingstone/Elsevier; 2006. p. 1005–39.
21. Attanoos RL, Gibbs AR. Pathology of malignant mesothelioma. Histopathology. 1997;30:403–18.
22. Baratti D, Kusamura S, Cabras AD, Laterza B, Balestra MR, Deraco M. Lymph node metastases in diffuse malignant peritoneal mesothelioma. Ann Surg Oncol. 2010;17:45–53.
23. Butnor KJ, Sporn TA, Hammar SP, Roggli VL. Well-differentiated papillary mesothelioma. Am J Surg Pathol. 2001;25:1304–9.
24. Baratti D, Kusamura S, Nonaka D, Oliva GD, Laterza B, Deraco M. Multicystic and well-differentiated papillary peritoneal mesothelioma treated by surgical cytoreduction and hyperthermic intra-peritoneal chemotherapy (HIPEC). Ann Surg Oncol. 2007;14:2790–7.
25. Churg A, Colby TV, Cagle P. The separation of benign and malignant mesothelial proliferations. Am J Surg Pathol. 2000;24:1183–200.
26. Attanoos RL, Griffin A, Gibbs AR. The use of immunohistochemistry in distinguishing reactive from neoplastic mesothelium: a novel use for desmin and comparative evaluation with epithelial membrane antigen, p53, platelet-derived growth factor-receptor, P-glycoprotein and Bcl-2. Histopathology. 2003;43:231–8.
27. Ordonez NG. Immunohistochemical diagnosis of epithelioid mesothelioma: an update. Arch Pathol Lab Med. 2005;129:1407–14.
28. Cerruto CA, Brun EA, Chang D, Sugarbaker PH. Prognostic significance of histomorphologic parameters in diffuse malignant peritoneal mesothelioma. Arch Pathol Lab Med. 2006;130:1654–61.
29. de Pangher V, Recchia L, Cafferata M, et al. Malignant peritoneal mesothelioma: a multicenter study on 81 cases. Ann Oncol. 2010;21:348–53.
30. Baratti D, Kusamura S, Martinetti A, Seregni E, Oliva DG, Laterza B, Deraco M. Circulating CA125 in patients with peritoneal mesothelioma treated with cytoreductive surgery and intraperitoneal hyperthermic perfusion. Ann Surg Oncol. 2007;14:500–8.
31. Bruno F, Baratti D, Martinetti A, Morelli D, Sottotetti E, Bonini C, Guaglio M, Kusamura S, Deraco M. Mesothelin and osteopontin as circulating markers of diffuse malignant peritoneal mesothelioma: a preliminary study. Eur J Surg Oncol. 2018;44:792–8.
32. Park JY, Kim KW, Kwon HJ, et al. Peritoneal mesotheliomas: clinicopathologic features, CT findings, and differential diagnosis. Am J Roentgenol. 2008;191:814–25.
33. Whitley N, Brenner D, Antman K, Grant D, Aisner J. CT of peritoneal mesothelioma: analysis of eight cases. Am J Roentgenol. 1982;138:531–5.
34. Yan TD, Haveric N, Carmignani CP, Bromley CM, Sugarbaker PH. Computed tomographic characterization of malignant peritoneal mesothelioma. Tumori. 2005;91:394–400.
35. Yan TD, Haveric N, Carmignani CP, Chang D, Sugarbaker PH. Abdominal computed tomography scans in the selection of patients with malignant peritoneal mesothelioma for comprehensive treatment with cytoreductive surgery and perioperative intraperitoneal chemotherapy. Cancer. 2005;103:839–49.
36. Dubreuil J, Giammarile F, Rousset P, et al. The role of 18F-FDG-PET/ceCT in peritoneal mesothelioma. Nucl Med Commun. 2017;38:312–8.
37. Laterza B, Kusamura S, Baratti D, Oliva GD, Deraco M. Role of explorative laparoscopy to evaluate optimal candidates for cytoreductive surgery and hyperthermic intraperitoneal chemotherapy (HIPEC) in patients with peritoneal mesothelioma. In Vivo. 2009;23:187–90.
38. Rogoff EE, Hilaris B, Huvos AG. Long-term survival in patients with malignant peritoneal mesothelioma treated with irradiation. Cancer. 1973;32:656–64.

39. Jones DEC, Silver D. Peritoneal mesothelioma. Surgery. 1979;86:556–60.
40. Chahinian AP, Pajak TF, Holland JF, et al. Diffuse malignant mesothelioma. Prospective evaluation of 69 patients. Ann Intern Med. 1982;96:746–55.
41. Antman KH, Osteen R, Klegar K, et al. Early peritoneal mesothelioma: a treatable malignancy. Lancet. 1985;2:977–81.
42. Kirmani S, Cleary SM, Mowry J, et al. Intracavitary cisplatin for malignant mesothelioma: an update. In: Proc Am Clin Oncol, vol. 7, 1988. (Abstract 1057).
43. van Gelder T, Hoogsteden HC, Versnel MA, et al. Malignant peritoneal mesothelioma: a series of 19 cases. Digestion. 1989;43:222–7.
44. Markman M, Kelsen D. Efficacy of cisplatin-based intraperitoneal chemotherapy as treatment of malignant peritoneal mesothelioma. J Cancer Res Clin Oncol. 1992;118:547–50.
45. Neumann V, Muller KM, Fischer M. Peritoneal mesothelioma-incidence and aetiology. Pathologe. 1999;20:169–76.
46. Eltabbakh GH, Piver MS, Hempling RE, et al. Clinical picture, response to therapy, and survival of women with diffuse malignant peritoneal mesothelioma. J Surg Oncol. 1999;70:6–12.
47. Sugarbaker PH. Peritonectomy procedures. Ann Surg. 1995;221:29–42.
48. Antman K, Shemin R, Ryan L, et al. Malignant mesothelioma: prognostic variables in a registry of 180 patients, the Dana-Farber Cancer Institute and Brigham and Women's Hospital experience over two decades, 1965-1985. J Clin Oncol. 1988;6:147–53.
49. Chahinian AP, Antman K, Goutsou M, et al. Randomized phase II trial of cisplatin with mitomycin or doxorubicin for malignant mesothelioma by the cancer and Leukemia group B. J Clin Oncol. 1993;11:1559–65.
50. Carteni G, Manegold C, Garcia GM, et al. Malignant peritoneal mesothelioma - results from the international expanded access program using pemetrexed alone or in combination with a platinum agent. Lung Cancer. 2009;64:211–8.
51. Vogelzang NJ, Rusthoven JJ, Symanowski J, et al. Phase III study of pemetrexed in combination with cisplatin versus cisplatin alone in patients with malignant pleural mesothelioma. J Clin Oncol. 2003;21:2636–44.
52. Jänne PA, Wozniak AJ, Belani CP, et al. Open-label study of pemetrexed alone or in combination with cisplatin for the treatment of patients with peritoneal mesothelioma: outcomes of an expanded access program. Clin Lung Cancer. 2005;7:40–6.
53. Simon GR, Verschraegen CF, Jänne PA, Langer CJ, Dowlati A, Gadgeel SM, et al. Pemetrexed plus gemcitabine as first-line chemotherapy for patients with peritoneal mesothelioma: final report of a phase II trial. J Clin Oncol. 2008;26:3567–72.
54. Hesdorffer ME, Chabot JA, Keohan ML, et al. Combined resection, intraperitoneal chemotherapy, and whole abdominal radiation for the treatment of malignant peritoneal mesothelioma. Am J Clin Oncol. 2008;31:49–54.
55. Baratti D, Kusamura S, Cabras AD, Dileo P, Laterza B, Deraco M. Diffuse malignant peritoneal mesothelioma: failure analysis following cytoreduction and hyperthermic intraperitoneal chemotherapy (HIPEC). Ann Surg Oncol. 2009;16:463–72.
56. Deraco M, Baratti D, Hutanu I, Bertuli R, Kusamura S. The role of perioperative systemic chemotherapy in diffuse malignant peritoneal mesothelioma patients treated with cytoreductive surgery and hyperthermic intraperitoneal chemotherapy. Ann Surg Oncol. 2013;20:1093–100.
57. Kepenekian V, Elias D, Passot G, et al. Diffuse malignant peritoneal mesothelioma: evaluation of systemic chemotherapy with comprehensive treatment through the RENAPE database: multi-institutional retrospective study. Eur J Cancer. 2016;65:69–79.
58. Jaquet P, Sugarbaker PH. Current methodologies for clinical assessment of patients with peritoneal carcinomatosis. J Exp Clin Cancer Res. 1996;15:49–58.
59. Baratti D, Kusamura S, Guaglio M, Deraco M. Peritoneal metastases: challenges for the surgeon. Minerva Chir. 2015;70:195–215.
60. Baratti D, Kusamura S, Cabras AD, Deraco M. Cytoreductive surgery with selective versus complete parietal peritonectomy followed by hyperthermic intraperitoneal chemotherapy in patients with diffuse malignant peritoneal mesothelioma: a controlled study. Ann Surg Oncol. 2012;19:1416–24.
61. Deraco M, Baratti D, Kusamura S, Laterza B, Balestra MR. Surgical technique of parietal and visceral peritonectomy for peritoneal surface malignancies. J Surg Oncol. 2009;100:321–8.
62. Bijelic L, Stuart OA, Sugarbaker PH. Adjuvant bidirectional chemotherapy with intraperitoneal pemetrexed combined with intravenous cisplatin for diffuse malignant peritoneal mesothelioma. Gastroenterol Res Pract. 2012;2012:1–6. Article ID 890450.
63. Blackham AU, Shen P, Stewart JH, et al. Cytoreductive surgery with intraperitoneal hyperthermic chemotherapy for malignant peritoneal mesothelioma: mitomycin versus cisplatin. Ann Surg Oncol. 2010;17:1720–7.
64. Robella M, Vaira M, Mellano A, et al. Treatment of diffuse malignant peritoneal mesothelioma (DMPM) by cytoreductive surgery and HIPEC. Minerva Chir. 2014;69:9–15.
65. Elias D, Bedard V, Bouzid T, et al. Malignant peritoneal mesothelioma: treatment with maximal cytoreductive surgery plus intraperitoneal chemotherapy. Gastroenterol Clin Biol. 2007;31:784–8.
66. Chua TC, Yan TD, Morris DL. Outcomes of cytoreductive surgery and hyperthermic intraperitoneal chemotherapy for peritoneal mesothelioma: the Australian experience. J Surg Oncol. 2009;99:109–13.
67. Gilani SNS, Mehta A, Garcia-Fadrique A, et al. Outcomes of cytoreductive surgery with hyperthermic intraperitoneal chemotherapy for peritoneal mesothelioma and predictors of survival. Int J Hyperth. 2018;34:578–84.

68. Yan TD, Deraco M, Baratti D, et al. Cytoreductive surgery combined with hyperthermic intraperitoneal chemotherapy for peritoneal mesothelioma—a multi-institutional registry study. J Clin Oncol. 2009;27:6237–42.
69. Alexander HR Jr, Bartlett DL, Pingpank JF, et al. Treatment factors associated with long-term survival after cytoreductive surgery and regional chemotherapy for patients with malignant peritoneal mesothelioma. Surgery. 2013;153:779–86.
70. Hommell-Fontaine J, Isaac S, Passot G, et al. Malignant peritoneal mesothelioma treated by cytoreductive surgery and hyperthermic intraperitoneal chemotherapy: is GLUT1 expression a major prognostic factor? A preliminary study. Ann Surg Oncol. 2013;20:3892–8.
71. Magge D, Zenati MS, Austin F, et al. Malignant peritoneal mesothelioma: prognostic factors and oncologic outcome analysis. Ann Surg Oncol. 2014;21:1159–65.
72. Ihemelandu C, Bijelic L, Sugarbaker PH. Iterative cytoreductive surgery and hyperthermic intraperitoneal chemotherapy for recurrent or progressive diffuse malignant peritoneal mesothelioma: clinicopathologic characteristics and survival outcome. Ann Surg Oncol. 2015;22:1680–5.
73. Malgras B, Gayat E, Aoun O, et al. Impact of combination chemotherapy in peritoneal mesothelioma Hyperthermic Intraperitoneal chemotherapy (HIPEC): the RENAPE study. Ann Surg Oncol. 2018;25:3271–9.
74. Yan TD, Deraco M, Elias D, Glehen O, Levine EA, Moran BJ, Morris DL, Chua TC, Piso P, Sugarbaker PH, Peritoneal Surface Oncology Group. A novel tumor-node-metastasis (TNM) staging system of diffuse malignant peritoneal mesothelioma using outcome analysis of a multi-institutional database. Cancer. 2011;117:1855–63.
75. Schaub NP, Alimchandani M, Quezado M, et al. A novel nomogram for peritoneal mesothelioma predicts survival. Ann Surg Oncol. 2013;20:555–61.
76. Cao C, Yan TD, Deraco M, Elias D, Glehen O, Levine EA, Moran BJ, Morris DL, Chua TC, Piso P, Sugarbaker PH, Peritoneal Surface Malignancy Group. Importance of gender in diffuse malignant peritoneal mesothelioma. Ann Oncol. 2012;23:1494–8.
77. Pillai K, Pourgholami MH, Chua TC, Morris DL. Ki67-BCL2 index in prognosis of malignant peritoneal mesothelioma. Am J Cancer Res. 2013;3:411–23.
78. Votanopoulos KI, Sugarbaker P, Deraco M, et al. Is cytoreductive surgery with hyperthermic intraperitoneal chemotherapy justified for biphasic variants of peritoneal mesothelioma? Outcomes from the peritoneal surface oncology group international registry. Ann Surg Oncol. 2018;25:667–73.
79. Krasinskas AM, Borczuk AC, Hartman DJ, et al. Prognostic significance of morphological growth patterns and mitotic index of epithelioid malignant peritoneal mesothelioma. Histopathology. 2016;68:729–37.
80. Valmary-Degano S, Colpart P, Villeneuve L, et al. Immunohistochemical evaluation of two antibodies against PD-L1 and prognostic significance of PD-L1 expression in epithelioid peritoneal malignant mesothelioma: a RENAPE study. Eur J Surg Oncol. 2017;43:1915–23.
81. Huang Y, Alzahrani NA, Liauw W, Morris DL. Effects of sex hormones on survival of peritoneal mesothelioma. World J Surg Oncol. 2015;13:210.
82. Pillai K, Pourgholami MH, Chua TC, Morris DL. MUC1 has prognostic significance in malignant peritoneal mesothelioma. Int J Biol Markers. 2013;28:303–12.
83. Singhi AD, Krasinskas AM, Choudry HA, et al. The prognostic significance of BAP1, NF2, and CDKN2A in malignant peritoneal mesothelioma. Mod Pathol. 2016;29:14–24.
84. Li YC, Khashab T, Terhune J, et al. Preoperative thrombocytosis predicts shortened survival in patients with malignant peritoneal mesothelioma undergoing operative Cytoreduction and Hyperthermic Intraperitoneal chemotherapy. Ann Surg Oncol. 2017;24:2259–65.
85. Chua TC, Yan TD, Deraco M, Glehen O, Moran BJ, Sugarbaker PH. Multi-institutional experience of diffuse intra-abdominal multicystic peritoneal mesothelioma. Br J Surg. 2011;98:60–4.
86. Nizri E, Baratti D, Guaglio M, et al. Multicystic mesothelioma: operative and long-term outcomes with cytoreductive surgery and hyperthermic intra peritoneal chemotherapy. Eur J Surg Oncol. 2018;44:1100–4.
87. Baratti D, Kusamura S, Cabras AD, et al. Diffuse malignant peritoneal mesothelioma: incorporation of a simple pathological grading into recently proposed TNM classification improbe out come prediction. In: 9th International Congress on peritoneal Surface malignancies. Amsterdam, ND. 9-11 October 2014.

22 Rare Localizations of Mesothelioma

Marta Betti and Federica Grosso

22.1 Introduction

Malignant Mesothelioma (MM) commonly arises in the pleura and peritoneum but also occurs most rarely at pericardium, Glisson's capsule, and in males in the tunica vaginalis testis (TVT). In the early somite stage of the development embryo, multiple coelomic spaces are formed. Each of these spaces is enclosed by mesoblasts, which are derived from the intra-embryonic mesoderm.

The pericardium is a double-layered sac, which surrounds and acts as mechanical protection for the heart. The outer sac is called fibrous pericardium and the inner one is called serous pericardium. The serous pericardium is divided into the parietal pericardium, which is directly fused with the fibrous pericardium, and the visceral pericardium, which adheres directly to the heart. The two layers of the serous pericardium are separated by the pericardial cavity, a virtual space, which contains the serous fluid [1].

M. Betti
Infrastruttura Ricerca, Formazione, Innovazione, Azienda Ospedaliera SS. Antonio e Biagio e Cesare Arrigo, Alessandria, Italy
e-mail: marta.betti@ospedale.al.it

F. Grosso (✉)
Mesothelioma Unit – Oncology, Azienda Ospedaliera SS. Antonio e Biagio e Cesare Arrigo, Alessandria, Italy
e-mail: federica.grosso@ospedale.al.it

The tunica vaginalis is a serous membrane that surrounds the testis or epididymis (visceral lamina) or the spermatic cord and internal wall of the scrotum (parietal lamina) [2]. During embryologic development, the tunica vaginalis derives from the closure of the superior portion of the processus vaginalis, a socklike evagination of the peritoneum. This structure normally covers the entire testis except from the posterior border. It has a visceral layer and an outer parietal layer that lines the internal spermatic fascia of the scrotal wall. These layers and the potential membrane they delimit may be affected by a wide variety of pathologic processes, including neoplastic disorders [3]. Histologically, the cells that line the tunica vaginalis are similar to those that line the pleura, peritoneum, and pericardium, thus are at risk of developing mesothelioma [4].

The Glisson's capsule extends into the liver, as a layer of connective tissue surrounding the liver and sheathing the hepatic artery, portal vein, and bile ducts within the liver. In literature, the capsule composition has been debated. Some authors believe that Glisson's capsule is characterized by collagen fibers including type I and type III collagen, fibroblast cells and small blood vessels, and no mesothelial cells of its own, suggesting that malignant peritoneal mesothelioma could invade the liver [5]. By contrast, other authors speculate that Glisson's capsule is covered by mesothelial cells and exactly these cells are the origin of the primary intrahepatic mesothelioma [6].

G. L. Ceresoli et al. (eds.), *Mesothelioma*, https://doi.org/10.1007/978-3-030-16884-1_22

22.1.1 Incidence

The extra pleural malignant mesotheliomas (EPMMs), i.e., pericardial mesothelioma (PM), mesothelioma of the tunica vaginalis testis (MTVT), and primary intrahepatic malignant mesothelioma (PIHMM), are very rare tumors. In the Italian National Mesothelioma Registry (ReNaM), between 1993 and 2012, PM and MTVT accounted for 51 (0.2%) and 65 (0.3%) of 21,463 MMs diagnosed, respectively [7] (Table 22.1). The ReNaM reported that PM and MTVT each made up to 0.3% of all MMs in the country between 1993 and 2012, with estimated standardized incidence rates of 0.003 and 0.01 (per 100,000 person-year), respectively [7]. The United States SEER program reported incidence rates of 0.36 and 0.54 (per 10,000,000 person-year) in 1973–2013 for PM and MTVT, respectively [8].

Cases of PIHMM are only sporadically reported. To the best of knowledge, only 15 cases of PIHMM have been so far reported in the published literature [9] (Table 22.2).

Table 22.1 Malignant mesothelioma cases collected in the Italian National Mesothelioma Register (ReNaM) by anatomical site (from V Rapporto ReNaM 1993–2012 [7])

	Pericardium ($N = 51$)	Tunica vaginalis testis ($N = 65$)
Sex, n (%)		
M	35 (69%)	65 (100%)
F	16 (31%)	–
Age		
0–24	1 (2%)	1 (1.5%)
25–34	2 (3.9%)	3 (4.6%)
35–44	4 (7.8%)	5 (7.7%)
45–54	8 (15.7%)	7 (10.8%)
55–64	8 (15.7%)	7 (10.8%)
65–74	19 (37.2%)	21 (32.3%)
75–84	8 (15.7%)	19 (29.2%)
85+	1 (2%)	2 (3.1%)
Histotype		
Epithelioid	17 (33.3%)	35 (53.8%)
Biphasic	9 (17.6%)	9 (13.8%)
Sarcomatous	5 (9.8%)	4 (6.2%)
Not specified	14 (27.5%)	16 (24.6%)
Not available	6 (11.8%)	1 (1.5%)
Asbestos exposure		
Occupational	22 (43.1%)	35 (53.9%)
Household	–	1 (1.5%)
Environmental	1 (2%)	–
Leisure-related	–	1 (1.5%)
Unknown or improbable	13 (25.5%)	16 (24.6%)
To define	10 (19.6%)	8 (12.3%)
Not classified	5 (9.8%)	4 (6.2%)
Standardized incidence rates (per 100,000 person-year)	0.003	0.01

22.1.2 Asbestos Exposure

The International Agency for Research on Cancer (IARC) asserted that all types of asbestos are carcinogenic and may cause MM at any site [10]. However, the etiological role of asbestos exposure in EPMMs has not formally been demonstrated in case-control epidemiological studies. Thus, the potential role of asbestos exposure in PM and MTVT development has been suspected. In large occupational cohorts with heavy asbestos exposures, no cases of PM and MTVT have been reported, by contrast, 30% of case reports published have some potential, assumed, or confirmed history of asbestos exposure [8].

Table 22.2 PIHMM cases collected from literature review

	PIHMM ($N = 15$)
Sex, n (%)	
M	7 (46.7%)
F	8 (53.3%)
Age	
0–24	–
25–34	–
35–44	1 (6.7%)
45–54	3 (20%)
55–64	7 (46.7%)
65–74	3 (20%)
75–84	1 (6.7%)
85+	–
Histotype	
Epithelioid	10 (66.7%)
Biphasic	4 (26.7%)
Sarcomatous	1 (6.7%)
Asbestos exposure	
Yes	1 (6.7%)
No	11 (73.3%)
Not recorded	3 (20%)

In the ReNaM, 45% of the PM cases and 57% of the MTVT cases diagnosed between 1993 and 2012 were identified and classified as definitely, probably, or possibly due to asbestos exposure in occupational setting, or otherwise, i.e., household, environmental, or leisure-related exposure [7]. Moreover, the presence of asbestos bodies in the pericardium has been debated. Several studies reported the absence of the asbestos in the examined tissues, only two studies reported the presence of asbestos bodies in the lung tissues of PM patients [11, 12], and one study reported the presence of asbestos fibers in the pericardium [13].

The association between asbestos exposure and PIHMM has not yet been demonstrated. Only one patient out of 15 (6.7%) had a history of asbestos exposure [9].

22.2 Pericardial Mesothelioma

PM is the most common malignant primary of the pericardium [14]. The diagnosis is difficult because of the nonspecific clinical signs and symptoms. The symptoms and clinical signs may be nonspecific, such as cough, shortness of breath, weight loss, chest pain, and night sweats or more specific, such as edema, pericardial effusion, constrictive pericarditis, and heart failure. Fever may be among the initial symptoms, potentially misleading to inflammatory or infective pericarditis often responsible for delayed diagnosis. Unlike mesotheliomas of the pleura and peritoneum, radiography may not contribute to correct diagnosis for PM patients showing only an enlargement of the mediastinum [15] (Fig. 22.1). Citologically, the pericardial fluid is

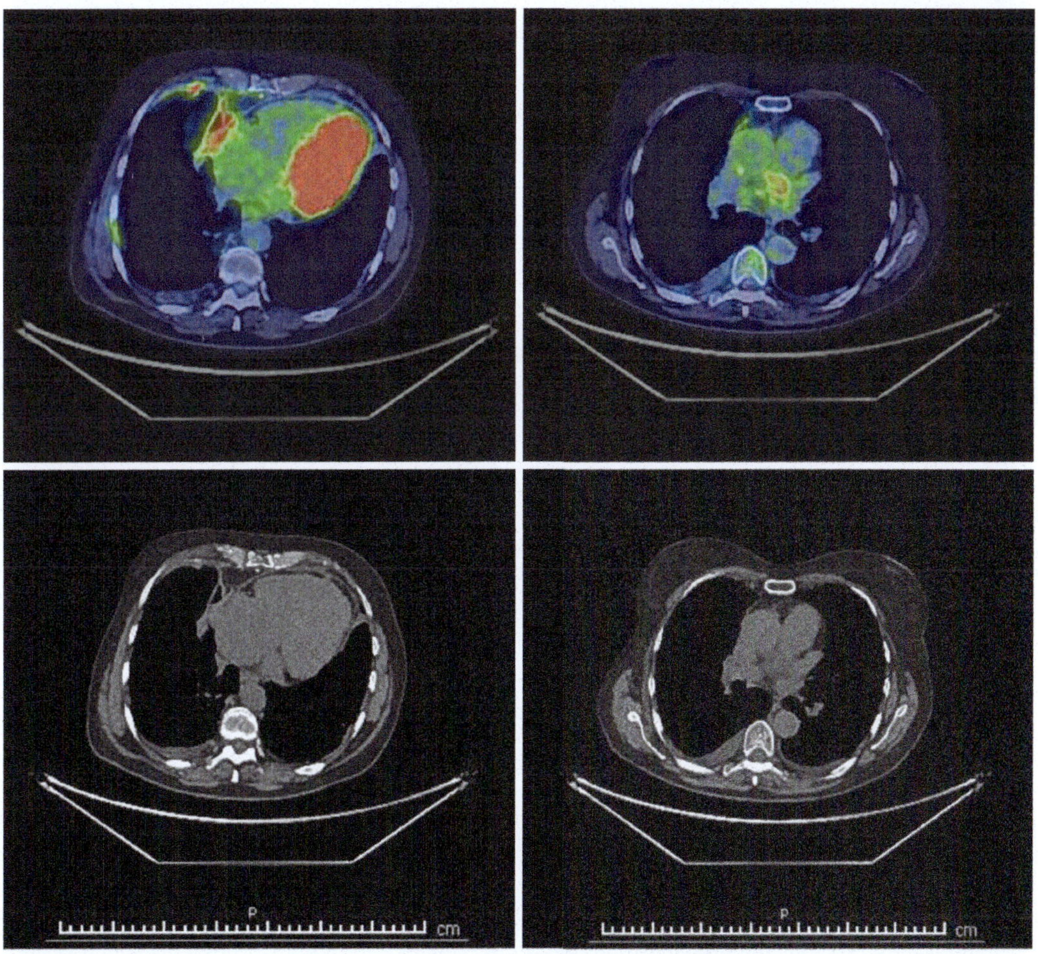

Fig. 22.1 Positron emission tomography (PET) and computed tomographic (CT) imaging of a pericardial mesothelioma

often negative for malignant cells and shows only signs of inflammation, mainly activated mesothelial cells aggregated in papillary structures. Therefore, most of PM are diagnosed postmortem [4]. As for pleural and peritoneal mesotheliomas, also for PM three histological subtypes have been recognized, i.e., epithelial, sarcomatous, and biphasic, being the epithelioid histotype the most common as for the other primary sites.

The median age at diagnosis is 55.5 years (range 22–87) with a male-to-female ratio of 3:1 at all ages [16]. PM tended to be diagnosed in younger patients with respect to pleural mesothelioma. The prognosis is dismal and the median survival is approximately 5–7 months [8].

PM may spread locally, invading the myocardium and the surrounding tissues, such as the pleura and lungs, or can metastasize to lymph nodes and distant organs (e.g., liver, bone, and brain). Treatment is mostly palliative and may include surgery approaches, i.e., pericardiotomy that may result in immediate, but temporary, relief of constrictive symptoms, pericardiectomy, surgical excision of the macroscopic tumor (frequently incomplete), radiotherapy, and chemotherapy according to the protocols adopted in malignant pleural mesothelioma providing only little clinical benefit [17].

The etiology is rarely investigated, thus the potential role of risk factors for PM development has been only suspected. Smoking habits, therapeutic ionizing radiation, chemotherapeutic treatment, and cardiovascular disease were deduced from the patient's clinical history as potential risk factors [8]. Moreover, factors that may play a role include genetic predisposition, immune impairment, infections, dietary factors, and recurrent serosal inflammation.

22.3 Primary Intrahepatic Malignant Mesothelioma

PIHMM has not been yet included in the World Health Organization (WHO) classification of hepatic tumors [18]. The PIHMM clinic pathological characteristics remain to be elucidated. Pain and weight loss are common at presentation while cough can be caused by the irritation of the diaphragm. Fever usually occurs secondary to tumor necrosis and the lesion has been sometimes confused with hepatic abscesses. Preoperative anemia affects at least one-third of patients (5/15). This finding represents a new and important association and is likely due to intra-lesional bleeding. Imaging studies (Fig. 22.2) and tissues biopsies with histology examination (in particular positive immunohistochemistry for calretinin and vimentin) should be included as preoperative evaluation to perform a correct diagnosis. Although difficult, it is important to establish a differential diagnosis preoperatively between primary and secondary hepatic cancer (i.e., hepatocellular carcinoma, cholangiocarcinoma, and adenocarcinoma that metastasized from an unknown site) because many cancers with the metastatic liver lesions usually need chemotherapy prior to surgery [9].

Histologically, three different patterns can be distinguished for PIHMM: epithelial, sarcomatous, and biphasic. Two-third (66.7%) of the patients show epithelioid histology, while the rest is biphasic (26.7%) and only one is sarcomatoid. Approximately, 50% of patients with PIHMM are male and the mean age at onset is 60.4 (range 41–83 years) [9].

PIHMM is usually located peripherally and invades deeper into the liver as it continues to grow. It may involve the diaphragm. Surgery when technically feasible is the mainstay of treatment. Radiation therapy can be only delivered in selective patients with localized tumor and systemic treatment with pemetrexed-based chemotherapy can only achieve partial remission and as only a palliative role.

22.4 Mesothelioma of the Tunica Vaginalis Testis

MTVT was described for the first time in 1957 [19]. It is often a fatal type of testicular malignancy. The clinical presentation is non-specific; insidious and painless enlargement of the scrotum with recurrent hydrocele occurs in more than half of patients and testicular or paratesticular mass is

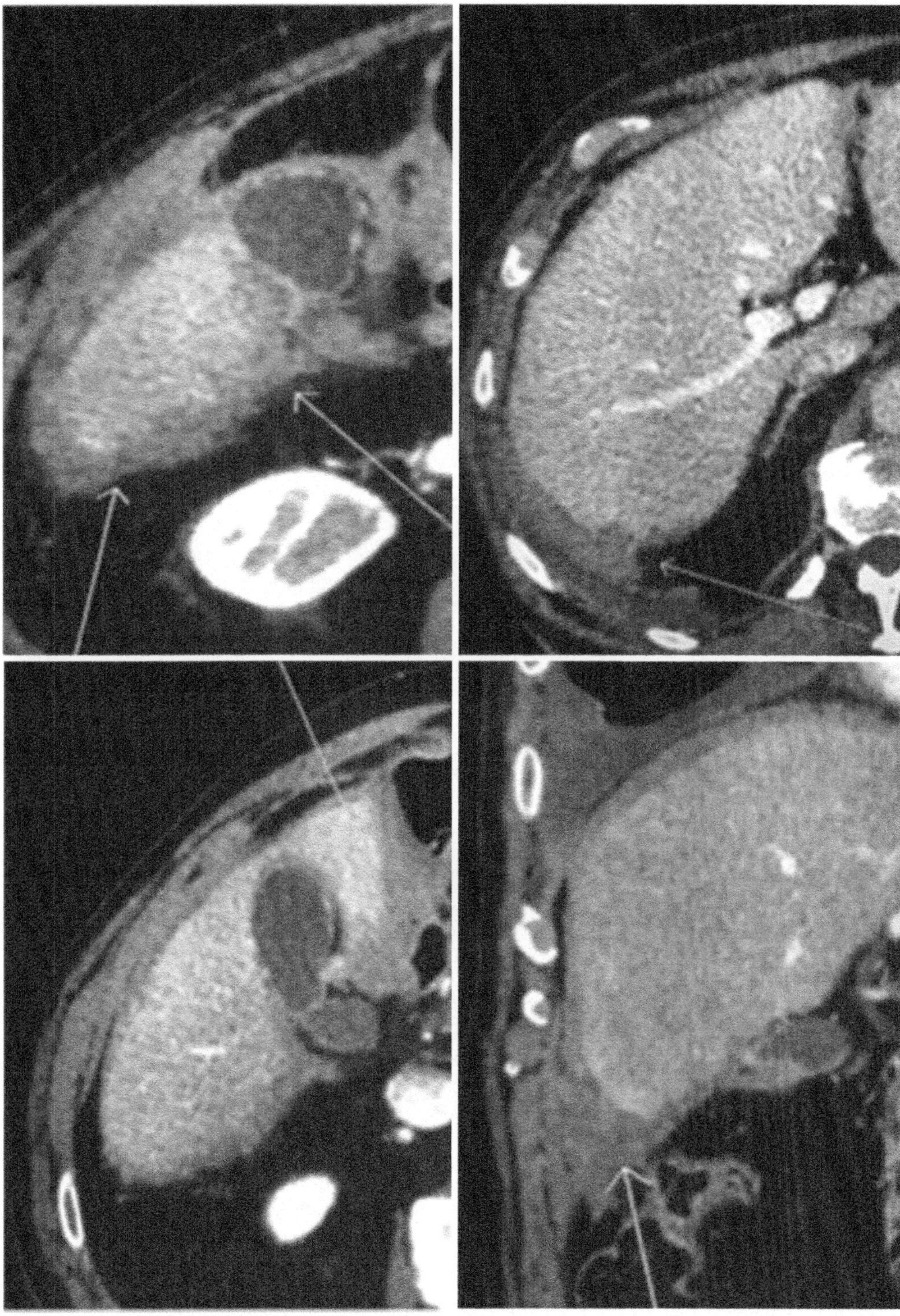

Fig. 22.2 CT imaging of a mesothelioma arising from Glisson's capsule

present in approximately one-third. Thickening of the tunica vaginalis is an important sign of this disease. Most of MTVTs are unilateral.

As with PM, cytological analysis has low sensitivity, thus a preoperative diagnosis is rarely obtained. Immunohistochemistry shows positivity to the same tumor markers that are used to diagnose pleural mesothelioma, i.e., calretinin, Wilms tumor antibody, D2-40, epithelial membrane antigen, thrombomodulin, and cytokeratin 7. Moreover, MTVTs are usually negative for immunohistochemical markers Ber-EP4, carcinoembryonic antigen (CEA), Leu-M1, and tumor-associated glycoprotein (TAG-72). Ultrasound plays an important role for preoperative diagnosis because ultrasonographic imaging shows specific features, i.e., focalized thickening of tunica vaginalis with nodules, multiple paratesticular nodular masses, multiple nonhomogeneous nodular masses attached to the tunica vaginalis, and tumor with mixed echogenicity associated with hydrocele [20]. Actually, most of the cases are identified intra-operatively on the basis of hemorrhagic hydrocele fluid, white-yellow nodules or papillary excrescences of the TVT, or fibrotic thickening of the TVT.

MTVT is mainly epithelial with papillary, tubule-papillary, or solid pattern and sometimes is biphasic and sarcomatoid. The mean age at diagnosis is 58 years and the median is 63.5 (range from 7 to 91 years) [8].

MTVT may invade the testis and frequently extends to the internal ring. Retroperitoneal or inguinal metastasis may occur if the testis is invaded or if vascular invasion is present.

Surgery, radiotherapy, and chemotherapy are the main treatment options for MTVTs and the multimodal treatment approaches are often offered to patients with advanced disease. Surgical intervention represents the treatment of choice and consists of radical orchiectomy and complete excision of the spermatic cord and hemiscrotum [21]. Cisplatin and pemetrexed may be used as chemotherapy. The prognosis is poor, with median survival of 23 months (range 2–64 months) [22].

The pathogenesis is still unclear. History of prior condition in the testicular area, i.e., long-term inguinal hernia or herniorrhaphy, long-standing hydrocele, or long-term spermatocele has been reported as potential risk factors. Trauma, inguinal inflammation, long-term epididymitis, orchitis, herniorrhaphy, inguinal infection, and tobacco smoking have all been also implicated as predisposing factors. As with PM, localized ionizing radiation and genetic predisposition have been proposed as potential risk factors for MTVT [8]. However, as with other EPMMs, no epidemiological studies of risk factors for MTVT have been so far identified.

22.5 Conclusions

PM, PIHMM, and MTVT are very rare tumors and account for less than 1% of all mesothelioma cases, according to registry data and the literature review. The Italian ReNaM and the United States SEER program reported the estimated standardized incidence rates only of PM and MTVT. These rare localizations of mesothelioma have not been much investigated because of their low prevalence. In literature, only a limited number of review, case reports, and case series have been found. The epidemiology of rare cancers is still poorly studied and the treatment of these exceptional presentations of MM poses many challenges and difficulties to clinicians. To date, no epidemiological case-control studies or cohort studies have been performed in order to identify their incidence and etiological risk factors.

The etiological role of asbestos exposure has been hypothesized for EPMMs. They share the same embryological origin (mesothelium) of pleura and peritoneum. Thus, it was speculated that asbestos fibers might reach the anatomical sites in two different ways: penetrating the pleura after inhalation and then being transported by lymphatic flow or reaching the blood stream and subsequently being distributed to the whole body [23]. The literature rarely reports asbestos exposure in patients with these malignancies. For PM, 30% of case reports published have some potential, suspected, or confirmed history of asbestos exposure although few details are provided [8]. Based on Italian ReNaM, patients with PM, and

MTVT mainly show occupational asbestos exposure (approximately 43 and 54%, respectively). In spite of this, there are no cases in asbestos-cement industry, in shipbuilding and railway industries and there is only a case of MTVT in national defense (i.e., the highest risk economic sectors in which asbestos exposure is significant and in which the highest rates of pleural mesothelioma are seen). The absence of exposures in these traditional sectors is evident and not easy to explain, thus it needs to be confirmed in a larger sample. Therefore, the available evidences are not sufficient to suggest an association between inhaled asbestos exposure and the development of PM and MTVT [24]. Review of the literature disclosed only 15 previously reported adult cases of PIHMM. Only one patient showed occupational exposure to asbestos [9].

As with pleural mesothelioma, other risk factors are discussed in the etiology of these EPMMs (e.g., exposure to therapeutic ionizing radiation and genetic predisposition). Radiation therapy is mentioned as part of the medical history for few patients presenting with either PM or MTVT [8]. Patients received irradiation for previous malignancies (e.g., breast cancer, Hodgkin, and non-Hodgkin lymphomas). A germline predisposition to mesothelioma has been previously described [25]. Patients with germline mutations at the *BAP1* gene show a large risk of developing an inherited cancer syndrome that includes different tumors, among which pleural and peritoneal mesotheliomas [26–29]. Although these mutations have not yet been found in patients with EPMM, it is not unreasonable to expect that they may play a role in the pathogenesis of these tumors.

Because of the low sensitivity and the poor specificity of the diagnosis, EPMMs can be extremely challenging to diagnose for clinicians, often resulting in numerous physician visits, misdiagnoses, and substantial delays in diagnosis. The National Comprehensive Cancer Network evidence-based cancer guidelines made no recommendations for their management. EPMMs have a non-specific and atypical clinical presentation, thus the diagnosis may be demanding and often establish post-operative or post-mortem. Physical examination, imaging studies, pathological examination, and immunohistochemical staining are required to confirm the diagnosis of EPMMs. Information about asbestos exposure is important because it could raise the possibilities of a correct mesothelioma diagnosis.

A standard treatment does not exist and the vast majority of cases with advanced disease can be treated with palliative systemic treatment only using the same regimen as for malignant pleural mesothelioma. Locoregional approaches can have a role in palliating symptoms in PM whereas more extensive surgeries with curative intent should be offered within multimodal approaches to patients with localized PIHMM or MTVT.

Global efforts, such as prospective registry for these exceptional presentations should be strongly encouraged to improve clinical knowledge about their clinical history, prognostic, and predictive factors and to help clinicians to choose the best treatment for each patient.

Acknowledgments We wish to thank Misischi Francesca for PET and CT imaging.

References

1. Volpe JK, Makaryus AN (2018) Anatomy, chest, heart and pericardial cavity.
2. Recabal P, Rosenzweig B, Bazzi WM, Carver BS, Sheinfeld J. Malignant mesothelioma of the tunica Vaginalis testis: outcomes following surgical management beyond radical orchiectomy. Urology. 2017;107:166–70.
3. Garriga V, Serrano A, Marin A, Medrano S, Roson N, Pruna X. US of the tunica vaginalis testis: anatomic relationships and pathologic conditions. Radiographics. 2009;29:2017–32.
4. Hassan R, Alexander R. Nonpleural mesotheliomas: mesothelioma of the peritoneum, tunica vaginalis, and pericardium. Hematol Oncol Clin North Am. 2005;19:1067–87. vi.
5. Su S-S, Zheng G-Q, Liu Y-G, Chen Y-F, Song Z-W, Yu S-J, Sun N-N, Yang Y-X. Malignant peritoneum mesothelioma with hepatic involvement: a single institution experience in 5 patients and review of the literature. Gastroenterol Res Pract. 2016;2016:1–12. 6242149.
6. Sasaki M, Araki I, Yasui T, Kinoshita M, Itatsu K, Nojima T, Nakanuma Y. Primary localized malignant biphasic mesothelioma of the liver in a patient with asbestosis. World J Gastroenterol. 2009;15:615–21.

7. Registro Nazionale dei Mesoteliomi - V Rapporto - Edizioni INAIL. 2015.
8. Mezei G, Chang ET, Mowat FS, Moolgavkar SH. Epidemiology of mesothelioma of the pericardium and tunica vaginalis testis. Ann Epidemiol. 2017;27:348–359.e11.
9. Ismael H, Cox S. Primary intrahepatic mesotheliomas: a case presentation and literature review. Int J Surg Case Rep. 2018;47:1–6.
10. Straif K, Benbrahim-Tallaa L, Baan R, et al. A review of human carcinogens--part C: metals, arsenic, dusts, and fibres. Lancet Oncol. 2009;10:453–4.
11. Rizzardi C, Barresi E, Brollo A, Cassetti P, Schneider M, Melato M. Primary pericardial mesothelioma in an asbestos-exposed patient with previous heart surgery. Anticancer Res. 2010;30:1323–5.
12. Fujiwara H, Kamimori T, Morinaga K, Takeda Y, Kohyama N, Miki Y, Inai K, Yamamoto S. An autopsy case of primary pericardial mesothelioma in arc cutter exposed to asbestos through talc pencils. Ind Health. 2005;43:346–50.
13. Churg A, Warnock ML, Bensch KG. Malignant mesothelioma arising after direct application of asbestos and fiber glass to the pericardium. Am Rev Respir Dis. 1978;118:419–24.
14. Warren WH. Malignancies involving the pericardium. Semin Thorac Cardiovasc Surg. 2000;12:119–29.
15. Tateishi K, Ikeda M, Yokoyama T, Urushihata K, Yamamoto H, Hanaoka M, Kubo K, Sakai Y, Nakayama J, Koizumi T. Primary malignant sarcomatoid mesothelioma in the pericardium. Intern Med. 2013;52:249–53.
16. Mensi C, Giacomini S, Sieno C, Consonni D, Riboldi L. Pericardial mesothelioma and asbestos exposure. Int J Hyg Environ Health. 2011;214:276–9.
17. Eren NT, Akar AR. Primary pericardial mesothelioma. Curr Treat Options in Oncol. 2002;3:369–73.
18. Haji Ali R, Khalife M, El Nounou G, Zuhri Yafi R, Nassar H, Aidibe Z, Raad R, Abou Eid R, Faraj W. Giant primary malignant mesothelioma of the liver: a case report. Int J Surg Case Rep. 2017;30:58–61.
19. Barbera V, Rubino M. Papillary mesothelioma of the tunica vaginalis. Cancer. 10:183–9.
20. Segura-González M, Urias-Rocha J, Castelán-Pedraza J. Malignant mesothelioma of the tunica Vaginalis: a rare neoplasm--case report and literature review. Clin Genitourin Cancer. 2015;13:e401–5.
21. DeVita VT, Lawrence TS, Rosenberg SA. DeVita, Hellman, and Rosenberg's cancer: principles & practice of oncology (vol. 2, p. lxxii, 1485, I-112), Philadelphia: Wolters Kluwer/Lippincott Williams & Wilkins; 2008.
22. Chekol SS, Sun C-C. Malignant mesothelioma of the tunica vaginalis testis: diagnostic studies and differential diagnosis. Arch Pathol Lab Med. 2012;136:113–7.
23. Miserocchi G, Sancini G, Mantegazza F, Chiappino G. Translocation pathways for inhaled asbestos fibers. Environ Health. 2008;7:4.
24. Marinaccio A, Binazzi A, Di Marzio D, et al. Incidence of extrapleural malignant mesothelioma and asbestos exposure, from the Italian national register. Occup Environ Med. 2010;67:760–5.
25. Testa JR, Cheung M, Pei J, et al. Germline BAP1 mutations predispose to malignant mesothelioma. Nat Genet. 2011;43:1022–5.
26. Betti M, Casalone E, Ferrante D, et al. Inference on germline BAP1 mutations and asbestos exposure from the analysis of familial and sporadic mesothelioma in a high-risk area. Genes Chromosomes Cancer. 2015;54:51–62.
27. Ribeiro C, Campelos S, Moura CS, Machado JC, Justino A, Parente B. Well-differentiated papillary mesothelioma: clustering in a Portuguese family with a germline BAP1 mutation. Ann Oncol Off J Eur Soc Med Oncol. 2013;24:2147–50.
28. Ohar JA, Cheung M, Talarchek J, Howard SE, Howard TD, Hesdorffer M, Peng H, Rauscher FJ, Testa JR. Germline BAP1 mutational landscape of Asbestos-exposed malignant mesothelioma patients with family history of cancer. Cancer Res. 2016;76:206–15.
29. Kittaneh M, Berkelhammer C. Detecting germline BAP1 mutations in patients with peritoneal mesothelioma: benefits to patient and family members. J Transl Med. 2018;16:194.

23 Unmet Needs and Future Outlook of Mesothelioma Management

Dean A. Fennell

23.1 Overcoming the Therapeutic Plateau in Mesothelioma

Despite all of the research efforts during the last one and a half decades, mesothelioma remains a cancer lacking effective therapy after first-line treatment. This is clearly a huge unmet need. This chapter will discuss how this problem is being currently addressed and some of the key clinical research trajectories being taken to meet this challenge.

There have been bold attempts to develop treatments in the relapsed setting in well-designed large randomized clinical trials. To date, none of these have been positive. A major hurdle in developing effective therapy is *phenotypic diversity*. Mesothelioma is a mosaic that comprises genomically diverse subtypes. Presently, molecular stratification of treatments for mesothelioma is in its infancy. However, targeted approaches are emerging that may provide important opportunities to selectively and effectively treat patients, based on protein, DNA, or methylation specific tests. Some of the more important advances will be discussed.

Third, our knowledge of mesothelioma and its biology is changing rapidly. This is driven by the informatics revolution and global collaborative efforts such as the tumour genome atlas (TCGA) and other large scale genomic profiling efforts. Coupled to platforms capable of screening for drug–gene interactions, exciting opportunities exist to not only lay bare the most promising molecular targets, but also to generate drug-gene interaction hypotheses that can be tested in the laboratory, in order to translate into the clinical setting.

Finally, the immunotherapy revolution has transformed the treatment of another thoracic cancer (non-small cell). Can this happen for mesothelioma? I believe that the answer is "Almost certainly"; the international consensus internationally being "yes." This is evident from the emerging early phase data for immunotherapy. However, to approve treatment, large well designed randomized phase III trials are needed, coupled with biomarkers capable of enriching patients likely to benefit.

23.2 Inter-Patient Genomic Heterogeneity: A Barrier to a One Size Fits All Approach

Identifying an approved therapy for mesothelioma in the relapsed setting has proven an insurmountable challenge to date. Three key reasons underpinning this failure are as follows.

Perhaps the most important factor has been insufficient efficacy across an unselected

D. A. Fennell (✉)
Leicester Mesothelioma Research Programme, University of Leicester and University Hospitals of Leicester NHS Trust, Leicester, UK
e-mail: df132@le.ac.uk

G. L. Ceresoli et al. (eds.), *Mesothelioma*, https://doi.org/10.1007/978-3-030-16884-1_23

population. Addressing this problem requires research investment, to deal with mesothelioma specific biological features and optimal ways to have them targeted. To date, there has been limited investment in mesothelioma drug-discovery research, increasing the level of challenge.

Second, inter-patient heterogeneity. Mesothelioma comprises three major morphological subgroups which exhibit a spectrum of aggressiveness, increasing from epithelioid through biphasic to sarcomatoid. By amalgamating these subtypes into a single group as has been the case in most studies historically, attempts to uncover efficacy signals may have been thwarted by dilutional effects of the inter-patient heterogeneity. For example, in the context of a well-designed randomized placebo-controlled clinical trials, patients with indolent or slow growing mesothelioma, may do relatively well in time-to-event analyses. Similarly, in the absence of an efficacious control arm, the paucity of double blind placebo or active symptom controlled randomised controlled trials may have contributed to a failure in identifying potentially active treatments. Looking back at early lung cancer development, for example, early incremental changes in therapy in the relapsed setting depended on this approach [1, 2].

Recent studies involving genomic interrogation have greatly increased our understanding of how somatic genomic landscape of mesotheliomas differ between individuals, the impact of these genetic changes on tumour behaviour [3], and the implications for drug-based interventions. Bueno et al. have conducted the largest genomic interrogation of mesothelioma to date [4], involving the analysis of 99 whole exomes, and 103 targeted exomes from 216 patients. In common with earlier, smaller, yet seminal studies of inter-patient genomic heterogeneity [5, 6], recurrent mutations, and copy number alterations were observed in consensus cancer genes *BAP1*, NF2 with evidence of high-frequency CDKN2A deletions, respectively. Based on the catalogue of somatic mutations in cancer (COSMIC) as well as mesothelioma specific transformation studies [7, 8] and transgenic mouse data [9], NF2, BAP1, and CDKN2A are among the most common genomic aberrations in mesothelioma, that are most likely cancer drivers for which targeted strategies could be applied. Gene-dosage effects are evident with concurrent involvement of more than driver conferring a more aggressive phenotype [9].

Studies reveal a complex genomic architecture of mesothelioma, with individual gene harbouring diverse alterations such as fusions, single nucleotide variants, fusions and copy number variation (including microdeletions); as exemplified by inactivation of BAP1. In this example, inactivation correlates with a loss of nuclear expression (or in the case of deletion, loss of expression). Accordingly, protein expression patterns revealed by immunohistochemistry may provide the most pragmatic single assay to assay putative function, in order to serve as a predictive biomarker [10–12] in stratified clinical trials. In the case of NF2, inactivation can occur by a two-hit mechanism involving both allelic loss and mutation [13]; furthermore, NF2 inactivation may be phenocopied by mutations in the same pathway involving LATS2, RASSF1, and SAV1 [14], again challenging the choice of biomarker for therapy stratification.

Availability of whole exome sequencing data has enabled exploration of therapeutically tractable subsets. For example, microsatellite instability (MSI) involving hypermutation caused by defects in the mismatch repair system has been reported to occur at low frequency (<3%), in mesothelioma [15] as estimated by the genomic tool, MANTIS. MSI is associated with a higher neoantigen burden, tumour inflammation, and higher sensitivity to anti-PD1 immunotherapy. Recent Federal Drug Administration approval for the PD1 inhibitor pembrolizumab in MSI-high tumours was the first such site-agnostic approval that could potentially benefit a small fraction of patients with mesothelioma. A recent report exploring MMR deficiency in mesothelioma has failed to identify MSI in a cohort of 329 mesotheliomas as inferred by combined immunohistochemistry and multiplexed microsatellite markers [16]. Collectively MSI appears to be a rare event, unlikely to explain the limited responses to immunotherapy, reported in mesothelioma and discussed in more detail below.

Homologous DNA repair deficiency (HRD) associated with inactivation of the tumour suppressor BRCA1 confers synthetic lethality to PARP inhibitors [17, 18]. Although not mutated in mesothelioma, BRCA1 protein expression is variable in mesothelioma, with loss seen in 38% of patients [19].

In the context of mesothelioma, a positive HRD has been found to correlate with poor prognosis, and in one study 10 out of 82 patients were found to have at least one core gene altered in the homologous repair pathway. It is not known whether such patients might exhibit sensitivity to PARP inhibition [20]. BAP1 has been implicated as a regulator of BRCA1, with mutation leading to lower expression [21]. Coupled to evidence implicating BAP1 in homologous recombination [21], this raises the possibility that BAP1 may confer a HRD phenotype in mesothelioma. Recent preclinical studies have shown that PARP inhibitors do in fact have significant single-agent activity in cell lines. The precise mechanisms underpinning this phenotype and whether or not this translates into the clinic have yet to be determined.

Hassan et al. have recently reported that 12% of patients (29 out of 239) with mesothelioma have a germline pathogenic defect in a core DNA repair gene (screening for 73). These included *BAP1* (*N* = 17 pts), *CHEK2* (*N* = 5), *PALB2* (*N* = 2), and BRCA1, MLH1, POT1, TP53, and MRE11A (*N* = 1 each). Notably, all patients harbouring the BAP1 germline mutations (7%) harboured a second mutation predicted to lead to complete inactivation. Based on this, the team has initiated a clinical trial to explore the efficacy of the PARP inhibitior olaparib in mesothelioma, NCT03531840.

23.3 Rare Genomic Events and Therapeutic Opportunity

A subset of cancer genes harbouring inactivation events arises at relatively high frequency in mesothelioma (CDKN2A, BAP1, NF2). Recent interrogation of the genomic landscape has revealed rare events that may be therapeutically tractable. Analysis of genes undergoing positive selection (dN/dS > 1) that are potentially involved in transformation as cancer drivers, revealed three cancer genes which were present below 10%; SETD2, LATS1, and protein patched homolog 1 (PTCH1). The latter having potential as a therapeutic target [22].

PTCH1 (protein patched homolog 1) is a tumour suppressor and receptor for sonic hedgehog, a secreted molecule involved in tumourigenesis, that upon binding PTCH1, leads to the release of the G protein-coupled receptor, smoothened protein (SMO) which then signals cell proliferation. PTCH1 normally suppresses the release of SMO. Pathogenic mutations in PTCH1 are frequently found in basal cell carcinoma and can be therapeutically targeted [23, 24] leading to significant tumour regressions. Accordingly, mesotheliomas harbouring PTCH1 might be susceptible to such inhibitors. Preclinical evidence of activity of the Hedgehog (Hh) antagonist vismodegib has been recently reported [25–27], consistent with other reports of constitutive Hh pathway signalling in mesothelioma. The potential role for PTCH1 driver mutations as a dependency on Hh signalling has yet to be explored. SMO and SUFO mutations involved in Hh signalling have been identified in preclinical models of mesothelioma, suggesting that Hh may be activated by mechanisms other than PTCH1 mutation [28].

Mutated epidermal growth receptor (EGFR) is an established molecular target for treatment of lung adenocarcinoma. Early studies of the EGFR tyrosine kinase inhibitor (TKI) in mesothelioma, failed to show activity, despite there being evidence of EGFR overexpression in 97% of patients. Pathogenic EGFR mutations confer addiction to EGFR TKI [29, 30]. In mesothelioma, such mutations are rare but have been described [31–33]. To date, there is no evidence to suggest that mutations of EGFR in mesothelioma exhibit addiction and clinical sensitivity to specific EGFR TKIs.

In common with EGFR, rearrangement of the Anaplastic lymphoma kinase (ALK) gene (most commonly, EML4-ALK) is an established molecular target for stratified therapy in lung adenocarcinoma [34–37]. Recent analysis of 88 patients with peritoneal mesothelioma has revealed 13% of patients with positive anaplastic lymphoma kinase (ALK). Strong expression was associated with ALK rearrangements comprising novel fusion partners STRN, TPM1, and ATG16L [38]. Interestingly, these mesotheliomas lacked common driver mutations in CDKN2A, BAP1, NF2, or SETD2 suggesting mutual exclusivity. ALK rearrangements were associated with younger women and not associated with pleural mesothelioma. As with EGFR there is no evidence reported to date to suggest that these novel rearrangements confer addiction to ALK inhibitors either in the laboratory or clinical settings; however, therapeutic potential is a possibility awaiting exploration.

The evolutionary timing of rare mutations is a major factor in determining therapeutic potential. Such mutations may occur late in the natural history and appear as a branch mutation [39]. Such mutations will not be present throughout the tumour and, therefore, targeting may not confer the significant therapeutic benefit seen in lung cancer in the case of EGFR or ALK, or basal cell carcinoma (PTCH1). Understanding the evolutionary timing of putative drugable mutations and their spatial heterogeneity will be crucial in defining potential as an oncogenic dependency. Such a study has been undertaken in non-small cell lung cancer and renal Cancer, prefixed TraceRx [40–43]. In the context of malignant pleural mesothelioma, systematic interrogation of the intratumour genomic heterogeneity is warranted to help catalogue and segregate clonal versus non-clonal events.

23.4 Emergence of Personalised Therapy for Mesothelioma

Examples of mesothelioma stratification are emerging and beginning to enter the clinical arena with some early signals of efficacy. Perhaps the most advanced in terms of drug development, is the targeting of argininosuccinate synthetase 1 (ASS1) negative mesothelioma. This enzyme is involved in the synthesis of arginine from citrulline, the penultimate step in the arginine biosynthesis pathway. Because normal cells can synthesize arginine via this route, it is termed a non-essential amino acid. It has been shown, however, that the ASS1 expression is lost in a significant proportion of mesotheliomas [44]. These mesotheliomas lose the ability to generate arginine and become auxotrophic, that is, it becomes an essential amino acid and a *metabolic dependency* or addiction.

Denying arginine from ASS1 negative mesotheliomas leads to induction of apoptosis. Early preclinical studies highlighted a potential therapeutic pathway based on pharmacological manipulation of circulating arginine [44]. This can be achieved by catalytic degradation using pegylated enzyme arginine deiminase (ADI PEG20). This concept was translated into the clinic in the ADAM study [45] in which patients were randomised to either ADI PEG20 or active symptom control. The study met its primary endpoint, progression-free survival with a hazard ratio of 0.56. Evidence of metabolic response was seen [46]. Loss of ASS1 was correlated with promoter methylation and the level of ASS1 silencing was correlated with efficacy. Subsequent studies revealed a correlation between loss of ASS1 expression and resistance to platinum (in ovarian cell lines) [47]. Based on the potential synergy with platinum, a phase 1 clinical trial (TRAP) was conducted confirming the safety of ADI-PEG20/pemetrexed-cisplatin [48]. Based on this study and the finding that ASS1 deficiency has its highest frequency in biphasic and sarcomatoid mesotheliomas, a global phase II/III randomised clinical trial has been initiated called ATOMIC, that has been designed to evaluate the additional benefit of ADI-PEG20 with chemotherapy (NCT02709512).

Targeting of ASS1 represents a rare example of a rational strategy for treating mesotheliomas that have progressed stepwise from the bench to the bedside. Loss of ASS1 expression occurs via an epigenetic mechanism. Demethylation of ASS1 is a key mechanism underlying acquired resistance demonstrating plasticity of the target. However, this resistance is accompanied by a switch in metabolic dependence from arginine to polyamine biosynthesis [49]. An increase in polyamine metabolites is seen in ASS1 deficient patients who become resistant to ADI-PEG20 and a synthetic lethal relationship exists between polyamine metabolism and ASS1 negativity, implicating a novel strategy for treating these cancers.

BAP1 mutation was originally identified in two seminal publications, which identified both germline and somatic inactivating events in this tumour suppressor gene [5, 6]. BAP1 cooperates with the polycomb complex PRC2, to modify the epigenome via trimethylation of histone H3 (at aspartate 23). Levine's group showed that this BAP1 mediated upregulation of PRC2 requires the methyltransferase activity of EZH2, and confers sensitivity to inhibition of EZH2 both in vitro and in vivo [50]. Based on these observations, a phase II clinical trial of the EZH2 inhibitor tazemetostat was enrolled in patients with BAP1 inactivated mesothelioma (evidenced by immunohistochemistry - NCT02860286). This study was recently reported at ASCO 2018 to have met its primary endpoint, 12-week disease control, suggesting that targeting EZH2 in mesothelioma may exhibit clinically meaningful activity. This study represents the first prospectively stratified clinical trial based on targeting of a commonly mutated tumour suppressor.

23.5 Leveraging Large Scale Informatics Data to Identify New Therapeutic Approaches

Large scale efforts are underway to decipher both novel cancer dependencies and drug-gene interactions that could serve as hypotheses for future proof-of-concept early clinical trials [51–54]. Such efforts have potential to reveal new ways to target common mutations present in mesothelioma. One prominent example of this is the discovery of protein arginine methyltransferase 5 (PRMT5) as a synthetic lethal target in methylthioadenosine phosphorylase (MTAP) deleted cancers [55–57]. This genomic event occurs frequently in mesotheliomas and several other cancers and is associated with homozygous deletion of a region of the short arm of chromosome 9 (9p21.1). This deletion carries not only CDKN2A which encodes the tumour suppressors p16ink4A (inhibitor of CDK4/6) and p14ARF (inhibitor of MDM2) along with MTAP. Complete deletion of MTAP was shown to perturb the metabolic levels of methylthioadenosine (MTA), inhibiting PRMT5 and increasing the susceptibility of PRMT5 to exogenous inhibition. In contrast to previous failed efforts to identify synthetic lethal strategies for MTAP deleted mesothelioma using L-alanosine [58, 59], an approach targeting the MTAP-PRMT5 synthetic lethal relationship, could be potentially exploited therapeutically.

Homozygous deletion of chromosome 9p21.2 CDKN2A2 leads to loss of expression of p16ink4a, the endogenous inhibitor of cell division kinase (CDK) regulators 4 and 6 [60]. CDK4/6 drive the cell cycle transition through the G1/S checkpoint by inhibiting the tumour suppressor, retinoblastoma protein (Rb) via its phosphorylation leading to dissociation of the E2F transcription factor. Accordingly, loss of p16inka enhances CDK4/6 mediated Rb phosphorylation and proliferation, contributing to transformation. CDKN2A deletion is negatively prognostic in mesothelioma [61, 62]. In contrast, large scale pan-cancer pharmacogenomics studies have revealed a statistically robust, strong association between CDKN2A deletion and sensitivity to CDK4/6 inhibition [52]. As expected, this interaction is blocked by Rb mutation, which carries a very low mutation rate of 1.22% in mesothelioma.

The use of pharmacogenomically profiled cell lines to reveal potential vulnerabilities has been applied recently in the context of mesothelioma. The DR5 receptor (TRAIL receptor) was shown to be a potential drug target in BAP1 mutated mesotheliomas in vitro, in vivo, and in ex vivo mesothelioma explants [63]. This raises the potential of a drug which has to date not demonstrated significant efficacy in unselected cancers.

Using this same high throughput screening approach, fibroblast growth factor receptor inhibition was also shown to be sensitized by BAP1 mutation [64]. Both of these strategies that target BAP1 are therapeutically tractable, increasing the potential for BAP1 to be leveraged as a predictive biomarker.

Collectively, the growth of data linking somatic mutations in mesothelioma to drug sensitivity provides the basis for expanding the repertoire of prospectively stratified clinical trials. One such model to explore multiple hypotheses in the clinical setting is the umbrella study [65], examples of which are currently underway in non-small cell lung cancer [66]. As an example, the British Lung Foundation funded MiST trial [67] will evaluate novel therapies in the context of BAP1, BRCA1, p16INK4A, and PDL1 stratification with the goal of acquiring early phase efficacy signals in a prospective molecularly stratified context.

23.6 The Immunotherapy Revolution and Mesothelioma: Key Challenges

Targeting PD1 and PDL1 has led to a paradigm shift in the treatment of multiple cancers including non-small cell lung cancer where there have been multiple changes in the standard of care in a record time interval [68–74]. Disabling the PD1 inhibitory checkpoint in mesothelioma has demonstrated encouraging activity in the relapsed setting. The first prospective report of anti-PD1 activity [75] in 25 patients with >1% PDL1 expression, showed a 20% objective response rate with a 76% disease control rate. Those patients exhibiting a response went on to have a median duration of 12 months. Similarly, the PD1 inhibitor Nivolumab exhibits single-agent activity in unselected mesothelioma [76]; in a single centre phase 2 trial, 34 patients were enrolled to receive nivolumab. Twelve-week disease control rate was 47% (the study met its primary endpoint) with an associated 24% partial response rate. Interestingly, PDL1 was not found to correlate with outcome.

Accordingly, in neither study (representing the only published prospective phase II studies of anti-PD1 therapy to date), there is no definitive verdict on the role of PDL1 as a biomarker. Randomised trials will be needed to rigorously establish the interaction between PDL1 expression and efficacy; this is because PDL1 is significantly associated with worse prognosis in mesothelioma [77]. If PDL1 is indeed positively predictive and negatively prognostic, this should increase the chances of detecting an efficacy signal. CONFIRM (NCT03063450) is an ongoing phase III trial evaluating nivolumab versus placebo in patients with relapsed mesothelioma [78] and PROMISE (NCT02991482) is comparing pembrolizumab versus chemotherapy (gemcitabine or vinorelbine). These large randomised studies will provide more robust evidence regarding efficacy of immunotherapy and also the value of PDL1 as a biomarker.

Recent studies have revealed synergistic interactions between anti-PD1 therapy and different combination treatments, leading to changes in the standard of care in other cancer settings such as melanoma [79] and lung cancer [80, 81]. Targeting CTLA4 alone in mesothelioma has been robustly demonstrated as being inactive in a large randomised phase III trial [72, 82]. However, there is compelling evidence to suggest that combining with anti-PD1 or anti-PDL1 therapy could be clinically useful. An early phase single arm trial has reported activity of CTLA4 PDL1 combination therapy in relapsed mesothelioma with durvalumab/tremelimumab [83] demonstrating a 28% response rate with a median response duration of 16 months. The MAPS2 (IFCT-1501) clinical trial randomised nivolumab and ipilimumab versus nivolumab alone, reported an incremental disease control rates (42.6% versus 51.9%), consistent with there being a synergistic interaction [84], which has led to an orphan drug designation by the US Food and Drug Administration.

Other combinations may show promise in the clinic. Vascular endothelial growth factor (VEGF) negatively regulates the infiltration of T lymphocytes and its inhibition is both rationale synergistic with anti-PD1 therapy [85]. In lung cancer, addition of bevacizumab incrementally increases the efficacy of anti-PDL1/chemotherapy [80]. In mesothelioma, studies are either enrolling (NCT03502746) or in development to explore anti-angiogenesis/PD1 or PDL1 combinations (including the MiST trial). Based on emerging evidence, clinical synergy may be a real possibility in mesothelioma.

Regulatory T cells mediate immune inhibitory activity and are augmented by focal adhesion kinase (FAK), leading to evasion of anti-tumour immunity [86]. Inhibition of FAK potentiates anti-PD1 [87] in preclinical models, and this has led to a phase I clinical trial evaluation pembrolizumab and defactinib in mesothelioma (NCT02758587). Modulating the immune microenvironment towards the anti-tumour phenotype is a major driver which has led to an increase in a diverse number of non-randomised combination studies that include the addition of antibody-dependent conjugate, hyperthermia, and arginase inhibition.

Perhaps the most promising combination strategy to emerge recently has been the impressive synergy observed when anti-PD1 or anti-PDL1 therapy is combined with chemotherapy [72, 80] in non-small cell lung cancer [72, 80]. Studies are now underway in mesothelioma (NCT02784171, NCT02899195, ACTRN12616001170415), which is capable of recapitulating the incremental benefits seen in lung, could transform outcomes for patients. This approach may be particularly important in lessening the requirement for upfront biomarker stratification.

23.7 Summary: A Rapidly Evolving Landscape of New Therapeutic Opportunities

The last 5 years have seen an extraordinary transformation of the mesothelioma research landscape. These changes spanning our understanding of the genomic landscape and interpatient heterogeneity is driving the emergence of stratified therapy, with early clinical signals of promise. The immunotherapy revolution has already transformed the lives of patients with a diverse range of cancers and mesothelioma is now in the firing line. There is an acceleration in the rate of new treatment paradigms being translated to mesothelioma from other cancers (combination immunotherapy and chemoimmunotherapy being two examples). Based on this pace of development, it is widely anticipated that the next half decade will see significant changes to the standard of care particularly in the relapsed setting, which is long overdue.

References

1. Shepherd FA, et al. Prospective randomized trial of docetaxel versus best supportive care in patients with non-small-cell lung cancer previously treated with platinum-based chemotherapy. J Clin Oncol Off J Am Soc Clin Oncol. 2000;18:2095–103. https://doi.org/10.1200/JCO.2000.18.10.2095.
2. Shepherd FA, et al. Erlotinib in previously treated non-small-cell lung cancer. N Engl J Med. 2005;353:123–32. https://doi.org/10.1056/NEJMoa050753.
3. Farzin M, et al. Loss of expression of BAP1 predicts longer survival in mesothelioma. Pathology. 2015;47:302–7. https://doi.org/10.1097/PAT.0000000000000250.
4. Bueno R, et al. Comprehensive genomic analysis of malignant pleural mesothelioma identifies recurrent mutations, gene fusions and splicing alterations. Nat Genet. 2016;48:407–16. https://doi.org/10.1038/ng.3520.
5. Bott M, et al. The nuclear deubiquitinase BAP1 is commonly inactivated by somatic mutations and 3p21.1 losses in malignant pleural mesothelioma. Nat Genet. 2011;43:668–72. https://doi.org/10.1038/ng.855.
6. Testa JR, et al. Germline BAP1 mutations predispose to malignant mesothelioma. Nat Genet. 2011;43:1022–5. https://doi.org/10.1038/ng.912.
7. Xu J, et al. Germline mutation of Bap1 accelerates development of asbestos-induced malignant mesothelioma. Cancer Res. 2014;74:4388–97. https://doi.org/10.1158/0008-5472.CAN-14-1328.
8. Altomare DA, et al. A mouse model recapitulating molecular features of human mesothelioma. Cancer Res. 2005;65:8090–5. https://doi.org/10.1158/0008-5472.CAN-05-2312.
9. Jongsma J, et al. A conditional mouse model for malignant mesothelioma. Cancer Cell. 2008;13:261–71. https://doi.org/10.1016/j.ccr.2008.01.030.
10. Walts AE, et al. BAP1 immunostain and CDKN2A (p16) FISH analysis: clinical applicability for the diagnosis of malignant mesothelioma in effusions. Diagn Cytopathol. 2016;44:599–606. https://doi.org/10.1002/dc.23491.
11. Hida T, et al. BAP1 immunohistochemistry and p16 FISH results in combination provide higher confidence in malignant pleural mesothelioma diagnosis: ROC analysis of the two tests. Pathol Int. 2016;66:563–70. https://doi.org/10.1111/pin.12453.
12. Hida T, et al. Immunohistochemical detection of MTAP and BAP1 protein loss for mesothelioma diag-

nosis: comparison with 9p21 FISH and BAP1 immunohistochemistry. Lung Cancer. 2017;104:98–105. https://doi.org/10.1016/j.lungcan.2016.12.017.
13. Cheng JQ, et al. Frequent mutations of NF2 and allelic loss from chromosome band 22q12 in malignant mesothelioma: evidence for a two-hit mechanism of NF2 inactivation. Genes Chromosomes Cancer. 1999;24:238–42.
14. Miyanaga A, et al. Hippo pathway gene mutations in malignant mesothelioma: revealed by RNA and targeted exon sequencing. J Thorac Oncol. 2015;10:844–51. https://doi.org/10.1097/JTO.0000000000000493.
15. Bonneville R, et al. Landscape of microsatellite instability across 39 cancer types. JCO Precision Oncol. 2017;2017:1–15. https://doi.org/10.1200/PO.17.00073.
16. Arulananda S, et al. Mismatch repair protein defects and microsatellite instability in malignant pleural mesothelioma. J Thorac Oncol. 2018;13:1588–94. https://doi.org/10.1016/j.jtho.2018.07.015.
17. Farmer H, et al. Targeting the DNA repair defect in BRCA mutant cells as a therapeutic strategy. Nature. 2005;434:917–21. https://doi.org/10.1038/nature03445.
18. Fong PC, et al. Inhibition of poly(ADP-ribose) polymerase in tumors from BRCA mutation carriers. N Engl J Med. 2009;361:123–34. https://doi.org/10.1056/NEJMoa0900212.
19. Busacca S, et al. BRCA1 is an essential mediator of vinorelbine-induced apoptosis in mesothelioma. J Pathol. 2012;227:200–8. https://doi.org/10.1002/path.3979.
20. Knijnenburg TA, et al. Genomic and molecular landscape of DNA damage repair deficiency across the cancer genome atlas. Cell Rep. 2018;23:239–254 e236. https://doi.org/10.1016/j.celrep.2018.03.076.
21. Hakiri S, et al. Functional differences between wild-type and mutant-type BRCA1-associated protein 1 tumor suppressor against malignant mesothelioma cells. Cancer Sci. 2015;106:990–9. https://doi.org/10.1111/cas.12698.
22. Martincorena I, et al. Universal patterns of selection in cancer and somatic tissues. Cell. 2018;173:1823. https://doi.org/10.1016/j.cell.2018.06.001.
23. Von Hoff DD, et al. Inhibition of the hedgehog pathway in advanced basal-cell carcinoma. N Engl J Med. 2009;361:1164–72. https://doi.org/10.1056/NEJMoa0905360.
24. Rudin CM, et al. Treatment of medulloblastoma with hedgehog pathway inhibitor GDC-0449. N Engl J Med. 2009;361:1173–8. https://doi.org/10.1056/NEJMoa0902903.
25. Meerang M, et al. Antagonizing the hedgehog pathway with Vismodegib impairs malignant pleural mesothelioma growth in vivo by affecting Stroma. Mol Cancer Ther. 2016;15:1095–105. https://doi.org/10.1158/1535-7163.MCT-15-0583.
26. You M, et al. Targeting of the hedgehog signal transduction pathway suppresses survival of malignant pleural mesothelioma cells in vitro. J Thorac Cardiovasc Surg. 2014;147:508–16. https://doi.org/10.1016/j.jtcvs.2013.08.035.
27. Shi Y, et al. Role of hedgehog signaling in malignant pleural mesothelioma. Clin Cancer Res. 2012;18:4646–56. https://doi.org/10.1158/1078-0432.CCR-12-0599.
28. Lim CB, et al. Mutational analysis of hedgehog signaling pathway genes in human malignant mesothelioma. PLoS One. 2013;8:e66685. https://doi.org/10.1371/journal.pone.0066685.
29. Mok TS, et al. Gefitinib or carboplatin-paclitaxel in pulmonary adenocarcinoma. N Engl J Med. 2009;361:947–57. https://doi.org/10.1056/NEJMoa0810699.
30. Paez JG, et al. EGFR mutations in lung cancer: correlation with clinical response to gefitinib therapy. Science. 2004;304:1497–500. https://doi.org/10.1126/science.1099314.
31. Enomoto Y, et al. Epidermal growth factor receptor mutations in malignant pleural and peritoneal mesothelioma. J Clin Pathol. 2012;65:522–7. https://doi.org/10.1136/jclinpath-2011-200631.
32. Kim JE, et al. Mutational profiling of malignant mesothelioma revealed potential therapeutic targets in EGFR and NRAS. Transl Oncol. 2018;11:268–74. https://doi.org/10.1016/j.tranon.2018.01.005.
33. Schildgen V, et al. Low frequency of EGFR mutations in pleural mesothelioma patients, Cologne, Germany. Appl Immunohistochem Mol Morphol. 2015;23:118–25. https://doi.org/10.1097/PDM.0b013e3182a3645e.
34. Butrynski JE, et al. Crizotinib in ALK-rearranged inflammatory myofibroblastic tumor. N Engl J Med. 2010;363:1727–33. https://doi.org/10.1056/NEJMoa1007056.
35. Kwak EL, et al. Anaplastic lymphoma kinase inhibition in non-small-cell lung cancer. N Engl J Med. 2010;363:1693–703. https://doi.org/10.1056/NEJMoa1006448.
36. Peters S, et al. Alectinib versus Crizotinib in untreated ALK-positive non-small-cell lung cancer. N Engl J Med. 2017;377:829–38. https://doi.org/10.1056/NEJMoa1704795.
37. Soda M, et al. Identification of the transforming EML4-ALK fusion gene in non-small-cell lung cancer. Nature. 2007;448:561–6. https://doi.org/10.1038/nature05945.
38. Hung YP, et al. Identification of ALK rearrangements in malignant peritoneal mesothelioma. JAMA Oncol. 2018;4:235–8. https://doi.org/10.1001/jamaoncol.2017.2918.
39. McGranahan N, et al. Clonal status of actionable driver events and the timing of mutational processes in cancer evolution. Sci Transl Med. 2015;7:283ra254. https://doi.org/10.1126/scitranslmed.aaa1408.
40. Jamal-Hanjani M, et al. Tracking genomic cancer evolution for precision medicine: the lung TRACERx study. PLoS Biol. 2014;12:e1001906. https://doi.org/10.1371/journal.pbio.1001906.
41. Jamal-Hanjani M, et al. Tracking the evolution of non-small-cell lung cancer. N Engl J Med. 2017;376:2109–21. https://doi.org/10.1056/NEJMoa1616288.

42. Mitchell TJ, et al. Timing the landmark events in the evolution of clear cell renal cell cancer: TRACERx renal. Cell. 2018;173:611–623 e617. https://doi.org/10.1016/j.cell.2018.02.020.
43. Turajlic S, et al. Deterministic evolutionary trajectories influence primary tumor growth: TRACERx renal. Cell. 2018;173:595–610 e511. https://doi.org/10.1016/j.cell.2018.03.043.
44. Szlosarek PW, et al. In vivo loss of expression of argininosuccinate synthetase in malignant pleural mesothelioma is a biomarker for susceptibility to arginine depletion. Clin Cancer Res. 2006;12:7126–31. https://doi.org/10.1158/1078-0432.CCR-06-1101.
45. Szlosarek PW, et al. Arginine deprivation with pegylated arginine deiminase in patients with argininosuccinate synthetase 1-deficient malignant pleural mesothelioma: a randomized clinical trial. JAMA Oncol. 2017;3:58–66. https://doi.org/10.1001/jamaoncol.2016.3049.
46. Szlosarek PW, et al. Metabolic response to pegylated arginine deiminase in mesothelioma with promoter methylation of argininosuccinate synthetase. J Clin Oncol. 2013;31:e111–3. https://doi.org/10.1200/JCO.2012.42.1784.
47. Nicholson LJ, et al. Epigenetic silencing of argininosuccinate synthetase confers resistance to platinum-induced cell death but collateral sensitivity to arginine auxotrophy in ovarian cancer. Int J Cancer. 2009;125:1454–63. https://doi.org/10.1002/ijc.24546.
48. Beddowes E, et al. Phase 1 dose-escalation study of pegylated arginine Deiminase, Cisplatin, and Pemetrexed in patients with argininosuccinate synthetase 1-deficient thoracic cancers. J Clin Oncol. 2017;35:1778–85. https://doi.org/10.1200/JCO.2016.71.3230.
49. Locke M, et al. Inhibition of the polyamine synthesis pathway is synthetically lethal with loss of Argininosuccinate synthase 1. Cell Rep. 2016;16:1604–13. https://doi.org/10.1016/j.celrep.2016.06.097.
50. LaFave LM, et al. Loss of BAP1 function leads to EZH2-dependent transformation. Nat Med. 2015;21:1344–9. https://doi.org/10.1038/nm.3947.
51. Garnett MJ, et al. Systematic identification of genomic markers of drug sensitivity in cancer cells. Nature. 2012;483:570–5. https://doi.org/10.1038/nature11005.
52. Iorio F, et al. A landscape of pharmacogenomic interactions in cancer. Cell. 2016;166:740–54. https://doi.org/10.1016/j.cell.2016.06.017.
53. Tsherniak A, et al. Defining a cancer dependency map. Cell. 2017;170:564–576 e516. https://doi.org/10.1016/j.cell.2017.06.010.
54. Boehm JS, Golub TR. An ecosystem of cancer cell line factories to support a cancer dependency map. Nat Rev Genet. 2015;16:373–4. https://doi.org/10.1038/nrg3967.
55. Marjon K, et al. MTAP deletions in cancer create vulnerability to targeting of the MAT2A/PRMT5/RIOK1 Axis. Cell Rep. 2016;15:574–87. https://doi.org/10.1016/j.celrep.2016.03.043.
56. Mavrakis KJ, et al. Disordered methionine metabolism in MTAP/CDKN2A-deleted cancers leads to dependence on PRMT5. Science. 2016;351:1208–13. https://doi.org/10.1126/science.aad5944.
57. Kryukov GV, et al. MTAP deletion confers enhanced dependency on the PRMT5 arginine methyltransferase in cancer cells. Science. 2016;351:1214–8. https://doi.org/10.1126/science.aad5214.
58. Illei PB, Rusch VW, Zakowski MF, Ladanyi M. Homozygous deletion of CDKN2A and codeletion of the methylthioadenosine phosphorylase gene in the majority of pleural mesotheliomas. Clin Cancer Res. 2003;9:2108–13.
59. Kindler HL, Burris HA 3rd, Sandler AB, Oliff IA. A phase II multicenter study of L-alanosine, a potent inhibitor of adenine biosynthesis, in patients with MTAP-deficient cancer. Investig New Drugs. 2009;27:75–81. https://doi.org/10.1007/s10637-008-9160-1.
60. Russo AA, Tong L, Lee JO, Jeffrey PD, Pavletich NP. Structural basis for inhibition of the cyclin-dependent kinase Cdk6 by the tumour suppressor p16INK4a. Nature. 1998;395:237–43. https://doi.org/10.1038/26155.
61. Lopez-Rios F, et al. Global gene expression profiling of pleural mesotheliomas: overexpression of aurora kinases and P16/CDKN2A deletion as prognostic factors and critical evaluation of microarray-based prognostic prediction. Cancer Res. 2006;66:2970–9. https://doi.org/10.1158/0008-5472.CAN-05-3907.
62. Dacic S, et al. Prognostic significance of p16/cdkn2a loss in pleural malignant mesotheliomas. Virchows Arch. 2008;453:627–35. https://doi.org/10.1007/s00428-008-0689-3.
63. Kolluri KK, et al. Loss of functional BAP1 augments sensitivity to TRAIL in cancer cells. elife. 2018;7:e30224. https://doi.org/10.7554/eLife.30224.
64. Quispel-Janssen JM, et al. Comprehensive pharmacogenomic profiling of malignant pleural mesothelioma identifies a subgroup sensitive to FGFR inhibition. Clin Cancer Res. 2018;24:84–94. https://doi.org/10.1158/1078-0432.CCR-17-1172.
65. Billingham L, Malottki K, Steven N. Research methods to change clinical practice for patients with rare cancers. Lancet Oncol. 2016;17:e70–80. https://doi.org/10.1016/S1470-2045(15)00396-4.
66. Middleton G, et al. The National Lung Matrix Trial: translating the biology of stratification in advanced non-small-cell lung cancer. Ann Oncol. 2015;26:2464–9. https://doi.org/10.1093/annonc/mdv394.
67. Yap TA, Aerts JG, Popat S, Fennell DA. Novel insights into mesothelioma biology and implications for therapy. Nat Rev Cancer. 2017;17:475–88. https://doi.org/10.1038/nrc.2017.42.
68. Reck M, et al. Pembrolizumab versus chemotherapy for PD-L1-positive non-small-cell lung cancer. N Engl J Med. 2016;375:1823–33. https://doi.org/10.1056/NEJMoa1606774.
69. Brahmer J, et al. Nivolumab versus Docetaxel in advanced squamous-cell non-small-cell lung

cancer. N Engl J Med. 2015;373:123–35. https://doi.org/10.1056/NEJMoa1504627.
70. Langer CJ, et al. Carboplatin and pemetrexed with or without pembrolizumab for advanced, non-squamous non-small-cell lung cancer: a randomised, phase 2 cohort of the open-label KEYNOTE-021 study. Lancet Oncol. 2016;17:1497–508. https://doi.org/10.1016/S1470-2045(16)30498-3.
71. Garon EB, et al. Pembrolizumab for the treatment of non-small-cell lung cancer. N Engl J Med. 2015;372:2018–28. https://doi.org/10.1056/NEJMoa1501824.
72. Gandhi L, et al. Pembrolizumab plus chemotherapy in metastatic non-small-cell lung cancer. N Engl J Med. 2018;378:2078–92. https://doi.org/10.1056/NEJMoa1801005.
73. Soria JC, et al. Osimertinib in untreated EGFR-mutated advanced non-small-cell lung cancer. N Engl J Med. 2018;378:113–25. https://doi.org/10.1056/NEJMoa1713137.
74. Forde PM, et al. Neoadjuvant PD-1 blockade in resectable lung cancer. N Engl J Med. 2018;378:1976–86. https://doi.org/10.1056/NEJMoa1716078.
75. Alley EW, et al. Clinical safety and activity of pembrolizumab in patients with malignant pleural mesothelioma (KEYNOTE-028): preliminary results from a non-randomised, open-label, phase 1b trial. Lancet Oncol. 2017;18:623–30. https://doi.org/10.1016/S1470-2045(17)30169-9.
76. Quispel-Janssen J, et al. Programmed death 1 blockade with Nivolumab in patients with recurrent malignant pleural mesothelioma. J Thorac Oncol. 2018;13:1436–7. https://doi.org/10.1016/j.jtho.2018.05.038.
77. Mansfield AS, et al. B7-H1 expression in malignant pleural mesothelioma is associated with sarcomatoid histology and poor prognosis. J Thorac Oncol. 2014;9:1036–40. https://doi.org/10.1097/JTO.0000000000000177.
78. Fennell DA, et al. CONFIRM: a double-blind, placebo-controlled phase III clinical trial investigating the effect of nivolumab in patients with relapsed mesothelioma: study protocol for a randomised controlled trial. Trials. 2018;19:233. https://doi.org/10.1186/s13063-018-2602-y.
79. Larkin J, et al. Combined Nivolumab and Ipilimumab or monotherapy in untreated melanoma. N Engl J Med. 2015;373:23–34. https://doi.org/10.1056/NEJMoa1504030.
80. Socinski MA, et al. Atezolizumab for first-line treatment of metastatic nonsquamous NSCLC. N Engl J Med. 2018;378:2288–301. https://doi.org/10.1056/NEJMoa1716948.
81. Hellmann MD, et al. Nivolumab plus Ipilimumab in lung cancer with a high tumor mutational burden. N Engl J Med. 2018;378:2093–104. https://doi.org/10.1056/NEJMoa1801946.
82. Maio M, et al. Tremelimumab as second-line or third-line treatment in relapsed malignant mesothelioma (DETERMINE): a multicentre, international, randomised, double-blind, placebo-controlled phase 2b trial. Lancet Oncol. 2017;18:1261–73. https://doi.org/10.1016/S1470-2045(17)30446-1.
83. Calabro L, et al. Tremelimumab combined with durvalumab in patients with mesothelioma (NIBIT-MESO-1): an open-label, non-randomised, phase 2 study. Lancet Respir Med. 2018;6:451–60. https://doi.org/10.1016/S2213-2600(18)30151-6.
84. Dual checkpoint blockade takes aim at relapsed mesothelioma. Cancer Discov. 2017;7:OF7. https://doi.org/10.1158/2159-8290.CD-NB2017-087.
85. Manegold C, et al. The potential of combined immunotherapy and antiangiogenesis for the synergistic treatment of advanced NSCLC. J Thorac Oncol. 2017;12:194–207. https://doi.org/10.1016/j.jtho.2016.10.003.
86. Serrels A, et al. Nuclear FAK controls chemokine transcription, Tregs, and evasion of anti-tumor immunity. Cell. 2015;163:160–73. https://doi.org/10.1016/j.cell.2015.09.001.
87. Jiang H, et al. Targeting focal adhesion kinase renders pancreatic cancers responsive to checkpoint immunotherapy. Nat Med. 2016;22:851–60. https://doi.org/10.1038/nm.4123.

The manufacturer's authorised representative in the EU is Springer
Nature Customer Service Centre GmbH, Europaplatz 3, 69115 Heidelberg,
Germany. If you have any concerns regarding our products, please
contact ProductSafety@springernature.com

Printed and bound by CPI Group (UK) Ltd, Croydon, CR0 4YY
13/08/2026
02195497-0004